D1087327

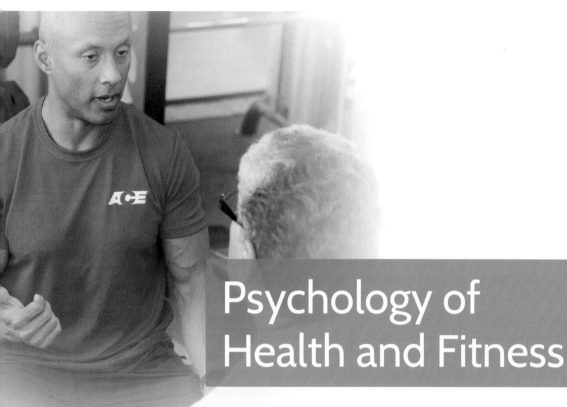

Psychology of Health and Fitness

Barbara A. Brehm, EdD

Professor

Department of Exercise and Sport Studies

Smith College

Northampton, MA

F.A. Davis Company • Philadelphia

F.A. Davis Company
1915 Arch Street
Philadelphia, PA 19103
www.fadavis.com

Copyright © 2014 by F.A. Davis Company

Copyright © 2014 by F.A. Davis Company. All rights reserved. This product is protected by copyright. No part of it may be reproduced, stored in a retrieval system, or transmitted in any form or by any means, electronic, mechanical, photocopying, recording, or otherwise, without written permission from the publisher.

Printed in the United States of America

Last digit indicates print number: 10 9 8 7 6 5 4 3 2 1

Publisher: Quincy McDonald
Manager of Content Development: George Lang
Developmental Editor: Joanna Cain
Art and Design Manager: Carolyn O'Brien

As new scientific information becomes available through basic and clinical research, recommended treatments and drug therapies undergo changes. The author(s) and publisher have done everything possible to make this book accurate, up to date, and in accord with accepted standards at the time of publication. The author(s), editors, and publisher are not responsible for errors or omissions or for consequences from application of the book, and make no warranty, expressed or implied, with regard to the contents of the book. Any practice described in this book should be applied by the reader in accordance with professional standards of care used with regard to the unique circumstances that may apply in each situation. The reader is advised always to check product information (package inserts) for changes and new information regarding dose and contraindications before administering any drug. Caution is especially urged when using new or infrequently ordered drugs.

Library of Congress Cataloging-in-Publication Data

Brehm, Barbara A.
  Psychology of health and fitness / Barbara A. Brehm, EdD, professor, Department of Exercise and Sport Studies, Smith College, Northampton, MA.
      pages cm
  Includes index.
  ISBN 978-0-8036-2827-4
  1. Clinical health psychology. 2. Health attitudes. 3. Physical fitness—Psychological aspects.
4. Behavior modification. I. Title.
  R726.7.B74 2014
  613.7—dc23
                        2013045758

Authorization to photocopy items for internal or personal use, or the internal or personal use of specific clients, is granted by F.A. Davis Company for users registered with the Copyright Clearance Center (CCC) Transactional Reporting Service, provided that the fee of $.25 per copy is paid directly to CCC, 222 Rosewood Drive, Danvers, MA 01923. For those organizations that have been granted a photocopy license by CCC, a separate system of payment has been arranged. The fee code for users of the Transactional Reporting Service is: 978-0-8036-2827-4/14 0 + $.25.

For my parents, Lois Williams Brehm and Carl T. Brehm, in memoriam, with gratitude for encouraging me to follow a path with a heart.

On ne voit bien qu'avec le cœur. L'essentiel est invisible pour les yeux.
(It is only with the heart that one can see rightly; what is essential is invisible to the eye.)
Antoine de Saint-Exupéry

Le Petit Prince

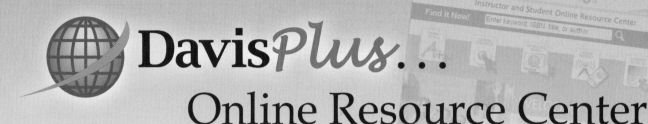

DavisPlus...
Online Resource Center

DavisPlus is your online source for a wealth of learning resources and teaching tools, as well as electronic and mobile versions of our products.

STUDENTS

Unlimited FREE access.
No password.
No registration.
No fee.

INSTRUCTORS

Upon Adoption.
Password-protected library of title-specific, online course content.

Visit http://davisplus.fadavis.com

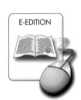

WELCOME   CLINICAL SCENARIOS   INTERACTIVE MEDIA   MOBILE PRODUCT   LEARNING ACTIVITIES   E-EDITION

Explore more online resources from F.A.Davis...

DAVIS'S DRUG GUIDE.com
powered by
Unbound Medicine®

www.drugguide.com
is Davis's Drug Guide Online, the complete Davis's Drug Guide for Nurses® database of over 1,100 monographs on the web.

Taber's Online
powered by
Unbound Medicine®

www.tabersonline.com
delivers the power of Taber's Cyclopedic Medical Dictionary on the web. Find more than 60,000 terms, 1,000 images, and more.

DAVIS'S Laboratory and Diagnostic Tests with Nursing Implications
powered by
Unbound Medicine®

www.LabDxTest.com
is the complete database for Davis's Comprehensive Handbook of Laboratory and Diagnostic Tests with Nursing Implications online. Access hundreds of detailed monographs.

www.FADavis.com

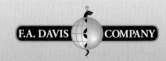
F.A. DAVIS COMPANY

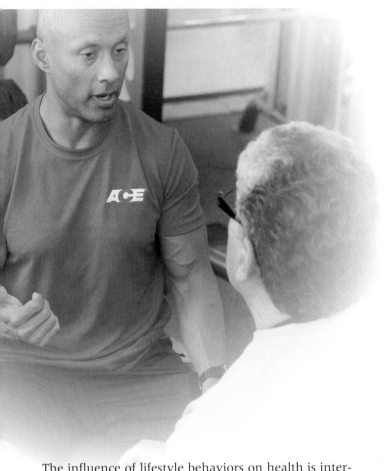

Preface

The influence of lifestyle behaviors on health is interesting and relevant for every individual, whether one takes a public-health perspective focused on the prevention of chronic illness for the majority of citizens or a personal perspective while pondering what to have for lunch. It has become clear over the past 50 years that behavior and health are inseparably entwined. Research supports the notion that the way people live their lives, including their activity levels, eating habits, stress-management practices, and substance-use habits, strongly influences their likelihood of developing many of the most-common health problems. Scientists have discovered which lifestyle behaviors generally serve to prevent chronic illness and injury, as well as to optimize quality of life on a daily basis. In fact, most people have a rough idea of what they should eat and how much they should exercise, and they know they should drink less alcohol or quit smoking. What is the final frontier in public health and medical care? Motivating and guiding people to do what they already know they should do.

I have been fascinated with health and exercise psychology since I designed my first health behavior course in the Department of Exercise and Sport Studies at Smith College in 1985. In that same year, I started writing articles featuring concepts in applied exercise science for health and fitness professionals, translating scientific research into more-accessible language. Since that time, I have had the pleasure of working with

hundreds of students and professionals who have sought to better understand exercise adherence and other applications of health and exercise psychology and behavior change theory. As a group exercise instructor, personal trainer, lifestyle coach, and fitness program director, I have coached hundreds of clients to adopt new behaviors and resolutions and been inspired by the effort and strategies they bring to the behavior-change process.

Many students in the allied health sciences and in exercise science fields study health and exercise psychology for their degrees and for their work. The more we learn about health, the more experts agree that an interdisciplinary approach yields the best understanding about topics in health and health behavior. Health psychology helps clinicians figure out what makes their patients sick and clients tick. Exercise psychology provides fascinating knowledge about the psychophysiological benefits of physical activity and the many factors related to exercise adherence. This text draws from both fields to create an applied psychology perspective most helpful for understanding health behavior.

Health and fitness professionals recommend lifestyle change to prevent and treat illness and injury. Professionals need to know not only which lifestyle changes to recommend but also how to communicate these recommendations to patients in ways that are understandable and that motivate patients to follow them. For example, exercise science students hoping to work as health and fitness professionals need more than knowledge of exercise physiology to help their clients design effective lifestyle interventions for disease prevention and the promotion of optimal health. Students studying athletic training or physical therapy must acquire not only knowledge and skills in the assessment and treatment of injury and illness but also the behavioral-counseling skills that enable them to connect with their patients. This connection is essential to better understand the patient's medical needs and then design and deliver treatment recommendations in ways most likely to lead to successful engagement in the rehabilitation program. Coaching education students must be masters not only of their sport in terms of teaching motor skills and playing strategy and structuring effective conditioning and training programs but also of motivating their athletes to train for peak performance.

Psychology texts can be difficult reading for some students whose primary interests are the physical sciences. Such students often find that psychological variables are more difficult to "see" than physical characteristics such as muscle strength, blood pressure, or body composition. Psychologists must go to great lengths to define and manipulate variables to establish relationships among the many intangible factors that explain behavior. Many students have a hard time visualizing the complex psychological models of behavior. They respond more readily to an instructional approach that links theory and application. Students learn more from textbooks that stimulate their interest while presenting theoretical explanations. This applied health and fitness psychology textbook not only teaches students about the current theories in health psychology and exercise psychology, but it also anchors this learning in real-life application. This link to application engages students more deeply in learning and increases the depth of their understanding, as well as their effectiveness in their future lives and work.

Barbara A. Brehm

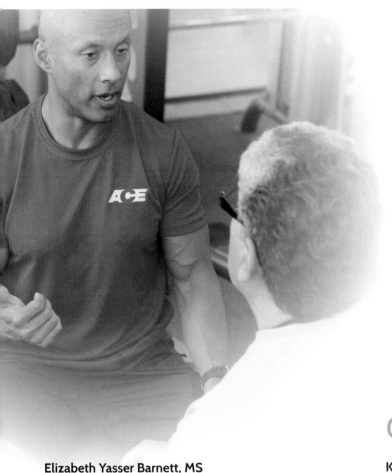

Contributors

Elizabeth Yasser Barnett, MS
Doctoral student
Harvard School of Public Health
Boston, MA

Kristina Bell
Research Assistant, Department of Psychology
Fort Lewis College
Durango, CO

Brent Bode, MS, CSCS
Head Coach, Youth Competitive Rowing
Community Rowing Inc., Boston
Brighton, MA

Brian Burke, PhD
Associate Professor of Psychology
Fort Lewis College
Durango, CO

Abigail Clarke, CYT 500
Certified Embodyoga® Teacher
Yoga Center Amherst
Amherst, MA

Kelly Coffey
Personal Trainer
Strong Coffey Personal Training
Northampton, MA

Mike Durham, BSSW, LSW, LICDC
Substance Abuse Counselor and Educator
Kenyon College
Gambier, OH

Sarah Keyes, MSW
Post-Graduate Fellow
Cambridge Health Alliance
Cambridge, MA

Ashley Niles, MAT
Wilderness Therapy Guide
Pacific Quest
Big Island, HI

John O'Sullivan, PT, OCS, ATC
Physical Therapist
Valley Medical Group
Florence, MA

Helene M. Parker, ACSM-CPT
Personal Trainer and Research Assistant
Smith College
Northampton, MA

Rosalie Peri, RN
NSCA Certified Personal Trainer
Fluid Motion Pilates and Yoga Studio
Haydenville, MA

Sharon R. Sears, PhD
Associate Professor of Psychology
Licensed Clinical Psychologist
Fort Lewis College
Durango, CO

Tom Stabile, MA, CSCS
ACE Certified Personal Trainer
ACSM Certified Clinical Exercise Specialist
Stability Fitness
Mount Vernon, OH

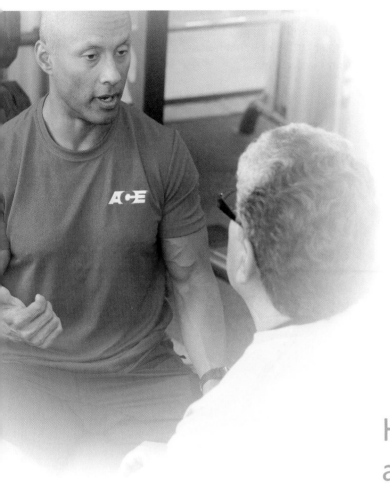

Health Psychology
at Work Contributors

CHAPTER 1
Elizabeth Yasser Barnett, MS
Doctoral student
Harvard School of Public Health
Boston, MA

CHAPTER 2
Tom Stabile, MA, CSCS
ACE Certified Personal Trainer
ACSM Certified Clinical Exercise Specialist
Stability Fitness
Mount Vernon, OH

CHAPTER 3
Rosalie Peri, RN
NSCA Certified Personal Trainer
Fluid Motion Pilates and Yoga Studio
Haydenville, MA

CHAPTER 4
Brian L. Burke, PhD
Associate Professor of Psychology
Fort Lewis College
Durango, CO

CHAPTER 5
Sarah Keyes, MSW
Post-Graduate Fellow
Cambridge Health Alliance
Cambridge, MA

CHAPTER 6
Abigail Clarke, CYT 500
Certified Embodyoga® Teacher
Yoga Center Amherst
Amherst, MA

CHAPTER 7

Ashley Niles, MAT
Wilderness Therapy Guide
Pacific Quest
Big Island, HI

CHAPTER 8

John O'Sullivan, PT, OCS, ATC
Physical Therapist
Valley Medical Group
Florence, MA

CHAPTER 9

Brent Bode, MS, CSCS
Head Coach, Youth Competitive Rowing
Community Rowing Inc., Boston
Brighton, MA

CHAPTER 10

Kelly Coffey
Personal Trainer
Strong Coffey Personal Training
Northampton, MA

CHAPTER 11

Mike Durham, BSSW, LSW, LICDC
Substance Abuse Counselor and Educator
Kenyon College
Gambier, OH

CHAPTER 12

Helene M. Parker, ACSM-CPT
Research Patient Coordinator
Center for Human Nutrition
Washington University School of Medicine
St. Louis, MO

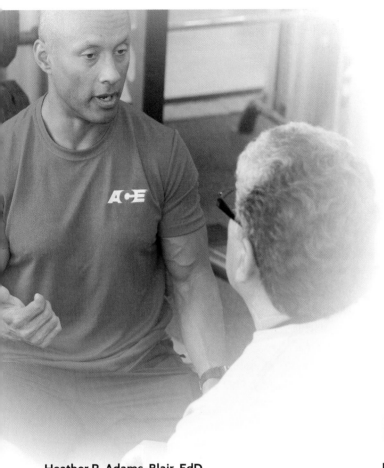

Reviewers

Heather R. Adams-Blair, EdD
Associate Professor and Graduate Coordinator
Eastern Kentucky University
Richmond, KY

John B. Bartholomew, PhD
Professor and Graduate Advisor
University of Texas
Austin, TX

Jeffrey A. Beer, ATC, LAT, CEAS
Assistant Professor, Department of Exercise
   and Sports Sciences
Program Director, Undergraduate Athletic Training
   Education
Manchester College
North Manchester, IN

Stacey Buser, MS, ATC, LAT
Program Director, Athletic Training
Senior Clinical Instructor
University of Akron
Akron, OH

Lee J. Cohen, MS, ATC
Head Athletic Trainer/Clinical Instructor
College at Brockport
Brockport, NY

Daniel R. Czech, PhD
Professor
Georgia Southern University
Statesboro, GA

Zachary J. Dougal, MA, ATC, LAT
Clinical Education Coordinator-ATEP/Assistant Professor
Manchester College
North Manchester, IN

Rebecca Ellis, PhD
Associate Professor
Georgia State University
Atlanta, GA

Mary Ann Erickson, PhD
Professor/Chair, Department of Exercise Science
Fort Lewis College
Durango, CO

Jennifer Farroll, MS, ATC, LAT
Assistant Professor/Associate Athletic Trainer
Union University
Jackson, TN

Erin Foreman, MS, ATC, LAT
Head Athletic Trainer/Assistant Professor
Manchester University
North Manchester, IN

Noah Gentner, PhD, CC-AASP
Assistant Professor/Sport Psychology Graduate Program
    Coordinator
Georgia Southern University
Statesboro, GA

Brendon S. Hale, PhD
Assistant Professor
Mississippi State University
Mississippi State, MS

Michelle Hamilton, MS, ATC
Assistant Athletic Director/Head Athletic Trainer
California State University
San Marcos, CA

Michael James Hanley, MS, LAT, ATC
Assistant Director, Athletics for Medical Services
East Carolina University
Greenville, NC

Kristin Hoffner, BA, MS
Lecturer
Kinesiology Department
Arizona State University
Tempe, AZ

Peter Koehneke, MS, ATC
Professor, Department of Kinesiology
Director, Athletic Training Education
Canisius College
Buffalo, NY

Gerald Larson, PhD
Chair/Assistant Professor
Avila University
Kansas City, MO

Chelsea Marie Lohman, MAT, ATC, LAT, CSCS
Teaching Assistant
Texas Tech University
Lubbock, TX

Meghan H. McDonough, PhD
Assistant Professor
Purdue University
West Lafayette, IN

Valerie Jean Moody, PhD, ATC, LAT, CSCS, WEMT-B
Associate Professor /Co-Program Director,
    Athletic Training Education Program
University of Montana
Missoula, MT

Jamie Moul, EdD, LAT, ATC
Director, Athletic Training Education Program
Appalachian State University
Boone, NC

Joseph M. Murphy, PhD, ATC
Assistant Professor
Salem State University
Salem, MA

Mikiko A. Nakajima, EdD, ATC
Assistant Professor
California State University
Long Beach, CA

Meredith Petschauer, PhD, ATC
Senior Lecturer
University of North Carolina
Chapel Hill, NC

Tiffany M. Reiss, PhD
Associate Professor
Bastyr University
Kenmore, WA

Eric Scibek, MS, ATC, CSCS
Clinical Assistant Professor
Sacred Heart University
Fairfield, CT

John Daniel Shields, MEd, ATC, LAT
Adjunct Instructor
Cedar Valley College
Lancaster, TX

Jeremy Sibold, EdD, ATC
Assistant Professor
University of Vermont
Burlington, VT

Robert C. Sipes, EdD, ATC, CSCS
Assistant Professor
University of Wisconsin
Oshkosh, WI

Melissa Snyder, PhD, ATC, CSCS
Assistant Professor
Ashland University
Ashland, OH

Corrie Struble, PhD, ATC
Clinical Education Coordinator/Assistant Professor
Shaw University
Raleigh, NC

Bradley L. Tripp, PhD, ATC
Clinical Assistant Professor, Director, Graduate Athletic
  Training Program
University of Florida
Gainesville, FL

Benito J. Valesquez, DA, ATC, LAT
Associate Professor/Department Chair, Department
  of Athletic Training and Exercise Physiology
Midwestern State University
Wichita Falls, TX

Nicole Anne Wilkins, MS, ATC, LAT
Assistant Athletic Trainer/Adjunct Faculty
St. Edwards University
Austin, TX

Krista Wolfe, DPT, ATC
Director, PTA Program
Central Penn College
Summerdale, PA

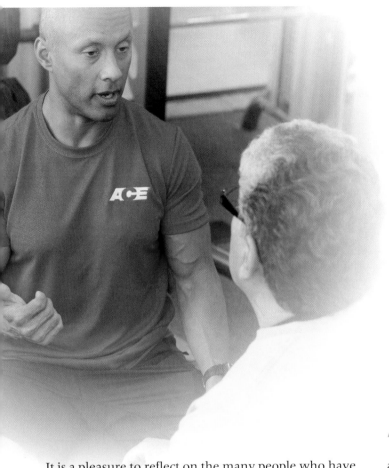

Acknowledgments

It is a pleasure to reflect on the many people who have inspired my journey as a teacher and a writer and helped to shape this book. My opening acknowledgment goes to the many students and health and fitness professionals I have had the pleasuring of knowing over the years. Your thought-provoking questions and perspectives have helped to expand my ideas about fitness, health, and behavior. I would also like to thank the students who will be using this book as they prepare for careers helping people to become healthier and more active. Your work as change agents is crucial in our world at this time, as the barriers to healthy activity levels, eating behaviors, and stress management often discourage behavior-change efforts. Your guidance and support will help people develop the lifestyle behaviors that optimize health and well-being.

Special thanks to my graduate school advisors of long ago. Eugene Evonuk at the University of Oregon sharpened my understanding of physiology and biochemistry, and William McArdle of Queens College inspired my interest in applied physiology. Over the years, my appreciation for Bernard Gutin's unflagging intellectual curiosity, good humor, and fascination with the complexity of the human experience continues to grow, and I have tried to bring these qualities to my own work in the world.

My colleagues in the Department of Exercise and Sport Studies and in the Department of Athletics and Recreation have supported and informed my growth as a teacher and as a writer over the years, and they taught me much about the world of athletics and sport. Smith College's faculty development program, the Kahn Institute, has helped to support my scholarly work on a number of levels, and my participation in its interdisciplinary seminars has broadened my understanding of many issues in the areas of health, psychology, and human behavior.

I am deeply appreciative of the time and effort given by the many professionals who contributed essays for the "Health Psychology at Work" feature that appears in each chapter. These individuals provided fresh and interesting perspectives on a variety of health psychology topics and their application to behavior-change work. Their names are in the Contributors list. I thank psychologist Sharon R. Sears for her helpful perspectives on behavior-change models in Chapter 4 as well as for her ideas on several other topics.

A number of Smith students have served as research assistants throughout the course of this project. Psychology major Sarah Billian left no stone unturned while sifting through research on all of the chapter topics during the initial stages of this project; Alex Cheng and Helene Parker expanded the search on several topics and helped with many other tasks. Patricia Cipicchio's assistance with searches, art manuscripts, and other projects was especially invaluable during the final year of work. Many thanks to Smith College for funding these student assistants. In addition, our department's administrative assistants, Michelle G. Finley and Alexandra Fox, also assisted in the forward motion of this undertaking.

I wish to thank Cedric X. Bryant and Daniel Green at the American Council on Exercise for their good work in developing effective health and fitness professionals and for believing in the important role health and exercise psychology plays in professional development. Special thanks go to Quincy McDonald at F.A. Davis Publishers for helping to craft a vision for this book. Developmental editor Megan Klim Duttera worked to shape the manuscript in its early days. Joanna Cain, Pamela Speh, Gayle Crist, and the editorial crew at Auctorial Pursuits, Inc. guided this early work into the editorial process that develops a book, ferreting out reviewers and smoothing the rough edges of my writing. Pamela Speh was especially helpful in getting the manuscript through its final stages and into production. Thanks also to George Lang and Stephanie Rukowicz at F.A. Davis for their work.

Many people provided extensive and multifaceted support during the writing of this book. The generosity of spirit shown by my sister Susan K. Hall and my friend Karen Buchwald Wright is deeply appreciated. Heartfelt gratitude to my husband Peter for his steady assistance on the home front—you were there when I needed you most, uphill and downhill, in headwinds and tailwinds, and I thank you. Our amazing and delightful sons, Ian and Adam, give me hope and energy each day.

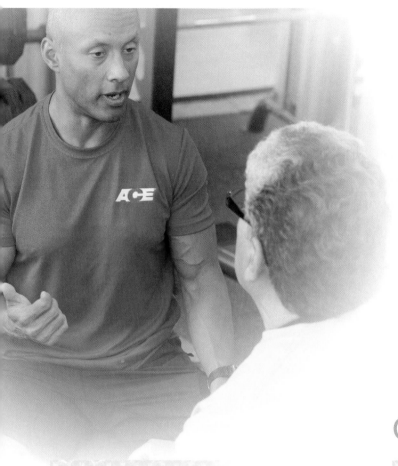

Contents

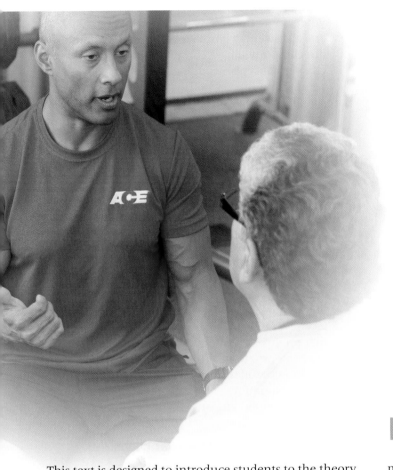

Introduction

This text is designed to introduce students to the theory and application of health and exercise psychology, especially in the context of how people form and change health behaviors. The first section presents foundational knowledge essential for understanding associations between behavior and health. Chapter 1 situates the book's interdisciplinary approach in relation to the fields of psychology, exercise science, and health science and briefly reviews the important influence that a variety of health behaviors have on the development of the most-common chronic diseases. Chapter 1 also discusses how researchers and professionals use the scientific method to develop theories and models about health, behavior, and behavior change. Chapter 2 summarizes the physiological systems that play important roles in mind–body communication and in the maintenance of health. Chapter 3 introduces students to the psychophysiological effects of physical activity. The physical and psychological benefits of regular physical activity can be motivational for people embarking on behavior-change programs.

The second section explores the psychology of health behavior and behavior change. Chapter 4 presents the behavior-change models that have proven to be most applicable for changing health behaviors, along with an exploration of the nature of motivation for behavior change. Chapter 5 discusses some basic skills that can help health and fitness professionals move from a directive style of communicating with clients to

more of a guiding style that enables clients to access the meaningful motivation required to sustain lasting change. Chapter 5 also describes the behavior-change skills shown to be most effective for people transforming an intention to change a behavior into actual lifestyle change. Because feelings of stress and the stress response are such an intricate part of health, motivation, and behavior, Chapter 6 goes into some detail on the nature of stress, the stress response, and coping. This chapter explores the relationship between stress and health and concludes with current ideas about the qualities that enhance people's ability to cope effectively with stress and to resist the negative health effects associated with excess stress. No health psychology text would be complete without a discussion of the roles played by culture and life stage in the formation of health behaviors and in the behavior-change process. Chapter 7 encourages students to consider the diversity of human experience and the special issues that influence the context of behavior because of people's cultural backgrounds and life stage.

The last section of this book examines behavior change for specific applications. Chapter 8 explores behavior-change strategies for increasing exercise adherence. Chapter 9 discusses nutrition and dietary change, focusing on behavior-change strategies for improving eating behaviors. Chapter 10 takes on issues related to weight control, especially behavior-change recommendations for preventing obesity and promoting healthy body composition. Chapter 11 presents perspectives on changing negative health behaviors, including both substance-use disorders and behavioral addictions. Disordered eating and pathogenic weight-control measures are discussed in this context. Chapter 12 looks at behavior change from a clinical perspective and the issues important to consider when trying to understand and apply behavior change theory in a clinical setting. It is likely that health and fitness professionals will work with all kinds of people throughout their careers, including people coping with chronic illness and/or injury. The information in Chapter 12 echoes the more-theoretical links between behavior and chronic illness discussed in Chapter 1 and so brings the book full circle to the big picture of behavior and health.

Features

This textbook strives to connect theoretical knowledge to practical applications, in order to help students find the theoretical material interesting, understandable, and relevant. Several special features in each chapter are designed to enhance student learning, including the following:

- Motivating Change Sections: Several Motivating Change application sections are strategically placed throughout each chapter. These summarize applications useful to the health and fitness professional for the theoretical material presented in the chapter. The Motivating Change sections help students develop a context for the chapter information and see how the theoretical material is important and relevant.
- What's the Evidence? Each chapter presents a brief summary of a research study that examines important chapter concepts. This feature gives students a critical perspective on the link between research and theory, with an eye to understanding the phrase "evidence-based practice."
- Game Changers: The Game Changers box features important historical figures in the exercise and health sciences whose work has changed the way that experts and students alike view the subject matter in these fields. This feature not only provides an interesting historical context in diverse areas, but it also illustrates the nature of model building in science and how researchers can radically transform thinking on their topics of expertise.
- Health Psychology at Work: This feature consists of essays from health and fitness professionals who are actively using chapter material in their work. Professionals featured include personal trainers, exercise and yoga instructors, educators, psychotherapists, a physical therapist, a youth sport coach, a wilderness therapy guide, and a university employee-wellness program director. Providing a context for the use of chapter concepts will hopefully motivate students considering careers in the helping professions to see that learning the material will be relevant for their future work and employment opportunities.
- Health Psychology and You: These boxes feature activities that invite student participation to encourage students to see chapter concepts in personally relevant and interesting ways.
- Critical Thinking Questions: Several questions at the end of each chapter encourage students to apply chapter material in new ways to deepen their understanding of chapter material and the issues to which the material applies.
- Running Scenario: Each chapter opens with a fictitious but plausible scenario featuring one or more young health and fitness professionals who face several situations throughout the chapter that provoke questions about the application of chapter material. This feature is designed to encourage student thinking and discussion of real-life situations where chapter concepts might provide helpful guidance.

Additional Online Features at DavisPlus

Additional learning-support features are available at the F.A. Davis Online Resource Center, including the following:

- Sample Multiple-Choice Questions: These practice questions help students review their knowledge and prepare for quizzes and exams.
- Video Scenarios: These scenarios present typical situations encountered by health and fitness professionals. Students view the first portion of the scenario in which a challenge related to chapter concepts is presented. Students are encouraged to imagine themselves as the professional in the scenario situations and think about how they might respond. After watching the first part of the scenario, students are presented with a decision-point multiple-choice question to direct student thinking and discussion and encourage students to explore how they might deal with the situation. Students then view one possible resolution to the scenario. Four additional multiple choice questions helps students explore how the scenario is related to chapter concepts.

Psychology of Health and Fitness

CHAPTER OUTLINE

LEARNING OBJECTIVES

After reading this chapter, you will be able to:

1. Describe the range of topics included in the field of psychology.

2. Discuss the relationship of health and fitness.

3. Explain the range of topics included in the field of health psychology.

4. Summarize the topics studied in the field of exercise psychology.

5. Explain how people's lifestyle behaviors affect their health.

6. Describe the relationship between health behavior and risk of heart disease and other leading causes of death.

7. Identify which health behaviors have the greatest impact on health.

8. Describe the process of science and the scientific method.

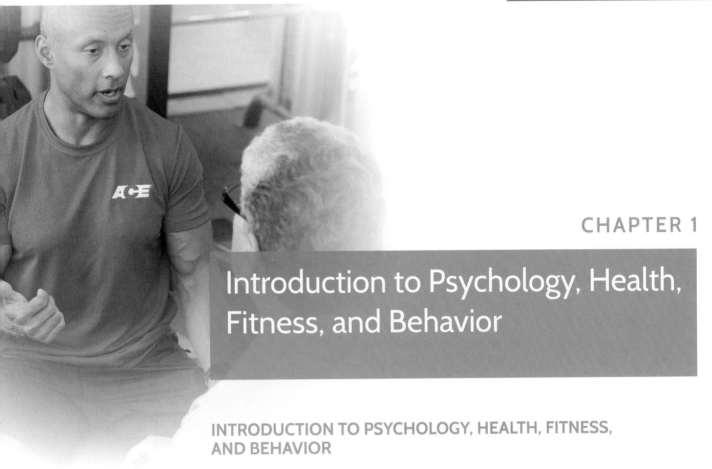

CHAPTER 1

Introduction to Psychology, Health, Fitness, and Behavior

INTRODUCTION TO PSYCHOLOGY, HEALTH, FITNESS, AND BEHAVIOR

◼ *September, a brand-new school year. Evan is beginning his senior year of college and a required internship at a medical fitness center for his kinesiology degree. Evan loves sports and exercise, and he has always dreamed of opening his own club. Working in the medical fitness center is not at all what he expected to be doing when he chose his kinesiology major, but he learned in his program that medical fitness is an expanding market. As people live longer, they are dealing with more chronic illness, and exercise is recommended as part of their treatment. His advisor urges him to give this internship his best effort and to gain a deeper understanding of this area of employment.*

One of his required courses this semester is "Psychology of Health and Fitness." Evan has excelled in exercise physiology and exercise prescription but does not know much about psychology. He hopes the course will help him "figure out" his new clients. Frankly, they puzzle him. Evan has had no problem telling people which exercises will build what muscles and can describe every possible exercise that can be done on each piece of equipment in the fitness center, but he does not feel like he is connecting very well with the clients. In fact, Carla, his supervisor, has moved him from the front desk to folding towels after several clients complained that Evan talked so fast they often could not follow what he was saying.

Folding towels is not what Evan wants to be doing tomorrow for his next shift at the medical fitness center. His internship is supposed to help him land his first real job in the fitness world. How is he going to make a better impression on Carla? How is he going to learn how to better connect with the clients? ◼

Most health and fitness professionals have heard their clients say, "I know what to do; I just can't get myself to do it." Part of becoming a successful health and fitness professional involves helping clients understand what they should do, in terms of changing their behavior to promote health and prevent disease.

The other part consists of teaching clients the skills and helping them find the motivation necessary to sustain health-promoting lifestyles. The study of psychology can help professionals understand and apply successful behavior change strategies.

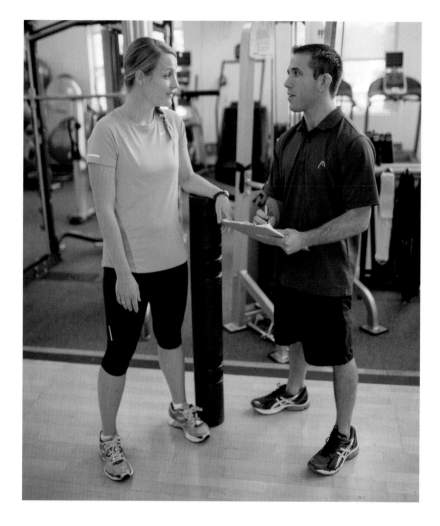

This chapter introduces the field of psychology as well as the subdisciplines of health psychology and exercise psychology. Behavior change theory draws from research and practice in these areas (Fig. 1-1). The first section of this chapter helps acquaint readers with the exciting range of topics explored by health psychologists and exercise psychologists.

The second part of this chapter provides a brief overview of the relationship between lifestyle and long-term health. The majority of health problems faced by citizens around the globe are strongly influenced by lifestyle factors such as cigarette smoking, diet, and activity level. Chronic, noncommunicable diseases consume exorbitant resources in every country and diminish quality of life for those suffering from illness and often for those caring for them.

The last section of the chapter introduces readers to the scientific process used by psychologists to improve the understanding of thoughts, emotions, and behavior, and to formulate guidelines for effective practice. Health and fitness professionals must continually strive to incorporate evidence-based practices into their work. An understanding of the research process helps readers understand where evidence-based guidelines come from, and why they continually evolve and change.

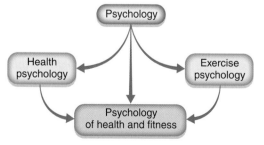

Figure 1-1. The psychology of health and fitness.

FOUNDATIONS OF THE PSYCHOLOGY OF HEALTH AND FITNESS

Psychology is the scientific study of the mind, particularly thoughts, emotions, and behavior. The word "psychology" comes from the Greek word *psyche*, which refers to the soul, spirit, or life force of a person. The ancient Greeks used the word "psyche" to refer to the inner force that motivates behavior. Psychologists study the many aspects of mental function and how mental function is related to behavior.

The Field of Psychology

Psychology has a long and interesting history (Box 1-1). Psychologists investigate phenomena like perception and thinking: how people take in and process information from the environment and construct ideas about the world and their lives. They explore questions such as why people viewing the exact same scenario interpret events in different ways, how mood disorders such as depression affect the way people construct meaning in different situations, and

how spiritual beliefs influence a person's response to a health threat.

Psychologists also study personality, the distinctive qualities of character that can be used to describe individuals' patterns of thinking and behavior. For example, psychologists might investigate the relationship between traits such as perfectionism and low self-esteem, and risk of developing an eating disorder. Researchers have explored whether people who are fearful and anxious are more prone to stress-related health problems than people who are more relaxed. Psychologists have studied the personality traits associated with success in competitive sports.

People are social by nature, and understanding relationships is an important aspect of psychology. Psychologists investigate how people form relationships with one another and behave in groups, a field of study known as social psychology. Social psychologists often apply information and theories from the field of sociology. Sociology is the study of social structure and function, and sociologists explore how humans behave in groups. Sociologists study how social groups and institutions affect behavior and how social

---

Box 1-1. Psychology: Evolution of a Science

Psychology attributes its beginnings as a science to Wilhelm Wundt, a German physiologist who published a book called *Principles of Physiological Psychology* in 1874. Wundt created what is regarded as the first psychology laboratory at the University of Leipzig in 1879. His work on the study of human consciousness continued under the leadership of his most famous student, Edward B. Titchener. Titchener and psychologists of his day focused on breaking down human consciousness into its separate parts. Trained subjects used introspection to describe the workings of the mind.

Psychologists call William James the "father of American psychology." James helped construct theories of human consciousness, thought, and behavior. He published a leading text of the time, *The Principles of Psychology*, in 1890.

Sigmund Freud shifted psychology's focus in ways shocking to his Victorian peers, by proposing that behavior is motivated in large part by inner impulses, both conscious and subconscious, rather than by rational thought alone. Freud believed that many psychological disorders resulted from early childhood experiences and unbalanced subconscious drives. Freud theorized that unconscious motives could be revealed through dreams and errors of speech (when people mistakenly say the wrong word but the word may reveal an unconscious motive, known as a Freudian slip).

In response to psychology's emphasis on the conscious and subconscious mental processes, the next wave of psychologists strived to bring the science of psychology back to the realm of measurable variables. These psychologists focused on observable phenomena, primarily behavior, and developed a movement in psychology known as behaviorism. In the early 1900s, Russian scientist Ivan Pavlov demonstrated the classical conditioning process, which showed that behaviors could be changed by teaching animals new associations. He showed that dogs that repeatedly received food after a bell was rung would begin to salivate after hearing the bell, even when food did not appear. B.F. Skinner later investigated how behavior could be shaped by punishments and rewards delivered after a behavior occurs, a process called operant conditioning. Reward and punishment are still used in many instances to shape behavior, especially when training animals and children.

Psychology's focus shifted again in the second half of the 20th century, with a renewed interest in mental processes. This new focus became known as humanism and emphasized the conscious experience of human beings. The humanist psychologists believed that behavior was more than a conditioned response shaped by reward and punishment; that human beings possessed free will and the ability to make decisions. Carl Rogers and Abraham Maslow are two of the best known of the humanist psychologists.

relationships develop and become structured according to social rules, or norms. Social psychologists are interested in the way individuals are affected by social influences and interactions, and how social position in a group or larger community influences thoughts, emotions, and behavior. They study such topics as the effect of a person's gender on child-rearing behavior and the relationship of a person's socioeconomic status to level of perceived stress.

People tend to talk about the mind as though it is somehow separate and distinct from the body. In the 17th century, philosopher-scientist René Descartes popularized the notion that the body and mind were separate entities, a concept called dualism. Scientists today believe that the idea of dualism is too simplistic. Over the years, as psychologists have conducted research to better understand how the mind works, researchers have developed experimental techniques to evaluate some of the physiological processes that accompany thinking, emotions, and behaviors. Scientists have found it impossible to totally separate body and mind. Psychophysiology describes the study of physiology as it relates to thoughts, emotions, and behaviors. One might call psychophysiology the physiology of psychology. Research in this area has illuminated many interesting phenomena, including some of the physiological events that accompany the stress response and some of the ways in which participation in physical activity may increase feelings of relaxation. The nature of addiction is also an important topic in psychophysiology.

The structure and function of the brain and nervous system form the focus of a specialized area of study called neuroscience. Neuroscientists study topics such as how nerve cells communicate with one another and form connections (Fig. 1-2), which areas of the brain appear to be active under various conditions, and how substances and behaviors affect the nervous system. For example, psychologists in this area investigate which regions of the brain are active when people and other animals experience anger, pleasure, sleep, or exercise. Neuroscientists may study the relationship of chronic stress to memory loss, or how the intake of

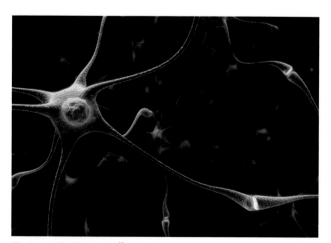

Figure 1-2. **Nerve cells.** © Thinkstock

certain nutrients affects the level of specific chemicals in the brain and how these nutrients and chemicals are in turn related to feelings of alertness or fatigue.

Research scientists are not the only people interested in psychology. Many people study psychology because they want to better understand the nature of human beings. Some people find psychology interesting because it helps them understand themselves. People who work with people increase their on-the-job effectiveness by improving their understanding of others. Anyone interested in human behavior will find the study of psychology interesting and helpful.

Changing Ideas About Health

The word health generally refers to level of well-being. In the early 1900s, people in the medical field used the word "health" to indicate the absence of illness and disease. Patients sought medical advice for symptoms, and medical professionals focused primarily on treating the sick and disabled. In 1948, the World Health Organization (WHO) was founded; as WHO worked to define its mission, it defined the word "health," and broadened the concept to go beyond absence of disease. WHO defined health as "a state of complete physical, mental and social well-being and not merely the absence of disease or infirmity" (WHO, 1948). This definition reflected the changing ideas about the nature of health in the middle of the 20th century, from a focus on physical health, including disease and disability, to a more-holistic notion that health involves the whole person: body, mind, and community. Some writers in the health psychology field refer to a biopsychosocial model of health to emphasize the biological, psychological, and social components of health and to distinguish this broader view of health from the biomedical model, which focuses primarily on the physical causes and symptoms of disease and other health problems.

Many readers will be familiar with the term holistic health, which like the biopsychosocial model of health emphasizes the fact that a person's state of health involves more than the physical body. Holistic health encompasses not only body, mind, and community but other realms of life as well, including spiritual well-being.

A concept similar to that of holistic health is wellness, which designates a dynamic state in which people strive to maximize their well-being in all areas of life, from physical, emotional, and spiritual health to occupational, economic, and environmental health. Wellness emphasizes the ideas of self-responsibility and self-care, working with health-care providers as necessary but also developing a lifestyle that helps prevent disease and makes the most of an individual's potential (Game changers 1-1).

Maximizing quality of life, the general well-being of a person, is a concept central to most definitions of health and has become increasingly recognized as an important goal of medical care. What's the difference between wellness and quality of life? The concepts are

Game Changers 1-1. Leaders in the Wellness Movement: Halbert Dunn, John Travis, Meryn Callander, and Donald Ardell

The term "wellness" is believed to have been coined and introduced by physician Halbert L. Dunn in the early 1960s. Dunn gave a series of talks on wellness and published a book of essays called *High Level Wellness*. Dunn promoted the idea that optimal health could not be attained solely by traditional medical treatment, but that people needed to cultivate wellness-promoting lifestyles. His writing struck a chord in many other physicians, as well as allied health professionals, health and physical educators, and the public at large.

The introduction of improved sanitation and personal hygiene and the development of antibiotic drugs led to dramatic declines in infectious disease during the first half of the 20th century. During that time, physicians were often lifesavers and could cure many patients with their powerful new drugs. But during the second half of the century, as patients began to live longer, physicians saw an increase in chronic diseases, such as heart disease, stroke, and lung disease, for which no curative drug existed. Dunn was one of the first physicians of his time to propose that lifestyle has a stronger influence on health than medical care, a radical shift in medical orientation. Dunn proposed putting more resources into the prevention of disease and the promotion of health.

Another physician, John W. Travis, agreed with Dunn. When Travis began seeing patients early in his practice, he was struck by the absurdity of patients expecting doctors to heal them from a lifetime of poor behavior choices. Travis could not cure the lung disease brought on by decades of heavy smoking or the liver disease that developed from excessive alcohol consumption. Yet such patients looked to him for a remedy, as though he could fix an unsolvable problem. Travis soon quit practicing medicine and began organizing, writing, and speaking to promote the wellness movement. He was joined in this endeavor by many, including his wife, Meryn Callander. The wellness model designed by Travis and colleagues is one of the most comprehensive. More information on the work of Travis and Callander can be found on their website, www.thewellspring.com.

Donald B. Ardell, PhD, was another early leader in the wellness movement. Ardell was an educator, speaker, and writer who helped to popularize the wellness lifestyle. He helped to promote many facets of wellness, including participation in regular physical activity, and has been himself a marathon runner. Ardell also focused on the importance of humor and creating meaning in one's life. More information on Ardell's eclectic and humorous approach to wellness can be found on his website, www.seekwellness.com/wellness.

very similar, but wellness tends to be used in a way that emphasizes lifestyle and personal responsibility. Perhaps because quality of life is more commonly used in medical parlance, it is more likely to refer to an individual's state of well-being, focusing more on product than process.

MOTIVATING CHANGE: A Positive Approach Improves Behavior Change Motivation

A wellness focus emphasizes making the most of each day and generating passion for life. Engagement in activities that give life meaning combined with experiencing positive emotions can motivate clients to persist in behavior change programs that improve their quality of life. The big picture of wellness is more interesting than trying to give up something enjoyable, like eating less dessert. When dietary and other changes are viewed as means to positive ends, client motivation is strengthened. Lizzie Yasser's employee wellness program (Health Psychology at Work 1-1) illustrates how a creative approach can help motivate clients to reduce stress and improve other health behaviors.

Health and Fitness

Just as the definition of health has evolved over the years, so has the meaning of fitness. Most people use the word fitness today to mean general good health and physical condition, usually as a result of a healthy lifestyle that includes regular physical activity and good eating habits. Today the concepts of health and fitness overlap considerably. It is hard to imagine someone having fitness without health, and health without at least a moderate level of physical fitness.

However, several decades ago, the concepts of health and fitness did not have much to do with each other. Health was mostly about not being ill, and fitness was about athletic and physical prowess. Fitness seems to have evolved from the concept of *fit*, to be the right shape. In the context of physical fitness, this meant being in shape for one's sport or one's occupation. Although average people were urged to have enough fitness to allow them to perform their jobs as well as any recreational activities they enjoyed, the physical demands of life were fairly low. The concept of fitness was mostly limited to physical strength and endurance.

HEALTH PSYCHOLOGY AT WORK 1-1: Worksite Wellness

Lizzie Yasser, M.S.

Lizzie directs a wellness program for employees on the University of California's Santa Cruz (UCSC) campus. Her program caters to UCSC's 4,500+ employees and 500+ retirees. Lizzie runs a large program that includes quarter-long classes as well as one-time events. Lizzie "loves to play" and came to worksite wellness from the sport world; she was a four-time All-American college tennis player and national champion at Trinity University in San Antonio, Texas. Her master's degree is in exercise and sport studies.

"My goal as program coordinator is to offer something for everyone, in all areas of wellness, including exercise, nutrition, and stress management. So I create many kinds of different activities and programs at various locations and times of day to attempt to draw out people across all areas of the wellness spectrum. My hope is that people will discover—or in some cases, rediscover—the joy of being healthy, and will spread that enjoyment to their co-workers, friends, and families.

"I try to make the wellness program welcoming and convenient for even the busiest people. One way to do this is to take wellness to the workers, to individual departments and work groups. If departments are hosting a training, orientation, or meeting, they can invite me to lead a free 5- to 20-minute wellness break during the day. I also visit departments and offer fun and interactive workshops, and give people practical ideas to improve health and reduce worksite injury. I always incorporate an activity at the end of the session that will make people laugh. I have found that after 75 people spend 2 minutes making monkey faces or practicing 'laughter yoga,' there is a real energy in the room that wasn't present before.

"In wellness, attitude is so important. If people in these classes have fun, and other people see or hear about them having fun, they might give the activity a try. Last year, I hosted a series of stress-free zones, a stress-management program that was part of our campus-wide wellness challenge. These 'zones' were actually just rooms where we set up arts and crafts supplies and played relaxing music. Over 50 people attended our Valentine-themed stress-free zone, and many participants called or e-mailed me later to tell me how much they enjoyed it. (I even received homemade cards from participants, thanking me for hosting the event!) I think adults really miss doing some of the things we did as kids, so I have started offering other programs that incorporate arts, crafts, and even some old recess games. Even people from our most stressed departments make time to attend these types of programs. Then, when they return to work, they find themselves in a much happier space.

"I am really proud of our employees for fully embracing this program, each in his or her own way. It has been especially neat to see how different activities resonate with different people. One of our participants who had been overweight for years recently lost 40 pounds, ultimately lowering her high blood pressure, too. She is a high-level administrator who works long hours and had put her health on hold for many years, gradually gaining weight and feeling more stressed. When she joined our "Slugs on a Stroll" walking program (our mascot is the Banana Slug), she really related to walking and enjoyed using the free pedometer that's part of the program. She logged 10,000 steps almost every day, made healthful changes in her eating, and felt so much better once she started exercising that she kept doing it. I don't take credit for her success—she was ready to make some major changes in her life, and I am thankful that the UCSC wellness program was there to support her."

As research in the second half of the 20th century began to reveal a link between physical activity and health, the concept of **health-related fitness** took shape. Health-related fitness refers to those fitness components most related to good health (Table 1-1). Researchers found that people with a higher exercise capacity (probably associated with a more active lifestyle) were found to have a lower risk of heart disease (Gibbons, Blair, Cooper, & Smith, 1983). Certain levels of muscular strength and flexibility were thought to be associated with lower risk of back and other problems. Researchers also began to find that a sedentary lifestyle and too much body fat were associated with **morbidity** (illness) and premature **mortality** (death)

(Marks, 1960). An interest in fitness moved from solitary confinement in the gym into the medical and public health arenas.

For most people, a moderate level of health-related fitness is considered an important part of general health (Box 1-2; Health Psychology in Your Life 1-1). Fitness is a key component in most models of wellness. The list of health benefits associated with regular physical activity is very long. As many parts of the world have seen a rapid rise in their rates of chronic illnesses related to a sedentary lifestyle, the importance of fitness as an essential component of health has gained new attention and, in the eyes of many, urgency.

Table 1-1. Components of Fitness

Health-related fitness components are most strongly related to overall good health and may reduce risk for chronic health problems such as high blood pressure, obesity, and osteoporosis. They also generally reflect participation in activities that improve health. Performance-related fitness components include health-related components, as well as additional variables related to athletic success. Performance-related fitness components vary with sport.

COMPONENT	DEFINITION	BENEFIT
Health-related fitness components		
Aerobic fitness (also known as cardiovascular endurance)	How well people are able to sustain high levels of continuous exercise	Aerobic fitness reflects the ability of the heart and lungs to deliver oxygen and nutrients to the muscles, and the muscles' ability to produce energy.
Muscle strength and muscle endurance	Muscle strength reflects how much weight a muscle group can move one time; muscle endurance reflects how many repetitions of the movement can be completed	Muscle strength and endurance prevent injury, and exercise to improve muscle strength and endurance improves blood sugar regulation and body composition.
Flexibility	Range of motion around a joint	A basic level of flexibility is necessary for good posture and ease of motion.
Body composition	Percentage of the body that is composed of fat tissue	Excess fat tissue, especially fat located in the abdominal area, is associated with several health risks, including poor blood sugar regulation, high blood pressure, and heart disease.
Balance	Ability of a person to maintain a position without falling, or to perform a series of movements without falling	Good balance prevents falling and is especially important in older adults.
Performance-related fitness components		
Motor skills	Specific movement patterns such as throwing a javelin, kicking a ball, or hitting a ball with a bat. Motor skills may include fine motor skills, which require small movements such as accurately firing a gun, or large movements such as most track events, including pole vaulting, other jumps, and the throws.	Motor skills are necessary to enjoy participation in a given activity.
Coordination	Ability to put movement sequences together accurately and quickly	A high level of coordination is required for most sports, from bowling and gymnastics to ice skating and team sports.
Reaction time	Speed of response to a stimulus	A fast reaction time is important in many sports, because sports require a quick response to situations. The faster the response, the more successful the athlete.
Speed	How fast a movement or a movement event is accomplished	Time is an important variable in many sports, and faster athletes win. Sprint performance in running and swimming events is all about speed. Speed is also important in every team sport.

Box 1-2. What Matters in Physical Education: Physical Fitness or Physical Activity?

Physical education used to be about teaching sports and improving performance on physical fitness assessments. Early interest in the assessment of physical fitness focused on measurable attributes. For example, muscle strength could be measured by finding out how much weight a person could lift, and agility by how quickly someone could move a couple of blocks from one side of the room to another. Flexibility was measured by how far a person could stretch. Endurance was measured by looking at how fast someone could run, walk, swim, or cycle a given distance. And so forth. (More information on fitness testing can be found in Chapter 8.) Many athletes enjoyed fitness testing because it established their exquisite fitness abilities and motivated them to continue training hard.

Then there was everyone else. Because fitness tests were scored according to test population norms, 50% of people scored below average, and only the top 10% were in the top 10%. Many people found fitness testing rather demoralizing, which left them even less motivated to exercise. Exercise scientists interested in the relationship between fitness and health realized that fitness test scores are due in great part to a person's heredity, and scores were higher when people chose their parents well. In fact, many young people could score fairly well on fitness tests yet were inactive, smoked, and over-ate, so physical fitness, as measured by the tests, did not correlate strongly with a healthful lifestyle.

Exercise scientists have worked to find a better way to evaluate the relationship between fitness and health. As research clarified the strong association between regular physical activity and many health variables, the focus of physical education shifted. More important than measurable fitness is simply being active throughout the day and participating in vigorous exercise that builds aerobic fitness and muscle strength and endurance. Although many people enjoy sports and working out, more do not, and physical educators are working hard to more effectively reach less-active people. One example is encouraging people to wear pedometers and count their steps every day. This may do more for people's health than subjecting them to a battery of tests.

HEALTH PSYCHOLOGY IN YOUR LIFE 1-1: Personal Interpretations of Health, Wellness, and Fitness

What do people mean by the words "health," "wellness," and "fitness"? First, consider what these words mean to you, and record your answers. Then briefly interview at least 10 people, asking them to define the three in their own words. Try to find a variety of people with different ages and backgrounds. Interview both men and women. Once you have completed your interviews, take a look at what you have found. Did people's definitions of health tend to be similar? If not, how did they differ? What about definitions of wellness? Fitness? Compare your findings to those of your classmates.

■ *Evan folds the towels at the front desk, shadowing Carla's best front desk worker, Jason. Carla has asked Evan to simply observe the clients who come and go and how Jason greets them and answers their questions. Evan has been thinking a lot about how health and fitness mean different things to different people. Working on health issues overrides physical fitness for most of the people at the medical fitness center. For most of the clients, muscle strength is not about looking good at the beach but is a matter of regaining enough strength after a period of bed rest to stay at home and not need assisted-living care. Many of the clients have transitioned from participation in cardiac rehabilitation and physical therapy to strength-training programs. The strength training most of the clients perform is focused on improving quality of life and regaining mobility. Evan sees how health-related fitness is synonymous with regaining health for many of the clients here.*

Evan also watches how Jason greets people as they come in. Jason has a ready smile and seems sincerely happy to see each person who comes through the door. He greets almost all of them by name, having worked at this fitness center for over a year. When people are in a hurry, Jason does not say much more than, "Hello Mr. Smith, how are you today?" But some of the people look really worried and even lonely. They seem glad to talk, even just about the weather. Jason seems able to pick up on their cues and make everyone feel welcome. ■

Health Psychology

Health psychology is an area of psychology concerned with the interactions of thoughts, emotions, and behavior with health and illness conditions and experiences. People have long been fascinated with psychology, behavior, and health (Box 1-3). Health psychologists investigate the many social and psychological factors that help people stay healthy and that contribute to illness, injury, and feelings of pain. They also study how people respond to the experience of being sick, how people cope with health-care systems, and how public health efforts influence behavior and health. Many health psychologists work in health and medical settings to help promote personal and community health. This section examines some of the most common areas of study within the field of health psychology.

Concepts Regarding Health

Definitions of health vary widely from person to person and from culture to culture. Health psychologists investigate how people form ideas about health and wellness and how cultural and social expectations influence people's perceptions of their own health and the health of family members. For example, they might explore the following:

- Why do some people view a decline in fitness as a normal part of the aging process and simply something one must live with, whereas others view loss of strength and endurance as a medical problem calling for intervention?
- Why do some people limit their definitions of health to simply "not being sick," whereas others seek high-level wellness?

Health psychologists are also interested in how concepts regarding health vary among groups of people. For example, some groups are less likely to include psychological well-being as a component of health, whereas others place as much importance on psychological well-being as on physical health. Health psychologists are interested in the ways in which people attribute health to various factors, from spiritual actions, including prayer and luck, to lifestyle measures, such as taking handfuls of dietary supplements each day.

Psychological Factors Associated With the Development of Illness

Many health psychologists study the role of psychological processes in the development of illness. Philosophers and cultures throughout time have observed that physical health problems often involve mental functions, especially feelings of stress, anxiety, and depression. For example, blood pressure is affected by many factors, including nutrition, body weight, and genetic predisposition. One might categorize these variables as physical factors. In addition, feelings of chronic, unrelenting, negative stress can also affect blood pressure (Harburg et al., 1976). When blood pressure tends to remain high throughout the day, even when a person is at rest, a diagnosis of high blood pressure, or hypertension, is made. Similarly, many musculoskeletal problems (disorders of the musculoskeletal system, which comprises the bones, muscles, and joint structures), such as back pain, are strongly influenced by psychological factors.

The observation that psychological factors sometimes influence the development of bodily illness led to creation of the term psychosomatic illness. With regard to illness, the word "psychosomatic" means having both psychological (psycho) and physical (somatic) causes. When an illness is psychosomatic, this does not mean that the causes are purely psychological; the illness is not "all in one's mind." It simply means that both psychological and physical factors contribute to its development or onset. As health psychologists have explored the psychological components of illness, especially chronic conditions such as hypertension, obesity, and pain syndromes, it has become clear that many chronic

---

Box 1-3. Early Philosophers: The First Western Health Psychologists

People have always been fascinated by the mind and health. Thinkers across culture and time have speculated on the nature of life, consciousness, and reality. The early Greek philosophers developed interesting and complex theories about the nature of the human being and the nature of thought and behavior. Because many psychological constructs are somewhat logical, reasoning led to many sound conclusions. For example, Aristotle wrote, "All human actions have one or more of these seven causes: chance, nature, compulsions, habit, reason, passion, desire." Modern psychologists might say that Aristotle provided a good start to explaining health behavior. Health behaviors such as exercise and eating behaviors can all be prompted by the seven factors that Aristotle listed.

The ancient Greek physician-philosopher Hippocrates, best known for the Hippocratic oath that physicians take when they begin practicing medicine, wrote, "If we could give every individual the right amount of nourishment and exercise, not too little and not too much, we would have found the safest way to health." Many readers and health professionals would agree.

illnesses have some psychosomatic characteristics. Feelings of stress are especially likely to worsen many chronic health problems, such as asthma, skin problems, digestive disorders, and heart disease (Thoits, 2010). The term psychosomatic illness is less commonly heard today because it does not particularly distinguish a special and definitive disease process.

Health psychologists study how psychological factors are related to health and illness. For example, they might ask the following:

- How is hostility related to increased risk for heart disease?
- How does depression increase risk of premature illness and death?

The Experience of Sickness and Health

Health psychologists are interested in how people experience health and health problems. They explore how people respond to their own health problems as well as the health problems of family members and friends. They might ask the following:

- How do people access health care?
- What kind of healers do they turn to for help (Fig. 1-3)?
- How do people help themselves when they experience health problems?

Health psychologists have done a great deal of research on people's interactions with medical-care systems. They have looked at provider-patient communication, the influence of social support on patient health outcomes, and the stressful nature of many hospital experiences. Patient adherence to medical advice has been a popular area of study. Some of the topics health psychologists explore include the following:

- Why do so many patients quit taking prescribed medication without informing their providers?
- Why do people diagnosed with diabetes often continue to eat too much of the wrong foods despite diabetes education?

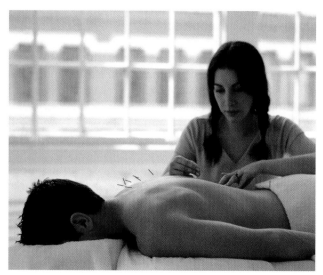

Figure 1-3. Acupuncture. © Thinkstock

Health psychologists explore how people cope with poor health, not only when treatments are available to speed recovery but also when no effective treatments are available. They study how people cope with pain and suffering and chronic and worsening illness, as well as death and dying. Questions include the following:

- How do people perceive death and interact with the health-care system in these challenging situations?
- How can hospice care be most effectively delivered?

Health-Promoting and Health-Damaging Behavior

Health psychologists study the relationship between behavior and health as well as the many factors that influence lifestyle choices. They are interested in why some people are motivated to develop healthful lifestyles that include good eating and physical activity behaviors. Health psychologists also study why some people develop habits that are likely to damage their health, whereas others do not. Health psychologists explore questions such as the following:

- Why do some people show a great deal of self-control and succeed at changing eating and exercise behaviors?
- Why do some people have more difficulty quitting smoking than others?
- What predisposes some people to addiction to alcohol or drugs? Work? Sex? Exercise?

Evaluation of Health Promotion Strategies

Some health psychologists study the effectiveness of health-promotion and disease-prevention strategies. They study issues such as the following:

- How do people respond to public health campaigns urging them to get a flu shot or wear seat belts?
- How can worksite health programs get more people to exercise?
- Which strategies are best at reaching the currently sedentary population?
- How can the medical system best advise people on preventing chronic illness?
- How can providers learn to communicate more effectively?
- How can providers help motivate patients to take action to improve their health and prevent disease?

Health psychologists are also concerned with improving health-care delivery systems and health-care policy. Areas of interest include the following:

- How could people learn to access health care through clinics rather the hospital emergency department?
- How can health-care services become more affordable, given a certain level of financial resources, and what services should be available?

- How can low-income families, who have a disproportionately high rate of health problems, be better supported in adopting behaviors that help with disease prevention?

Health Disparities Between Groups

Health psychologists are also interested in the health of communities and countries. Some health psychology researchers study the health disparities between nations and look for factors responsible for these differences. For example, although the United States spends more than any other country on health care, it has a fairly high rate of infant mortality, whereas other countries that spend less on health care have healthier babies (Murray & Frenk, 2010). Health psychologists might explore the following:

- Why is access to health care not always associated with good health?
- Why are some groups within the United States more prone to certain diseases than others?
- Are the observed differences due to ethnicity, socioeconomic status, or education? Dietary behaviors? Family structure or religious practices?

The Interdisciplinary Nature of Health Psychology

Health psychology is an expanding and increasingly interdisciplinary field. It draws information and methods from the fields of sociology, anthropology, biology and the health sciences, psychophysiology, economics, and public health. Health psychologists interested in stress management, health promotion, and disease prevention have become increasingly interested in the importance of exercise and frequently venture into the realm of exercise psychology and other exercise sciences as they explore issues such as motivation for exercise and the emotional health benefits of physical activity.

As Evan watches Jason interact with the people coming to the medical fitness center, Evan notices that Jason seems to listen more than talk. This is what his supervisor Carla meant when she directed Evan to slow down, connect and listen more, and talk less. Because Evan has been anxious to impress everyone with his exercise science background, he has had a tendency to say a lot and talk too fast to make sure everyone could see how knowledgeable he was about exercise physiology and exercise prescription.

But now Evan is beginning to understand that the people coming to the fitness center want more than advice. The picture of people's lives is so much larger than he had anticipated! These people want reassurance, support, a friendly face, and a smile. Some are uncertain about

their health and whether they are doing their exercises correctly. Many are retired and seem to have a lot of time on their hands; they move fairly slowly through their routines.

This week Evan is no longer folding towels but is shadowing the personal trainers as they work with new clients. It has been hard for him to listen without saying anything, but he believes that he is learning a lot. ■

Exercise Psychology

Exercise psychology studies the psychological factors related to the performance of exercise and physical activity. These include the psychological variables that are related to whether people are active, as well as the psychological effects of exercise. Exercise psychology emerged originally from the field of sport psychology, which focused primarily on the psychology of athletes and sport performance. This section examines some of the most common areas of study within the field of exercise psychology.

Motivation to Exercise

Exercise psychologists are interested in what motivates all kinds of people to participate in sport and exercise. For example, they explore the following:

- What motivates lifelong exercisers?
- Why do sedentary people decide to start an exercise program?
- How do people new to exercise make the decision to begin, and what steps do they take to begin exercising?

Exercise Adherence

Exercise adherence is following, and not dropping out of, an exercise program. Exercise adherence means sticking to a specified set of physical activity recommendations. Exercise psychologists try to tease out the factors associated with exercise program adherence and dropping out. They also study, design, and test strategies to enhance exercise adherence, including cognitive and behavioral skills that might help people continue to exercise in the face of difficulties. Some exercise psychologists work in the area of obesity treatment. They are concerned with adherence to lifestyle change programs that include both eating behaviors and exercise. Exercise adherence is a critical area of study for both disease treatment, as in the case of cardiac rehabilitation, and disease prevention.

Positive Psychological Effects of Exercise

One of the most fascinating areas of study in exercise psychology concerns the psychological effects of exercise. Exercise psychologists have studied the effects of exercise on many variables, including mood, fatigue, pain perception, self-concept, and emotional health. Exercise sometimes improves mood disorders, including depression and anxiety, as well as feelings of stress. Exercise has been explored as a tool for psychotherapy.

Exercise psychologists have also investigated the relationship between participation in physical activity and altered states of consciousness. Many committed exercisers have reported feelings of euphoria and enjoyment during exercise, known as the "runner's high." Exercise psychologists explore the psychophysiology of this euphoria as well as other reports of peak experience during exercise. Exercise psychologists study questions such as the following:

- What factors are associated with the experience of euphoric states during exercise?
- What types and amounts of exercise are most effective for treating depression?

Negative Effects of Exercise

Unfortunately, the effects of physical activity are not all positive. Exercise psychologists also study the negative effects of exercise participation, such as injury and compulsive behaviors. For example, they might explore the following:

- How do people committed to sport and physical activity cope with injuries that limit participation?
- How do people deal with catastrophic injury?
- What criteria differentiate between committed and compulsive exercisers?
- How do people with body image and eating disorders use exercise to purge calories and cope with disordered eating behaviors?

How Personality Interacts with Exercise Participation

Exercise psychologists study how personality is related to athletic achievement and sport performance. They investigate relationships among personality traits and exercise motivation, exercise adherence, and mood enhancement following exercise. They research questions such as the following:

- Are certain personality traits predictive for risk of developing exercise dependence?
- How can people develop stronger willpower in order to make regular physical activity a priority?

Exercise and Quality of Life

Exercise has a great deal to offer as a tool for disease treatment and prevention, helping people to stay healthy and recover from illness. But physical activity can also be helpful for people with debilitating and terminal illnesses by improving quality of life. Physical activity can improve quality of life for the very old, helping them to maintain functional capacity for as long as possible. Exercise psychologists examine the meaning of quality of life and the role that physical activity plays for people with a variety of conditions and limitations. Even when exercise may not prolong life, it can make life more enjoyable and delay dependence on others for help with the activities of daily living.

■ *Carla is impressed that Evan has toned down his talkativeness and decides he is ready to help clients get started using the fitness center. She gives Evan a folder of forms to help prepare him for working with his first client. Chester is a 68-year-old male who has just been diagnosed with type 2 diabetes. Chester's wife of 45 years died 2 years ago, and, since that time, Chester has gained 20 pounds. Chester runs a Christmas tree farm out in the country and is somewhat active. Chester's doctor would like the medical fitness staff to help Chester develop an exercise program to improve his blood sugar regulation; he will also be working with a dietitian on improving his eating habits. Carla instructs Evan to start Chester on 20 minutes of aerobic activity and a simple six-station weight-training program that works the major muscle groups.*

Evan wants to give Chester much higher volumes of exercise. He wonders, "How else will he get the diabetes under control?" Evan has learned that diabetes improves most with at least 45 minutes of exercise a day. And only six stations? How is he supposed to hit all the muscles with only six stations? This is going to be a challenge. ■

HEALTH AND BEHAVIOR

Both health psychologists and exercise psychologists study behavior. The term behavior refers to the way something acts, or behaves. Behavior related to or affecting health is called **health-related behavior** or **health behavior**. Health-related behaviors include those related to smoking, sleeping, drug use, exercising, eating, and sex. Many behaviors affect health, from looking both ways before crossing a road and walking carefully on icy sidewalks to resisting the urge to join the brawl in the pub and taking a hot bath to relax. In fact, almost everything affects health, when health is defined broadly to include physical, psychological, and social well-being.

Of course, some health-related behaviors have a greater impact than others. When public health officials are evaluating which health behaviors should be targeted in their educational and outreach efforts, they will look for the behaviors that have the greatest impact on the biggest health problems for the largest number of people. Impact can be judged by the costs, both monetary and other, attributed to a given behavior. For example, researchers might estimate the health-care costs associated with a particular behavior, such as smoking tobacco, or mortality rates for illnesses caused or contributed to by a given behavior, such as excessive alcohol consumption. Other costs may be considered as well, such as lost productivity from illness (days or even years that a person was unable to work because of illness or premature death).

Some important costs are difficult to measure, such as influence on quality of life.

The Impact of Behavior on Health

What is the impact of behavior on health? How can the effect be measured? How much does behavior matter? Should people really be concerned about their smoking, eating, or physical activity? Experts look at the impact of behavior on health in a variety of ways. One of the most common indicators used by epidemiologists is cause of death. Although cause of death alone does not capture the entire health picture, all countries keep track of these statistics, so they are readily available. Looking at cause of death provides a broad picture of a country's important health issues.

The leading causes of death in the United States have changed over time (Table 1-2). (For definitions of the causes of death not discussed in detail here, see Box 1-4.) In 1900, the top three causes of death were infections (pneumonia and influenza, tuberculosis, and diarrhea and digestive infections), whereas by 2010 the top three causes were chronic illnesses, most with no single clear causative agent: heart disease, cancer, and chronic lower respiratory diseases. As researchers have followed this changing picture of mortality rates in the United States, they have searched for explanations. The decline in infectious illness is attributed to improved sanitation in homes and communities, cleaner water supplies, better personal hygiene (including more hand

Table 1-2. Top 10 Causes of Death in the United States, 1900 and 2010

1900	2010
1. Pneumonia and influenza	Heart disease
2. Tuberculosis	Cancer
3. Diarrhea and digestive tract infections	Chronic lower respiratory disease
4. Heart disease	Stroke
5. Stroke	Accidents
6. Kidney disease	Alzheimer's disease
7. Accidents	Diabetes
8. Cancer	Kidney disease
9. Senility	Influenza and pneumonia
10. Diphtheria	Suicide

Information from the National Center for Health Statistics, Centers for Disease Control and Prevention.
Murphy, S. L., Xu, J., & Kochanek, K. D. (2012). Deaths: preliminary data for 2010. *National Vital Statistics Reports*, *60*(4). Retrieved from www.cdc.gov/nchs/data/nvsr/nvsr60/nvsr60_04.pdf

Box 1-4. Causes of Death: Definitions

Some of the causes of death listed in the tables in this chapter may be unfamiliar to many readers. The causes not otherwise discussed in this chapter are defined briefly here.

Chronic lower respiratory disease: Chronic diseases of the lower airways, including the bronchi and lungs. Usually refers to chronic bronchitis and emphysema. Same as chronic obstructive pulmonary disease.

Chronic obstructive pulmonary disease (COPD): Diseases involving persistent obstruction of airflow, usually chronic bronchitis and emphysema (as opposed to asthma, which is usually reversible). These diseases cause the airways to narrow, restricting airflow.

Coronary heart disease (CHD): Heart disease caused by insufficient circulation to the heart; the arteries supplying the heart are called the coronary arteries. Same as coronary artery disease.

Diarrhea and digestive tract infections: Diarrhea refers to frequent and watery bowel movements. Diarrhea can be caused by many things, including infectious bacteria and viruses. Diarrhea is usually one of the symptoms of digestive tract infections.

Diphtheria: Infectious disease characterized by fever, weakness, and difficulty breathing. People in higher-income countries are usually immunized against this illness, which often caused death in 1900.

HIV/AIDS: Human immunodeficiency virus (HIV) weakens certain immune cells, leading to acquired immune deficiency syndrome (AIDS), in which the body is unable to control infectious agents. HIV is spread through the exchange of bodily fluids, especially when sharing needles as in intravenous drug use, and during sexual intercourse.

Hypertensive heart disease: Problems with the heart associated with high blood pressure. High blood pressure leads to a thickening of the heart muscle and its arteries, which can lead to inefficient pumping action and heart failure.

Influenza (flu): A contagious viral infection that causes inflammation of the respiratory system, fever, chills, and muscle weakness and pain. The main cause of death from influenza is pneumonia.

Continued

Box 1-4. Causes of Death: Definitions–cont'd

Kidney disease: Diseases of the kidney impair kidney function. The two leading causes of kidney disease are hypertension and diabetes.

Lower respiratory infections: Infections of the bronchi and lungs, including pneumonia, bronchitis, and other infections.

Malaria: An infectious illness caused by a parasite spread by infected mosquitoes. Malaria is responsible for a million deaths each year, especially in sub-Saharan Africa.

Neonatal infections: Infections occurring in newborn infants.

Pneumonia: A disease of the lungs, where the lungs become inflamed and filled with excess fluid. Pneumonia can be caused by viruses or bacteria. Some categories of mortality list pneumonia and influenza together because the causes are hard to separate. In other words, flu can often lead to pneumonia.

Tuberculosis: Bacterial infection most commonly infecting the lungs. The body isolates the bacteria by creating nodules (tubercles) around them. Tuberculosis is characterized by fever, weight loss, and chest pain and was a leading cause of death in 1900. It is still dangerous today, although less prevalent, because antibiotic-resistant strains are developing.

washing), and improved methods of food preparation at home and outside the home. The discovery and development of antibiotics also has helped to reduce mortality from infectious disease.

The leading causes of death today are more complicated. Heart disease, cancer, and chronic lower respiratory diseases are said to be **multifactorial** in causation, meaning that many factors lead to their development. Some of these factors are uncontrollable, including genetics and aging. But scientists believe that many of these illnesses are caused in large part by health behaviors. Examining the factors associated with some of the leading causes of death provides a good illustration of the strong link between health and behavior.

Behavior and Heart Disease

Heart disease includes all diseases affecting the heart, including infections, irregular heartbeat, valve problems, and problems with the circulatory system of the heart. The leading cause of death from heart disease is **atherosclerosis**, also known as hardening of the arteries. Over time, the lining of the arteries becomes irritated and inflamed, a process thought to be triggered by blood fats and cholesterol in the form of damaged **low-density lipoproteins** (LDLs) building up on the arterial lining. Immune cells move in to destroy the damaged LDLs. The immune cells are unable to dissolve the material on the artery wall but instead trigger chronic inflammation. The material that accumulates from the process of atherosclerosis is called **plaque**. Plaque is composed of not only cholesterol and fats but also calcium and other minerals, immune cells, and blood clots.

Plaque does not always cause a problem. Often the plaque stabilizes and, in some cases, can even shrink (Ornish, 1998). Other times, the plaque may become increasingly inflamed, swell, and break open. When this happens, blood clots may form, and the clots and particles of plaque can lodge in the bloodstream and cut off

blood flow. When blockage occurs in an artery of the heart, the result is a heart attack, or **myocardial infarction** (Fig.1-4). When heart tissue does not receive an adequate supply of blood, the cells in that area die, and the heartbeat can be disrupted. **Coronary heart disease** refers to heart disease caused by disease in the coronary arteries, which supply blood to the heart muscle.

Initially, early changes in the artery walls may appear as **fatty streaks**, indicating the early stages of the atherosclerotic process. Fatty streaks may develop in adolescence or even earlier. As time goes by, the fatty streaks may become thicker and larger until the function of the artery lining is disrupted, and the plaques cause severe damage. Plaques can build in any artery and compromise blood flow in that region. Plaques in the arteries supplying the brain can cause **ischemic stroke**, brain damage caused by a lack of blood flow to a region of the brain. Ischemic stroke usually occurs when a blood clot and bits of plaque block the artery. (**Hemorrhagic stroke** is caused when a blood vessel in the brain bursts and disrupts normal circulation.) Plaque and blood clots can block blood flow in the blood vessels of the legs or arms or of the kidneys and other organs.

Scientists do not understand all of the factors that cause the development of plaque in the arteries; however, they have found that certain **risk factors** are associated with the likelihood of the development of atherosclerosis in an individual. A risk factor is a variable that helps to predict the likelihood of an event or disease process. Risk factors indicate probabilities only; they are not always causative in and of themselves. Instead, they may be related to another factor that operates to cause physiological changes that lead to disease. For example, poverty increases risk for atherosclerosis. Poverty, in and of itself, does not cause the plaque buildup. Other related risk factors, such as higher levels of stress hormones, harmful dietary patterns, inability to afford fruits and vegetables, poor environmental air quality, and smoking, contribute to the physical buildup of plaque.

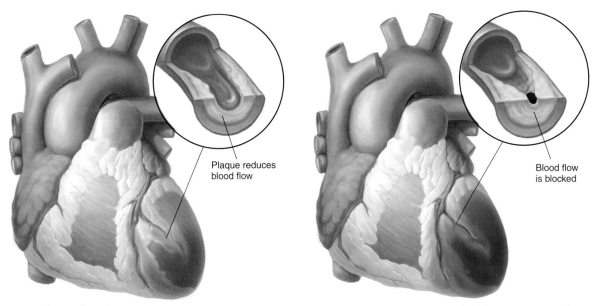

Plaque reduces
blood flow

Blood flow
is blocked

Figure 1-4. Atherosclerosis. *(Modified From Gylys,B. & Wedding, M.E.: Medical Terminology Systems. F.A. Davis, Philadelphia, 2009, p.198; with permission.)*

Dozens of risk factors for artery disease have been identified. Some of these are strong predictors of risk but cannot be changed and are often referred to as unmodifiable risk factors. For example, age and heredity both strongly influence risk, but a person is unable to change these. Other risk factors are at least somewhat modifiable and appear to be entirely or partly related to health behaviors. Behavior-related risk factors include the following:

- **Smoking:** Smoking tobacco seems to speed the process of atherosclerosis in several ways. Chemicals in the smoke may activate the LDL particles to begin sticking to the artery lining. Smoking may also lower the levels of various protective factors in the blood. The nicotine in tobacco smoke raises blood pressure, which in turn can accelerate plaque buildup. Heart disease is the leading cause of tobacco-related deaths.
- **Sedentary lifestyle:** A sedentary lifestyle means that people have very low levels of physical activity. Such low activity levels are harmful to health. Regular physical activity appears to maintain arterial health in many ways. It helps to reduce inflammation, improve blood cholesterol levels, reduce high blood pressure, and improve blood sugar regulation. Exercise burns calories and helps prevent excess body fat, in combination with appropriate food intake. If physical activity helps people feel happier and less stressed, it may reduce heart disease risk by reducing levels of harmful stress hormones. When frequent activity does not occur, artery disease is more likely to develop as the systems described earlier fail to function optimally.
- **Hypertension:** Hypertension appears to damage the artery lining and make the lining more susceptible to the process of atherosclerosis.

Hypertension is not a health behavior per se, but hypertension can be reduced somewhat with a good diet that is low in sodium but high in fruits, vegetables, and other healthful foods. Blood pressure can also be reduced with regular exercise, stress management, and reducing excess weight.

- **Diabetes:** Diabetes is a disorder marked by poor blood sugar regulation, resulting in elevated levels of blood sugar. There are several types of diabetes. The most common is type 2 diabetes, which begins with a problem in the body's response to the hormone insulin, which signals receptors on the cell membranes to direct cells to take up sugar from the blood. Like hypertension, type 2 diabetes is not a behavior but is strongly influenced by a variety of behaviors, including diet and physical activity. Excess body weight (which is also influenced by diet and activity) increases a person's likelihood of developing type 2 diabetes.
- **Harmful blood fat levels:** Higher blood levels of LDLs and lower levels of high-density lipoproteins (HDLs) are associated with increased risk for atherosclerosis. High-density lipoproteins are large compounds that carry cholesterol and fat in the bloodstream. The blood levels of these fats are influenced by a number of different factors, including sex (women have higher HDL levels than men, until they reach menopause), exercise (which raises HDLs), alcohol consumption (moderate consumption raises HDLs), genetics (some people inherit a defect in fat metabolism that raises LDLs), and obesity.
- **Obesity:** Some researchers believe that much of obesity's association with atherosclerosis risk is the fact that obesity can be a marker for other lifestyle factors, including poor diet and sedentary lifestyle. However, visceral obesity,

which refers to excess fat tissue located around the viscera (the abdominal organs), has a strong association with, and may contribute to the causation of, type 2 diabetes, hypertension, harmful blood fat levels, and atherosclerosis.

- **Poor diet:** Researchers continue to debate what is meant by a poor diet, and dietary recommendations for good health are discussed in more depth in Chapter 9. Most scientists agree, however, that poor eating habits often include too many calories, not enough vegetables and fruits, and too many processed foods high in added sugars and fats, and refined grains. Poor dietary habits may contribute to a number of heart disease risk factors, including obesity, harmful blood fat levels, hypertension, and diabetes.
- **Stress:** Stress is the most difficult to define of the heart disease risk factors, because moderate levels of stress are considered normal. Stress appears to become most harmful when stress hormone levels are elevated for long periods of time and when people perceive sources of stress to be negative, likely to have a harmful outcome, uncontrollable, and unrelenting. Elevated stress responses have been linked to hypertension and heart disease. Feelings of stress may also affect other important health behaviors, because people under stress may smoke more, exercise less, and make poorer food choices.

Modification of these behavior-related risk factors can lead to improved disease management/treatment.

■ *Evan is a little worried about getting started with Chester, but once he meets Chester, his fears evaporate. Chester is a friendly, talkative, easygoing man. Although he has never been in a fitness center before, he has a good attitude and has decided to do everything he can to improve his blood sugar regulation. Evan asks Chester a number of questions about his health concerns and fitness goals and gives Chester plenty of time to talk, resisting his impulse to jump in and start giving Chester advice. As Evan comes to see that Chester is truly a beginner at organized exercise programs, he understands why Carla recommended starting him off slowly. Evan does not want to scare Chester away with a program that is too complicated. In fact, teaching Chester how to use six strength-station machines may be too much! Evan's hour with Chester is almost up already, so Evan spends the rest of the time helping Chester get comfortable on the treadmill. After 10 minutes of walking, Chester is finally walking at a normal pace without grabbing onto the handrail every few seconds. Chester seems pleased that he has mastered his first machine. He thanks Evan warmly and promises to return in 2 days. Carla compliments Evan on his*

good listening skills and adapting his approach to Chester's personal needs. ■

Behavior and Cancer

Cancer refers to a group of diseases that are characterized by uncontrolled abnormal cell growth. Normal cells have a limited life span and die when they become old or damaged. Cancer cells somehow evade this process and continue to grow and multiply. Although cancer is driven by changes to a cell's genetic material, researchers believe that only 5% to 10% of cancers are caused by inherited genetic defects and that the majority of cancers are due to a combination of lifestyle and environmental factors, including exposure to carcinogens, substances that initiate and promote the development of cancer (Anand et al., 2008). Carcinogens can take the form of radiation (e.g., ultraviolet exposure from the sun that increases risk of skin cancer), viruses (e.g., some types of human papillomavirus increase risk for cervical cancer in women), and chemicals (e.g., many of the chemicals in tobacco smoke act as carcinogens in the body). Some of this exposure is the result of health behaviors, whereas much of it is simply a result of living in the modern world, where carcinogens appear in the water, air, and food supply as well as in common household and occupational chemicals. Although rates of cancers caused by infectious agents appear to be declining around the world, cancers related to lifestyle are expected to continue to rise (Bray, Jemal, Grey, Ferlay, & Forman, 2012).

Individuals can do a great deal to reduce their exposure to carcinogens and adopt behaviors that may reduce cancer risk. Some of the health behaviors most strongly related to risk of cancer include the following:

- **Tobacco use:** Use of tobacco products is thought to be the primary cause of many cancers. Cigarette smoking causes 80% to 90% of lung cancer, as well as many other types of cancer.
- **Alcohol consumption:** Alcohol increases risk of several cancers, especially cancers of the breast, liver, esophagus, stomach, colon, and rectum.
- **Diets:** Some chemicals in food, including certain chemicals produced when charring meats, increase risk. However, plenty of fruits and vegetables in the diet reduce cancer risk.
- **Sedentary lifestyle:** A sedentary lifestyle is associated with increased cancer risk. Regular physical activity has been associated with reduced risk of breast, colon, and prostate cancers. Physical activity helps to prevent obesity, another risk factor for cancer.
- **Unprotected sexual behavior:** Some sexually transmitted viruses increase cancer risk, especially human immunodeficiency virus (HIV), the virus that causes AIDS, and human papillomavirus.
- **Sun exposure:** Unprotected exposure increases skin cancer risk.

- **Poor sleeping behavior:** Irregular sleep patterns, as seen in people who work night shifts (and many college students), are associated with increased risk of breast and prostate cancers. Melatonin, a hormone that increases with exposure to darkness and enhances sleep, helps to prevent these cancers and may be in short supply in sleepless people.
- **Exposure to toxic chemicals and other carcinogens:** Exposure can be reduced in many ways. Obviously, avoiding carcinogenic chemicals is best, at home, at work, in the art studio, and in the chemistry lab. Wearing gloves, working in well-ventilated areas, and following other recommended protective procedures significantly reduce risk.

In addition, some types of cancer are highly curable if caught early. Regular screenings for skin, cervical, breast, prostate, and colorectal cancers can find cancers when they are most treatable.

Behavior and Other Leading Causes of Death

Smoking contributes to chronic lower respiratory diseases such as emphysema and chronic bronchitis. The process of atherosclerosis that leads to heart disease can cause ischemic stroke, so the relationship between lifestyle and artery disease in the heart is the same for artery disease in the brain. Hemorrhagic stroke risk increases with hypertension, so lifestyle factors that reduce hypertension risk reduce stroke risk as well.

Fatigue, alcohol use, and anger increase risk of fatal accidents. A balanced lifestyle with adequate rest, a nutritious diet, and physical activity keeps the immune system at its best and may help prevent infections such as pneumonia and influenza (the flu). Alzheimer's disease may be somewhat related to lifestyle. Compromised blood flow to the brain from atherosclerosis appears to be part of the disease, so the factors discussed previously in the section on heart disease apply to Alzheimer's disease as well. Smoking, poor diet, and sedentary lifestyle may affect brain health in additional ways, perhaps through the immune system and processes of inflammation. Hypertension and diabetes are two of the leading causes of kidney disease.

Understanding Applications of Risk Factor Data

It is important to note that these links between health behaviors and causes of death are in the long run "on-the-average" observations that may or may not apply to any given individual. Many people have multiple behavior-related risk factors for diseases yet are never afflicted, whereas others embrace all the right health behaviors but die at an early age. There is a great deal that researchers do not understand about health and disease.

It is also important to remember that the larger picture of an individual's life includes other risk factors such as education level, socioeconomic status, place of residence, occupation, and genetics that interact with the health behavior variables discussed previously. It is

important to not "blame the victims" for their diseases. For example, people dealing with heart disease, obesity, or lung cancer should not be blamed for their health problems. Risk factors may or may not have played a role; in any individual life, the complex interactions of heredity, environment, behavior, and luck are difficult to tease apart. Many factors influencing health are not under an individual's control.

MOTIVATING CHANGE Suspend Judgment and Praise Effort

Understanding the link between health behaviors and disease risk can easily lead you to become judgmental regarding the behaviors of clients with whom you are working. Such judgment is shortsighted and harmful to the therapeutic relationship that you are trying to establish. People are more likely to change their behaviors when they are feeling positive about themselves and strong. Judgment from others reinforces what they are doing wrong, paints a negative picture of them, and builds negative feelings. Judgment says, "You are a bad person. You are stupid for (fill in the blank: smoking, getting fat, not exercising). It is your own fault, and you should change." Imagine how you would feel if you knew that someone was thinking that way about you.

Health and fitness professionals themselves always have areas of their lives in which they could improve. For example, maybe your exercise program is good, but your desk is a mess and you tend to procrastinate. Having flaws is human; acknowledging your own shortcomings allows you to build empathy with your clients. Nobody is perfect; we are all on self-improvement journeys. We are trying to do our best with the cards that we have been dealt. The best way to improve your relationship with clients who are struggling with health behavior change is to acknowledge that change is difficult in your own life as well, that you try hard yourself to improve whatever area you are working on, and that you applaud the efforts your clients are making. Your faith in them, your hope for a better future, and your total immersion in the learning process and excitement about the progress you see them making will give them more effective motivation than negative judgments.

Calculating Risk: Which Behaviors Have the Greatest Impact on Health?

The previous discussion underlines the importance of health-related behavior. Certain behaviors, as seen previously, are risk factors for a number of causes of death. For example, smoking contributes to deaths from heart disease, cancer, stroke, respiratory disease, pneumonia, Alzheimer's disease, and kidney disease. Exercise level and diet made several appearances as well. Is there any way to quantify which behaviors have the greatest impact on health?

Researchers have attempted to do just that. Using available figures for how much different factors contribute to the various causes of death, Mokdad, Marks, Stroup, and Gerberding (2004) calculated what they called "actual causes of death" (rather than which organ or system failed, such as heart, lung, or kidney disease) (Table 1-3).

Although some researchers have questioned the methods for calculating the numbers in Table 1-3, they still provide interesting food for thought. Some (Blair, 2004) have criticized the method for estimated deaths due to poor diet and physical inactivity because these were estimated from data on obesity. Physical activity and diet can also contribute to death independent of their effects on obesity, and, of course, not all obese people are inactive. Nevertheless, Table 1-3, along with the earlier discussion of the relationship between behavior and causes of mortality, presents a compelling picture of the strong link between lifestyle and the leading causes of death in the United States. The analysis presented in Table 1-3 suggests that the risk factors most closely connected with mortality rates (of the risk factors analyzed) are tobacco, diet, and physical activity. According to the analysis, these three factors are responsible for about one-third of annual deaths in the United States.

Readers should also note that these lifestyle factors influence morbidity as well as mortality. Although the preceding analysis focused on causes of death, many people live with chronic illness that significantly limits quality of life. Health-related behaviors affect not only quantity but also quality of life.

Global Health: Health Behavior Around the World

When mortality data from around the world are examined, many similarities are apparent between the United States and other relatively high-income countries (Table 1-4). Some of the differences between the

Table 1-3. Actual Causes of Death in the United States, 2000

ACTUAL CAUSE	NUMBER OF DEATHS ATTRIBUTED TO THIS CAUSE	PERCENTAGE OF TOTAL DEATHS IN 2000
Tobacco	435,000	18.1
Poor diet and physical activity	365,000	15.2
Alcohol consumption	85,000	3.5
Microbial agents	75,000	3.1
Toxic agents	60,000	2.3
Motor vehicle	43,000	1.8
Firearms	29,000	1.2
Sexual behavior	20,000	0.8
Illicit drug use	17,000	0.7
Total	1,124,000	46.8

Adapted from Mokdad, A. H., Marks, J. S., Stroup, D. F., & Gerberding, J. L. (2004). Actual causes of death in the United States, 2000. *Journal of the American Medical Association*, *291*(10): 1238-1245; and Mokdad, A. H. (2005). Correction: actual causes of death in the United States, 2000. *Journal of the American Medical Association*, *293*(3): 293-294.

Table 1-4. Top 10 Causes of Mortality for All Countries in 2008, Grouped by Income Level

CAUSE OF DEATH	PERCENTAGE OF DEATHS
High-income countries	
Coronary heart disease	15.6
Stroke	8.7
Respiratory system cancers	5.9
Alzheimer's and other dementias	4.1
Lower respiratory infections	3.8
Chronic obstructive pulmonary disease	3.5
Colon & rectal cancers	3.3
Diabetes	2.6
Hypertensive heart disease	2.3
Breast cancer	1.9
Middle-income countries	
Coronary heart disease	13.7
Stroke	12.8
Chronic obstructive pulmonary disease	7.2
Lower respiratory infections	5.4
Diarrheal illness	4.4
HIV/AIDS	2.7
Road traffic accidents	2.4
Tuberculosis	2.4
Diabetes	2.3
Hypertensive heart disease	2.2

Table 1-4. Top 10 Causes of Mortality for All Countries in 2008, Grouped by Income Level—cont'd

CAUSE OF DEATH	PERCENTAGE OF DEATHS
Low-income countries	
Lower respiratory infections	11.3
Diarrheal illness	8.2
HIV/AIDS	7.8
Coronary heart disease	6.1
Malaria	5.2
Stroke and cerebrovascular disease	4.9
Tuberculosis	4.3
Prematurity and low birth weight	3.2
Birth asphyxia and birth trauma	2.9
Neonatal infections	2.6

World Health Organization. (2010). The top ten causes of death. Fact sheet 310. Retrieved from www.who.int/mediacentre/factsheets/fs310_2008.pdf

Table 1-5. Leading Causes of Global Mortality, 2004*

CAUSE OF MORTALITY	PERCENTAGE OF TOTAL DEATHS
High blood pressure	12.8
Tobacco use	8.7
High blood sugar	5.8
Physical inactivity	5.5
Overweight and obesity	4.8
High cholesterol	4.5
Unsafe sex	4.0
Alcohol use	3.8
Childhood underweight	3.8
Indoor smoke from solid fuels	3.3

*Data from low-, middle-, and high-income countries are combined.
World Health Organization (WHO). (2009). Global health risks: mortality and burden of disease attributable to selected major risks. Retrieved from www.who.int/healthinfo/global_burden_disease/GlobalHealthRisks_report_full.pdf

mortality rates presented in Table 1-2 and those for high-income countries in Table 1-4 are due to differences in causes of death classification between the U.S. Centers for Disease Control and Prevention and WHO. For example, cancers are separated by cancer site in the WHO data, whereas the CDC table puts all cancers together.

Leading the pack for the high-income countries are heart disease, stroke, and respiratory cancers, all heavily influenced by tobacco use and the whole panoply of heart disease risk factors discussed earlier in this chapter.

Behavior is also related to the leading causes of death in middle- and low-income countries. For middle-income countries, heart disease, stroke, and COPD are the top three. Chronic obstructive pulmonary disease (COPD) is similar to the classification "diseases of the lower respiratory system," and again, mortality rates partly reflect tobacco use. People in low-income countries also die of heart disease (fourth leading cause of death) and stroke (sixth leading cause) but more frequently die of infectious diseases, including lower respiratory infections such as pneumonia and influenza, diarrheal illnesses, and HIV/AIDS.

How much of the global disease burden is attributable to preventable or controllable risk factors? Data from WHO, for all countries combined—including low, middle, and high-income countries—are presented in Table 1-5. High blood pressure leads the list of modifiable

risk factors, followed by tobacco use. High blood sugar (diabetes), physical inactivity, overweight and obesity, and high cholesterol follow. These data demonstrate the strong association between health behaviors and modifiable risk factors (such as hypertension and obesity), and causes of death, not only in the United States but also around the world. It is interesting to note that of the top seven causes of death for high-income countries, six are related to physical activity and diet. One cannot help but wonder how a healthy lifestyle, if carried out by everyone in a country, would affect life expectancy. Several research groups have attempted such calculations. One group, from the United Kingdom, calculated that people who do not smoke but do exercise, eat an adequate amount of fruits and vegetables, and drink alcohol in moderation live an additional 14 years compared to the life expectancy of people who practice none of those four behaviors (Khaw et al., 2008).

Health Behavior and Quality of Life

These analyses are interesting from population perspectives, and they present a large picture of national and global health. But what about health conditions that may not show up on mortality data charts? Many health issues not mentioned are strongly related to health behaviors. Preventing or at least delaying these conditions greatly improves quality of life.

Osteoporosis, a disease characterized by progressive loss of bone mineral, is a good example. Like atherosclerosis, osteoporosis has both unmodifiable and modifiable risk factors. Risk increases with age, sex, and genetics: older, thin Caucasian and Asian women with strong family histories have greatest risk. But lifestyle factors can help preserve bone density, even in this group. Strength training and other weight-bearing exercise, along with a good diet that includes enough protein and plenty of fruits and vegetables, together with some sources of calcium and vitamin D, reduce risk of fracture.

Another example is back pain. Chronic back pain plagues many adults. Many cases of back pain are worsened by a combination of obesity and too much sitting. Appropriate exercise that strengthens core muscle groups, along with education on proper posture and body mechanics, helps reduce back pain for many people, as does moderate weight loss.

Several emotional health problems also respond to health behavior measures. Feelings of stress and mild to moderate anxiety and depression often improve with exercise and various stress management techniques, such as breathing exercises and meditation.

Beyond reducing risk of premature death and illness, health behaviors have the potential to increase high-level wellness and to help people feel more energetic, positive, and productive. A healthful lifestyle can give people the energy and enthusiasm they need to achieve their goals and get the most out of life (Fig. 1-5).

In 2 days, Chester returns for more exercise and some instruction on using the strength training equipment. Evan greets him warmly and asks Chester how he felt after his first session on the treadmill. "Like a million bucks! No problem," Chester booms back. Evan is pleased to see Carla smiling at them from the window in her office, which overlooks the workout room. Chester hops right onto the treadmill and looks quite comfortable during his 20-minute walk. Evan helps Chester check his heart rate with the sensors on the machine but also shows him how to take his pulse to double-check the automatic sensors.

After the treadmill session, Evan begins showing Chester several of the strength training machines. Chester is very slow to catch on and needs a great deal of assistance setting the seat position and figuring out how to work the machine. Evan knows that his relationship with Chester takes precedence over getting the workout done, so he forces himself to move slowly and patiently. He understands that the most important job right now is to listen carefully to Chester's questions, answer them clearly, and build Chester's confidence for working out at the fitness center. ■

Behavior Change: An Emerging Priority

It may seem simple. Improving a few behaviors helps to promote health, improve quality of life, and prevent disease. To feel great, and maybe even live longer, people just need to quit smoking, exercise, eat right, and manage stress. What is the problem, then? The problem is that even though the scientific evidence supporting the link between behavior and health grows stronger every day, people's health behaviors are not changing nearly as much as they need to. Figure 1-6 illustrates the dramatic increase in diabetes that has

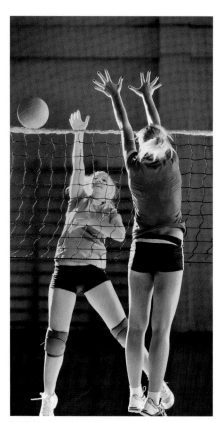

Figure 1-5. **High-level wellness.** © Thinkstock

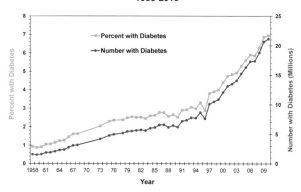

Number and Percentage of U.S. Population with Diagnosed Diabetes, 1958-2010

CDC's Division of Diabetes Translation. National Diabetes Surveillance System available at http://www.cdc.gov/diabetes/statistics

 CDC

Figure 1-6. Number and percentage of U.S. population with diagnosed diabetes, 1958-2010. *(Courtesy of CDC's Division of Diabetes Translation. National Diabetes Surveillance System.)*

occurred in the United States since 1958. The rate of diagnosed diabetes in the United States tripled from 1958 to 1998. Perhaps some of the increase can be explained by more-aggressive blood sugar testing and diagnosis, but it is unlikely that improvements in diagnosis would triple the rate. Since the mid 1990s, the rate of diabetes has doubled, so that in 2007, the rate was over six times higher than it was in 1958. Type 2 diabetes is often associated with low levels of physical activity and poor diet and is usually accompanied by obesity, so these high rates are a clarion call for health-behavior change on a national scale.

Figure 1-7 presents a similar picture. The rates of both obesity and diabetes are pictured for each state in the United States for the years 1994, 2000, and 2008. The maps present a striking picture of the increase in obesity and diabetes rates over this period. In 1994, less than 4.5% of the population was diagnosed with diabetes in many states. By 2008, the rate in many states had passed the 9% mark.

Behavior change for health promotion and disease prevention must become a priority for at least three reasons. First, behavior change can entirely prevent or at least significantly delay the development of many chronic illnesses, as discussed previously. Second, medications currently used to treat chronic illness are often expensive and frequently have undesirable side effects. They can certainly be helpful, especially when used in conjunction with behavior change. People often need less medication when improving their health behaviors. Third, U.S. health-care costs are rising dramatically, and the medical system simply cannot keep up with the increasing rates of chronic illness.

Given this knowledge and reasoning, why does behavior not change, or at least not change enough? Society at large deserves a great deal of the blame. People often do not have ready access to opportunities for physical activity. Healthy foods are more expensive than soft drinks containing high-fructose corn syrup made from subsidized corn. The pressures of jobs, family responsibilities, poverty, and other demands can pile up, and, for too many people, the easiest way to reduce feelings of stress is to turn on the television and grab a snack.

Can the medical system help? Many physicians have called for increased focus on the prevention of chronic illness and a better connection of medicine to public health, to include more prevention efforts in medical care (Marvasti & Stafford, 2012). Doctors can urge people to exercise, quit smoking, and eat well. But the current medical system is limited in its capacity to provide preventive care. The time and energy of doctors and other health-care providers is primarily spent on patients needing care for health problems, with little time left over to spend on efforts for prevention.

It is clear that social change is needed, along with medical reform. But individual responsibility for trying to make healthful choices must be a part of the health-care picture. Psychologists have discovered a great deal about how behavior change occurs, and this knowledge can help health and fitness professionals support behavior change efforts in their patients and clients. Research has already revealed a great of information about how people form the intention to change their behavior and go about making plans and exerting effort to exercise, eat better, or quit smoking (Johnson, Scott-Sheldon, & Carey, 2010; Lin, O'Connor, Whitlock, & Beil, 2010). Scientists know a great deal about successful motivation strategies, what factors are likely to best support people trying to change their health behaviors, and how to structure recreational, worksite, and educational programs to maximize adherence.

One thing is clear: giving advice is not enough. People have been given advice on health behaviors for years. Although some people do follow the advice, whether it

Age–Adjusted Prevalence of Obesity and Diagnosed Diabetes Among U.S. Adults Aged 18 years or older

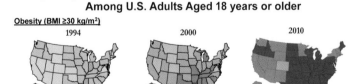

Obesity (BMI ≥30 kg/m²)

☐ No Data   ☐ <14.0%   ☐ 14.0% –17.9%   ☐ 18.0% – 21.9%   ☐ 22.0% – 25.9%   ■ ≥26.0%

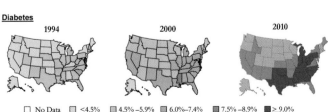

Diabetes

☐ No Data   ☐ <4.5%   ☐ 4.5% –5.9%   ☐ 6.0% –7.4%   ☐ 7.5% –8.9%   ■ ≥ 9.0%

Figure 1-7. **Percentage of U.S. adults who were obese or who had diagnosed diabetes.** *(Courtesy of CDC.)*

CDC's Division of Diabetes Translation. National Diabetes Surveillance System available at http://www.cdc.gov/diabetes/statistics

is from news reports, friends, or health-care providers, more do not. Health and fitness professionals are specially trained to work with people on an ongoing basis, to help guide people in positive ways to make their health and fitness a priority, and to help people realize that high-level wellness is worth the effort, because it gives people the energy to sustain a satisfying and fulfilling life.

■ *After 2 months of exercising and improving his diet, Chester has made progress with his diabetes control program. Evan is pleased when Chester informs him he has lost 10 pounds and that his morning blood glucose values are much better. So Evan is puzzled when Chester cancels several appointments at the fitness center in a row, saying he is too busy. Carla urges Evan to try calling Chester at home and remind him that one of the big reasons he was seeing such improvement was his exercise program. Chester sounds a little guilty over the phone and admits that the exercise program is getting pretty boring for him and that he has starting to walk more outdoors. Evan agrees to work with Chester to make some changes in the exercise recommendations to accommodate the outdoor walking.*

When Chester comes in a few days later, Evan greets him warmly, and the two of them sit down to discuss designing a new more-"outdoorsy" program for Chester. Evan opens the conversation by congratulating Chester again on his blood sugar improvements and weight loss, and then asks Chester if he realizes a lot of the improvements are because of the regular exercise. Chester seems surprised at the question and asks Evan to explain how exercise improves blood sugar values. This gives Evan a chance to provide Chester with more information about the effects of exercise on blood sugar regulation. He emphasizes how short-lived the exercise effects are and the importance of almost daily activity to keep the cells responding appropriately to insulin. Chester seems interested, and Evan gives him some information to read on exercise and diabetes.

Evan then works with Chester to set up an outdoor walking program. Chester is pleased that Evan is open to making these changes. He decides he will continue strength training twice a week with Evan because this type of exercise will help him with his work on his Christmas tree farm and because he now understands that strength training helps his blood sugar. Evan asks Chester if he would like more variety in the strength work, and Chester says that would be great. Evan is happy to have a chance

to use his exercise prescription skills to bring more ideas to Chester's program. ■

HOW PSYCHOLOGISTS STUDY HEALTH, EXERCISE, AND BEHAVIOR

Like all scientists, psychologists learn about health, exercise, and behavior by observing what goes on in the world, thinking about what they see, and then predicting what might happen, given certain situations. Sometimes they test their predictions by designing scientific experiments in which they set up a given situation and observe the outcome. Other times they measure different factors that occur in a group of people to see if a relationship exists among the factors. As they consider the outcomes of their studies, they revise their thinking and design more experiments (Fig. 1-8). This process of observing, thinking logically, predicting relationships, experimenting to test ideas, measuring variables, evaluating data, and drawing conclusions is called the scientific method. Scientists strive to be as objective as possible in their work in order to discover the truth, as far as humans can know it.

The Process of Science: Model Building

All of this observing and thinking leads to writing and description and to what scientists call theories. A theory is an explanation for things that scientists have observed. A theory usually outlines how one thing may cause another or how changes in one factor relate to changes in other factors. For example, a physician-scientist might observe that many of his heart disease patients seem angry, rushed, and controlling. He might theorize that people who are angry and impatient have higher rates of heart attack. This was exactly the case with Redford

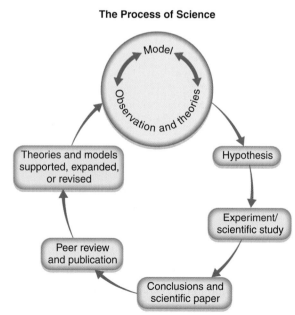

Figure 1-8. The process of science.

Williams and his colleagues Dahlstrom and Barefoot (What's the Evidence? 1-1).

Theories contribute to larger constructions that are referred to as models. A model is a representation, usually a simplification, of the subject of inquiry. The goal of science is to devise accurate models by testing theories. Using the process of science, the scientist speculating about the link between personality and heart attack comes up with his theory (one part of the explanation for heart disease causation). When he tests his theory, he contributes to the medical model that explains heart disease (the entire body of knowledge that explains the process of heart disease).

Psychologists use the scientific method to study health, exercise, and behavior. Researchers begin by reading everything published about the subject in which they are interested. The research groups described in "What's the Evidence? 1-1" read all the scientific papers that had ever been published on personality traits and risk of coronary heart disease. For example, they studied the research on Type A behavior pattern, one of the current (for their time) models that explained how personality traits might be related to risk of coronary heart disease (CHD). Type A behavior pattern is a theory created by cardiologists Meyer Friedman and Ray Rosenman (1974), who observed that their heart disease patients tended to share several personality traits. These patients were often highly competitive, hard driving, aggressive, and impatient. They were often "workaholics" with a high need for control. Barefoot and colleagues thought about the Type A research, as well as other research on stress and heart disease, and observed their own patients. They devised a new prediction: that the reason Type A behavior pattern increases risk of CHD is primarily the presence of feelings of hostility, distrust, and anger that are a part of the Type A profile. In other words, some of the characteristics (competitiveness, hardworking, and so forth) might not be harmful unless they generate negative feelings like anger. When scientists make a prediction like this, it is called a hypothesis. The hypothesis predicts the outcome of an experiment.

WHAT'S THE EVIDENCE? 1-1

Hostility Increases Risk of Death

Barefoot, J. D., Dahlstrom, W. G., & Williams, R. B. (1983). Hostility, CHD incidence, and total mortality: a 25-year follow-up study of 255 physicians. *Psychosomatic Medicine, 45*(1), 59-63.

■ PURPOSE

At the time of this study, research on the relationship between feelings of hostility, anger, and distrust was just beginning. Prior research on the relationship between hostility scores and CHD had demonstrated that in people undergoing coronary artery examination via angiograms, higher hostility scores were correlated with higher rates of artery blockage. The purpose of the study by Barefoot and colleagues was to look at the hostility-CHD relationship in a prospective manner, to see if hostility scores in young men were predictive of CHD 25 years later.

■ STUDY

Researchers were able to gather health and mortality data from 255 of 343 people who had taken a questionnaire measuring level of hostility while they were medical students at the University of North Carolina Medical School during the years 1954–1959. Responding subjects were divided into four groups based on the hostility scores. The death rate from CHD for subjects scoring highest on hostility was almost five times higher than that for subjects scoring in the lower two groups, supporting the idea that hostility is somehow associated with artery disease.

The researchers were also surprised by an unexpected result: hostility scores were strongly predictive of all-cause mortality in this group, not just mortality from CHD. Additional deaths were due to cancer, other cardiovascular problems, gastrointestinal illness, accidents, and suicide. The all-cause mortality rate for the two higher hostility groups was 6.4 times higher than for the lower two groups. The authors concluded, "Thus, it appears that high [hostility] scores not only contribute to the pathogenesis or progression of cardiovascular disease, but they also may affect one's ability to survive other disorders (p. 62)."

■ IMPLICATIONS

The researchers speculated that the link between feelings of anger, hostility, and distrust and CHD and other disease processes may be mediated partly by lack of social support. Feelings of anger, hostility, and distrust tend to push others away and lead to fewer social contacts and poorer social support. Social support is a powerfully protective factor. People need people; they need a social network that includes acquaintances, neighbors, colleagues, friends, and family.

Studies since 1983 have also demonstrated the negative impact of chronic tension and anger on the body. Helping people learn to better deal with negative thoughts and feelings is an important component of disease prevention. These observations underscore the important role that psychological factors play in health and disease.

Scientists then design an experiment in a way that tests the hypothesis, to find out if the hypothesis is true or false. Barefoot and colleagues did just that.

Once the experiment is done, the variables measured, and the conclusions drawn, the scientists write their report for a scientific journal. They send their article to the journal, and the journal reviews the new paper that they have received using the peer review process, in which scientific experts in the subject area scrutinize the article. The reviewers critique the article to be sure that the authors measured what they thought they were measuring, that the statistical methods were used appropriately, and that their conclusions are sound. Usually the journal editor sends the article back to the authors two or three times for clarifications; then, if the article passes muster, it is finally published. The article by Barefoot and colleagues was published in a peer-reviewed journal called *Psychosomatic Medicine* in 1983.

Results of a study are not accepted by the scientific community until the research reporting the findings has gone through the peer review process and have been accepted for publication. Even after publication, other scientists question the experimental methods, the statistics, and the results. Corrections are often printed, scientists argue at their professional meetings, and new experiments are conducted to challenge the existing research. New hypotheses are formed and tested. Theories are revised and expanded; models change. The process begins anew, with new arguments, thoughts, hypotheses, and experiments.

The Scientific Method: Solving Puzzles

Scientific studies take many different forms as they help expand and correct scientific models and theories. The scientific method uses logic, observation, and reasoning to determine relationships among variables. A variable is something that varies; in other words, it can take on two or more values. Minutes of exercise per week, height, age, and score on a measure of self-confidence are examples of variables. Scientists conduct investigations to try to understand how the change in one variable, typically called an independent variable or treatment variable, is related to or causes change in another variable, the dependent variable. To untangle these relationships, scientists use established research practices to identify the underlying truth as effectively as possible. The most common of these practices includes experimental studies, correlational studies, and qualitative studies.

Experimental Studies

Experimental studies have the most control over the subjects and variables involved. Typically an experimental situation is designed and administered, and results are observed. Some of the ways in which scientists conducting experimental studies strive to achieve accuracy in their results include the following.

Isolate the Effect of Independent Variables

To observe and understand the relationships between variables, researchers try to hold all nonexperimental variables as constant as possible, so that the independent and dependent variables are the variables that change during the experiment. For example, researchers are interested in the effect of exercise on certain chemicals in the brain. They might take two groups of rats and give one group exercise, while the other group does not get to exercise. To make differences in exercise level the only independent variable, researchers will try to keep all other conditions the same. They will use the exact same strain, age, and sex of rat in both groups and house, feed, handle, and care for all rats in identical ways. At the end of the experiment, when the chemical levels are compared, the scientists will be more certain that any changes in these chemicals will have been caused by differences in activity level.

Experiments with humans tend to present a different set of challenges. Sometimes researchers have little or no control over the variables in their studies. So instead of controlling outside variables, they will simply try to keep the variance of values for the outside variables as similar as possible for all groups. For example, if researchers want to find out whether students who learn and practice loving-kindness meditation report less stress and higher levels of well-being than other students, they might solicit a large group of volunteers. Obviously, the students will not be littermates with identical genetic material. They will have many other differences as well. To try to make groups as similar as possible, investigators use a process called random assignment. Random assignment to groups or treatments means that each subject has the same chance of getting into a given group. By assigning students randomly to groups (one group gets meditation, another gets an alternative treatment as similar as possible to meditation), researchers hope the groups vary in similar ways on factors such as health, sleep habits, diet, or anything else that might affect feelings of stress and well-being. Some students in each group will not be getting enough sleep, some will be breaking up with their romantic partners, and some will have parents going through a divorce. But the researchers hope that the level of background emotional distress will be similar for each group.

Control for the Expectations of Subjects and Researchers

Because expectations so strongly influence the way humans experience life, science tries to control these as much as possible. Subjects in the experiment should not know whether they are receiving a treatment that might cause a certain effect. The group receiving the actual experimental variable of interest is called the treatment group. A control group does not receive or undergo the treatment or variable that the experimenters are testing. Ideally, subjects in the control group often receive a dummy condition called a placebo. A placebo closely matches the treatment condition but lacks the ingredient believed to be exerting an effect. This group "controls for" the placebo effect (Box 1-5). The placebo effect refers to the fact that subjects in a study may demonstrate changes in the dependent variable simply because they are getting attention or expecting an effect, rather than because the independent variable itself is causing the change. In medicine, inert pills that look the same as the drug being tested are given. In a meditation study, one group will receive the real instructions, whereas another might simply discuss a related topic without actually meditating. Both groups will think that they are getting "the real thing." Even in animal studies, the control group receives a placebo. If the treatment groups receive an injection of a drug, the control group gets an injection of an inert substance, to control for the effect of the injection procedure.

The expectations of the researchers performing the experiment can also get in the way of accurate results. Even the most careful and well-meaning people tend to see what they expect or want to see. (This expectation can be strengthened when the researcher's income or grant money is dependent on experimental results.) Experimenters may throw out data that do not conform, thinking an error has occurred. They may miss certain observations that they were not expecting to see. So in the best experimental design, a double-blind study, neither the experimenters running the tests nor the subjects know who is in the experimental or placebo treatment groups. Of course someone knows, but that person assigns numbers to subjects and is not directly involved in administering the study. In the health sciences, a double-blind experimental study is typically used to test medical treatments or drugs. Many of these are called double-blind, randomized

---

Box 1-5. The Surprising Complexity of the Placebo Effect

Researchers have long known about the power of belief. When people believe a medicine or behavior will have a certain effect, the effect frequently occurs, even though the medicine or behavior may have no other actual therapeutic value beyond inspiring the person's belief. Dishonest "healers," supplement manufacturers, and all kinds of salesmen have often used the placebo effect to get people to endorse and buy their products.

The word placebo is Latin for "I please," and indeed placebos do please. The power of belief is so strong that researchers need to separate this power from the physiological effects of medicines in order to evaluate the benefit of a given drug, other substance, or treatment. For example, people with sham knee surgery fare as well as those who get real surgery (Kirkley, et al., 2008), and women receiving a placebo to treat sexual dysfunction still experience improvement in sexual satisfaction (Bradford & Meston, 2011). An even stranger experimental result: people who swill sports drinks around in their mouth but spit them out improve their aerobic endurance (Pottier, Bouckaert, Gilis, Roels, & Derave, 2010). Results that occur with the administration of a placebo are real results. For example, Pottier et al. have speculated that sports drinks stimulate carbohydrate receptors in the mouth, which then interfere with fatigue signals being sent to the brain. Such results are why placebo treatments are included in experimental studies whenever possible.

Another interesting study found that even when subjects knew they were receiving a placebo, their symptoms improved significantly. Eighty patients with irritable bowel syndrome (IBS) (a disorder of the lower intestinal tract marked by pain and irregular bowel movements) were randomly assigned to a placebo group or a no-treatment group (Kaptchuk, et al., 2010). Placebo treatments usually involve deceiving subjects into believing that they may be getting a helpful drug, but this group was told that they were not receiving a drug. They were told that they were receiving "placebo pills made of an inert substance, like sugar pills, that have been shown in clinical studies to produce significant improvement in IBS symptoms through mind-body healing processes." Both groups had the same amount of interaction with health-care providers. Nevertheless, the placebo group showed significantly better improvement (59% reported "adequate symptom relief") in their IBS symptoms than the no treatment group (35% reported relief). The researchers noted that this is similar to the results of many good drug treatment trials, where the drug is compared to a placebo control. They speculated that the ritual of taking a pill may send a message to the brain that results in symptom relief.

Another illustration of the power of belief is the nocebo effect. The nocebo effect occurs when people develop negative outcomes to a treatment after a clinician or researcher has suggested that such an outcome might occur. For example, patients told that they might experience a headache as a side effect of a drug may experience a headache even though they were not given the active drug, but an inactive placebo. Brain imaging studies have found that negative expectations can override a drug's typical actions. Researchers suggest that clinicians carefully word information about treatments and side effects to nurture positive expectations while not withholding relevant information (Collaca & Miller, 2011).

control trials, meaning that they use double-blind methods with subjects randomly assigned to groups. Such studies are considered the gold standard of experimental methods because they have the most experimental control.

Use Statistical Methods to Evaluate the Probability That Results Were Due to Chance

Statistical methods are based on mathematical models of probability. Statisticians use these methods to examine experimental data. They compare groups and look at how the values of one variable change in relationship to other variables or treatments. Because most variables vary somewhat, there is always the possibility that the variance observed between groups is due to random chance rather than being an effect of the independent variable. Scientists using statistical methods can calculate the likelihood that differences observed in experimental data are significant, which means that the results have a low likelihood of occurring purely by chance. Statistical methods are also used in correlational research and even parts of qualitative studies, described next.

Correlational Research

Many times experimental study designs are not feasible. For example, it may be unethical to administer the treatment variable of interest to subjects, such as smoking cigarettes or remaining sedentary, because health risks are associated with these behaviors. Instead, scientists must just observe what naturally occurs in people who choose these behaviors. Sometimes it is not possible for subjects or experimenters to be blinded to the treatment: people can figure out if they are exercising or not exercising, or consuming a low-calorie diet or not. The time course of the development of chronic disease is often an issue, as is the cost of following people for several years. Correlational research methods are commonly employed by scientists when a true experiment is not feasible or may not yield the best information. In correlational research, values on variables of interest are observed and recorded, and statistical methods are used to evaluate the relationship, or correlations, among variables. Such research methods allow investigators to draw conclusions about how the behavior of one variable is related to another. When two variables are associated with each other, or correlated, they vary together. When one increases, the other either increases or decreases. So, for example, because smoking is correlated with heart disease, epidemiological data should show that as the number of cigarettes smoked per day increases, so does the likelihood of heart disease. When an increase in one variable is associated with an increase in the other variable, the correlation is said to be positive. As the number of cigarettes smoked per day increases, life expectancy goes down. This is an example of a negative correlation, which means that as one variable increases, the other decreases (Fig. 1-9).

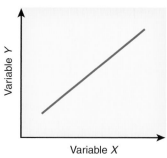

Positive correlation

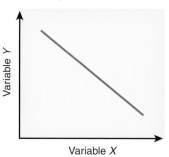

Negative correlation

Figure 1-9. **Positive and negative correlations.**

Epidemiological studies collect data on free-living populations and use statistical methods to observe associations and draw conclusions. Such studies may take several forms. Case-control studies are a type of correlational research commonly used by epidemiologists and medical researchers, in that naturally occurring disease patterns are observed. In case-control studies, researchers examine people with the variable of interest, such as lung cancer. They then select a comparable group of people without lung cancer as the "control" group. The researchers try to match the control group to the other group on as many variables as possible, including age, sex, socioeconomic status, and so forth. The groups are then compared on a number of variables of interest to the researchers. In the case of lung cancer, case-control studies helped to reveal the link between cigarette smoking and lung cancer. The people in the lung cancer groups had much high rates of smoking than people in the control group.

Most case-control studies are retrospective, in that they look back in time. Evidence and conclusions drawn from these studies are not considered to be as strong as prospective research, in which investigators gather data about the present, recording answers over time. This is because time, along with a disease diagnosis, can blur the memory. People trying to answer questions about what they did many years ago may err. They may misreport how much they smoked, what they ate, or how much stress they were under. Prospective research measures variables as they are occurring. For example, people are usually more accurate in reporting how much they smoked this week, or how much alcohol they drank yesterday, than in recalling how much they smoked or drank many years ago.

Sometimes epidemiological studies simply collect a large amount of information on a large number of people and analyze the data without forming case-control comparisons. For example, in 1948, a new study called the Framingham Heart Study began collecting data on 5,209 men and women between the ages of 30 and 62 from the town of Framingham, Massachusetts. The study's goal was to determine major risk factors for heart disease. This study was one of the first to find an association between lifestyle factors, including diet, smoking, and physical activity, and heart disease. These original volunteers are still being followed, and new groups have been added to this exciting study. More information about the Framingham Heart Study can be found on their website, www.framinghamheartstudy.org/about/history.html.

When evaluating the results of epidemiological studies or other studies that generate correlations, it is important to remember that correlations may not necessarily have a cause-and-effect relationship. Correlations only show that two (or more) variables vary together. They cannot demonstrate that one is causing the other to change. Sometimes there is a cause-and-effect relationship, but other times another factor may be causing both of the other variables to change together. For example, it has been observed that countries with a higher daily average intake of fat tend to have higher rates of breast cancer. However, as further studies have been done, total daily fat intake does not appear to cause most breast cancer. It is possible that a third factor—for example, higher intake of meat, lower intake of fruits and vegetables, or living in a polluted, industrialized country—is linked to both fat intake and breast cancer rate.

Epidemiological studies can, however, suggest causative relationships that are then explored with other studies. Experimental studies in laboratory animals may demonstrate a biologically plausible mechanism for causation. When a large number of epidemiological studies all find a similar association between two variables, scientists take note, especially when studies find the same result on different groups of people. Case-control studies can strengthen an observation as well. Often statistical techniques combine the data from several studies into a single large analysis, called a meta-analysis, to get a clearer picture of a correlation. But in the end, readers must always take care to never assume causation in correlational data.

Qualitative Research Methods

Qualitative research methods are often used when a study's goal is exploratory or when researchers are looking for in-depth information. Qualitative research can ask different types of research questions, such as how people think about a given topic, or interpret their experiences. Qualitative research typically focuses on a small group of participants and collects non-numerical data. Researchers may interview people extensively, asking open-ended questions to probe deeply into why they think, feel, or act in certain ways. Because the data are not numbers, statistical analyses are not performed. However, researchers using qualitative methods still strive for empirical rigor, combing their data in established ways for patterns and themes. Many research projects use a combination of both quantitative and qualitative methods. For example, a study of exercise adherence in a group of volunteers might collect data on frequency of exercise, ratings of stress, and other numerical data that are analyzed with statistical methods. However, researchers may also interview a select group of subjects and ask them about their adherence, to see if new factors emerge that had been hitherto unrecognized.

Research Ethics

The ethical conduct of scientists and their institutions sometimes comes under intense scrutiny, as reports of fraudulent data or inaccurate statistical calculations come to light. It is usually other scientists who discover the unethical behavior of their peers. Such behavior is, fortunately, fairly rare. And while scientists are human and do make mistakes (and even lie from time to time), on the whole, the process of science is eventually self-correcting and leads to improvements in long-term understanding.

All research institutions have strict guidelines concerning research ethics, and members are punished when the rules are broken, often losing their research funding and even their jobs. Guidelines spell out every detail of the research process. Especially important are the rules concerning the use of human subjects, and every institution has an independent board that reviews research proposals to be sure that people are treated ethically, that experimental protocols are not harmful, and that subjects are given as much information as possible about the potential benefits and costs of their participation. In addition, use of laboratory animals is strictly regulated.

Most journals and professional meetings ask researchers to give full disclosure of all special interests that might influence their work. For example, sources of funding from grants and the researcher's participation in other relevant organizations must be listed with the article.

Continued Questioning, Analysis, and Research

For scientists, the research process is never over because the results from one study always suggest more questions that lead to more thinking, hypotheses, testing, and analysis. Scientists avoid use of the words *prove* or *proof*, which imply that conclusions are unquestionable and beyond the shadow of a doubt. Science is built on doubt and critical analysis. When scientists evaluate the conclusions of their studies, they use a softer language. They say, "Our studies support the idea that . . ." or "Our data suggest that . . ." even when the results are very strong and meaningful.

The Art of Applying Science

Health and fitness professionals are often eager to apply the latest scientific results regarding human health and performance (Behavior Change in Action 1-1). Health and fitness professionals can keep up with exercise science by reading professional journals, taking continuing education classes, and discussing new ideas with coworkers. Professionals should be cautious when reading scientific reports about research in the popular media. Although the research may be very interesting, science reporters may overstate a study's conclusions in order to attract readers. For example, years ago when researchers found a link between consumption of tomato products and reduced risk of prostate cancer, headlines blared, "Pizza reduces cancer risk." Such headlines are misleading.

 Chester is pleased that he can take his walking program outdoors. He makes himself a route using the paths through his tree farm, and as his walking distance increases he begins hiking in nearby state parks. Evan gives

Chester the contact information for a local hiking club for older adults, and Chester starts walking with them almost every week. Chester admits to Evan that he had been pretty depressed after his wife died and was spending too much time alone. The hiking club proves to be a great way to get out and be with people.

Evan convinces Carla that many people might enjoy coming to the fitness center more if it were a more social environment. She lets Evan design a strength-training class that meets twice a week, where the group would gather for a warm-up, then do their workouts that he designed, ending with a brief stretch and educational/ motivational discussion. Chester becomes Evan's volunteer assistant and enjoys helping others learn new exercises.

As the year and Evan's internship draw to a close, Carla tells him that she is very impressed with his work, is sad to see him go, and offers him a part-time job. She knows Evan is looking for full-time jobs and offers to write him a great recommendation for his job hunt. Evan is happy to have Carla's strong recommendation and a part-time job to fall back on if a full-time job does not materialize. Working at the medical fitness center has taught him so much, and he tells Carla he is grateful for the internship opportunity. ■

BEHAVIOR CHANGE IN ACTION 1-1

Motivating Clients with Health Information

■ **Challenge**

What is the best way to discuss health information with clients in ways that motivate positive behavior change?

■ **Plan**

An overwhelming volume of information supporting the relationship between behavior and health is available. Some of it is complicated and confusing, and some studies contradict each other. Many times the experts cannot seem to agree, which makes it hard for health and fitness professionals to decide what advice to give. In addition, it can be difficult to know how much information should be given. Some clients seem ignorant about their health conditions, and you may long to give them more information. But too much information, especially disturbing information, can make clients defensive and even less likely to change behavior. When you think about discussing health information, make motivational messages your priority. The following suggestions can help you motivate clients with health information.

Give clients short articles on their health concerns. Some clients like written material, rather than verbal advice. They may need time to digest the thoughts. Follow up later with questions, such as, "What did you think about those suggestions for exercise to help reduce high blood pressure?" You might also ask, "Did you have any questions about what kind of exercise is best for reducing high blood pressure?"

Use client questions as your guide. If clients are interested in your answer, they are more likely to listen. Let them know that you are listening carefully to their questions by giving them your full attention, including good eye contact. Let them ask the entire question, without jumping in early and cutting them off.

Check in for understanding and interest every few sentences. As you answer their questions, stop periodically to be sure they are following. Ask, "Does that make sense? Do you see how smoking does that?" If they

BEHAVIOR CHANGE IN ACTION 1-1–cont'd

start looking around or looking distracted, or you sense that they are now only listening to be polite, wrap up your lecture with a one-sentence bottom line summary, such as, "That is why nutrition experts are urging people to eat at least five servings of vegetables a day."

Say the most important things first. Your clients may tune out after a short time, so you can skip the warm-up. If they have asked about helping their overweight kids, do not launch into a debate about the problems with physical education in the school system. That can come later, if there is time. Instead say, "Vigorous physical activity is critical for preventing more fat gain. What do your kids like to do?"

Let clients make concrete suggestions for implementing changes. If your conversations have come around to behavior change, and your clients want advice, start by asking what they think would work for them. You can help them make the suggestions as concrete as possibly by asking questions. When they say, "I guess I will try to exercise more," you might ask, "What kind of exercise would work best for you?" If they say, "Walking," you might ask, "What time of day would fit your schedule?" In this way, you may get clients to start envisioning the changes that they want to make.

Phrase suggestions for improving health in a positive fashion. If possible, explain how the changes will benefit the client, rather than how not changing will lead to harm. This is easy for some behaviors (listing exercise benefits) and harder for others (the strongest benefits of quitting smoking are often avoiding health problems). Some clients may be more motivated by avoiding harm, and if they are bringing up disease prevention, you don't need to avoid the subject. If they ask, "Would quitting smoking really reduce my risk of heart disease?," they probably could stand to hear about how smoking increases the deposition of arterial plaque. Then finish with the good news. "Quitting smoking will greatly lower your risk of heart disease."

Gauge their confidence in changing. Ask questions such as, "Does this seem reasonable to you? Do you think you could do this?" People are most likely to implement behavior change when they are confident that they can do so.

Express your confidence in clients' ability to change. Your confidence means a lot. Tell clients why you are confident. "I have been so impressed with the way you have gotten here every week. I am sure that you will be able to add that walk on Saturday afternoon with your friend at home."

Stick to advice that is widely endorsed. News about nutrition, exercise, and other health behaviors appears almost daily in the media. Before urging clients in your care to make lifestyle changes, check to see what the experts are saying about the news. Have other researchers found similar results? Are professional organizations publicizing the same news? Do expert panels appear to endorse the recommendation?

Stay within your scope of practice. Your certification organization and professional affiliations can guide you. For example, unless you are a licensed dietitian, the only dietary advice you can give is general-healthy eating advice. If your clients have health problems, they should have the guidance of a dietitian. Similarly, unless you are licensed to diagnose illness, send clients to their health-care providers when they start describing their aches and pains and asking you what is wrong.

Be sure your advice is reasonable. Consider the impact that your recommendations might have on your clients. Is the recommendation likely to have a significant positive effect? Often benefits are so small that it is not worth changing one's life around to fit the new behavior in. People who already spend enough time exercising (in their eyes) may not want to hear about the two more hours of additional training that they need to be doing each week. Clients may become paralyzed if they are overwhelmed with too much advice.

KEY TERMS

atherosclerosis	case-control studies	double-blind study	health
behavior	chronic obstructive pulmonary disease (COPD)	dualism	health behavior
behaviorism		epidemiological studies	health psychology
biomedical model of health	classical conditioning	exercise adherence	health-related behavior
	coronary heart disease	exercise physiology	health-related fitness
biopsychosocial model of health	correlational research	exercise psychology	hemorrhagic stroke
cancer	dependent variable	fatty streaks	high-density lipoproteins
carcinogens	diabetes	fitness	holistic health

KEY TERMS—cont'd

humanism	morbidity	plaque	scientific method
hypertension	mortality	prospective	social psychology
hypothesis	multifactorial	psychology	sociology
independent variable	myocardial infarction	psychophysiology	sport psychology
irritable bowel syndrome	neuroscience	psychosomatic	theory
ischemic stroke	nocebo effect	qualitative research methods	type 2 diabetes
low-density lipoproteins	operant conditioning		variable
lower respiratory infections	osteoporosis	quality of life	viscera
	peer review process	random assignment	visceral obesity
melatonin	personality	retrospective	wellness
meta-analysis	placebo	risk factors	
model	placebo effect		

CRITICAL THINKING QUESTIONS

1. Hospital environments have been accused of following only a biomedical model of health, focusing on treating the physical symptoms of disease without adequate regard to patients' emotional and social well-being. Describe some changes that hospitals might consider making to reflect more of a biopsychosocial model of health.

2. Take a look at the fitness components listed in Table 1-1. Which components might be most important for a 70-year-old woman with low bone density and a family history of bone fractures? Which might be most important for a young man who is overweight and has a family history of obesity? Which would be important for a college ice hockey player?

3. What are some of the factors that influence people to overeat, especially to eat too much of the wrong kinds of food? What factors lead to low levels of physical activity? What are some healthy influences that help people eat more fruits, vegetables, and other beneficial foods? That help people be active?

4. Some students experience more than the usual amount of anxiety when they take exams, and this anxiety can interfere with their ability to concentrate and their performance. You hypothesize that performing exercise before an exam can help such students feel less anxious during the exam. Design a study to test your hypothesis.

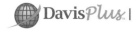 For additional resources log in to Davis*Plus* (**http://davisplus.fadavis.com**/ keyword "Brehm") and click on the Premium tab. (Don't have a *Plus*Code to access Premium Resources? Just click the Purchase Access button on the book's Davis*Plus* page.)

REFERENCES

Anand, P., Kunnumakara, A. B., Sundaram, C., Harikumar, K. B., Tharakan, S. T., Ois, O. S., . . . Aggarwal, B. B. (2008). Cancer is a preventable disease that requires major lifestyle changes. *Pharmaceutical Research*, 25(9), 2097-2116.

Barefoot, J. D., Dahlstrom, W. G., & Williams, R. B. (1983). Hostility, CHD incidence, and total mortality: a 25-year follow-up study of 255 physicians. *Psychosomatic Medicine*, 45(1), 59-63.

Blair, S. N. (2004). Letter in response to modifiable behavioral factors as causes of death. *Journal of the American Medical Association*, 291(24), 2942.

Bradford, A., & Meston, C. M. (2011). Behavior and symptom change among women treated with placebo for sexual dysfunction. *The Journal of Sexual Medicine*, 8(1), 191-201.

Bray, F., Jemal, A., Grey, N., Ferlay, G., & Forman, D. (2012). Global cancer transitions according to the Human Development Index (2008-2030): a population-based study. *The Lancet Oncology*, 13(8), 790-801.

Collaca, L., & Miller, F. G. (2011). The nocebo effect and its relevance for clinical practice. *Psychosomatic Medicine* 73(7), 598-603.

Friedman, M., & Rosenman, R. H. (1974). *Type A Behavior and Your Heart*. Greenwich, CT: Fawcett.

Gibbons, L. W., Blair, S. N., Cooper, K. H., & Smith, M. (1983). Association between coronary heart disease risk factors and physical fitness in healthy adult women. *Circulation*, 67, 977-983.

Harburg, E., Erfurt, J. C., Hauenstein, L. S., Chope, C., Shull, W. J., & Schorck, M. A. (1973). Socio-ecological stress, suppressed hostility, skin color, and black-white male blood pressure: Detroit. *Psychosomatic Medicine*, 35(4), 276-296.

Johnson, B. R., Scott-Sheldon, L. A. J., & Carey, M. P. (2010). Meta-synthesis of health behavior change meta-analyses. *American Journal of Public Health*, 100(11), 2193-2198.

Kaptchuk, T. J., Friedlander, E., Kelley, J. M., Sanchez, M. N., Kokkotou, E., Singer, J. P., . . . Lembo, A. J. (2010). Placebos without deception: a randomized controlled trial in irritable bowel syndrome. *PLoS ONE*, 5(12). e15591. doi: 10.1371/journal.pone.0015591

Khaw, K.-T., Wareham, N., Bingham, S. Welch, A., Luben, R., & Day, N. (2008). Combined impact of health behaviours and mortality in men and women: the EPIC-Norfolk Prospective Population Study. *PLoS Medicine*, 5(1), e12. doi:10.1371/journal.pmed.0050012

Kirkley, A., Birmingham, T. B., Litchfield, R. B., Griffin, J. R., Willits, K. R., Wong, C. J., . . . Fowler, P. J. (2008). A randomized trial of arthroscopic surgery for osteoarthritis of the knee. *New England Journal of Medicine*, 359(11), 1097-1107.

Lin, J. S., O'Connor, E., Whitlock, E. P., & Beil, T. L. (2010). Behavioral counseling to promote physical activity and a healthful diet to prevent cardiovascular disease in adults: a systematic review for the U.S. Preventive Services Task Force. *Annals of Internal Medicine*, 153(11), 736-750.

Marks, H. H. (1960). Influence of obesity on morbidity and mortality. *Bulletin of the New York Academy of Medicine*, 36(5), 296-312.

Marvasti, F. F., & Stafford, R. S. (2012). From sick care to health care—reengineering prevention into the U.S. system. *New England Journal of Medicine*, 367(10), 889-891.

Mokdad, A. H., Marks, J. S., Stroup, D. F., & Gerberding, J. L. (2004). Actual causes of death in the United States, 2000. *Journal of the American Medical Association*, 291(10), 1238-1245.

Mokdad, A. H. (2005). Correction: actual causes of death in the United States, 2000. *Journal of the American Medical Association*, 293(3), 293-294.

Murphy, S. L., Xu, J., & Kochanek, K. D. (2012). Deaths: preliminary data for 2010. *National Vital Statistics Reports*, 60(4). Retrieved from www.cdc.gov/nchs/data/nvsr/nvsr60/nvsr60_04.pdf

Murray, C. J. L., & Frenk, J. (2010). Ranking 37th — measuring the performance of the U.S. health care system. *New England Journal of Medicine*, 362(2), 98-99.

Ornish, D. (1998). Avoiding revascularization with lifestyle changes: the multicenter lifestyle demonstration project. *American Journal of Cardiology*, 18(10, suppl. 2), 72-76.

Pottier, A., Bouckaert, J., Gilis, W., Roels, T., & Derave, W. (2010). Mouth rinse but not ingestion of a carbohydrate solution improves 1-h cycle time trial performance. *Scandinavian Journal of Medicine and Science in Sports*, 20(1), 105-111.

Thoits, P. A. (2010). Stress and health: major findings and policy implications. *Journal of Health and Social Behavior*, 51(S), S41-S53.

World Health Organization (WHO). (2010). The top ten causes of death. Fact sheet 310. Retrieved from www.who.int/mediacentre/factsheets/fs310_2008.pdf

World Health Organization (WHO). (2009). Global health risks: mortality and burden of disease attributable to selected major risks. Retrieved from www.who.int/healthinfo/global_burden_disease/GlobalHealthRisks_report_full.pdf

World Health Organization (WHO). (1948). Preamble to the Constitution of the World Health Organization as adopted by the International Health Conference, New York, 19-22 June 1946; signed on 22 July 1946 by the representatives of 61 States (Official Records of the World Health Organization, no. 2, p. 100) and entered into force on 7 April 1948. Retrieved from www.who.int/about/definition/en/print.html

CHAPTER OUTLINE

LEARNING OBJECTIVES

After reading this chapter, you will be able to:

1. Explain how the various body systems contribute to communication between mind and body.

2. Understand the basic structure and function of the nervous system and describe how the nervous system orchestrates stress and relaxation responses.

3. Apply information about the endocrine system and its hormones to various health-related issues.

4. Conceptualize communication among the nervous, endocrine, and immune systems as they coordinate physiological function.

5. Explain how the digestive system is influenced by the nervous, endocrine, and immune systems and how it is affected by the stress response.

6. Describe the basic structure of the musculoskeletal system and how it communicates with the nervous, endocrine, and immune systems.

7. Explain the basic structure and function of the respiratory and cardiovascular systems.

8. Understand how health behaviors influence the various systems of the body and how these systems in turn influence health.

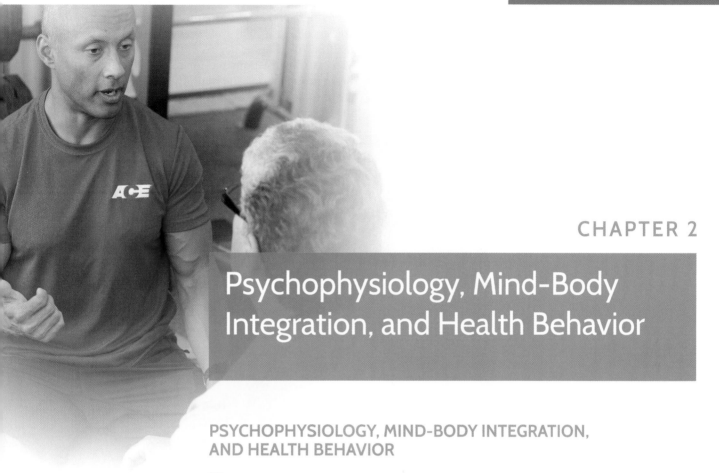

CHAPTER 2

Psychophysiology, Mind-Body Integration, and Health Behavior

PSYCHOPHYSIOLOGY, MIND-BODY INTEGRATION, AND HEALTH BEHAVIOR

■ *Maya has a taken a summer job working on a cruise ship. "Sunshine, vacation, here I come," she thinks. She will be teaching water aerobics, beginning yoga, and a morning "rise and shine" walking class. Maya anticipates that this will be a nice change from the four part-time jobs she has been working for the past several years. In 3 months, she will be starting a full-time job at the local community college, running the fitness center and teaching a variety of exercise classes.*

Little does she know that her cruise will offer little free time and that the fitness instructor will turn into the resident authority on every health-related topic in the book! Thankfully, her kinesiology coursework, her years of experience, and her continuing education classes have kept her up to date in the health field, so she can answer the deluge of questions she receives, refer clients appropriately, and make informed decisions about the situations she encounters.

Her first surprise client presents himself in her beginning yoga class on the afternoon of departure. Nick is several years older than the others in the class and stiff as a board, but, with the attitude of a man ready to conquer the world, he muscles his way through the postures, pushing himself to the point of straining, and ignoring Maya's instructions to the class to go slowly and gently. At the beginning of class, he told Maya that he has had back problems for many years but that his doctor told him yoga should be fine. Maya wonders where people get the idea that yoga is always safe for everyone. Nick's breathing is shallow and tense, and Maya is afraid he will hurt himself. Maya's first priority is to keep everyone free of injury. How is she going to connect with Nick and help him work with his body rather than against it? ■

Understanding and applying the psychology of health and fitness requires basic knowledge of psychophysiology and health. To understand health, one must understand both the body and the mind. Health and exercise psychologists are especially interested in how health behaviors impact body and mind and how change in one area may affect other areas. Health and exercise psychologists are interested, for example, in whether exercise or a certain eating style improves mood. If so, how do such improvements occur? Are there other ways to achieve these changes? Similarly, how are mood and motivation related?

The goal of this chapter is to highlight topics that will enhance understanding of health and exercise psychology and of the behavior-change process. This chapter also seeks to underscore the interrelatedness of these mind-body systems. Students can use this knowledge to educate clients about how behavior relates to health. This chapter begins with sections on the three systems most responsible for mind-body integration: the nervous, endocrine, and immune systems. Subsequent material on the digestive, musculoskeletal, respiratory, and cardiovascular systems also explores mind-body communication. In addition, this chapter presents common health-behavior issues related to each system that health and fitness professionals are likely to encounter in their work with clients.

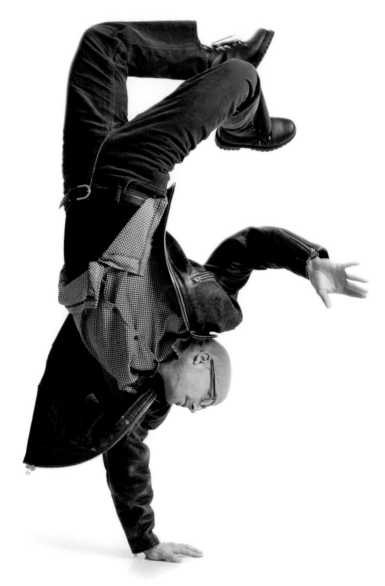

© Thinkstock

INTRODUCTION TO THE HUMAN MIND AND BODY

At the most basic level, the human organism is matter and energy. Scientists are just beginning to understand how this matter and energy generate thought. Does thought evolve from matter, from the cells, proteins, and other molecules in the brain? Does thought direct the action of matter, the activity of cells, and the many molecules that act as messengers between cells? The answer to both of these questions appears to be yes, and the deeper scientists probe into the realities of human psychophysiology, the fuzzier the line grows between mind and body.

Cells

Basic knowledge of the cells and how they function and communicate with one another provides a foundation for understanding psychophysiology. Cells are the most basic structural and functional unit of life. They carry on many of the basic life processes common to all organisms: ingesting nutrients, generating energy to power their functions, excreting waste, manufacturing the proteins needed to produce energy and perform other cellular functions, and replicating themselves. In addition to these activities, cells are specialized to perform specific functions, depending upon cell type. For example, muscle cells are designed to produce a great deal of energy to fuel the shortening of specialized proteins that cause muscle contraction. Specialized tasks are determined by which genes, segments of the cell's genetic material that help direct cell function, are activated in that particular cell.

MOTIVATING CHANGE: Health Behavior Often Trumps Genetics

Understanding that the predisposition for many chronic illnesses can be weakened by appropriate health behaviors is motivating for many people (Box 2-1). Clients may decide to manage stress, change their eating habits, or begin exercising because they have a family history of hypertension, type 2 diabetes, or other chronic illness. Prevention, or at least delaying the onset of illness, can be especially motivational for people who have watched parents or other relatives cope with the effects of disease. Health and fitness professionals often take a family history to evaluate an individual's risk of coronary heart disease and other illnesses when beginning their work with a new client. This is a good time to explore whether or not clients may find risk reduction a motivating factor for behavior change. While you cannot promise clients you can help them live forever, it is reasonable to suggest that appropriate behavior change can reduce risk for certain chronic diseases.

Each cell includes many specialized structures known as organelles, with each structure playing a special role (Fig. 2-1):

- **Nucleus:** Contains the cell's genetic material (DNA, see below).
- **Deoxyribonucleic acid (DNA):** Provides a master plan for all the proteins the body needs to make. The proteins, in turn, carry out many important functions of the cell and of the body.
- **Ribosome:** Produces proteins. Some ribosomes make proteins needed by the cell; others make proteins for specialized functions, such as chemicals the cell secretes.
- **Rough endoplasmic reticulum:** Sorts and processes the proteins with other substances to make larger molecules such as neurotransmitters

Box 2-1. Genetics, Epigenetics, and Health Behavior: Which Has the Most Influence on Health?

A great deal of research is exploring which genes predispose people to which health problems. Some health disorders are entirely caused by errors in genetic coding that lead to the manufacture of problematic proteins, which in turn fail to perform their proper function. For example, sickle-cell anemia produces a poorly shaped hemoglobin molecule. Hemoglobin is responsible for binding oxygen and carbon dioxide in the red blood cells. While normal red blood cells are smooth and disk shaped, the misshapen hemoglobin molecule produced with sickle-cell anemia causes the red blood cells to fold and produce a flat, sickle-like shape that has difficulty flowing through the capillaries. When the capillaries become blocked, tissues are deprived of oxygen and nutrients and cannot get rid of waste products. In this case, genetic predisposition plays a very important role in health.

Fortunately, the majority of health problems result primarily from an interaction of genetics and health behaviors. Researchers have found that the leading chronic health problems (such as heart disease, obesity, type 2 diabetes, hypertension, stroke, and most cancers) seem to be related to many different genes, with these genes having only low to moderate predictive value (Chakravarti, 2003; Lettre et al., 2011). Thus, researchers have turned their attention to the mechanisms by which genes are expressed and the many factors that influence these mechanisms, a field called epigenetics (Rodenhiser, 2006). DNA is part of a larger structure called chromatin, and this structure influences the operation of the DNA. Chromatin is a complex structure of DNA and proteins that makes up the chromosomes. In addition, cellular activity, including the activity of cell membrane receptors, influences the action of a variety of molecules responsible for activating specific genes. Research suggests that chromatin and genetic expression are influenced by many lifestyle factors, including diet and exercise, that influence which genes get turned on and off (Davis & Ross, 2007; Simopoulos, 2008).

While genetics is important, one must recognize that environment and health behaviors interact with genetics to produce an individual's state of health. Many people may manage to escape, or at least delay, a genetic predisposition to chronic disease by avoiding environmental toxins and carcinogens and developing a healthful lifestyle.

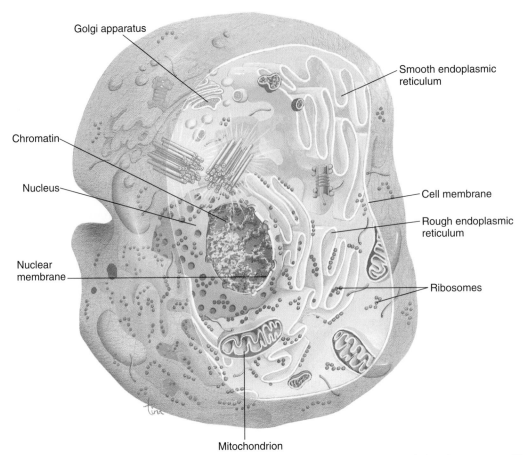

Figure 2-1. **Basic cell structure.** *(Modified from Scanlon, V.C. & Sanders, T. (2011). Essentials of Anatomy and Physiology. F.A. Davis, Philadelphia, p. 54; with permission.)*

- **Smooth endoplasmic reticulum:** Produces fatty acids and hormones such as estrogens and testosterone, along with many other substances
- **Golgi complex:** Receives most of the proteins processed by the rough endoplasmic reticulum for further processing; the Golgi complex often makes molecules that will be secreted by its cell (e.g., lipoproteins that carry triglycerides and cholesterol in the bloodstream).
- **Cell membrane:** Surrounds the cell and is composed primarily of fats and proteins (Fig. 2-2). Special channels and proteins embedded in the membrane help control which substances pass through the membrane.
- **Receptor sites:** Proteins embedded in the cell membrane where signaling molecules may bind; each receptor site binds with signaling molecules of a particular structure.

Organs

In the human body, many cells are part of larger structures called organs, such as the eyes, stomach, and muscles. Within an organ, there are many types of specialized cells that help the organ perform its functions and communicate with the rest of the body. Consider the skin. The skin contains not only the cells that can be seen on the surface of the body but other types of cells as well. The skin includes special glands that produce sweat,

which is secreted through small pores. Hair follicles produce hair, and small muscles can make the hair stand up, producing "goose bumps" when a person is cold.

Systems

In order to understand the structure and function of the human body, physiologists group organs into systems. A system is a group of organs that work together to accomplish a specific task, such as digestion or delivering oxygen to all the body's cells. Systems overlap considerably, and some organs participate in several systems. Some systems, such as the immune system, contain cells that are not part of organs. The rest of this chapter presents some of the systems most commonly involved in discussions of health behavior change.

THE NERVOUS SYSTEM: Wired for Communication

When people think about the systems that connect body and mind, the first thing they usually think of is the nervous system (Fig. 2-3). The nervous system is composed of the central nervous system and the peripheral nervous system. The central nervous system contains the brain and spinal cord. The brain is a dense concentration of nerve cells contained in the skull, and

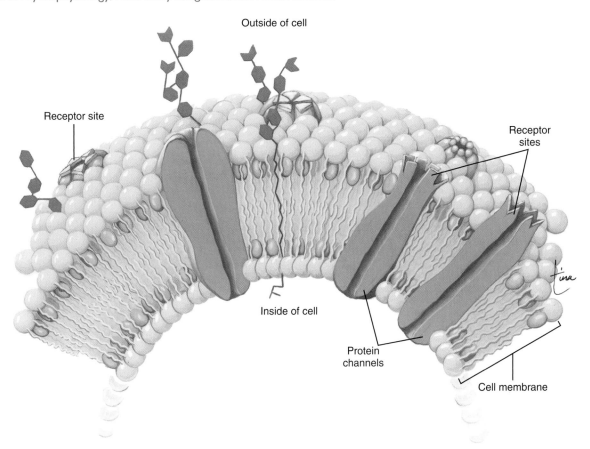

Figure 2-2. Cell membrane. *(Modified from Scanlon, V.C. & Sanders, T. (2011). Essentials of Anatomy and Physiology. F.A. Davis, Philadelphia, p. 53; with permission.)*

the spinal cord is a thick band of nervous tissue that is contained within the vertebrae, the bones that form the spinal column. The peripheral nervous system consists of the peripheral nerves, which spread from the spinal cord to all parts of the body. All these structures are composed of nervous tissue, collections of specialized cells that contribute to the communication abilities of the nervous system. The nervous system coordinates all parts of the body so that they work together.

Nerve Cell Structure and Function

The nervous system is comprised of cells that are exquisitely designed for communication with one another. Two basic types of cells are found within the nervous system: neurons and neuroglia. Neurons communicate by sending electrical signals to adjacent neurons. They are capable of activating muscles, other organs, and glands; carrying information from the sensory organs, such as the eyes and ears, to the brain; and carrying out psychological functions such as thinking and remembering. Neuroglia are cells that support and nourish the neurons, maintaining a good environment for neuron function. There are many different types of neuroglia that serve a variety of functions in keeping the nervous system up and running.

Neurons have a cell body, dendrites, and an axon (Fig. 2-4). The cell body contains the structures typical of body cells, including the nucleus that holds the cell's genetic material. Many dendrites and a single axon reach out from the cell body. The cell body and the dendrites receive input from other neurons, while the axon transmits information to other cells, including neurons, muscles cells, and gland cells.

The place where two neurons communicate is called a synapse (Fig. 2-5). Neurons communicate by releasing special chemicals called neurotransmitters, which travel across the minute space between the two cells, called the synaptic cleft. The neuron releasing the neurotransmitter is referred to as the presynaptic neuron, and the neuron receiving the neurotransmitter is called the postsynaptic neuron. The neurotransmitters cross the synaptic cleft to the postsynaptic neuron (or sometimes another type of cell) and bind with matching receptor sites on that cell's surface. This binding activates the postsynaptic neuron and can trigger various actions in that cell. For example, activation may lead to a nerve impulse, helping to spread a message along a whole chain of neurons. Neurotransmitters can also *block* nerve transmission. When certain neurotransmitters bind with receptors on the adjacent cells, the postsynaptic neuron becomes inhibited and is less likely to be activated and to pass along a message. This may be beneficial, for example, when the message is pain, and neurotransmitters and receptors that lessen the pain message are often welcome.

After the neurotransmitter has activated its receptor, it can be removed in several ways. Sometimes, the neurotransmitter is broken down by special enzymes. Other times, it is transported back to the cell from which it came.

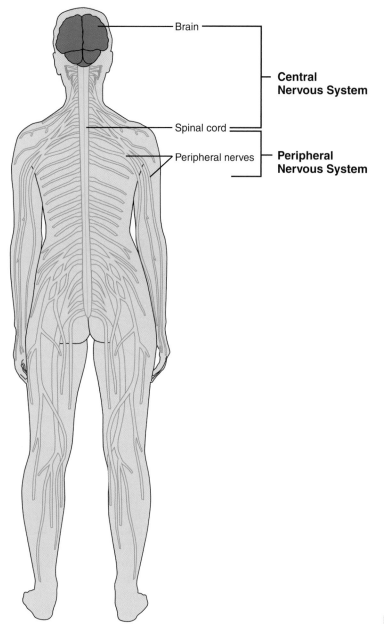

Figure 2-3. The nervous system.

Several medications work by blocking the movement of a neurotransmitter out of the synapse and away from its receptor. For example, the selective serotonin reuptake inhibitor (SSRI) drugs keep levels of serotonin higher in the synapse and are used to treat some forms of depression. Other types of antidepressants inhibit the reuptake of other neurotransmitters.

Researchers have discovered over a hundred chemicals that serve as neurotransmitters. Readers may be familiar with some of these. For example, presence of the neurotransmitter dopamine is associated with pleasant emotional states. Addictive drugs such as amphetamines and opiates appear to increase dopamine concentrations in the central nervous system. Parkinson's disease is marked by reductions in dopamine.

A particular neurotransmitter may have different effects on the postsynaptic neuron, depending upon which actions are triggered by the receptor site. For example, serotonin has effects on mood in the brain but also helps to regulate digestive processes in the digestive system. Many lifestyle variables, including physical activity, affect the behavior of neurotransmitters such as serotonin.

The next morning during the walk around the ship, a participant in Maya's walking group, Claire, confides to Maya that she has come on the cruise to deal with depression. Claire has been on depression medication for several years and has found it only moderately effective. Claire has read that exercise is as effective as medication for the treatment of mild-to-moderate depression, so she did not take her medicine this morning and has decided to go cold turkey. Maya praises Claire's decision to change her lifestyle to reduce symptoms of stress. However, she warns Claire that she really should stay on her medication during the cruise, while starting the lifestyle changes, and check with

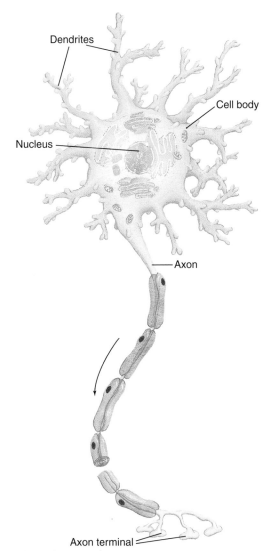

Figure 2-4. Neurons. *(Modified from Scanlon, V.C. & Sanders, T. (2011). Essentials of Anatomy and Physiology. F.A. Davis, Philadelphia, p. 177; with permission.)*

her doctor about tapering the medicine when she is back home, so she has a smooth transition to life without the medicine. After some discussion, Claire finally agrees to Maya's suggestion to resume her regular medical treatment while on board. As they walk around the ship, Maya advises Claire on her exercise program and encourages her to eat well, get enough sleep, and have fun. "Don't forget to come for salsa dancing lessons tonight after dinner! You can exercise and have fun at the same time!" ■

Communication Networks

Neurons form connections throughout the body, creating a complex and highly structured communication network. Neuroscientists have classified groups of neurons in a variety of ways that help model how the nervous system works (Fig. 2-6). The afferent nervous system consists of the nerve cells that receive information from the external and internal (inside the body) environments and conduct this information to the brain, where it is processed at both conscious and subconscious levels. Sensory signals originate in specialized organs and cells and are responsible for the senses of sight, sound, taste, and smell. Proprioceptors send information about the internal environment. For example, receptors in the skin send information about temperature, pressure, and chemical changes. Receptors in the joints and muscles send information about the body's position in space, the degree of contraction in muscles, and the amount of force being placed on tendons.

The afferent nervous system is constantly sending information to the brain, which sorts the input and decides which input is relevant and needs attention. For

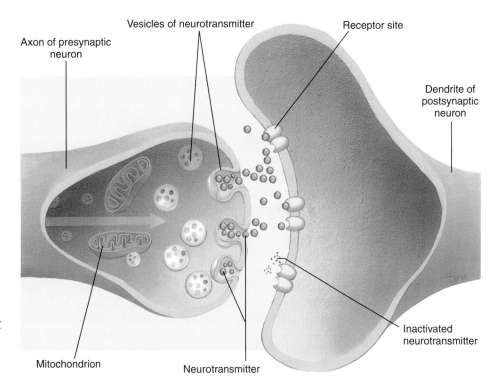

Figure 2-5. **Nerve synapse.** *(Modified from Scanlon, V.C. & Sanders, T. (2011). Essentials of Anatomy and Physiology. F.A. Davis, Philadelphia, p. 180; with permission.)*

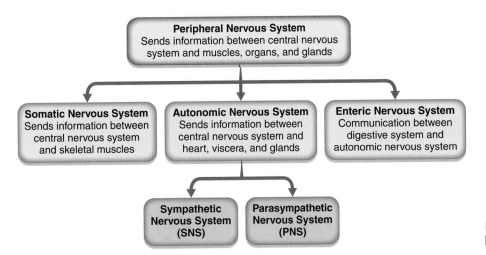

Figure 2-6. Classification of the branches of the nervous system.

example, much of the time, people are not consciously aware of background noise in their environments or the sensations of clothing next to their skin. But, if a snarling, vicious dog comes lunging toward a person, he would perceive the dog through information transmitted to his brain by afferent neurons. His ears would send information about the growling and barking sounds of the dog, his eyes would send information about the dog's appearance and movement, and his proprioceptors would send his brain information about his body's position and level of muscle tension. (If he fails to move quickly, sensory organs in his skin would receive input perceived as pain if the dog bites him.) His brain would integrate all this information, recall past experiences, and decide what to do. He might decide to run away, fast. In this case, his brain would sound the alarm and send messages to all systems of the body via the efferent nervous system, which carries messages from the brain to the rest of the body.

The peripheral nervous system is subdivided into three parts: the somatic, autonomic, and enteric nervous systems. The somatic nervous system sends impulses between the central nervous system and skeletal muscles. It allows the body to produce movement. This system is considered to be at least partly under conscious control. In the example above, the man decides to run, and his brain coordinates muscular contraction to produce a personal best in running time. The neurons that carry messages to the skeletal muscles are known as motor neurons. The autonomic nervous system (ANS) sends information between the central nervous system and nonmusculoskeletal systems, such as the circulatory system (heart and blood vessels), respiratory system (lungs and airways), digestive system, and endocrine system (glands that produce hormones). Scientists generally regard the activity of the ANS as outside of voluntary control, although biofeedback research has shown people can learn to control many autonomic functions, including heart rate, stomach acidity, and blood pressure (Box 2-2). The third branch

of the peripheral nervous system is the enteric nervous system (ENS), which has been called "the brain in the gut." Once considered part of the autonomic nervous system, this extensive nervous system network now rates its own category. With over 100 million neurons, the ENS monitors activity in the stomach and intestines and signals these organs to produce the muscular contractions that move food through the system. It regulates the secretion of enzymes and other chemicals essential for digestion from the digestive organs. The ENS communicates with the central nervous system through neuronal connections with the autonomic nervous system.

The autonomic nervous system can either speed up or slow down the activity of the organs and systems it innervates. The two branches of the ANS that perform these functions are the sympathetic nervous system (SNS) and the parasympathetic nervous system (PNS). Most organs are innervated by, or have input from, both the sympathetic and parasympathetic branches of the autonomic nervous system. The sympathetic nervous system is activated when the body needs to move, such as when it needs to perform physical activity and to respond to threats. Emotions such as anger, fear, and embarrassment activate the SNS. The SNS is most widely known as the activator of the stress response, often called the "fight-or-flight" response, which speeds up those functions necessary for immediate survival. For example, to help the man successfully evade the snarling dog, his liver releases sugar into the bloodstream to fuel his working muscles, and his heart beats faster and harder to circulate blood. The SNS suppresses such functions as digestion, which can be postponed until the emergency has passed. Table 2-1 lists some of the important physiological effects of SNS activation.

After getting safely away from the dog, the man slows his pace and heaves a sigh of relief. He gets home and collapses onto the couch. His brain and body have done a fine job of communicating, and he has escaped the threat of the dog. At this point, his brain decreases

Box 2-2. Biofeedback: Tuning in for Health and Rehabilitation

Biofeedback means feedback, or information, given to a person about his or her body. Biofeedback occurs when measures are taken that provide information about one's physical state. Biofeedback technology has more sensitivity than most people do, so this technology can enhance awareness and the learning of alternative responses. Biofeedback helps the central nervous system tune in to information already present in the body at a subconscious level. If a body response can be monitored, biofeedback training can be applied. Biofeedback technology can measure many variables, including muscle tension, brain wave activity, skin temperature, blood pressure, heart rate and rhythm, and stomach acid secretion. When health professionals use biofeedback technology to treat health problems, the goal is not only to help patients become more aware of their physical state but also to help them actually gain some control of that variable (Norris, 2006). For example, some people, by becoming more aware of muscle tension levels in their foreheads, can relax these muscles and reduce headache incidence. Hypertension has been called the "silent killer" because most people are unable to sense their blood pressure; however, biofeedback training can teach people this awareness and how to reduce blood pressure when they feel it creeping up (Nolan et al., 2010; Wang et al., 2010). Biofeedback can help stroke patients trying to recover muscle function learn new motor patterns. Biofeedback therapy has been shown to be effective for treating digestive system disorders, such as ulcers, irritable bowel syndrome, and incontinence, since the ENS is so responsive to training. Insomnia, chronic pain, and anxiety disorders often respond to biofeedback treatment. People with attention deficit disorders have used biofeedback to alter brain activity patterns.

No one knows exactly how autonomic functions are brought under voluntary control. People learning to reduce forehead muscle tension are hooked up to electrodes that measure muscle electrical activity. A beeping sound or other signal indicates tension level: more beeps, more tension. People try to slow the beeps, and most are able to do so. When asked how they do it, they reply with answers such as "I make my arms feel heavy and warm," or "I imagine I am on the beach," or they will say they breathe in a certain way.

People learning to use biofeedback usually work with a therapist who adjusts the instruments and gives suggestions. When biofeedback is used to decrease sympathetic arousal, people usually practice some kind of relaxation technique during the session, while tuning in to the biofeedback response. An important part of biofeedback training is learning to transfer the skills learned during practice sessions to real-life situations. A person must be able to regulate blood pressure while driving in traffic, talking to friends, and performing a job, not just when meditating in a quiet room hooked up to biofeedback instruments.

SNS activity while increasing parasympathetic output. One of the psychological states associated with activation of the PNS is called the relaxation response, the opposite of the stress response. The PNS is also said to be the nervous system for "rest and digest." Heart rate and blood pressure return to normal, muscles relax, and the digestive system resumes the task of digesting the last meal. Some of the actions of the PNS are listed in Table 2-1. This table shows that often the actions of the SNS are balanced by the actions of the PNS. For example, while the SNS increases heart rate, the PNS decreases heart rate (Health Psychology in Your Life 2-1).

Maya has been wondering how to get Nick to be more mindful during yoga practice, if he attends the next yoga class. Several of the participants have complained of difficulty sleeping, so Maya decides to lead a restorative yoga class, which employs very simple, relaxing postures held for longer periods. Maya knows the slow movements and deep breathing will help bring the parasympathetic nervous

system into play and reduce the sympathetic response that beginners like Nick, who are nervous about their performance, often bring to their practice.

Sure enough, here comes Nick, ready to go. As Maya turns on the gentle music and begins to lead the class in the first poses, explaining the goals of restorative yoga, she sees a look that appears to be annoyance cross Nick's face. He mutters something about "coming here for a workout!" but then settles into the pose. Maya moves from person to person, correcting alignment and pressing on tight shoulder muscles. When she gets to Nick, she draws his shoulders back and quietly advises him to avoid back problems by lengthening his spine rather than allowing his torso to collapse. Throughout the class, Maya gets everyone breathing deeply, and as the class moves along she can feel the tension in the room ease, as everyone's breathing, including Nick's, begins to slow down. At the end of class, she draws Nick aside and praises his progress in breathing and focus

Table 2-1. Activities of the Autonomic Nervous System

SITE	EFFECT OF SYMPATHETIC STIMULATION	EFFECT OF PARASYMPATHETIC STIMULATION
Eye	Dilates pupil; improves distance vision	Improves near vision
Arteries to skin	Constricts arteries	Dilates arteries
Arteries to skeletal muscle	Dilates arteries to active muscle groups and constricts arteries to other muscle groups	None
Arteries to abdominal organs	Constricts arteries	None
Fat cells	Increase breakdown and release of fats into bloodstream	None
Heart	Increases rate and strength of contraction; dilates coronary arteries	Decreases rate and strength of contraction; constricts coronary arteries
Lungs	Dilate airways	Constrict airways
Liver	Increases conversion of protein and starch into blood sugar	Increases synthesis of starch (glycogen)
Stomach and intestines	Decrease motility and tone; decrease secretion of digestive juices	Increase motility and tone; increase secretion of digestive juices
Kidney	Constricts blood vessels, resulting in decreased urine volume	none

HEALTH PSYCHOLOGY IN YOUR LIFE 2-1: Fluctuations in Resting Heart Rate

Many factors affect your heart rate. In this exercise, you will observe your heart rate under various conditions during the day. To take your heart rate, press two fingers over the pulse on the inside of your forearm, just below your wrist. Take your pulse in a seated position. Count how many times your heart beats in 15 seconds and then multiply by four. Record your results.

Take your heart rate at several times during the day, such as: in the morning after you wake up; after a stimulant, such as coffee or tea or smoking a cigarette; before an exam or when you are nervous; listening to peaceful music; thinking of something that makes you angry; and when you are sleepy before falling asleep.

Some people find they can cause a decrease in their resting heart rate by breathing very slowly. Measure your normal resting heart rate. Then close your eyes and allow your breathing to become slow and relaxed. Draw out your exhalation, breathing in for three counts and out for six. Some people can also feel their pulse speed up slightly as they inhale and slow down as they slowly exhale.

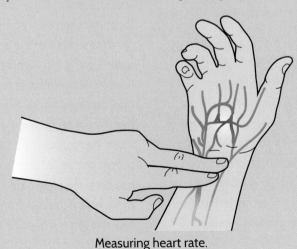

Measuring heart rate.

and hands him an article on yoga for the prevention of back problems. He gives her a smile, and his face is more relaxed than she has ever seen it. "Building core strength and improving posture are important for the muscles of the back. But so is being able to let go of stress and tension," she says. She urges Nick to see her if he has any questions. "Score one for the teacher!" she thinks. ■

MOTIVATING CHANGE: Habits of Stress and Perception Are Difficult to Change

When people perceive themselves to be facing a stressful situation, the effect on the nervous system is instantaneous. People vary in the ways they "decide" whether a given situation is threatening or not. People also create stressful thoughts in their minds that trigger a full-blown stress response, even when the stressful thoughts have no basis in reality and are simply irrational fears and worries. Stress-response patterns are deeply ingrained in everyone and very resistant to change. While it may be tempting to point out to clients how silly their fears and worries are and to let them know how much damage all this imagined stress is doing to their bodies, keep in mind that these worry patterns are an important part of the client's personality. It is not helpful to tell people stress is "all in their mind" or to just "think happy thoughts." Such advice is not helpful and will often turn clients off. Instead educate clients about the effects of chronic stress (more information on this can be found in Chapter 6) and encourage them to reduce feelings of stress with regular physical activity, a healthy lifestyle, and simple stress-reduction techniques like breathing exercises and to seek professional counseling if they find stress is interfering with their quality of life.

Brain Psychophysiology: Command Central for Mind-Body Integration

The brain acts as command central of the nervous system. It is the major location of conscious thought and awareness, memory, judgment, and planning. The brain also plays an important role in the generation and processing of emotions. Additionally, parts of the brain regulate physical functions such as breathing, heart rate, digestion, and the physical reflexes. Any injury to the brain can disrupt these vital functions. Even repeated minor blows to the head may have long-term negative consequences (Box 2-3).

The brain is composed of a high concentration of nervous tissue, with approximately 100 billion neurons and 100 trillion synapses. Human beings have the largest brain for their size of all mammals. While researchers can measure the electrical, blood flow, and metabolic activity of the brain, the ways that the brain manages to think, remember, and use language are still mostly a mystery.

Box 2-3. Concussion: Lifelong Impact

The skull provides a protective covering for the brain. Because the skull feels so solid, people have long had the impression that it can handle quite a bit of impact or even be used as a blunt instrument, as when soccer players hit the ball with their head. However, the skull cannot fully protect the brain from injury.

A century ago, observations of boxers suggested suffering severe blows to the head may lead to impairment. The term for boxers who show cognitive decline is *"punch-drunk syndrome."* More-recent evidence suggests that one need not experience repeated strong punches to the head to suffer from this form of dementia in later life. While the skull is strong, the brain tissue inside is somewhat fragile. A history of concussion may cause early dementia in some people. Concussion is a brain injury that occurs due to shaking or hitting that may or may not involve loss of consciousness. People with concussion exhibit short-lived impairments that eventually resolve on their own over time. Symptoms of concussion include headache, confusion, emotional changes, delayed reaction time, and drowsiness. Impairments are functional; no structural changes appear on brain scans.

Recent autopsy data suggest that people who have suffered from repeated concussions show similar brain tissue changes to people with Alzheimer's disease, including increased abnormal deposition of tau protein (McCrory, 2011). Tau protein normally serves to support nerve cells in the brain, but abnormal clumps of the protein indicate pathology. The disorder is now called chronic traumatic encephalopathy (CTE), and it has been observed in athletes, soldiers, and others who have experienced numerous head injuries.

At this time, it is unclear exactly how much trauma is required to produce CTE. Sports medicine organizations and the military have responded by putting new regulations into effect regarding return to play or service after concussion (Covassin, Elbin, & Stiller-Ostrowski, 2009; McCrory, 2009). Sports equipment designers are developing better head protection for athletes who experience a great deal of head trauma, such as football players who may receive hundreds of hits to the head during a single season.

The brain is one of the heaviest organs in the body. It is protected by the skull, covered with a connective tissue that bathes it in nourishing cerebrospinal fluid, and fed by a rich network of blood vessels.

The brain has four major parts: the cerebrum, the cerebellum, the diencephalon, and the brainstem (Fig. 2-7). The cerebrum is the largest brain area. The

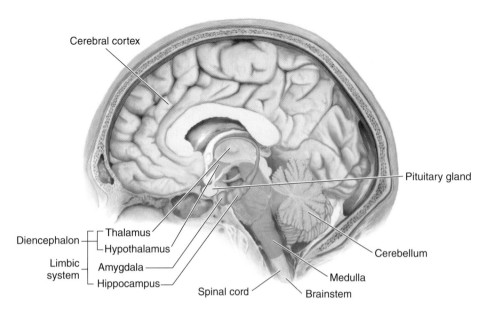

Figure 2-7. **The brain.** *(From: Gylys, B.A., & Wedding, M.E. (2009). Medical Terminology Systems, 6th edition. Philadelphia: F.A. Davis, p. 430, Figure 14-3., with permission.)*

outer layer of the cerebrum is called the cerebral cortex. It is responsible for higher mental functions, such as thinking, self-control, planning, and memory. Sensory areas in the cerebral cortex interpret sensory nerve impulses, motor areas control movement, and association areas are involved with emotional and intellectual processes.

The cerebellum aids in the regulation of movement. It integrates input from the cerebral cortex, where the brain plans movement, and information from the proprioceptors and sensory organs. The cerebellum helps turn the movement plan into the effective muscle contractions that produce movement. The cerebellum also helps regulate balance and posture.

Deeper areas of the brain are involved in many regulatory processes. The diencephalon is primarily made up of the thalamus, hypothalamus, and pineal gland. The thalamus integrates and relays sensory information to the cerebral cortex. It helps interpret sensations of pain, temperature, and pressure; it is also involved in emotion and memory. The hypothalamus is an important control center for many physiological functions. It controls the ANS, regulates the pituitary gland, and secretes several hormones and other chemical factors. The hypothalamus appears to be the center for the learned control of autonomic functions that occurs during relaxation and biofeedback training. The hypothalamus helps to regulate eating behavior through feelings of hunger and satiety (feeling like one has had enough to eat). The pineal gland secretes the hormone melatonin, which helps to regulate the body's biological clock. Melatonin levels increase with darkness and promote feelings of sleepiness. Melatonin may also play roles in memory and other processes.

The thalamus and hypothalamus are parts of an area of the brain called the limbic system, which also includes part of the cerebral cortex and other areas, such as the hippocampus and the amygdala, which play important roles in memory formation. The limbic system lies above

and around the brainstem and is involved with motivation and emotion; it also contributes to memory. Researchers have observed that memories associated with strong emotions are often easier to access. Because of its functions in emotions such as pain, pleasure, anger, fear, sorrow, sexual feelings, and affection, the limbic system is sometimes referred to as the "emotional" brain.

The deepest area of the brain is the brainstem. It contains structures that automatically regulate essential life functions such as breathing, heart action, and digestion through the sympathetic and parasympathetic branches of the autonomic nervous system. Although these functions are considered involuntary, psychological factors such as stress can affect them. An example is anxiety hyperventilation, in which breathing becomes very fast and interferes with the normal regulation of blood gas (oxygen and carbon dioxide) concentrations, resulting in dizziness, shortness of breath, pounding heart, and even fainting. Anxiety hyperventilation is uncomfortable and even frightening, and many experiencing this condition interpret it an impending heart attack. Breathing and relaxation practice are often effective treatments for anxiety hyperventilation, as people learn to interrupt the hyperventilation.

The nerve fibers of the reticular formation (RF) run through the middle of the brainstem up into the diencephalon and act as a major communication pathway between the brain and the rest of the body, an important mind-body connection. The RF acts as a gatekeeper, continuously scanning the sensory information entering the brain and evaluating its importance. It alerts higher centers to critical information, thus stimulating arousal and consciousness. It also blocks information deemed "less important" or irrelevant. The RF may be responsible for those stories of soldiers whose legs or arms are lost in battle, yet the soldier feels no pain until after the battle has ended, or athletes who continue to compete with broken bones and other severe injuries. On the other hand, the RF may become sensitized to low-level input that higher centers deem important and may amplify signals, increasing sensations such as pain that the cortex wants to focus on.

Health Behavior and the Nervous System

A number of health behaviors have been shown to affect the health of the brain and the rest of the nervous system (Box 2-4). The same behaviors discussed in Chapter 1 in relation to artery disease influence the arteries that supply the brain and influence stroke risk. Health behaviors have also been linked to changes in cognitive function, including risk of Alzheimer's disease and other forms of dementia.

Stroke

Stroke results when blood supply to the brain is interrupted. Plaques in the arteries supplying the brain can cause ischemic stroke, brain damage caused by a lack of blood flow to a region of the brain. Ischemic stroke usually occurs when a blood clot and bits of plaque block the artery. The many factors that affect risk of artery disease also affect risk of stroke. Smoking, sedentary lifestyle, high blood lipid levels, obesity, diabetes, and hypertension increase risk. Exercise, a healthy diet, and good stress management decrease risk.

Hemorrhagic stroke happens when a blood vessel in the brain bursts and disrupts normal circulation. High blood pressure can increase the risk of hemorrhagic stroke in susceptible people. High blood pressure can be controlled with many lifestyle measures as well as medications if necessary.

Changes in Cognitive Function

With aging, the number of neurons and synapses in the brain declines. This appears to be an inevitable part of the aging process, although this decline accelerates with various diseases. Along with this loss of neurons comes a delay in conduction velocity of the remaining neurons, so that the rate of information processing slows. Some of this slowdown seems to occur because of degeneration in the connections between nerve cells.

Of particular concern to many people is the gradual decline in short-term memory that begins in adulthood. When memory problems begin to occur, many people fear the onset of Alzheimer's disease, the most common form of dementia. Dementia is a term that refers to groups of symptoms, marked not only by memory impairment but also by an extreme decline in mental abilities such as judgment and abstract thinking, as well as changes in personality. Only severe memory loss, such as getting lost in familiar areas or the inability to recognize family members, is considered a symptom of dementia. But a decline in memory can be a source of frustration even for people who are not worried about dementia. Alzheimer's disease is the most common cause of dementia. Alzheimer's disease is marked by abnormal clumps of protein deposits in the brain. Dementia can also be caused by other disorders. Vascular dementia is caused by inadequate blood supply to the brain. While a stroke involves the larger arteries, vascular dementia involves blockage in the smaller arteries. Inadequate blood supply, over time, leaves neurons less healthy and functioning at lower levels.

Researchers studying Alzheimer's disease, other forms of dementia, and the aging brain have discovered many interesting links between lifestyle and brain health, just as research on artery disease has given us clues to lifestyle and atherosclerosis (Tyas, Snowdon, Desrosiers, Riley, & Markesbery, 2007). The aging and disease processes in the brain, as in other organs, are strongly influenced by genetics. But, like the heart and the arteries, the brain is also shaped by its environment and by factors such as exercise, stress, and nutrition.

This combination of genetics and lifestyle affects many variables, including the adequacy of the circulation to the brain, the rate of neuronal connections established and broken down, and the rate of neuron death with aging. This combination of genetics and lifestyle also has significant effects on a person's level

---

Box 2-4. For College Students: Maximizing Brain Power

The brain is an amazing organ. But it is also just a bunch of fairly fragile nervous tissue. The physical brain has physical needs: good nutrition, rest, exercise, and the avoidance of harmful substances. This sounds simple, but many college students take the brain for granted and fail to give their brains the conditions they need to work at maximal power.

Brains do best with 7 to 8 hours of sleep a night. Sleep is essential for memory, which is a big part of learning (Diekelmann & Born, 2010). Sleep is also essential for stress management and the ability to concentrate and focus on class lectures, reading, and homework. Most students know that time does not equal productive output. A paper that normally takes only a few hours to write can take days if the student is sick, exhausted, or depressed.

The brain needs an adequate blood sugar level, so food is essential (Smith, Riby, van Eekelen, & Foster, 2011). Big meals can leave people feeling tired, so several smaller meals during the day usually work best for the brain. Exercise improves memory, energy level, and focus, so it makes a good study break (Hillman, Erickson, & Kramer, 2008). Exercise also counteracts the bane of student existence: sitting in class, in front of the computer, or in lab.

Caffeine in moderation is fine for most people. However, too much caffeine can lead to the jitters, anxiety, and sleepless nights. Alcohol kills brain cells, makes people sleepy, and interferes with judgment, not to mention studying.

of daily function in the presence of the physiological changes in the brain that signify Alzheimer's disease.

The brain has a rich circulatory system that supplies the brain cells with oxygen and nutrients and removes wastes. While the brain comprises only 2% of the body's weight, it consumes about 20% of the oxygen used at rest. (This is why it is important to wear a hat in cold weather: a high level of circulation in the head can lead to heat loss.)

Researchers have found that factors that interfere with blood flow to the brain interfere with brain function (Tyas et al., 2007). Thus, all the lifestyle factors that are known to increase risk of artery disease increase risk of memory loss as well. Smoking, hypertension, sedentary lifestyle, poor blood lipid profile, and diabetes all accelerate arterial aging and compromise blood flow. Exercise can help keep blood vessels supplying the brain healthy by improving blood sugar regulation, blood pressure, and blood lipid profile.

Regular physical activity has been shown to increase blood levels of an important protein called brain-derived neurotrophic factor (BDNF). Higher levels of BDNF have been correlated with larger increases in hippocampal volume in both humans and laboratory animals. BDNF plays a role in stimulating the formation of new brain cells, a process called neurogenesis, from stem cells or precursor cells in the brain (Wu et al., 2008). Exercise appears to enhance signaling molecules, promoting new cell production and blocking other factors that inhibit neuron production and maturation (Gobeske et al., 2009).

Exercise may also prevent memory loss by reducing feelings of stress, anxiety, and depression. Studies in both animals and humans have shown that high levels of severe chronic stress are associated with significant nerve cell death in the hippocampus (Sapolsky, 1996). This region of the brain is especially important for memory. Depression, anxiety, and stress hinder memory in other ways as well, such as by interfering with the ability to concentrate. Memory functions do not work as well when people are distracted and unable to focus on the material they are supposed to remember.

Maintaining good health prevents the acceleration of the aging process. Conditions such as hypertension and diabetes should be aggressively controlled with lifestyle changes and medications, if necessary. Medications can be a double-edged sword, however, and contribute to memory loss. People on medications who seem to experience a change in memory should check with their physicians to see whether this is a medication side effect, in which case medications can be changed or dosages adjusted.

A heart-healthy diet with plenty of fruits and vegetables provides phytochemicals, vitamins, and minerals that may help prevent oxidative damage to body cells. Studies have found that memory problems in some adults are linked to nutrient deficiencies; memory improved when these were corrected (Ahmed &

Haboudi, 2010). Older adults with inadequate diets may benefit from supplementation.

Good emotional health practices may help keep the brain healthy. Controlling stress, depression, and anxiety and maximizing emotional health with a positive outlook and healthy pleasures may help the brain and will certainly improve quality of life as well. Social connections, spirituality, and altruism may help the brain as well as the heart.

The phrase "use it or lose it" applies to the brain just as it does to muscles, joints, and bones. Challenging the brain to learn new information by taking a class, learning a new language, reading, doing crossword puzzles, or engaging in other creative and challenging work encourages the growth of brain cells and the connections among them. A college education is one of the strongest protective factors for the prevention of dementia. Researchers theorize that lifelong learning helps to create a brain reserve, so that, even as some capacity is lost with aging and disease, people remain functional and have a higher quality of life for a longer period of time (Snowdon, 2001).

Adequate sleep is critically important for cognitive function and emotional well-being (What's the Evidence 2-1). Good sleep habits support good health in many ways. On the other hand, fatigue increases feelings of stress and can contribute to emotional health problems. Fatigue can also erode the energy available for self-control and make it more difficult for people to follow through with their behavior-change plans (Behavior Change in Action 2-1).

THE ENDOCRINE SYSTEM: Hormones Facilitate Mind-Body Communication

While the nervous system facilitates mind-body communication through its network of nerve cells, the endocrine system produces chemicals called hormones that originate in one part of the body but exert actions on tissues and organs that are often in other areas of the body. Hormones are similar to neurotransmitters in that they function by binding to receptors located on the membranes of target cells. Thus, hormones convey their messages in this act of binding with receptors. In some cases, the same chemical, such as norepinephrine, can function as both a neurotransmitter and a hormone. Norepinephrine is produced by neurons and sent as a neurotransmitter to adjacent neurons. Norepinephrine is also produced by the adrenal glands, which release it into the bloodstream, where it binds with receptor sites on various cells throughout the body. The endocrine system and its hormones are important players in mind-body communication (Fig. 2-8).

Hormone Production

Specialized cells within the glands produce hormones. For example, the pineal gland, discussed earlier in this

WHAT'S THE EVIDENCE? 2-1

Sleep, Emotion, and Self-Regulation

Yoo, S-S., Gujar, N., Hu, P., Jolesz, F. A., & Walker, M. P. (2007). The human emotional brain without sleep–a prefrontal amygdala disconnect. *Current Biology. 17*(20):R877-R878.

■ PURPOSE

Seung-Schik Yoo and colleagues were familiar with the psychological research showing a relationship between sleep deprivation and emotional imbalance and were curious to understand what parts of the brain might explain this association.

■ STUDY

Yoo, Gujar, Hu, Jolesz, & Walker (2007) recruited 26 male and female participants who were assigned to either a sleep-deprivation group or a sleep-control group. Subjects in the sleep-deprivation group missed an entire night of sleep and had been awake for about 35 hours in a row before laboratory testing. The control group slept normally at home.

In the laboratory, subjects were shown 100 images ranging in emotional tone from neutral to aversive while undergoing functional magnetic resonance imaging (fMRI). Functional magnetic resonance imaging measures blood flow to functioning areas of the brain; more blood flow means more activity in that region.

The researchers found that although amygdala activation increased in both groups when viewing aversive images, activation in the sleep-deprived group was about 60% higher than activation in the control group. In addition to greater activity in the amygdala, the area activated in the sleep-deprived group was about three times as large as the area activated in the control group. Because the amygdala is highly involved in processing emotions, this difference suggests that the sleep-deprived subjects were experiencing a stronger aversive response to the negative images.

In addition, the researchers found more coactivation of other emotional centers in the brain, such as the limbic system, in the sleep-deprived subjects, suggesting a much stronger emotional response. The sleep-deprived subjects showed little medial prefrontal cortex (MPFC) area activation during testing, whereas the control subjects showed high levels of activation in the MPFC. The MPFC is believed to exert an inhibitory control over the amygdala, to help people appropriately regulate their emotional responsiveness.

■ IMPLICATIONS

Sleep deprivation may lead to more emotional responsiveness with less self-regulatory control. This research helps explain the relationship between lack of sleep and mood disorders. It also reinforces the importance of adequate sleep for emotional self-regulation.

BEHAVIOR CHANGE IN ACTION 2-1

Help Clients Make Adequate Sleep Part of Every Behavior-Change Plan

■ Challenge

Poor sleep leads to feelings of fatigue, stress, and other negative emotional states, putting people at risk for relapse in their behavior-change programs. When people feel bad, they have stronger desires to return to behaviors that provide comfort: overeating, smoking, drinking alcohol, or sitting in front of the television.

■ Plan

Most people know the recommendations for good sleep: at least 7 to 8 hours per night. If sleep is a problem, health and fitness professionals can recommend commonsense lifestyle measures. When clients do not respond to lifestyle measures, they should seek the advice of their health-care providers because sleep problems can be an indication of another underlying disorder that would improve with treatment.

Ask clients about levels of fatigue. Fatigue feels bad and may motivate clients to make lifestyle changes to feel better. If clients experience fatigue, then ask them about their sleep patterns. Clients often know what they should do; talking to you may get them thinking about changes they want to make in their schedules so that they can get adequate sleep. Some clients will want to reduce fatigue with changes in eating and exercise behaviors. Although exercise and a healthy diet can improve energy levels, they are not a substitute for good sleep.

Ask clients about caffeine and alcohol consumption. Many clients do not know that caffeine stays in the body a relatively long time and may interfere with sleep quality many hours after consumption. Although alcohol may cause sleepiness, it also interferes with sleep quality.

Continued

BEHAVIOR CHANGE IN ACTION 2-1–cont'd

Encourage clients to notice whether they sleep better on exercise days. Many people find this to be the case. If clients find that exercise improves sleep quality, they may be motivated to exercise regularly. Some people find that exercising too close to bedtime is energizing and may interfere with sleep. Help these clients find a better time to work out.

Educate clients about good sleep hygiene. If clients ask for advice about improving their sleep, give them advice on good sleep habits. Encourage them to develop a soothing before-bed ritual for winding down. Most people sleep better with a regular sleep schedule, going to bed and rising at the same times each day. Clients should try to create a comfortable sleep environment that is cool, dark, and quiet.

Teach clients simple relaxation exercises that they can use at home. The breathing exercise on pages 66–67 and the relaxation exercises presented in Chapter 6 are easy to use and can reduce sympathetic arousal.

Encourage clients to address sources of stress that lead to wakefulness. Some clients may tell you that a certain issue is worrying them and keeping them awake. Rather than counseling clients on how to deal with particular problems, refer them to a professional.

Note: Health and fitness professionals should also practice what they preach in regard to adequate sleep.

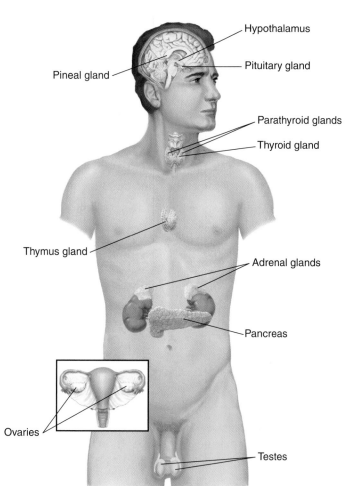

Figure 2-8. The endocrine system. *(Modified from Gylys, B. & Wedding, M.E. (2009). Medical Terminology Systems. F.A. Davis, Philadelphia, p. 395; with permission.)*

chapter, produces the hormone melatonin (Box 2-5). Melatonin travels in the bloodstream and binds with receptor sites on a variety of cells, including cells in the hypothalamus and pituitary gland. Another organ, the pancreas, releases hormones that help regulate blood sugar level. For example, the pancreas releases insulin into the bloodstream. The insulin binds with cells throughout the body, signaling the cells to allow blood sugar (glucose) to enter the cell from the blood.

The pineal gland and the adrenal glands are examples of endocrine glands, which release their hormones directly into the bloodstream without special ducts. Other major endocrine glands are presented in Figure 2-8, and their functions are summarized in Table 2-2.

Box 2-5. Jet Lag: Resetting the Pineal Gland

The natural cycles of the earth reflect the rhythm of day and night. Over evolutionary time, animals, including humans, have adapted to the 24-hour cycle of light and dark. All physiological functions are governed by this 24-hour cycle, known as the circadian ("about a day") rhythm. Everything from bowel function and body temperature to mental alertness and reaction time fluctuates in this 24-hour pattern. The pineal gland, located near the brain, helps regulate circadian rhythm.

Although the light-dark cycle changes gradually with the seasons, it has only been in very recent history that people have had to adjust to sudden changes in this cycle. Some people seem to adapt to time zone changes more easily than others, but almost everyone experiences a feeling of being out of sync when traveling through more than a time zone or two. People who work varying shifts, sometimes working at night and other times during the day, undergo the same stress.

The best way to reset one's circadian rhythm is with outdoor physical activity and plenty of exposure to daylight. Early-morning exposure to daylight helps reset the pineal gland. (Judicious use of caffeine can also be helpful.) The pineal gland is very sensitive to light and dark. To help the pineal gland know that it is night, it is best to maintain a dark environment and avoid blue light from computer screens close to bedtime.

Table 2-2. Major Endocrine Glands and Organs That Produce Hormones

GLAND	ACTIONS
Hypothalamus	• Integrates endocrine and nervous systems • Controls pituitary gland
Pituitary gland - anterior lobe	• Releases growth hormone to regulate growth of bone and other tissues and metabolism of nutrients • Releases prolactin to stimulate milk production in nursing mothers • Releases thyrotropic hormone to stimulate the thyroid gland to produce hormones • Releases adrenocorticotropic hormone to stimulate the adrenal gland to produce hormones • Releases follicle-stimulating hormone and luteinizing hormone which regulate the menstrual cycle • Releases endorphins to reduce feelings of pain
Pituitary gland - posterior lobe	• Releases antidiuretic hormone to help regulate water balance • Releases oxytocin, which facilitates uterine contractions in childbirth, milk release for breastfeeding, and interpersonal bonding
Thyroid gland	• Releases thyroid hormones to regulate metabolic rate, growth in children • Releases calcitonin to help regulate blood calcium level
Parathyroid glands	• Release parathyroid hormone, which works with calcitonin to regulate blood calcium level
Adrenal glands - adrenal cortex	• Release corticosteroid hormones to assist the stress response. Corticosteroids influence water balance, metabolism of nutrients, immune system, and sexual development and function.
Adrenal glands - adrenal medulla	• Release hormones epinephrine and norepinephrine which promote the stress response, increasing heart rate and blood pressure
Pineal gland	• Releases melatonin to regulate circadian rhythm
Gonads	• In females, the ovaries secrete hormones that participate in the menstrual cycle, pregnancy, and childbirth. • In males, the testes release hormones to regulate reproductive function.

Continued

Table 2-2. Major Endocrine Glands and Organs That Produce Hormones–cont'd

GLAND	ACTIONS
Digestive system	• Releases hormones that stimulate the secretion of digestive enzymes and other chemicals that assist with digestion • Releases ghrelin to stimulate feelings of hunger
Pancreas - islet cells	• Produce insulin and glucagon to regulate blood sugar level
Kidneys	• Release erythropoietin to increase the rate of red blood cell production
Heart	• Releases atrial natriuretic peptide to decrease blood pressure
Adipose tissue	• Releases leptin to help regulate appetite; may play a role in menstrual cycle regulation

Glands that release hormones to their target organs via ducts (small tubes) are known as exocrine organs. The salivary glands located near the mouth are examples of exocrine organs. The salivary glands produce and secrete saliva, a watery fluid that helps moisten food in the mouth and contains enzymes that begin the chemical breakdown of food.

Hormones are also produced by gland cells in organs that have other functions. For example, specialized cells in the stomach produce a hormone called gastrin that in turn helps to regulate the production and secretion of stomach acid. Other cells produce the hormone ghrelin that stimulates feelings of hunger and the drive to eat. The stomach also holds and churns food, so its major role as an organ assigns it to the digestive system.

Stress Response

A brief overview of some of the hormones that help regulate the "fight-or-flight" response provides an instructive example of how hormones work together and with the nervous system to coordinate important psychophysiological responses. When the brain perceives the need to deal with a source of stress, neurons in the hypothalamus activate the sympathetic nervous system and set the "fight-or-flight" response in motion. The nervous system responds immediately, and, because the stress response is so essential for survival, the endocrine system reinforces this response and helps to maintain arousal as long as necessary.

Activation of the SNS stimulates several important hormone pathways. One of these raises adrenaline, the hormone famous for the "adrenaline rush." Another name for adrenaline is epinephrine. Epinephrine is secreted by the adrenal glands, which are located on top of the kidneys. The adrenal glands are really two glands in one. The outside layer is called the adrenal cortex, while the inner portion is the adrenal medulla. The adrenal medulla is activated by direct nerve connection with the hypothalamus. When stimulated, it secretes the hormones epinephrine and norepinephrine. These two hormones are collectively referred to as the

catecholamines. They are sympathomimetic, meaning they mimic the action of the sympathetic nervous system. They increase heart rate, contractile force of the heart, and blood pressure. They dilate the airways, increasing the flow of air to the lungs. The catecholamines increase blood sugar, so the body has fuel for muscle contraction. And, like the SNS, the catecholamines slow the digestive processes, putting digestion on hold until the immediate stressful situation is dealt with.

Another hormone pathway raises the level of a hormone family known as the glucocorticoids, produced by the adrenal cortex. Cortisol, corticosterone, and cortisone are three glucocorticoids involved with the stress response. Glucocorticoids affect several metabolic processes, increasing energy availability and inhibiting processes unnecessary for immediate survival. For example, these hormones decrease the immune response to cold viruses, which explains why so many students get sick at the end of the semester, typically a high-stress time.

More detail on the psychophysiology of the stress response and the effects of stress on health and behavior change will be explored in Chapter 6. The psychophysiology of the stress response contributes to many health problems, such as high blood pressure, that are likely to arise when people experience chronic activation of the "fight-or-flight" response.

Health Behavior and the Endocrine System

Many common health behaviors exert strong effects on endocrine balance. Some of the endocrine functions most affected by health behaviors include the stress response, reproductive function, and the disruption of normal blood sugar regulation that leads to type 2 diabetes.

Stress-Related Illness

The stress response has far-reaching actions on many parts of the endocrine system, not to mention the mind and body in general, so health behaviors that affect the stress response affect almost everything. For example, chronic overactivation of the "fight-or-flight" response interferes with normal growth in children, sexual function in adults, and blood pressure regulation. Many health behaviors increase the stress response. Smoking delivers nicotine, a sympathomimetic substance, to the bloodstream, increasing the stress response. Caffeine is also a sympathomimetic drug and increases the stress response.

On the other hand, behaviors that lead to feelings of relaxation reduce the "fight-or-flight" response and the risk for stress-related disorders. Practices such as meditation, breathing exercises, or even a hot bath help turn off the "fight-or-flight" response and allow the parasympathetic functions of rest and digest to exert their beneficial effects. Appropriate levels of physical activity can also calm the "fight-or-flight" response and increase parasympathetic nervous system output.

With her classes done for the day, Maya stretches out in the sun to read her romance novel. But before she has read more than a few paragraphs, a shadow falls across her book. She looks up to see a woman she has noticed at meals but who has not been in any of Maya's classes. The woman asks Maya if she has a minute for a question. Maya reluctantly closes the book, smiles, and says, "Yes, of course." The woman, Harriet, is a lawyer, who has been working 60-hour weeks for many years, rarely taking a vacation. She has recently been diagnosed with hypertension and wants Maya's advice on reducing stress. Maya wonders where to begin but launches into her standard advice regarding regular exercise, rest and relaxation, and trying to cultivate a balance in life. "What a great idea to come on this cruise," she says. As they talk, Maya notices Harriet never smiles and seems preoccupied with her worries. Maya gently mentions that everyone can use professional support from time to time in coping with sources of stress. Maya also suggests that Harriet speak with a dietitian about making dietary changes to reduce her blood pressure. Maya encourages Harriet to join the early morning walk, and she agrees to give it a try. ■

Reproductive Function and Bone Density

Dietary choices, exercise levels, and stress can affect hypothalamic-pituitary-gonad communication in men and women. Reproductive function, especially in women, is dependent upon having adequate energy stores so that the body can support pregnancy and breastfeeding. When living conditions are too stressful and especially when food is scarce, the body may reduce or shut down reproductive function in order to prevent pregnancy and conserve energy.

In men, suppressed reproductive function manifests as lower reproductive hormone levels and reduced sex drive. Lower levels of the reproductive hormones such as testosterone over a long period can in turn lead to reduced muscle and bone mass and even premature osteoporosis in males with eating disorders (Mehler, Sabel, Watson, & Andersen, 2008).

In women of childbearing age, suppression of reproductive function results in a loss or disruption of the menstrual cycle. Amenorrhea refers to the absence of menstrual periods. Oligomenorrhea means fewer than the normal number of periods or abnormally light menstrual blood flow but some menstrual cycle activity. (Eumenorrhea is the term for normal cycling.)

A syndrome that came to be called the female athlete triad caught the attention of researchers in the 1980s when several young amenorrheic females were found to have a condition of low bone density typical of osteoporosis (Nattiv et al., 2007). Some females had even sustained vertebral compression fractures, fractures of the vertebrae responsible for the dowager's hump sometimes seen in older adults (Fig. 2-9). These fractures are not reversible and are painful and difficult to treat. Further studies suggested that, while some young women gained a little bone density following treatment with reproductive hormones, bone density failed to reach normal levels. This loss of bone density appears to be secondary to the low levels of reproductive hormones seen in young women with disordered eating behaviors that result in the intake of too little energy. Low body fat levels result in low levels of the hormone leptin. Low leptin levels appear to signal the hypothalamus that not enough energy or body fat is present to support the menstrual cycle and reproduction (Kelesidis, Kelesidis, Chous, & Mantzoros, 2010). The hypothalamus stops secreting the hormones that stimulate the pituitary gland to send out the hormones that regulate the menstrual cycle. Thus, the triad refers to three concurrent conditions: disordered eating, amenorrhea, and osteoporosis (Fig. 2-10).

Exercise does not usually cause a suppression of reproductive function, unless levels are excessive and inadequate calories are consumed. While the original subjects observed to have the triad syndrome were athletes (distance runners), the syndrome can also occur in people who are not athletes.

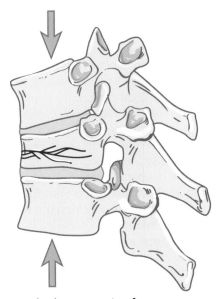

Figure 2-9. **Vertebral compression fracture.**

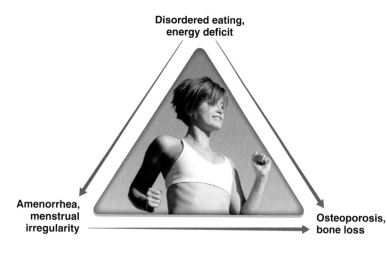

Disordered eating, energy deficit

Amenorrhea, menstrual irregularity

Osteoporosis, bone loss

Figure 2-10. **The female athlete triad.** Photograph © Thinkstock

MOTIVATING CHANGE: Preventing the Female Athlete Triad

Many exercise and sports organizations have worked hard to raise awareness about the dangers of disordered eating and the prevalence of disordered eating among athletes and recreational exercisers. While males are less likely to be affected, boys and men with eating disorders and those participating in sports that have weight restrictions, such as wrestling and lightweight rowing, may develop low energy intakes that can disrupt endocrine function.

Girls and women are exposed to multiple influences that may promote disordered eating and a drive for thinness that leads to the triad syndrome. Some sports favor athletes with low body fat levels, and females may strive to achieve an unrealistically thin physique, urged on by teachers, parents, and coaches. Many female athletes wear revealing attire that motivates them to lose weight to look better. Social norms regarding body size often promote an unrealistically thin body type for girls and women, a type unachievable for most, even with stringent dieting. It is easy for girls to become fixated on their appearance and to worry excessively about how they look.

Health and fitness professionals must be careful to reinforce positive reasons for behavior change. Help clients change exercise, eating, and other behaviors for the right reason: for good health. Try to promote the idea that good looks require good health, as does emotional well-being, the most important health component of all. Remember that your word may carry a lot of weight, especially with young people. A joke about too much belly flab may be the straw that breaks the proverbial camel's back, pushing a vulnerable young person to dangerous dieting.

If you become aware that a client seems to be developing an eating disorder, follow procedures for referring her or him to a professional. Referral procedures for eating disorders are discussed in Chapter 11. The eating disorder anorexia has the highest mortality rate of all psychological disorders, so it is important to intervene as soon as possible. However, if a female client mentions that she has developed menstrual irregularities, it is important not to assume these are the result of the triad. The menstrual cycle can become disrupted for many reasons, so refer clients back to their health care providers for a diagnosis.

Obesity and Type 2 Diabetes

Obesity poses a significant challenge to the endocrine system. As discussed in Chapter 1, North Americans have seen a sharp rise in type 2 diabetes rates over the last few decades. While the causes of type 2 diabetes are not completely understood, the observation that type 2 diabetes is reversible with weight loss provides strong evidence for a role of overeating as a cause. Excess storage of triglyceride in the liver and around the viscera interferes with normal insulin response, and blood sugar regulation is compromised (Taylor, 2008). Physical activity helps to improve insulin sensitivity in many people, with or without fat loss.

THE IMMUNE SYSTEM: Messengers, Soldiers, and Base Camps

Like the nervous system and the endocrine system, the immune system consists of cells spread throughout the body that carry on extensive communication to coordinate proteins, cells, tissues, and organs in various parts of the body. It coordinates the body's efforts to protect itself against pathogens, invaders such as viruses, bacteria, fungi, and other agents that can cause harm. The lymphatic system provides a home to high concentrations of immune cells that serve as messengers and soldiers as they guard the body from infection. Immune cells also circulate in the bloodstream.

The Lymphatic System

The lymphatic system (Fig. 2-11) provides the base camp (and nursery) for immune system messenger and

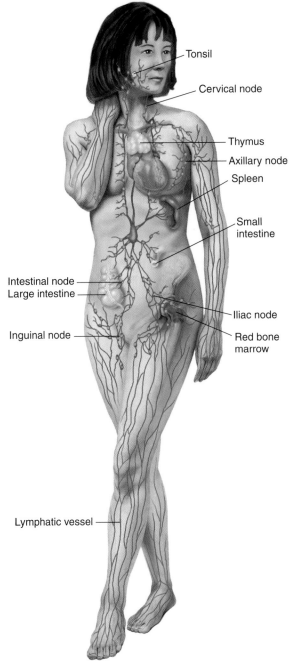

Figure 2-11. **The lymphatic system.** *(Modified from Gylys, B. & Wedding, M.E. (2009). Medical Terminology Systems. F.A. Davis, Philadelphia, p. 234; with permission.)*

soldier cells. Immune cells are most highly concentrated in the lymphatic system, which includes the lymph nodes and vessels that run throughout the body in parallel to the circulatory system's network of arteries and veins. The lymphatic system also includes the organs and tissues that help produce immune cells, including the spleen, thymus gland, and bone marrow.

The white blood cells or leukocytes are important immune cells. Leukocytes circulate throughout the body in the blood vessels and lymphatic system. Phagocytes are a type of leukocyte that attacks and breaks down invading organisms. Another important group includes the lymphocytes. The lymphocytes fall into two categories. The B lymphocytes arise from cells in the bone marrow and mature there, before finding their way into the blood and lymphatic vessels. These cells carry memories of past invaders and mount an immune response when these invaders reappear. The B lymphocytes identify invaders the body has previously been exposed to, producing antibodies that mark the invaders for destruction. Antibodies in turn activate a complex network of proteins called complement that disable pathogens. The T lymphocytes begin life as stem cells in the bone marrow but mature in the thymus gland (hence the T). The T cells attack pathogens that the B cells have identified as invaders. Because the immune system develops the ability to recognize and attack pathogens over time from exposure to various agents, these activities are referred to as acquired immunity (as opposed to innate immunity, discussed below).

Psychoneuroimmunology

At one time, physiologists thought the immune system functioned independently without much input from other physiological systems. Scientists now know that the immune system communicates extensively with the nervous and endocrine systems. The field of **psychoneuroimmunology** studies the interrelationships of these three systems that serve as communication networks in the maintenance of health (Game Changers 2-1). Researchers have found, for example, that psychological states such as depression can affect the synthesis and behavior of various immune cells, including various types of white blood cells such as leukocytes and macrophages that attack foreign invaders. Immune cells have receptor sites for and thus respond to neurotransmitters and hormones. For example, at low concentrations, norepinephrine stimulates the immune system. Elevated cortisol levels act to inhibit immune system activity, perhaps one of its energy-conservation effects. An elevation in cortisol has been observed with depression, so endocrine effects may help explain the link between depression and decreased immune response.

Immune cells do not merely eavesdrop on the nervous and endocrine systems; they talk back. Immune cells manufacture a variety of messenger substances classified as cytokines, which are similar to hormones. Cytokines are small proteins released by cells. These molecules then bind to receptors on the same cell, nearby cells, or cells in other parts of the body. Cytokines allow immune cells to communicate with other immune cells and a variety of other systems. The neuroglia of the nervous system also produce cytokines. As with neurotransmitters, each cytokine has matching cell surface receptors. Binding triggers a cascade of intracellular signaling and upregulation or downregulation of genes that produce specific proteins that affect cell behavior and function.

The Immune Response to Pathogens

The body protects itself from pathogens in many ways. Innate immunity refers to these nonspecific mechanisms and includes the barriers provided by the skin and

Game Changers 2-1. Candace Pert and the Molecules of Emotion

Candace Pert's work on opiate receptor biochemistry in the 1970s was able to demonstrate in the laboratory a phenomenon previously only speculated (Pert & Snyder, 1973). Scientists had wondered how drugs such as heroin and nicotine exerted their effects on the nervous system. Pert's lab found an opiate receptor in several regions of the brain in rats, guinea pigs, and mice and demonstrated its binding activity. Later work on endorphins (opiate look-alikes manufactured by the body itself) and the receptors and messenger molecules of the immune system propelled Pert and others to establish the field of psychoneuroimmunology. Pert and colleagues observed that the brain, endocrine system, and immune system were in constant communication with one another.

In 1997, Pert compiled her research, the research of others, and her own theories about mind-body communication into a book, *Molecules of Emotion*. In it, she set forth a description of how the biochemistry of the nervous, endocrine, and immune systems manifests the psychological experiences of people: emotions, sensations, and even thoughts. Pert explained how research on peptides from the nervous, endocrine, and immune systems and their receptors demonstrates the oneness of mind and body. "We know that the immune system, like the central nervous system, has memory and the capacity to learn. Thus, it could be said that intelligence is located not only in the brain but in cells that are distributed throughout the body and that the traditional separation of mental processes, including emotions, from the body is no longer valid" (Pert, 1997, p 187).

Pert, C. B. & Snyder, S. H. (1973). Opiate receptor: demonstration in nervous tissue. *Science*. 179(4077):1011-1014.
Pert, C. B. (1997). *Molecules of Emotion*. New York: Scribner.

mucous membranes that keep out pathogens. Innate immunity also includes a variety of internal defense mechanisms. For example, when certain immune cells become infected with viruses, they produce proteins called interferons. Interferons spread into neighboring cells and stimulate those cells to produce proteins that block the process of viral replication, thus limiting the damage that invading viruses can do.

One important immune system activity is the process of inflammation. Inflammation is a response mounted by the immune system when reacting to an injury. Injured cells produce cytokines that trigger the dilation of blood vessels in the injured area and call for leukocytes to come and disable pathogens. Symptoms of inflammation include redness and swelling, caused by increased blood flow and the migration of phagocytes to the injured area. Inflammation can help the body destroy foreign invaders and speed the healing of wounds.

But, unfortunately, sometimes inflammation only makes a bad situation worse. In the case of artery disease, white blood cell activity in the artery only increases the size of the plaques. Inflammation may also result from an inappropriate immune response, as when the immune system mistakenly attacks when it should not; examples include allergies and autoimmune responses. In the case of allergies, harmless substances such as dust mites or pollen may trigger respiratory inflammation, along with sneezing, runny nose and eyes, and a great deal of misery. The skin may also exhibit an allergic response, with redness, swelling, and itching.

Many serious illnesses are caused by an autoimmune response. Ordinarily, the immune system does a good job of distinguishing between pathogens and the body's own cells and tissues. Researchers do not yet fully understand what prompts the immune system to

attack the body's own cells. Such attacks are the cause of autoimmune disorders such as rheumatoid arthritis (inflammation of the joints), asthma (airway inflammation), and psoriasis (inflammation of the skin).

Health Behavior and the Immune System

The immune system communicates actively with the nervous and endocrine systems, so anything affecting these two systems affects immune response as well.

Inflammation

Inflammation appears to play an important role in triggering the negative health consequences of obesity (Mathieu, Lemieux, & Despres, 2010). As adipocytes (fat cells) pump into overdrive to store excess calories that have been turned into fat (triglyceride), the cellular machinery required to store this excess fat may not keep up with the storage demand. This might be visualized as a factory floor, where there are not enough workers to handle all the raw material coming in, and thus faulty products are made because the workers are working too quickly. In the case of adipocytes, the faulty products appear to be damaged proteins, which lead to a signaling for the immune system to break down these faulty proteins and malfunctioning adipocytes. Unfortunately, the immune cells that are called in, a type of phagocyte called *macrophages*, are unable to break down the fat cells, and so inflammation is triggered instead and persists at low levels as long as extra calories are being consumed.

In a similar way, excess fats lead to inflammation in the artery lining. In this case, the fats are part of large molecules called lipoproteins. Lipoproteins shuttle cholesterol and triglycerides around in the bloodstream. When low-density lipoproteins (LDLs) become oxidized, they stick to the artery lining. The body calls for help from the immune system, and macrophages are drawn to the sticky lipoproteins. Again, the macrophages are unable to adequately break down these large molecules, and, instead of cleaning up the damage, a larger mess is created, as the macrophages and the inflammation process trigger the formation of arterial plaque. As discussed in Chapter 1, avoiding chronic overconsumption of excess calories reduces this inflammatory response and the risk for artery disease.

Smoking increases low-level inflammation in the body. One proposed mechanism for smoking's effects is that some of the chemicals in smoke oxidize molecules in the body, such as LDL cholesterol. On the other hand, exercise is associated with lower levels of inflammation (Mathur & Pedersen, 2008). Some studies have suggested stress-reduction techniques such as yoga and meditation decrease measures of inflammation (Kiecolt-Glaser et al., 2010). Diet also appears to affect chronic low-level inflammation. Certain nutrients and foods, such as fish, fish oils, and plant foods, tend to be anti-inflammatory, while processed fats and high intakes of red meat seem to increase inflammation (Galland, 2010).

MOTIVATING CHANGE: Working With Clients Trying to Lower C-reactive Protein Levels

Many health and fitness professionals see clients who have been checked for systemic inflammation with a blood test that measures C-reactive protein (CRP). C-reactive protein is produced by the liver, and its blood level provides a reflection of a person's systemic inflammation. Testing for CRP is sometimes performed for people already at a higher risk of artery disease, such as people with several risk factors and those who have already had a heart attack or undergone surgery to repair clogged arteries. Other clients have been reading about inflammation, and many are taking fish oil and other supplements to prevent inflammation. They may not know their CRP levels but are still motivated to pursue lifestyle behaviors that reduce inflammation.

Clients interested in reducing inflammation should be educated about the important inflammation-reducing effects of exercise. Regular exercise is one of the best ways to reduce CRP. Weight loss in people who are overweight also reduces CRP level. Luckily, the advice for reducing CRP is the same as the advice for reducing risk of artery disease: manage chronic health conditions like hypertension and diabetes, do not smoke, eat well, and be active.

Lifestyle and the Common Cold

Most students can attest to the effects of stress and lack of sleep on immune system function. Students tend to develop more upper respiratory tract infections (colds) at the end of the semester, when stress peaks and hours of sleep decline as they scramble to write papers and keep up with the other obligations in their lives. The stress hormone cortisol suppresses immune function, one of

its energy-conservation effects. Too much stress can mean low immune response to pathogens. Similarly, the immune system relies on adequate sleep for its work, and lack of sleep lowers resistance. On the other hand, regular exercise, good eating habits, and adequate rest and relaxation allow the immune system to achieve peak performance.

Health behavior measures for cold prevention also include infection prevention: frequent hand washing and avoiding touching the mucous membranes of the nose and eyes. If possible, it is good to avoid sick people and to wash hands after touching anything they have touched: telephones, doorknobs, and the serving spoons in the cafeteria lines.

THE DIGESTIVE SYSTEM: A Gut Response

The digestive system includes a series of organs through which food passes, becoming broken down and absorbed along the way (Fig. 2-12). Food not absorbed is excreted as waste. The digestive system also includes other organs that assist in the digestive process. Many people experience problems with their digestive systems, and these problems may be exacerbated by stress, diet, exercise, and other health behaviors. Many health

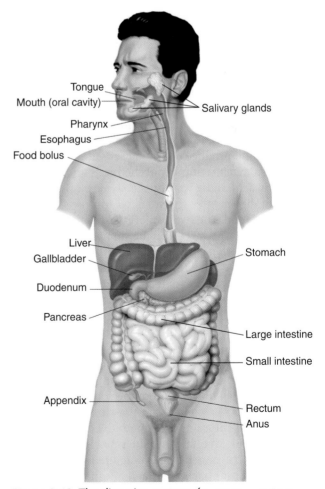

Figure 2-12. **The digestive system.** *(Modified from Gylys, B. & Wedding, M.E. (2009). Medical Terminology Systems. F.A. Davis, Philadelphia, p. 109; with permission.)*

and fitness professionals encounter clients on crazy diets that affect the health of the digestive tract or clients recovering from bariatric surgery designed to facilitate weight loss, in which the digestive system is surgically altered in ways (like making the capacity of the stomach smaller) that discourage overeating or reduce the absorption of calories from a meal. Problems with the digestive system can lead to malabsorption of nutrients, causing a variety of health challenges when nutrients are not available as needed. It is important to have a general understanding of the digestive system in order to understand nutrition, obesity, and the many health behavior issues involving this system.

Digestion and Absorption of Nutrients

The digestive system is responsible for converting food into molecules that can be used by the body. Food is ingested through the mouth, where it begins to be broken down by chewing and mixing with saliva, a watery fluid secreted by the salivary glands. Saliva moistens the food, making it easier to swallow. Saliva also contains digestive enzymes that begin the chemical breakdown of the carbohydrate and fat in food. After the food is chewed, it is swallowed into the esophagus, a tube that runs from the mouth to the stomach. The esophagus is located behind the trachea, which carries air to the lungs. The smooth muscle of the esophagus carries the food to the stomach with wave-like contractions. A sphincter, a tight band of muscle, is located between the esophagus and the stomach. This sphincter opens to allow food to pass into the stomach and then closes to prevent the stomach contents from backing up into the esophagus. Heartburn occurs when this sphincter relaxes and allows the acidic contents of the stomach to enter the esophagus and produce a burning sensation (Box 2-6).

In the stomach, a number of chemicals, including hydrochloric acid and a variety of enzymes, continue the process of digestion as the stomach contracts to churn and mix the food. The hydrochloric acid is manufactured and secreted by special cells in the stomach lining. It creates an extremely acidic environment in the stomach, which is ideal for breaking down food and killing many of the pathogens that may have entered the body with the meal. Very little nutrient absorption occurs in the stomach, which is why the stomach can be downsized with bariatric surgery and have minimal negative effect on nutrient absorption. As the stomach mixes the food, a sphincter between the stomach and small intestine opens and closes to allow small amounts of the mixture to enter the small intestine from the stomach.

When the acidic contents of the stomach enter the small intestine, messages are sent to the pancreas to secrete sodium bicarbonate into the small intestine to reduce acidity. The pancreas is an organ located near the junction of the stomach and small intestine (Fig. 2-13). In addition to secreting sodium bicarbonate, the pancreas secretes hormones that regulate blood sugar. The pancreas also secretes a mixture of digestive enzymes

---

Box 2-6. Stomach Acid: A Good Thing or a Bad Thing?

Heartburn is a name for gastroesophageal reflux disease (GERD). When stomach contents are not digesting properly, fermentation begins, gas builds up, and the expanding stomach contents can press against the sphincter that separates the stomach from the esophagus. If this sphincter opens, the stomach contents, which are very acidic, can back up into the esophagus, causing pain, irritation, and even erosion of the esophageal lining.

Stomach acid is actually a good thing, so the impulse to reach for antacids or proton pump inhibitors, drugs that reduce the stomach's production of hydrochloric acid and are marketed for GERD, should be carefully considered. The highly acidic environment of the stomach disables many pathogens. Some research suggests that by reducing stomach acid, people are at increased risk for stomach cancer, initiated by the presence of bacteria in the stomach (Waldum, Gustafsson, Fossmark, & Ovigstad, 2005). Bacteria also increase risk of stomach ulcers.

Stomach acid increases the breakdown of food, facilitating separation of important nutrients so that they will be readily absorbed when they reach the small intestine. For example, stomach acid aids in the digestion of protein. A highly acidic environment also helps calcium ions separate from food, thus making calcium more available in the small intestine. Studies suggest that people on long-term acid-reducing therapies decrease their absorption of calcium and thus increase their risk of osteoporosis (Sipponen & Harkonen, 2010).

Before reaching for products to reduce GERD, it is important to first try lifestyle measures. Indigestion is often caused by eating too much too quickly, not chewing food enough, eating while feeling stressed, and consuming alcohol. Many people find that they have better digestion when they avoid high-fat meals, eat in a relaxing environment, chew their food thoroughly before swallowing, and consume smaller meals. Omitting alcohol can also aid digestion because alcohol can irritate the stomach. Meals should be consumed several hours before lying down so that gravity can assist stomach emptying. Some people also find relief with digestive enzymes such as papain and bromelain, which come from the fruits papaya and pineapple, respectively (McCormick, 2008).

---

into the small intestine to continue the breakdown of carbohydrates, proteins, and fats. The liver manufactures a substance called bile that helps to emulsify the fats in the food being digested. Emulsify means to break the big globules of fat into smaller particles, in

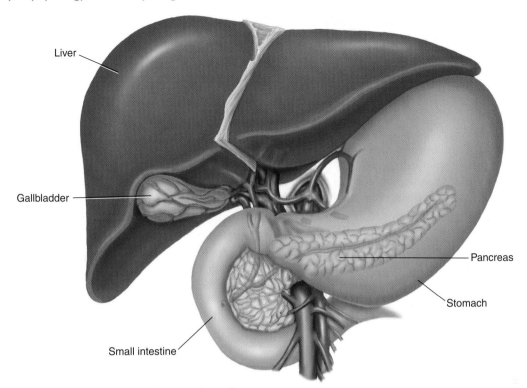

Figure 2-13. **The pancreas, gallbladder, liver, and small intestine.** *(Modified from Gylys, B. & Wedding, M.E. (2009). Medical Terminology Systems. F.A. Davis, Philadelphia, p. 110; with permission.)*

order to increase the surface area of the fat exposed to digestive enzymes. The bile manufactured by the liver is stored in an organ called the gallbladder, which in turn secretes the bile into the small intestine when the presence of fat is detected.

Digestion occurs both inside the small intestine itself and in the small cells, called absorptive cells, that line the small intestine. These cells line the surface of fingerlike projections that extend from the inner surface of the small intestine. These absorptive cells take in small molecules from the digestive tract and break them down even further, ultimately passing nutrients along into the lymphatic system or into the circulatory system for distribution to the rest of the body. Components of food that are not broken down remain in the small intestine and are passed along to the large intestine or colon. These remains are mostly fibers, plant structures such as cellulose that are not digestible by humans. The colon absorbs some water and a few minerals and then passes the waste to the rectum, which stores the feces until the urge to eliminate triggers the anal sphincter to open and expel the waste. The anal sphincter is a band of muscle whose function is to control elimination of the feces.

The Brain in the Gut

The activity of the digestive system is regulated by the rich network of nerves found in the enteric nervous system. The enteric nervous system also communicates with the brain via the ANS. A variety of hormones regulate all the digestive processes, from the movement of the smooth muscles of the digestive organs that push

food through the system to the release of enzymes that perform the chemical breakdown of food. The digestive system also has an extensive network of lymphatic tissue and immune cells ready to disable pathogens that find their way into the body via the mouth.

Food Allergies, Intolerances, and Sensitivities

Food allergies involve activation of an immune response. For example, people who are allergic to foods such as nuts and shellfish may experience swelling of the throat and airways when they consume the offending food. True allergies such as these can be life threatening, as swelling airways make it difficult or impossible to breathe. These allergies can progress to anaphylaxis and even death. Anaphylaxis is a severe reaction to an allergen. Symptoms include difficulty swallowing or breathing, itching, swelling, nausea and vomiting, and anxiety and confusion. Anaphylaxis is a medical emergency, and help should be sought immediately.

Celiac disease is an autoimmune disease activated by the presence of a protein called gluten that is found in wheat, rye, and barley. For some unknown reason, gluten triggers the immune cells to attack the lining of the small intestine. Celiac disease symptoms include abdominal pain, gas, bloating, diarrhea, constipation, malnutrition, fatigue, and weight loss. Celiac disease is difficult to diagnose, since many of these symptoms are very common. Blood tests may show antibodies to gluten, but these are not always clear. An examination of the lining of the small intestine can reveal the presence of damage and lead to a definitive diagnosis. But many people forego this test, opting instead to try a gluten-elimination diet to see if symptoms resolve. The only treatment for celiac disease is to follow a gluten-free diet. It is important to treat celiac disease because, if the lining of the small intestine is not functioning properly, malabsorption of nutrients can lead to malnutrition and disorders such as iron-deficiency anemia and osteoporosis.

Food intolerance refers to a situation in which the ingestion of a certain food or food component creates uncomfortable digestive symptoms, such as bloating or diarrhea. Food intolerances are different from food allergies in that they are not triggered by the immune system. A common food intolerance is lactose intolerance. People with lactose intolerance lack or have low levels of the enzyme lactase that is required to break down the milk sugar lactose. Lactose that is not digested ferments in the stomach and small intestine, causing gas, bloating, pain, and diarrhea. People with lactose intolerance can buy lactase pills to take with milk products or simply avoid milk products. Some people with lactose intolerance find they are able to consume small amounts of some dairy products, such as yogurt or cheese, without discomfort.

People with food sensitivities find that certain foods "disagree" with them. They may feel they have difficulty digesting the food, and they get a stomachache after eating it. For example, people who have been on low-fat diets may find eating a high-fat food such as quiche, French fries, or a fatty burger disagrees with them, feeling heavy and uncomfortable in the stomach. While food sensitivities are milder than food intolerances, food sensitivities can be a real problem for some people. People with food allergies, celiac disease, or food intolerances and, in fact, people who find eating difficult for any reason should work with a dietitian to figure out a nutritious diet that works for them.

Maya's coworker, a personal trainer who runs the weight room, is sick with a high fever today. Maya delivers a bowl of broth to his room and then runs upstairs to cover the afternoon shift in the weight room. A line of people stream through the doors as Maya flicks on the lights and checks the list at the desk to review what she is supposed to do. Once she has gotten set up, she wanders from person to person to see if they have any questions or need assistance.

Greg, a thin young man getting off the treadmill, asks if she has any advice on gaining weight. His expression looks worried, and Maya senses he wants to talk. They sit down at the desk, and Maya gives him her standard weight-gain advice. As she probes a little, Greg tells Maya he has lost a great deal of weight over the past several years and has just been diagnosed with celiac disease. He is having difficulty eating on the cruise, as he has not yet learned what not to eat. Maya has worked with clients with celiac disease before,

and she sends Greg to a good website that gives very specific eating and food preparation instructions. She learns he has not talked to the kitchen staff, so it is not surprising he is not feeling well. She sends him to the kitchen with a printout of the instructions to meet with the executive chef to be sure he is getting a gluten-free diet. She also reminds him to meet with a dietitian for more help with diet planning when he gets home. ■

Health Behavior and the Digestive System

A variety of health behaviors impact the digestive system. Digestive system sensitivity varies greatly from person to person, but some general observations can be made for both healthy digestive tracts and for people with digestive disorders.

Digestive System Health
Diet is the most obvious health behavior that impacts the digestive system. The healthy digestive system does best with a well-balanced diet that contains plenty of fruits, vegetables, and other sources of fiber. These foods support and encourage a mix of healthy bacteria that live in the intestines and help keep the digestive tract healthy. Fiber helps to prevent constipation, and it may also prevent a variety of digestive disorders such as diverticulitis, where inflammation and infection occur in the colon because of trapped particles of feces. Food with carcinogens, such as processed meats, and high-meat/low-fiber diets increase risk of colon cancers. Exercise reduces risk of colon cancer and speeds transit time, the time it takes food to move from the mouth, through the digestive system, and out of the system through the anus. A faster transit time means lower exposure to any carcinogens in the food. Feelings of stress have an enormous impact on the digestive system, as discussed in the section on the nervous system, above. For example, many people have had the experience of feeling hungry and preparing to eat but then getting into an argument and losing their appetite in a few short moments, as the anger and emotional effects of the argument set in.

The digestive system can be irritated and damaged by alcohol intake, resulting in liver disease and pancreatitis (inflammation of the pancreas). Alcohol and smoking in combination increase risk of esophageal cancer.

Irritable Bowel Syndrome
An example of a digestive disorder that is often helped by health behaviors is irritable bowel syndrome (IBS). IBS affects the colon and consists of a group of symptoms that include gas, bloating, cramping, diarrhea, and/or constipation. It is unknown why some people experience IBS. It may be that the nerves and muscles of the colon are especially sensitive in people with IBS. IBS can be a frustrating disorder to live with, especially if diarrhea and cramping inhibit daily activity. Some people with IBS reduce their symptoms by being

careful about what they eat. Some are helped by high-fiber diets and probiotic supplements and by avoiding foods that cause gas. Relaxation techniques can be very helpful for calming "the brain in the gut." Getting enough rest, managing stress, and exercise help some people with IBS.

MOTIVATING CHANGE: Exercising With Digestive Disorders

Digestive disorders such as IBS can be very painful, and clients with these disorders may be reluctant to try anything that might make their pain worse. Many have established eating behaviors that are working to some extent as well as some sort of daily routine. People with digestive disorders may hesitate to add physical activity to their lives, even though, like everyone, they need exercise. Exercise may feel uncomfortable, and, if diarrhea is part of the digestive disorder, clients may want to be near a bathroom at all times. Some times of the day may be better than others. Health and fitness professionals should listen carefully to the clients' concerns, even though digestive problems can be embarrassing to discuss. These clients may prefer low-impact activities to begin with, perhaps indoors near a bathroom. Cycling or rowing machines may work best for some. Running-type activities may be too much stress on the digestive tract. Strength training may be well tolerated. Be sympathetic, start slowly, and build gradually to increase client confidence along with fitness.

THE MUSCULOSKELETAL SYSTEM: Made to Move

The musculoskeletal system includes muscles, bones, joints, and the various other tissues that enable this system to produce voluntary movement. Movement is achieved when groups of muscle cells contract, causing a shortening of the muscles. The muscle contraction causes movements of the bones to which muscles are attached. These movements are finely regulated by the nervous system, and, while the movements are called "voluntary," their regulation, in terms of which exact muscles move when, is unconsciously controlled for the most part.

Muscles and Tendons

Muscular tissue is comprised of specialized cells containing proteins that slide into one another to produce a shortening of the cell that results in muscular contraction. These cells are called muscle fibers. Each muscle is composed of hundreds to thousands of muscle fibers, and their patterns of activation or recruitment determine the force and speed of the contraction. Groups of muscle fibers communicate with nerve cells known as motor neurons. One motor neuron plus the fibers that it innervates is known as a motor unit. A motor unit in a very small muscle, such as one of the muscles that moves the eye, may have as few as 10 to 20 muscle fibers. Large muscles, such as those in the thigh, that need to generate a great deal of force may have as many as 2000 to 3000 muscle fibers in a single motor unit. When the motor neuron sends a nerve impulse to the motor unit, all fibers in that unit contract fully. The force of contraction in a muscle is regulated by the nervous system, which decides how many motor units to activate, or recruit.

Individual muscle fibers are enclosed in a thin layer of connective tissue. Similarly, bundles of fibers are surrounded by connective tissue, and the entire muscle is supported in the same fashion. These layers of connective tissue join together at the ends of the muscles and insert into the bone and are called tendons. Tendons attach muscles to bone, and the layers of connective tissue provide structure for the muscle.

Muscle Fiber Types

Human muscles are composed of a mixture of muscle fiber types (Table 2-3). These fiber types fall into three main categories based on their speed of contraction and dominant method of energy production. The type I, or slow-twitch oxidative (SO) muscle fiber, is recruited for aerobic exercise—activity requiring a sustained elevation of metabolic rate and muscle contraction. Compared with other fiber types, the SO fibers are somewhat slower in contractile speed and somewhat lower in force production, but more resistant to fatigue.

Table 2-3. Muscle Fiber Types

FIBER TYPE	DESCRIPTION	SPEED	FORCE	ENERGY SYSTEM	FATIGUE RESISTANCE
I	Slow-twitch oxidative	Slow	Low	Aerobic	High
IIA	Fast-twitch oxidative-glycolytic	Fast	High	Aerobic & Anaerobic	Medium
IIB	Fast-twitch glycolytic	Fast	High	Aerobic	Low

They have a higher density of capillaries, since they rely on oxygen to produce energy. The SO fibers are also recruited for long sprint-type activity, exercise that occurs at maximal intensity for longer than a few minutes.

Type IIB, or fast-twitch glycolytic (FG) muscle fibers, are larger than SO fibers and are capable of producing more force faster. They rely on anaerobic energy systems to produce energy quickly. They also fatigue quickly, however, and need the SO fibers to help maintain intense physical activity that lasts longer than 10 to 30 seconds. Type IIA, or fast-twitch oxidative-glycolytic (FOG) fibers, are intermediate fibers that contract quickly but have greater endurance than the FG fibers. These fibers can produce energy from both anaerobic and aerobic pathways. They contribute to both sprint and endurance exercise, as needed.

Specificity of Training: Muscle Response

In response to exercise training, the muscle fiber types called upon for the production of movement become conditioned. They increase their energy-production machinery, including the concentration of enzymes needed to produce energy. They also increase their energy-storage capacities. Fibers that produce energy from the aerobic pathway grow more capillaries and other blood vessels and increase the size and number of the mitochondria in the cells. The mitochondria are organelles that turn glucose and oxygen into energy, carbon dioxide, and water. Athletes must train the specific muscle fibers and energy systems needed for performance. Simply strengthening the arms, for example, may not translate directly into better swim race times. Plenty of swimming at race pace will have a more direct effect on race performance.

Bones and Ligaments

The bones are organs made of dense mineralized tissues that comprise the skeleton and provide a structural framework for the body. The bones of the body come in a variety of shapes and sizes to fit their many functions. They are comprised of metabolically active tissues that are continuously responding to the internal environment of the body and to the forces being placed on the body. In response to these forces, bones are continuously being broken down and rebuilt. Bones also contain cartilage, the smooth tissue that reduces friction where bones come together at joints, to facilitate movement and protect the ends of the bones. Some bones contain tissue called red bone marrow that produces red blood cells, white blood cells (discussed above in the section on the immune system), and platelets, which facilitate the blood-clotting process. Yellow bone marrow is made primarily of adipocytes, which store triglycerides. In babies, all bone marrow is red bone marrow. With age, more yellow bone marrow develops. The reasons for this change are unclear.

Tendons attach muscles to the bones, and muscular contraction produces skeletal movement. The bones also serve many other functions. They protect internal organs. For example, the skull protects the brain. Bone tissue allows the body to maintain the correct blood concentrations of several minerals, including calcium and phosphorus, the two minerals most highly concentrated in bone tissue. When blood levels of these minerals become too low, hormones signal the bone to release minerals into the bloodstream, bringing their concentrations back to normal. The red bone marrow, mentioned above, is important for blood and immune function.

Bone structure varies with bone function. Compact bone tissue (Fig. 2-14) has a dense network of bone tissue with few spaces. Bone units called osteons are packed tightly together. Osteons are arrangements of different types of bone cells around a central canal occupied by blood and lymphatic vessels and nerves, which supply the bone with nutrients and deliver hormones and other chemical messengers that help direct bone activity. Trabecular bone tissue, also known as spongy bone tissue, has large spaces between columns of bone tissue. In some places, this space is filled with red bone marrow. Trabecular bone is lighter than compact bone and contributes less weight to the skeleton.

Bone tissue deposition and resorption (the break down of bone tissue) are directed by specialized bone cells. Osteoblasts arise from stem cells in the bone. Osteoblasts build new bone and eventually become bone

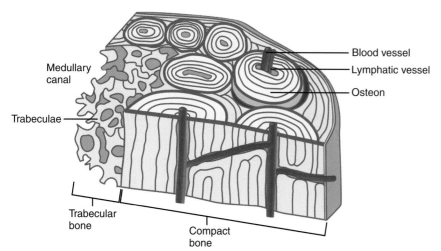

Medullary canal

Trabeculae

Trabecular bone

Compact bone

Blood vessel
Lymphatic vessel
Osteon

Figure 2-14. Compact and trabecular bone tissue.

cells (osteocytes) in the bony matrix. Osteoclasts help break down bone tissue to enhance the remodeling of the bones in response to the forces being placed on them and to release minerals into the bloodstream. With remodeling, the bones structure themselves to best support the forces being placed on them, due to body weight and physical activities (Box 2-7).

Ligaments are strong tissues that connect bones to each other and help form joints. Ligaments have poor blood supply and thus heal slowly. Anyone who has ever sprained an ankle or other joint has experienced damage to ligaments. Physical therapy for sprains involves strengthening exercises, which not only strengthen the muscles around the joint but improve ligament strength as well.

Synovial Joints

Because bones themselves do not bend, movement can only occur where bones come together to form joints. Joints are points of connection between bones or, in some cases, between bones and cartilage. There are several different types of joint structures in the human body, and not all allow movement. Synovial joints (Fig. 2-15) allow for the greatest range of motion. Bones connected by a synovial joint are surrounded by a dense joint capsule, whose lining generates synovial fluid, a thin, viscous fluid that lubricates the joint structures. Synovial fluid reduces friction, supplies joint structures with nutrition, and removes wastes. When a synovial joint is not moved for a long time, the synovial fluid becomes thicker. Movement stimulates the production and secretion of synovial fluid, helping joints move more easily. This is why appropriate exercise is recommended for joint health.

Cartilage covers the surface of the bones in a synovial joint. Ligaments provide supportive structure. Extra pads of fibrous cartilage help absorb impact forces in some joints, such as the knee and wrist. Some joints have one or more bursae (singular, bursa), saclike structures filled with fluid to help reduce friction. Fat pads around the joint also serve to reduce friction and cushion the joint.

Most joint structures are vulnerable to problems, especially with overuse and aging. Inflammation of the tendons is called tendonitis; of the bursa, bursitis. Arthritis refers to a group of disorders involving the joint. Osteoarthritis affects the cartilage that covers the bones in the joint. With osteoarthritis, this cartilage becomes damaged, thinner, or lost entirely. Rheumatoid arthritis is an autoimmune condition that attacks the joint lining, producing inflammation and pain.

It's a beautiful day, and Maya decides to sneak in a swim in the outdoor pool. But, before she can even get in the water, a woman she has never noticed before comes limping over to speak with her. Maya gives the woman a smile, as the woman launches into a 15-minute description of her knee pain. Maya listens sympathetically and asks questions, knowing full well she is not going to be giving much advice on this issue. She has noticed over her many years of work

Box 2-7. Mechanical Stressors Direct Bone Cell Activity

The bones rely on messages from the rest of the body to direct their cellular activity. Nature is a conservative force, especially when it comes to bone metabolism, and hates to waste unnecessary energy. When the bones do not hear messages of demand, they quit building up and strengthening the bone tissue. In situations such as space flight, bed rest, paralysis, or even very sedentary lifestyles, the stem cells in the bone stop making osteoblasts and instead die or develop into other cell types, such as adipocytes that form the yellow bone marrow (Ozcivici, Luu, Rubin, & Judex, 2010). On the other hand, mechanical stimulation of bone increases the activity of the osteoblasts and strengthens the bone through increased mineral deposition and improvement in bone quality.

Mechanical stimulation results from anything that puts force on the bones. Gravity itself stimulates bone metabolism. The forces of jumping, running, and punching provide mechanical stimulation. Tennis players have greater bone density in their playing arms than in their nondominant arms, the result of repeated force on the bones of the dominant arm. Nonexercise sources of mechanical stimulation include the use of vibration technology. Mechanical vibration stimulates bone formation and is increasingly part of orthopedic rehabilitation technology (Ozcivici, et al., 2010).

Physical activity is essential for preserving bone density, which gradually declines during the aging process. Weight-bearing activities, in which the body carries its own weight, such as walking, running sports, tai chi, and weight lifting, place more force on the bones than weight-supported activities, such as cycling and swimming. Activities that produce constantly changing forces result in greater bone strength than activities that provide continuous force. For example, walking and running provide changing forces, whereas using an elliptical trainer provides more of a continuous force. The more irregular forces of running sports, such as basketball, soccer, and racquet sports, provide even more bone stimulation. Relatively high-impact movements such as jumping, sprinting, hopping, and skipping are great for bones, if they can be done safely. Walking quickly provides more stimulation than walking slowly.

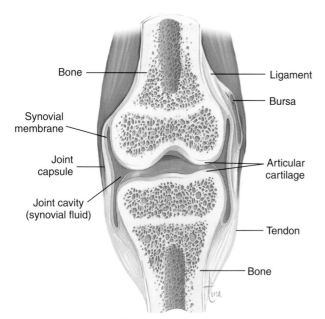

Figure 2-15. Synovial joints. *(Modified from Scanlon, V.C. & Sanders, T. (2011). Essentials of Anatomy and Physiology. F.A. Davis, Philadelphia, p. 140; with permission.)*

that people love to talk about their injuries and seem to figure that anyone in the fitness area knows everything about the body. Sometimes Maya privately guesses the correct diagnosis, as she finds out when clients come back after they have seen their health-care providers or specialists. When the woman has told her story, Maya expresses concern and urges her to check with the physician available on the ship. In the meantime, Maya suggests that she rest while on board, so as not to make her injury or condition worse. While the ship's doctor can give the client emergency treatment, the doctor will probably suggest that the woman see her doctor as soon as she gets home for more testing and a more-thorough evaluation and treatment. Maya tells the woman where to find ice and instructs her on using ice to help reduce pain and swelling. The woman seems a little disappointed but thanks Maya for her time. ■

Vertebral Column

One of the most complex (and most problematic) musculoskeletal structures in the human body is the spine, known as the vertebral column (Fig. 2-16). The spine is composed of a column of 26 individual bones called vertebrae (vertebra, singular). Between the vertebrae are the intervertebral discs, fibrocartilaginous structures with a soft, shock-absorbing interior. Surrounding the vertebrae and disks are strong, tough ligaments that hold the vertebral column together. The spinal cord is contained inside the vertebral column, and the spinal nerves pass through small openings between vertebrae (Fig. 2-17). When the vertebrae or disks press upon nerves, sensations of numbness, tingling, or pain may occur. Additionally, damage to the spinal nerves may

interfere with information delivery to target tissues. For example, if motor neurons to the leg are affected, the muscle strength of the leg may decline.

Mind-Body Communication in the Musculoskeletal System

Proprioceptors are the sensory organs in the tendons, joints, and muscles that communicate information to the brain. The nerves in the muscles also send information about the state of the muscles and contribute to sensations such as muscle tension and fatigue.

With exercise, muscles release peptide (protein) molecules traditionally classified as cytokines into the bloodstream. Some researchers have proposed that these peptides be called myokines, as they originate from muscle (Pedersen, 2011). These molecules help the muscles communicate with the nervous, endocrine, and immune systems. Some have an anti-inflammatory effect on the body and appear to contribute to many exercise benefits, such as better blood sugar regulation, less artery disease, and increased blood flow to the brain, along with the creation of new neurons in the brain (Pedersen, 2011).

Health Behavior and the Musculoskeletal System

Appropriate types and levels of physical activity help increase and maintain the integrity of all structures in the musculoskeletal system and serve to stimulate the production of helpful myokines. With inactivity, bones lose mineral. A lack of activity leads to atrophy (shrinking) of muscle tissue and to joint stiffness. Muscle weakness contributes to joint weakness as well because the muscles provide support for most joint structures.

The vertebral column is especially vulnerable to poor body mechanics. It is often harmed by years of poor posture, especially sitting posture, which places stress on disks in ways that push the disk to press on sensitive nerves. Appropriate strengthening exercises for the abdominal and back muscles can help prevent back problems.

The postural muscles include muscles of the lower and upper back, shoulders, neck, and face. During the "fight-or-flight" response, tension increases in the postural muscles, as the body prepares for action. Chronic tension in these muscles may become a habit with overactivation of the sympathetic nervous system and contribute to a variety of pain syndromes.

A healthy diet with enough protein and plenty of fruits and vegetables helps to maintain the health of the musculoskeletal system. Muscles and bones need adequate potassium, magnesium, and calcium, found in plant foods and dairy products. Obesity, especially excess fat in the abdominal region, can place extra stress on joints and contribute to back, hip, knee, and foot problems. Good footwear is essential for maintaining healthy joints and bones in the feet. Women generally have more foot problems than men (Menz, Jordan, Roddy, & Croft, 2010). This difference is likely due to footwear

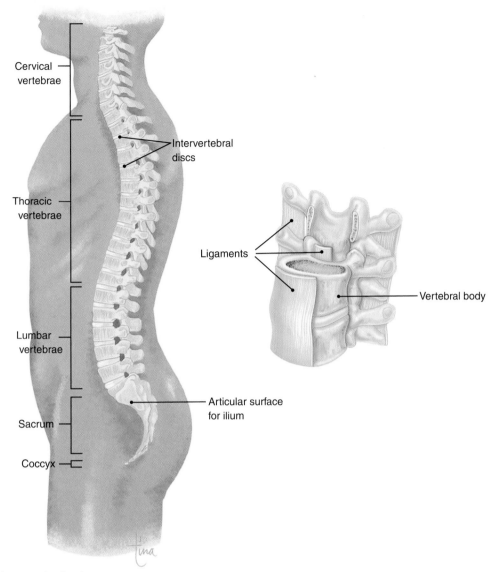

Figure 2-16. **The vertebral column.** *(Modified from Scanlon, V.C. & Sanders, T. (2011). Essentials of Anatomy and Physiology. F.A. Davis, Philadelphia, p. 129; with permission.)*

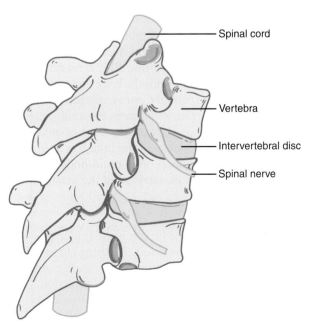

Figure 2-17. **The spinal nerves.**

with a narrow toe box and an elevated heel. Shoes that fit too tightly and high heels stress the bones and joints in the feet while they are supporting body weight.

THE CARDIORESPIRATORY SYSTEM: Vital Support for Every Cell

The cardiorespiratory system refers collectively to the respiratory and cardiovascular systems, which work together to supply all the body's cells with oxygen and nutrients and to take away the waste products of cellular metabolism. The respiratory system includes the organs that provide for the exchange of oxygen and carbon dioxide. The cardiovascular system includes the heart, blood vessels, and blood.

The Respiratory System

Along with the organs for respiration, or breathing, the respiratory system includes sensors for smell and the structures for voice production (Fig. 2-18). Air enters

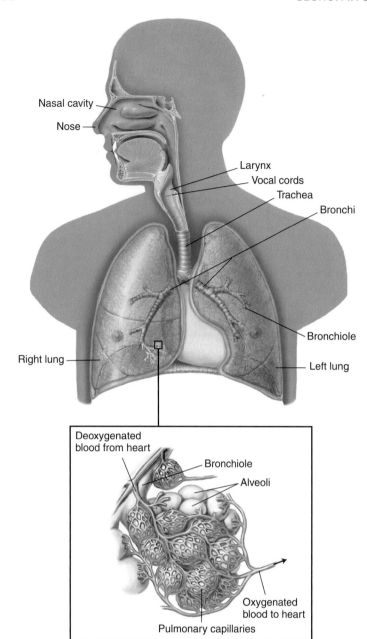

Figure 2-18. **The respiratory system and alveoli.** *(Modified from Gylys, B. & Wedding, M.E. (2009). Medical Terminology Systems. F.A. Davis, Philadelphia, p. 150; with permission.)*

the respiratory tract through the nose and mouth and then passes through the trachea and bronchi into the lungs. The actual exchange of oxygen and carbon dioxide occurs in the tiny air sacs of the lungs, called the alveoli (singular, alveolus). The lungs contain roughly 300 million alveoli. Gases diffuse readily across the thin alveolar and capillary membranes. Oxygen passing into the bloodstream binds with the hemoglobin molecule in red blood cells to be carried to other parts of the body. Hemoglobin also picks up the carbon dioxide generated by energy-production processes in the cells. The carbon dioxide then diffuses readily out of the blood, across the capillary and alveolar membranes, and into the air. Carbon dioxide also travels in the blood in other forms.

Regulation of Breathing

Many factors influence breathing rate, including anxiety and stress, exercise, and airway irritation. Most of the

time, breathing is regulated by groups of neurons in the brainstem. At rest, inhalation lasts about 2 seconds, and exhalation lasts about 3 seconds. The cerebral cortex also has nerve connections with the respiratory center, so breathing rate may be brought under voluntary control. Slowing the breathing rate voluntarily, especially extending the exhalation phase of breathing, is associated with feelings of relaxation. Control of the breath is used with many relaxation techniques and mind-body exercise forms, such as yoga, Pilates, tai chi, and the martial arts.

MOTIVATING CHANGE: Breathing Exercises for Stress Reduction

It has been said that the breath is the bridge between the body and the mind. Teaching clients to gradually slow their breathing is an effective and easy way to introduce them to stress-reduction practices. Try it yourself first. Either sit in a chair or lie on the floor. Lying down is more relaxing, although some clients may be uncomfortable lying on the floor. If you are sitting, use good sitting posture, with a nice long back and your head balanced over your shoulders. Become mindfully aware of your breathing, feeling the air coming in through your nose and filling your lungs. Feel the muscles lifting your ribs to make room for the air and the natural pause that occurs once your inhalation is complete. Then, allow the muscles to relax and the air to exhale slowly. Enjoy the pause at the end of the exhalation, before you feel a spark of energy urging you to breathe again. If you are seated and become dizzy, try the exercise lying down.

Now put your hand on your abdomen, below your waist. Allow the abdomen to relax and rise as you inhale. Feeling the abdomen rise and fall is much easier when you are lying down. If you are sitting, you may at least be able to feel your stomach (under your ribs) moving in and out. Allowing the breathing rate to be as comfortable as possible, count how many slow counts (approximately one count a second, but do not look at your watch) it takes for the inhalation. Then count the exhalation. Allow the exhalations to become slower and slower, until they are taking about twice as long as the inhalations. Try to do this exercise in a way that feels relaxed rather than forced.

Clients can practice this exercise any time of day to reduce nervous tension. Even just a minute or two of mindful breathing can disrupt the frantic energy of the "fight-or-flight" response. Performing some slow breathing before bed aids relaxation and sleep.

Health Behavior and the Respiratory System

As discussed in Chapter 1, smoking tobacco products is the single most preventable cause of death and disability worldwide. In addition to its effects on the cardiovascular system, smoking wreaks havoc on the respiratory system. Smoking increases risk of emphysema, a progressive destruction of the sensitive alveoli of the lung, and eventually the collapse of the respiratory bronchioles. Gas exchange becomes increasingly difficult.

Smokers are also more likely than nonsmokers to develop chronic bronchitis, an inflammation of the bronchioles. "Smoker's cough" is a symptom of chronic bronchitis, where inflammation produces excess mucus as the airways attempt to heal themselves. Between 80% and 90% of lung cancers are attributable to smoking. Tobacco smoke contains a number of carcinogens, which not only affect organs of the respiratory system but also are transported in the bloodstream to other organs as well. Cancers of the esophagus, stomach, kidney, pancreas, colon, and urinary bladder are more common in smokers than nonsmokers.

The Cardiovascular System

The cardiovascular system includes the heart, blood vessels, and blood (Fig. 2-19). This system circulates blood to every cell in the body, delivering oxygen, fuel,

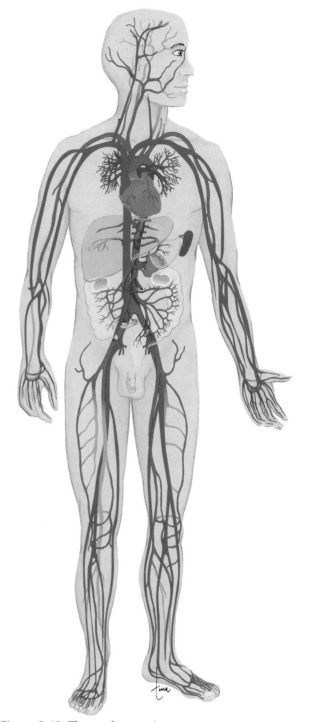

Figure 2-19. The cardiovascular system. *(Modified from Scanlon, V.C. & Sanders, T. (2011). Essentials of Anatomy and Physiology. F.A. Davis, Philadelphia, p. 321; with permission.)*

and messenger molecules such as peptides and hormones and removing waste products. The heart has four chambers, separated by valves to prevent backflow. Blood returning to the heart from the rest of the body enters the right atrium, which pumps the blood on to the right ventricle. From there, the blood is sent to the lungs for gas exchange. Once it has passed through the lungs, the oxygen-rich blood returns to the heart and enters the left atrium, which pumps the blood on to the left ventricle. The left ventricle sends the blood out to the rest of the body.

The blood vessels carrying oxygen-rich blood from the heart to the body are called arteries. The arteries branch like a tree, as they reach into all parts of the body. The smaller arteries are called arterioles. The arterioles send blood to the capillaries, the smallest blood vessels, where gas and nutrient exchange with cells actually occurs. Just as gases cross the capillary membrane, nutrients and waste products cross capillary and cell membranes, often with the help of transporter or membrane proteins. After their communication with the cells, the capillaries merge together into venules (little veins) and then into larger vessels known as veins which eventually return the blood to the right atrium.

Health Behavior and the Cardiovascular System

Health behaviors have a large impact on the cardiovascular system. The relationship of lifestyle factors to the development of artery disease was summarized in Chapter 1. Many health and fitness professionals study the relationship of lifestyle to cardiovascular disease and work in this field, at least for part of their career (Health Psychology at Work 2-1). Lifestyle change is important both for the prevention of heart disease and for the treatment of heart disease after it has been diagnosed. Smoking, physical activity, diet, and body composition are all related to the development of artery disease. In addition, chronic illnesses such as diabetes and hypertension, which are influenced by health behaviors, strongly increase risk of artery disease.

Chronic stress exerts a negative impact on the cardiovascular system. Sympathetic stimulation and the endocrine stress response cause an increase in heart rate and blood pressure. While it is normal for heart rate and blood pressure to go up and down throughout the day, it is hard on the heart and blood vessels when blood pressure remains elevated day after day. Some people experience irregular heartbeat patterns in response to stress.

Chronic stress, sedentary lifestyle, smoking, and a poor diet increase the clotting speed of the blood, making blood clots more likely to form within the circulatory system and on the artery linings. Blood clots on top of plaque can lead to artery blockage and, in turn, to heart attack or stroke.

◼ *It is almost time to disembark. Maya is looking forward to getting home and preparing for her new job. It was nice to get away, although it did feel like she worked more hours*

HEALTH PSYCHOLOGY AT WORK 2-1: Professional Education and Expertise Inspire Client Confidence

Tom Stabile, M.A., Exercise Physiologist and Personal Trainer

Tom Stabile works privately as a personal trainer in his own facility, Stability Fitness, in Mount Vernon, Ohio. In his undergraduate education, Tom followed the 6-year plan, studying dietetics, psychology, and other subjects. Later, Tom received his M.A. in Exercise Physiology. His first job was in cardiac rehabilitation, working with people recovering from heart disease. Tom holds three certifications: ACE Personal Trainer, NSCA Certified Strength and Conditioning Specialist, and ACSM Clinical Exercise Specialist. Tom has been employed in several hospital settings, which included work in cardiac and pulmonary rehabilitation and wellness. He has also worked in sports-enhancement settings. Tom loved working out even as a child and became a bodybuilder in his teens, winning the title of Mr. Teenage Youngstown in a bodybuilding contest.

"I love variety in my work, and I enjoy working with all kinds of people—from young athletes to the very old and frail. In order to work with such a wide range of clients and effectively individualize their exercise programs, I have had to keep current in many different areas of health and fitness. I love to learn; you never stop learning. I think my wide range of clinical experience and strong exercise science background strengthen my reputation and give clients confidence that they are in good hands. My previous work in cardiac rehab helped prepare me for many of the clients I work with today.

"I think I motivate people well because I am constantly upgrading my knowledge and staying current with the field. I do a lot of continuing education self-study courses, conferences, and classes, more than my three certifications require, plus I am constantly reading. My clients love seeing exercises and equipment on Oprah or other television shows after they have been doing these exercises or using that equipment in their workouts with me. Exercise science is constantly advancing which makes it such an exciting field.

"Along with a good background in exercise physiology and lots of good experience, you have to relate well to people. I had to learn this early in life, since I am fifth of eight kids. My mother was always telling us, 'Get along,' so I did. I meet all of my clients with an open mind and try to understand what they are looking for. I never assume anything, and I am constantly looking for feedback on how the exercise program is working for them. The hardest part is when they come in with the unrealistic goals and techniques that are so widespread in the media. I spend a lot of time educating them, stressing injury prevention, and entertaining them along the way. My goal is to make people leave feeling better mentally and physically than when they came in."

than she had anticipated. She is grateful that no one got in-jured on her watch and that she was able to help so many people stay active while on board. Maybe they will even keep exercising once they are home! ■

KEY TERMS

absorptive cells

acquired immunity

adrenal cortex

adrenal glands

adrenal medulla

afferent nervous system

alveoli (alveolus, singular)

Alzheimer's disease

amenorrhea

amygdala

anal sphincter

anaphylaxis

anxiety hyperventilation

arteries

arterioles

arthritis

atrophy

autoimmune response

autonomic nervous system (ANS)

B lymphocytes

bariatric surgery

bile

brain

brainstem

brain-derived neuro-trophic factor (BDNF)

bursa (bursae, plural)

bursitis

C-reactive protein (CRP)

capillaries

cardiorespiratory system

cardiovascular system

cartilage

catecholamines

celiac disease

cell membrane

central nervous system

cerebellum

cerebral cortex

cerebrum

chromatin

chronic traumatic encephalopathy (CTE)

circadian rhythm

colon

compact bone tissue

complement

concussion

corticosterone

cortisol

cortisone

cytokines

dementia

deoxyribonucleic acid (DNA)

diencephalon

diverticulitis

efferent nervous system

emphysema

emulsify

endorphins

enteric nervous system (ENS)

epigenetics

epinephrine

esophagus

eumenorrhea

exocrine organs

fast-twitch glycolytic (FG) muscle fibers

fast-twitch oxidative-glycolytic (FOG) muscle fibers

female athlete triad

food allergy

food intolerance

food sensitivity

functional magnetic resonance imaging (fMRI)

gallbladder

gastrin

gastroesophageal reflux disease (GERD)

genes

ghrelin

glands

glucocorticoids

gluten

Golgi complex

heartburn

hemoglobin

hippocampus

hormone

hydrochloric acid

hypothalamus

immune system

inflammation

innate immunity

innervated

interferons

intervertebral disks

irritable bowel syndrome (IBS)

joint

joint capsule

lactose intolerance

leukocytes

ligaments

limbic system

lymphatic system

lymphocytes

medial prefrontal cortex (MPFC)

melatonin

mitochondria

motor neurons

motor unit

muscle fibers

myokines

nervous system

nervous tissue

neuroglia

neuron

norepinephrine

nucleus

neurogenesis

neurotransmitter

oligomenorrhea

organ

organelle

osteoarthritis

osteoblasts

osteoclasts

osteocytes

osteons

pancreas

pancreatitis

parasympathetic nervous system (PNS)

pathogens

peripheral nervous system

phagocytes

pineal gland

platelets

postsynaptic neuron

postural muscles

presynaptic neuron

proprioceptors

psychoneuroimmunology

receptor sites

recruitment

rectum

red bone marrow

respiratory system

reticular formation (RF)

rheumatoid arthritis

ribosome

rough endoplasmic reticulum

saliva

satiety

slow-twitch oxidative (SO) muscle fibers

smooth endoplasmic reticulum

somatic nervous system

sphincter

spinal cord

spongy bone tissue

sympathetic nervous system (SNS)

sympathomimetic

synapse

synaptic cleft

synovial fluid

synovial joints

KEY TERMS–cont'd

T lymphocytes	trabecular bone	type IIB muscle fibers	vertebral column
tau protein	tissue	vascular dementia	vertebral compression
tendonitis	trachea	veins	fracture
tendons	type I muscle fibers	venules	white blood cells
thalamus	type IIA muscle fibers	vertebrae	yellow bone marrow

CRITICAL THINKING QUESTIONS

1. Tests that give you your "genetic barcode" are becoming widely available. If someone offered to let you take the test and get your results for free, would you take advantage of this offer? Why or why not?

2. The purpose of vaccines is to introduce a harmless dose of a pathogen (or parts of a pathogen) to the immune system, so that it will remember and attack the pathogen in the future. Do vaccines stimulate innate or acquired immunity? Explain.

3. Describe the health behaviors commonly associated with the college student lifestyle that contribute to the high prevalence of digestive disorders seen in this population. Describe the psychophysiological effects of each behavior.

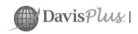 For additional resources login to Davis*Plus* (http://davisplus.fadavis.com/ keyword "Brehm") and click on the Premium tab. (Don't have a *Plus*Code to access Premium Resources? Just click the Purchase Access button on the book's Davis*Plus* page.)

REFERENCES

Ahmed, T. & Haboudi, N. (2010). Assessment and management of nutrition in older people and its importance to health. *Clinical Interventions in Aging. 5,* 207-216.

Chakravarti, A. & Little, P. (2003). Nature, nurture, and human disease. *Nature. 421,* 412-414.

Covassin, T., Elbin, R., & Stiller-Ostrowski, J. L. (2009). Current sport-related concussion teaching and clinical practices of sports medicine professionals. *Journal of Athletic Training. 44* (4), 400-404.

Davis, C. D. & Ross, S. A. (2007). Dietary components impact histone modifications and cancer risk. *Nutrition Reviews. 65*(2), 88-94.

Diekelmann, S. & Born, J. (2010). The memory function of sleep. *Nature Reviews Neuroscience. 11*(2), 114-126.

Galland, L. (2010). Diet and inflammation. *Nutrition in Clinical Practice. 25*(6), 634-640.

Gobeske, K. T., Das, S., Bonaguidi, M. A., Weiss, C., Radulovic, J., Disterhoft, J. F., & Kessler, J. A. (2009). BMP signaling mediates effects of exercise on hippocampal neurogenesis and cognition in mice. *PLoS ONE. 4*(10), e7506.

Hillman, C. H., Erickson, K. I., & Kramer, A. F. (2008). Be smart, exercise your heart: exercise effects on brain and cognition. *Nature Reviews Neuroscience. 9*(1), 58-65.

Kelesidis, T., Kelesidis, I., Chous, S., & Mantzoros, C. S. (2010). Narrative review: the role of leptin in human physiology: emerging clinical applications. *Annals of Internal Medicine. 152*(2), 93-100.

Kiecolt-Glaser, J. K., Christian, L., Preston, H., Houts, C. R., Malarkey, W. B., Emery, C. F., & Glaser R. (2010). Stress,

inflammation, and yoga practice. *Psychosomatic Medicine. 72*(2), 113-121.

Lettre, G., Palmer, D.C., Young, T., Ejebe, K. G., Allayee, H., Benjamin, E. J., . . . Boerwinkle, E. (2011). Genomewide association study of coronary heart disease and its risk factors in 8,090 African Americans: The NHBLI CARe Project. *PLoS Genetics. 7*(2), e1001300.

Mathieu, P., Lemieux, I., & Despres, J.-P. (2010). Obesity, inflammation, and cardiovascular risk. *Clinical Pharmacology and Therapeutics. 87*(4), 407-416.

Mathur, N. & Pedersen, B. K. (2008). Exercise as a mean to control low-grade systemic inflammation. *Mediators of Inflammation. 2008*:109502. doi:10.1155/2008/109502

McCormick, R. K. (2008). *The Whole-Body Approach to Osteoporosis.* Oakland, CA: New Harbinger.

McCrory, P. (2011). Sports concussion and the risk of neurological impairment. *Clinical Journal of Sports Medicine. 21*(1), 6-12.

McCrory, P., Meeuwisse, W., Johnston, K., Dvorak, J., Aubry, M., Molloy, M., & Cantu, R. (2009). Consensus statement on concussion in sport—the Third International Conference on Concussion in Sport held in Zurich, November 2008. *The Physician and Sportsmedicine. 37*(2), 141-159.

Mehler, P. S., Sabel, A. L., Watson, T., & Andersen, A. E. (2008). High risk of osteoporosis in male patients with eating disorders. *International Journal of Eating Disorders. 41*(7), 666-672.

Menz, H. B., Jordan, K. P., Roddy, E., & Croft, P. R. (2010). Characteristics of primary care consultations for musculoskeletal foot and ankle problems in the UK. *Rheumatology.* 49(7), 1391-1398.

Nattiv, A., Loucks, A. B., Manore, M. M., Sanborn, C. F., Sundgot-Borgen, J., Warren, M. P., & American College of Sports Medicine. (2007). American College of Sports Medicine position stand. The female athlete triad. *Medicine and Science in Sports and Exercise.* 39(10), 1867-1882.

Nolan, R. P., Floras, J. S., Harvey, P. J., Kamath, M. V., Picton, P. E., Chessex, C., . . . Chen, M. H. (2010). Behavioral neurocardiac training in hypertension. *Hypertension.* 55(4), 1033-1039.

Norris, P. (2006). Biofeedback applications. In: Rakel, D. P. & Faass, N. (eds.). *Complementary Medicine in Clinical Practice.* Sudbury, MA: Jones & Bartlett, 159-167.

Ozcivici, E., Luu, Y. K., Rubin, C. T., & Judex, S. (2010). Low-level vibrations retain bone marrow's osteogenic potential and augment recovery of trabecular bone during reambulation. *PLoS.* 5(6), e11178.

Pedersen, B. K. (2011). Muscles and their myokines. *Journal of Experimental Biology.* 214, 337-346.

Pert, C. B. & Snyder, S. H. (1973). Opiate receptor: demonstration in nervous tissue. *Science.* 179(4077), 1011-1014.

Pert, C. B. (1997). *Molecules of Emotion.* New York: Scribner.

Rodenhiser, D. & Mann, M. (2006). Epigenetics and human disease: translating basic biology into clinical applications. *Canadian Medical Association Journal.* 174(3), 341-348.

Sapolsky, R. M. (1996). Why stress is bad for your brain. *Science.* 273(5276), 749-750.

Simopoulos, A. P. (2008). The importance of the omega-6/omega-3 fatty acid ratio in cardiovascular disease and other chronic diseases. *Experimental Biology and Medicine.* 233(6), 674-688.

Sipponen, P. & Harkonen, M. (2010). Hypochlorhydric stomach: a risk condition for calcium malabsorption and osteoporosis. *Scandinavian Journal of Gastroenterology.* 45(2), 133-138.

Smith, M. A., Riby, L. M., van Eekelen, J. A. M., & Foster, J. K. (2011). Glucose enhancement of human memory: a comprehensive research review of the glucose memory facilitation effect. *Neuroscience and Biobehavioral Reviews.* 35(3), 770-783.

Snowden, D. (2001). *Aging with Grace; What the Nun Study Teaches Us About Leading Longer, Healthier, and More Meaningful Lives.* New York: Bantam Books.

Tyas, S. L., Snowdon, D. A., Desrosiers, M. F., Riley, K. P., & Markesbery, W. R. (2007). Healthy ageing in the Nun Study: Definition and neuropathologic correlates. *Age and Ageing.* 36(3), 650-655.

Waldum, H. L, Gustafsson, B., Fossmark, R., & Qvigstad, G. (2005). Antiulcer drugs and gastric cancer. *Digestive Diseases and Sciences.* 50(Suppl 1), S39-S44.

Wang, S. Z., Li, S., Xu, X. Y., Lin, G. P., Shao, L., Zhao, Y., & Wang, T. H. (2010). Effect of slow abdominal breathing combined with biofeedback on blood pressure and heart rate variability in prehypertension. *Journal of Alternative and Complementary Medicine.* 16(10), 1039-1045.

Wu, C.-W., Chang, Y.-T., Yu, L., Chen, H. I., Jen, C. J., Wu, S. Y., . . . Kuo, Y. M. (2008). Exercise enhances the proliferation of neural stem cells and neurite growth and survival of neuronal progenitor cells in dentate gyrus of middle-aged mice. *Journal of Applied Physiology.* 105(5), 1585-1594.

Yoo, S.-S., Gujar, N., Hu, P., Jolesz, F. A., & Walker, M. P. (2007). The human emotional brain without sleep—a prefrontal amygdala disconnect. *Current Biology.* 17(20), R877-R878.

CHAPTER OUTLINE

LEARNING OBJECTIVES

After reading this chapter, you will be able to:

1. Explain the words "exercise," "sport," and "physical activity" and the various terminologies used to describe exercise.

2. Summarize the physical effects of exercise training.

3. Discuss the effects of exercise on mood and stress reactivity and describe the possible reasons for these effects.

4. Understand the effects of exercise on sleep and discuss possible reasons for these effects.

5. Summarize the effects of exercise on self-esteem and body image and list possible mechanisms for these effects.

6. Explain the effects of exercise on memory and cognitive function and describe possible reasons for these effects.

7. Discuss the effects of exercise on symptoms of anxiety and depression—both for people diagnosed with mood disorders and for people occasionally experiencing symptoms of these disorders—and explain possible mechanisms for these effects.

8. Summarize public health recommendations for physical activity and discuss how these may differ from individualized recommendations.

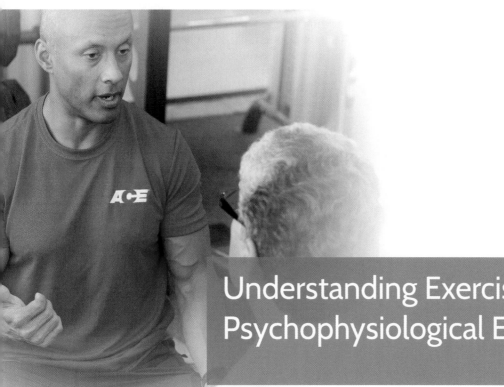

CHAPTER 3

Understanding Exercise and Its Psychophysiological Effects

UNDERSTANDING EXERCISE AND ITS PSYCHOPHYSIOLOGICAL EFFECTS

One fine afternoon in early spring, Melissa leaves her sedentary lifestyle to join a line-dancing class at a local community center. Although her three sons have always been active, playing sports at school and in community programs, Melissa has never felt she could afford the time for or costs of taking an exercise class herself. But, at her last physical exam, her health-care provider pointed out that she has steadily gained weight over the years and is now 20 pounds heavier than she was in her 20s. Melissa realizes she has put her own health on hold long enough. If she doesn't start improving her health now, turning the weight gain around in future years only becomes more difficult. She will be turning 40 in a few weeks, and she has always heard that it gets harder to lose weight as you get older.

Melissa is also ready for a change. Her teenage boys are gone a lot now, with activities after school and work during the summer. Melissa has sometimes thought she should take a walk after work to get more exercise. But her job as an administrative assistant is often emotionally exhausting, so she arrives home too tired to do anything but watch television, catch up on housework, and make dinner. Maybe now is the time to think about losing weight. Melissa's health-care provider has given her a flyer listing the exercise classes at the community center near her. A line-dancing class catches her eye. Melissa has always loved to dance. Maybe dance would not feel like exercise! The class is offered at 5 p.m., so Melissa can go right after work. The center offers the chance to try the class for free before registering. Melissa decides to give the class a try. ■

Regular physical activity contributes to physical and psychological health and well-being. Like other species, humans evolved to accommodate, expect, and require a certain level of physical activity. Until about a hundred years ago, most people were physically active for a significant amount of time each day. In the dawn of primate and human evolution, the activities of hunting and gathering food demanded several hours of physical movement most days. Finding and building shelters, migrating to areas with more food, and other survival activities demanded physical activity. Evolution favored survival of the fittest, both physically and psychologically. Strength and endurance, along with intelligence, cunning, and perseverance, helped early humans find food, deal with predators, find mates, and bear and raise young.

For most North Americans, the physical and psychological demands of modern lifestyles bear little resemblance to Stone-Age conditions, for which most people are extremely grateful. More to eat, less time searching for food, and low demands for physical exertion have meant greater comfort and the ability to expend physical and psychological energy on other things, such as designing space stations, writing symphonies, obtaining a college education, and pondering the meaning of life.

But, just as the human body still needs food and water, it continues to need physical activity. Over time, too little movement leads to loss of musculoskeletal mass, deposition of excess visceral fat, impaired blood sugar and fat regulation, hypertension, damaging levels of chronic inflammation, and premature artery disease. Changes in the nervous system appear to result as well, since sedentary lifestyles have been associated with mood disorders, memory loss, and other symptoms of cognitive decline. Recent studies suggest that even people who exercise regularly may experience the negative effects of a sedentary lifestyle if they spend too much continuous time on the couch or at their desks (Healy, Matthews, Dustan, Winkler, & Owen, 2011). In a study of 4,757 adults with an average age of 46.5 years, researchers found an association between uninterrupted minutes of inactivity each day and several variables associated with poor health, including insulin resistance (an indication of poor blood sugar control), lower levels of blood HDL cholesterol, higher levels of blood triglycerides, and higher levels of C-reactive protein (Healy, et al., 2011).

Many jobs, however, require long periods of seated work. Exercise scientists and public health officials continue to struggle with ways to make the Stone-Age genes and biochemistry of the human body compatible with modern lifestyles. To better understand the psychological and physical health challenges that result from sedentary lifestyles and the effects of exercise on the human mind and body, some knowledge of the psychophysiology of exercise is helpful.

The first section in this chapter provides a brief overview of how scientists measure and discuss physical activity. The next section reviews the most important physiological benefits of physical activity and discusses how these contribute to a person's state of health. The third section explores the many psychological benefits of physical activity and the psychophysiological processes that may help explain them. This chapter concludes with a brief summary of public health recommendations regarding participation in regular physical activity.

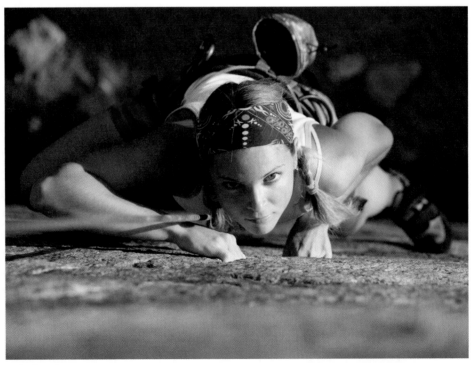

© Thinkstock

DESCRIBING AND MEASURING EXERCISE AND PHYSICAL ACTIVITY

From time to time, newspapers, magazines, and other media feature attention-grabbing headlines such as "Exercise Effective in Treating Depression" and "Exercise Slows Cognitive Decline." In order to interpret and apply these headlines and the underlying research to behavior-change work, it is important to understand what is meant by terms such as exercise and physical activity (Fig. 3-1). Because there are so many types of exercise and physical activity, the dose of exercise or physical activity that leads to a specific outcome must be clear and measurable. Also, because physical activity can sometimes have negative consequences, health and fitness professionals must be careful to avoid making recommendations likely to cause harm.

Differentiating Among Exercise, Physical Activity, and Sport

Physical activity refers to any bodily movement, especially movement involving large muscle groups and an elevated (above resting) level of energy expenditure. Most of the time, when researchers use the term "physical activity," they are referring to activities such as walking, raking leaves, climbing stairs, dancing, and participating in sports, rather than lifting a forkful of food to one's mouth or walking from the couch to the refrigerator. In scientific studies, researchers must always define what they mean by physical activity because the term is so broad.

Exercise is a type of physical activity performed with the intention of improving physical fitness and/or sport performance. People who swim laps during their lunch hour, take a group exercise class, or walk regularly after

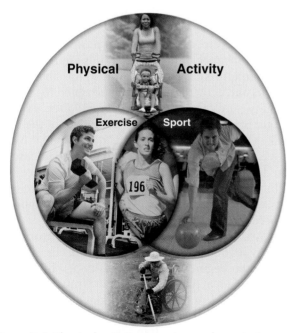

Figure 3-1. Physical activity, exercise, and sport. Photograph © Thinkstock

work would probably refer to these activities as exercise. Athletes often refer to their sport conditioning programs as exercise. Activities such as walking to school, biking to work, chopping wood for the fireplace, or washing windows are considered by most people to be physical activities, but, unless these activities are performed primarily for the purpose of increasing fitness, they are not usually called "exercise."

Sport is generally defined as a physical activity that is performed according to rules and customs. Sports are usually highly structured and take the form of a contest between individuals or teams. Sports almost always involve competition, and the goal is to win. Colloquially, people sometimes refer to recreational activities as sports. Sometimes such references include activities that consist mostly of training, with occasional competitions thrown in. For example, people might say they participate in the sport of rowing, yet they rarely compete. Many sports require a great deal of energy expenditure and high levels of physical fitness. These include team sports such as soccer, hockey, and lacrosse and individual sports such as running, track and field events, swimming, and racquet sports. Such sports certainly fall under the category of physical activity. Some sports, however, require fairly low levels of energy expenditure, although they often require high levels of coordination and skill and years of practice. Such sports include shooting, archery, darts, and bowling. Sport training and participation can increase fitness and confer many health benefits, depending on practices and competitions. Even participation in sports requiring fairly low energy levels can be enjoyable and reduce feelings of stress, and thus offers many health benefits.

Describing Exercise and Physical Activity

When discussing the effects of exercise on health, it is important to describe what is meant by exercise. Because exercise can refer to everything from gentle stretching while sitting in one's chair to running at maximal intensity, the term requires a more-precise description. Several terms are useful for describing exercise.

Exercise Type or Mode

Exercise mode refers to the type of activity. Examples of exercise modes are cycling, swimming, running, walking, and just about any exercise and sport activity. Some research studies must measure physical activity very precisely, down to the calorie and heartbeat, and use measurable exercise modes with reproducible workloads so that researchers can calculate how much energy the user expends per minute. Activity in these studies may take the form of cycling on a special ergometer, a stationary piece of exercise equipment on which researchers can apply a very precise workload. Other pieces of equipment such as some treadmills also allow for the accurate reproduction of exercise workload.

Depending on the project, researchers might employ a number of other exercise modes. Walking on a track or path, swimming, bicycling, and other activities are easy to define in terms of intensity, distance, and other variables that allow workload to be described. In epidemiological studies, people may self-report all types of physical activities, including flights of stairs taken, blocks walked, and household chores/yard work completed. Recreational physical activities such as folk dancing, bowling, horseback riding, and hiking are all types of exercise modes.

A number of exercise modes are extremely variable. For example, research has been done on hatha yoga. Anyone who has ever practiced yoga knows that yoga sessions may be very intense, such as those performed in Vinyasa style, where participants move quickly from pose to pose, working up a sweat and really challenging muscular strength and endurance. But some yoga classes, such as a session of restorative yoga, may be performed in a very gentle style that is mostly stretching, holding poses for long periods of time with little observable movement. Sport practices present a similar variety of movement types. The activity of a soccer forward is very different from the activity of the goalkeeper. In research studies, the activities performed within these exercise modes might need to be described in more detail, depending on the purpose of the research.

Exercise is often categorized into exercise type based on which energy production systems or fitness components are being activated. Cardiovascular exercise or aerobic exercise refers to activities that involve movement of the large muscle groups at a moderately vigorous level, leading to sustained elevation in metabolic rate. Intensity level is submaximal, however, so that the activity can continue for at least 10 minutes and often longer. The terms cardiovascular exercise and aerobic exercise are somewhat vague and can be used interchangeably. Cardiovascular exercise indicates that the exercise provides a conditioning effect for the cardiovascular system, thus improving cardiovascular health over time. Aerobic exercise means that the primary energy system relied on for the production of energy for muscular contraction is aerobic. Aerobic means "with oxygen." The body's aerobic energy system makes energy from the fuels that come from foods: carbohydrate, fat, and protein. Energy is captured from the chemical bonds in these fuels, with the help of the mitochondria, specialized energy-producing organelles contained in cells. Aerobic exercise is popular because it is usually performed at intensities that provide a conditioning effect but are fairly comfortable, or at least not too painful.

Anaerobic describes the body's energy production pathways that do not require the immediate presence of oxygen. The term anaerobic energy production is used for high-intensity exercise. Exercise at maximal intensity can only continue for a few minutes, at which point fatigue limits performance. Most high-intensity exercise, such as sprints, strength training, and many sports, rely on a combination of aerobic and anaerobic energy systems. Anaerobic exercise generally refers to high-intensity exercise. Athletes and other very fit people engage in anaerobic training to improve energy production pathways and increase speed, strength, and power. Because anaerobic exercise involves high exercise intensities, it may not be appropriate for beginners or those with health risks. People who do not like to exercise usually interpret the physical sensations occurring with anaerobic exercise as unpleasant and painful.

Interval training is a form of exercise where short bursts of high-intensity anaerobic exercise are combined with longer periods of aerobic exercise that allow the muscles time to recover. For example, someone might run at maximal speed for 30 seconds, and then jog at a more-moderate pace for 90 seconds. Several intervals are usually performed in a row.

Strength training refers to exercise performed to increase muscle strength. Strength refers to how much force muscles can exert against an object and is often measured by how much weight can be moved in various positions. Strength training can take the form of lifting weights, such as free weights, or using specialized equipment that enables the muscles to exert force against resistance. Strength training can also be performed using one's own body weight as resistance, as in abdominal curls or push-ups. Resistance can be applied to muscles when moving against water, especially with equipment that increases resistance. Strength training exercise is often described in terms of weight, repetitions, and sets. Repetitions (reps) refer to the number of times a given exercise is performed. A strength training session is usually comprised of a number of different exercises for a variety of muscle groups. One series of exercises is called a set. The effect of a strength-training workout varies according to all variables discussed above: weight, repetitions, and number of sets.

Stretching refers to exercise that pushes joints to the edge of their range of motion and thus improves range of motion, also known as flexibility. Special exercise positions and activities have been designed to increase flexibility and are often performed after exercise sessions. Stretching acts on the soft tissues of the musculoskeletal system, especially the muscles and the connective tissues surrounding muscles, called fasciae. Some types of activity, such as gymnastics, dance, and fencing, include quite a bit of stretching exercise in their training programs, since flexibility is important for successful performance.

Many styles of group fitness programs incorporate several types of exercise into each session. For example, classes often begin with low-intensity aerobic activity that builds to a higher intensity. Strength-training exercises for the major muscle groups may also be included. The intensity of the class may be lower near the end of the class. Classes often finish with some stretching exercises.

Frequency and Duration

Frequency and duration help describe the amount of exercise. Exercise frequency refers to how often the exercise is performed and is usually expressed as number of exercise sessions per week. In the case of rehabilitation exercises, or exercise programs for people with a low tolerance for physical activity, frequency may be expressed as sessions per day. For example, following injury or surgery, prescribed sets of exercise may be performed two or more times each day.

Exercise duration refers to time—usually how long an activity lasts. Duration is measured in hours, minutes, and/or seconds, depending on what makes the most sense. The duration of a sprint interval might be 20 seconds, whereas the duration of the entire workout might be 2 hours and 20 minutes.

Exercise Intensity

Intensity is a more-difficult variable to describe and measure. Conceptually, exercise intensity refers to the level of exertion and how hard a person is working. Exertion has both physical and psychological components, and both can be measured.

Exercise Heart Rate and Oxygen Consumption

For cardiovascular exercise of all intensity levels, exercise heart rate (HR) generally reflects exercise intensity (Fig. 3-2). A more-precise measure of metabolic activity is obtained by measuring how much oxygen is used by the body to produce energy, a measure called volume of oxygen consumed ($\dot{V}O_2$). Oxygen is taken in from the air and exhaled by the person exercising. The difference between these two concentrations can be calculated and used to estimate the level of aerobic energy production. This method requires special equipment and is not readily available unless the exerciser has access to an exercise physiology laboratory. HR and

oxygen consumption have a fairly linear relationship until very high exercise levels (Fig. 3-3). Therefore, because exercise HR provides a fairly good estimate of intensity, this variable is the one most commonly used.

Exercise HR is often expressed as a percentage of a person's maximal or estimated maximal HR. Maximal heart rate is the highest HR a person can achieve and is measured while a person is exercising at maximal intensity. Working at maximal intensity is difficult for most people and dangerous for some, so maximal HR is often estimated with the formula 220 – age. For example, using this formula, someone who is 20 years old would be predicted to have a maximal HR of about 200 (220 – 20 = 200). This formula is only a rough estimate, however, as about a third of all people have maximal HRs that are at least 10 beats higher or lower than predicted. Exercise intensity may also be estimated by calculating a percentage of HR reserve (the difference between maximal HR and resting HR) and adding this to resting HR.

Perception of Effort

Exercise intensity is sometimes estimated from people's subjective perceptions of how hard they are working. Perception of effort is based on many things: perception of local muscle fatigue (e.g., legs hurting while bicycling), the effort of breathing, and feelings of temperature and thirst as well as cognitive evaluations. The exploration of how the central nervous system perceives and rates exercise effort is a fascinating topic in the field of exercise psychology, and it continues to generate interesting research (Borg, 2010; Marcola, 2009).

The most commonly used scale to measure perception of effort is the Borg Scale, which measures a person's rating of perceived exertion (RPE) (Fig. 3-4), developed by researcher Gunnar Borg (1982). The scale runs from 6 to 20 because it was originally designed to

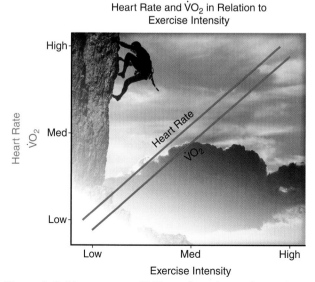

Figure 3-2. Heart rate and VO₂ as functions of exercise intensity. Photograph © Thinkstock

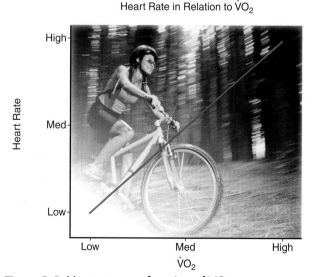

Figure 3-3. Heart rate as a function of VO₂. Photograph © Thinkstock

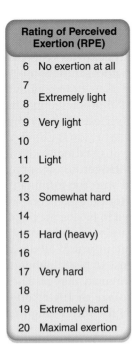

Figure 3-4. Rating of perceived exertion. *Scales with instruction available from www.borgperception.se. Used with permission.*

correspond to exercise HR, so that multiplying each level by 10 provided a rough guess of exercise HR. Because exercise HR is highly variable, the scale does not reliably predict HR. But it works well as a tool to describe exercise effort.

> **MOTIVATING CHANGE: People's Perceptions of Effort Are Important**
>
> Knowing people's perceptions of exercise intensity is just as important as knowing exercise HR. For example, some people have a naturally low HR; yet, the exercise might feel fairly difficult to them. Unless clients are very fit and athletic, it is usually a good idea to avoid exercise that is very high in intensity. Injuries are more likely to occur and people are more likely to drop out of exercise programs that feel uncomfortable.
>
> People may have some difficulty picking a number to represent their level of exertion at first but once they get used to the scale, they catch on quickly. Clients like to know you care how they are feeling, and you can use their response to adjust exercise intensity.

Exercise intensity is also described using common words, without a numbered rating scale attached. For example, people are often urged to exercise at a "moderately vigorous" intensity. Other phrases such as "exercise hard enough to work up a sweat" can help describe exercise intensity in ways people can understand. A common piece of advice regarding exercise intensity is the talk-sing test. If people are exercising at a level that accommodates the breath control required for singing, the intensity is very low. A moderate intensity allows people to talk but not sing. A very high intensity makes simple conversation difficult.

Although researchers require accurate measures of exercise intensity and thus need to measure intensity, most exercise recommendations for the general public discuss exercise intensity in these conceptual terms, such as "moderately intense," because trying to calculate and take exercise HR is confusing and bothersome to many people.

Exercise Volume

Exercise volume refers to "how much" exercise is done. While this may sound like a simple thing to measure, exercise volume must take into account exercise frequency, intensity, and duration in order for exercise volume measures to be compared and evaluated. Are 20 minutes of high-intensity exercise the same as an hour of low-intensity exercise? How can these be compared?

Exercise volumes or amounts are never totally comparable. The closest researchers come is to compare total caloric expenditure. But, because intensity is such an important factor in terms of the physiological effect of exercise, comparing 100 calories of high-intensity exercise to 100 calories of low-intensity exercise is like comparing apples and oranges. But sometimes a rough estimate is still helpful.

Epidemiological and other types of studies often use exercise volume measures to examine the relationship between physical activity and various measures of health. These exercise measures are usually estimated from self-report questionnaires. Exercise studies may also have subjects wear pedometers, which count the number of steps people take during a given period of time. Accelerometers are also used to give an indication of activity level. Accelerometers measure acceleration (changes in speed of movement) to estimate physical activity volume and can provide useful data for a variety of population groups (Freedson, Pober, & Janz, 2005; Harris, Owen, Victor, Adams, Ekelund, & Cook, 2009).

Evaluating the Effect of Physical Activity on Fitness and Health

Thousands of experiments have examined the effect of physical activity on fitness and health. The effects of exercise on many fitness and health variables are often examined with experimental studies. Training studies typically take a group of subjects, divide them into groups, and give each group a different treatment. After a certain period, the groups are compared, and results are published. Over time, these studies have led to recommendations for how much of which types of exercise help change specific variables. For example, studies have examined the best types of exercise for increasing bone density, reducing high blood pressure, or improving blood sugar regulation. In a similar fashion, experimental studies reveal relationships between exercise training and performance variables. Such studies help coaches design the best programs to decrease sprint time or improve jump height. Animal studies help elucidate physiological mechanisms behind the effects of physical activity on fitness and health.

The effects of physical activity on long-term health are often complex. Many health problems take years to develop, and the effects of exercise on such problems may be difficult to capture in a short study. Epidemiological studies can reveal relationships between physical activity and health by observing large groups of people over fairly long periods of time.

Studies often produce different conclusions about certain variables. As discussed in Chapter 1, models describing relationships among variables change over time as evidence accumulates to improve knowledge. It is easy to see why it took decades to reach some sort of consensus on how much exercise should be recommended in public health guidelines. The effect of physical activity varies with type of exercise, frequency, duration, and intensity. It varies with program length. It varies depending on fitness level, health, age, and sex of the subjects. Even for people of the same size, age, sex, and fitness level, a variety of responses are usually observed.

The relationship between exercise and physical health variables has been easier to study than the effect of exercise on psychological variables. Part of the reason is that physical variables are easier to "see" and measure in many cases. In addition, scientists' models of physical health adopted the exercise training variables more readily, and researchers have studied the training effects of exercise on variables such as strength and body composition for a longer time. As psychologists have devised questionnaires, scales, and other methods for measuring variables such as mood, self-concept, and level of depression and anxiety, studies have examined the relationship between physical activity and psychological variables as well.

EXERCISE AND PHYSICAL HEALTH

A number of important points regarding the physical health benefits of regular exercise are discussed in the first two chapters of this book. Because physical and psychological health are so closely linked, in order to understand the psychology of health and fitness, it is important to have some understanding of the physical health benefits of physical activity. Basically, as exercise stresses the body, the body responds to that stress by strengthening the systems being stressed. The response of the body to exercise varies somewhat with the type of exercise. This section provides a brief review of the most studied health benefits of physical activity.

Cardiovascular/Aerobic Exercise

Beneficial health effects occur after even one session of aerobic exercise. For example, the cell membrane receptors for insulin become more sensitive to insulin for

a day or two following exercise, enhancing the ability of cells to take up glucose from the bloodstream. This effect disappears rapidly, however, so regular activity is required to produce a significant change in blood glucose regulation. Some of the most important health effects of regular physical activity are discussed in following subsections.

Cardiovascular and Metabolic Health

Regular physical activity:
- Promotes artery health
- Helps to lower high blood pressure
- Improves blood lipid levels, raising HDL levels and lowering serum triglycerides
- Helps to prevent obesity by contributing to energy balance
- Improves insulin sensitivity
- Slows progression of dementia

The items in this array of metabolic benefits are often related, and most are affected not only by volume of physical activity but also by diet and stress levels as well. Exercise exerts its effect on these metabolic variables through a number of different pathways, as described in Chapter 2. Part of the big picture is that calorie expenditure helps prevent the hypertrophy of visceral adipocytes, a condition that some researchers have dubbed "adiposopathy" (Hays, Galassetti, & Coker, 2008), which leads to inflammation, insulin resistance, risky blood lipid levels, and high blood pressure. However, exercise exerts health-promoting effects independent of its prevention of excess visceral obesity. It increases concentration of HDL cholesterol and reduces blood markers of inflammation, such as C-reactive protein (Pedersen, 2011). (Inflammation occurs for many reasons, not just because of obesity.) Regular aerobic activity slows the clotting speed of the blood, decreasing the likelihood of blood clots forming in the arteries. Such clots can precipitate a heart attack or stroke. Insulin sensitivity, mentioned above, can help prevent type 2 diabetes. Factors that speed the progression of artery disease increase risk of dementia. Exercise is thought to slow the progression of dementia partly through promoting good arterial health and reducing systemic inflammation. This large picture suggests that exercise normalizes many metabolic pathways.

An interesting link between exercise and artery health highlights the importance of a substance called nitric oxide (NO), a compound that performs a variety of helpful roles in the body and is important for the normal function of arteries. Exercise increases the production of an enzyme called nitric oxide synthase. This enzyme stimulates the lining of arteries to release NO. NO, in turn, causes the little muscles lining the arteries to relax. This opens the arteries, allowing for greater blood flow and thus lowering blood pressure (Denvir & Gray, 2009). NO enhances arterial function and slows the progression of artery disease in a number of ways, such as by preventing blood cells from sticking to the artery lining (Allen et al., 2009). Exercise also appears to reduce oxidative stress in the arterial lining by increasing the activity of the body's innate antioxidant enzyme pathways (Durrant et al., 2009).

Cellular Health and Aging

In Chapter 2, mind-body integration was discussed in terms of several systems of the body, especially the nervous, endocrine, and immune systems. These three systems have received the most attention in terms of coordinating physiological homeostasis and cellular activity. However, even fat and muscle cells send messages to each other and other parts of the body. These messages are sent by small molecules such as the cytokines, myokines, and adipokines. These molecules have wide-ranging effects on all cells in the body.

One of the most interesting effects at the cellular level is the effect of exercise on the length of telomeres. Telomeres are structures found on the ends of chromosomes (Fig. 3-5). Nobel Prize winner Elizabeth Blackburn describes telomeres as being "like the tips of shoelaces. If you lose the tips, the ends start fraying (Dreifus, 2007)." Chromosomes contain long chains of DNA that are found in cell nuclei. Each time a cell divides, some of the telomere material is lost, and the telomeres become shorter. Blackburn and colleagues found that stress accelerates telomere loss, whereas exercise increases concentration of an enzyme, telomerase, which helps restore telomere length. Studies from Blackburn's laboratory found that higher fitness levels and higher activity levels seem to help buffer the effect of stress on telomere length. One study measured fitness levels in 944 patients with stable coronary heart disease (CHD) (Krauss et al., 2011). Previous research has shown that telomere length helps in predicting the mortality rate in people with CHD. Krauss et al. (2011) found that exercise capacity was significantly related to telomere length in these patients, with fitter subjects showing longer telomeres. In the

same laboratory, Puterman et al. (2010) examined the stress–telomere length relationship in 63 healthy post-menopausal women. The women were categorized into two groups—those meeting public health recommendations for physical activity and those who did not (and who were thus considered sedentary). While stress level was related to telomere length in the sedentary group, no relationship between stress and telomere length was observed for the active group.

Bone and Joint Health

Some types of aerobic exercise promote bone and joint health. Exercise that applies optimal levels of stress, such as those that occur during weight-bearing exercise such as walking, skipping, and running, helps increase bone quality and density. Studies on aerobic exercise and joint health suggest that the best type of exercise depends on the current state of joint health. Healthy joints do not seem harmed, and are usually helped, by moderate amounts of aerobic activity. However, high-impact activities such as running and jumping can worsen joint health and pain in joints that have sustained some level of damage, such as that which occurs with osteoarthritis. Appropriate levels of low-impact activities may improve well-being for people with joint pain from osteoarthritis (Devos-Comby, Cronan, & Roesch, 2006; Mendelson, McCullough, & Chan, 2011). People with osteoarthritis and joint injuries should work carefully with a physical therapist or experienced personal trainer to find the level and type of exercise that improve joint health.

The negative effects of exercise on joint health, through injury caused by participation in physical activity, should not be underestimated. One survey of children and young adults aged 5 to 24 years old estimated that sports injuries cause 2.6 million visits to hospital emergency departments each year in the U.S. alone (Goldberg, Moroz, Smith, & Ganley, 2007). Most injuries caused by exercise are mild and heal quickly, allowing injured people to eventually resume prior levels of physical activity; however, some injuries result in higher risk of osteoarthritis in later years, long-term disability, and even death.

Quality of Life

Quality of life reflects both physical and psychological levels of well-being. The psychological benefits of physical activity are discussed in the next section. Quality of life is listed in this section because an adequate level of physical fitness and health also helps promote feelings of well-being and satisfaction with one's quality of life. This is especially true the older people get. While most young people take for granted their ability to rise from a chair or carry groceries, in older adults, the inability to perform the activities of daily living (ADLs) can lead to loss of independent living. A good level of basic fitness allows people to enjoy activities that require walking, climbing stairs, lifting, and carrying. A decent level of aerobic fitness

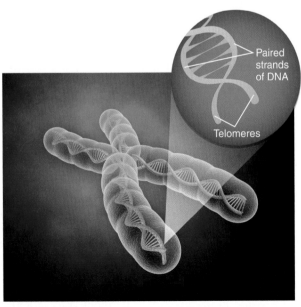

Figure 3-5. Telomeres. Photograph © Thinkstock

is required for traveling, dancing, and many other enjoyable pastimes.

■ *It is the day before the first dance class, and Melissa keeps talking herself in and out of going. She is tired and stressed and has so much to get done today. As she starts making her to-do list, she decides that she might skip the class today. Maybe she could start with the next class.*

As she drinks her morning tea, her sons enter the room talking about their camping trip next week. They have always enjoyed the science camp their school offers during vacation week. They remind Melissa that family members are invited for the hike on Sunday morning at the end of the camping trip. Will she be coming? Melissa would love to go on the hike with the kids, but she wonders how she could possibly keep up with her sons. She skipped the hike last year and remembers feeling sad that she did not join in the fun. When the students and their family members returned from the hike, their faces were shining, and they were joking and laughing. The hike is only 3 or 4 miles. "People should be able to walk that far," she thinks. As she looks at the enthusiasm on her sons' faces, she makes up her mind to go to the class after all and also to hike on Sunday. What is more important than spending time with her family? Her boys would be grown in a few short years. And, if she cannot keep up with her sons now, how in the world would she be able to enjoy active grandchildren when they come along? ■

How Much Exercise?

The amount of aerobic exercise that generates the many health benefits described above varies enormously from person to person, which is why exercise recommendations are best when they are individualized. In general, benefits begin to accrue with at least 30 minutes of aerobic activity per day. Metabolic and cardiovascular variables respond best to even larger amounts of exercise, up to 60 to 90 minutes of exercise per day. To some extent, longer periods of lower-intensity exercise can be exchanged for shorter periods of high-intensity exercise for people in good health who enjoy high intensity levels. People unaccustomed to physical activity usually balk at large amounts of activity, which is partly why public health recommendations tend to put forth a more-doable duration of 30 minutes per day. Public health recommendations for exercise are summarized at the end of this chapter.

Strength Training

As the name implies, strength training increases the strength of the muscles exercised. Strength training stimulates the muscle motor units being recruited to perform a given exercise. A motor unit includes a nerve fiber and the muscle fibers it innervates (Fig. 3-6). With training, the nervous system becomes better at recruiting the right number of motor units of the right type of muscle fibers to produce the strength of contraction required by the strength exercise. This means that part of the strength increase observed with training is due to a better nervous system response. In addition, the muscle fibers become better at making energy by increasing the concentration of enzymes in the mitochondria that produce energy. The muscles also increase the size and number of mitochondria. Over time, muscles even grow more capillaries and other blood vessels to enhance the delivery of oxygen and nutrients to muscle cells and to get rid of wastes.

Strength training also increases the strength of the joint structures, as discussed in Chapter 2. Tendons, ligaments, and joint capsules become stronger with appropriate levels of strength training. Exercise improves joint health by stimulating the secretion of synovial fluid from the joint capsule. This is why strength-training exercise is often part of physical therapy following injury—it helps strengthen joints. Strength training also puts force on bones and can signal bone-building osteoblasts to lay down more bone mineral.

Strength training has many other health benefits. Stronger muscles translate into lower risk of muscle

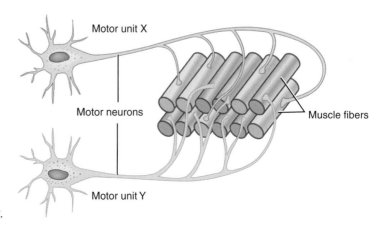

Figure 3-6. Motor unit.

strain from the ADLs. Stronger core muscles prevent back injury. In older adults, strength training may improve balance and reduce risk of falls that can lead to broken bones and disability.

Because of the increased metabolic rate of working muscles during strength training, many of the benefits described above for cardiovascular exercise accrue with strength training as well. These include better cell receptor response to insulin, release of anti-inflammatory myokines, improved blood lipid levels, and reduced risk of resting hypertension. If strength training contributes to energy balance, lifters experience less risk of obesity and excess visceral fat stores.

How much strength training is required to produce these benefits? Response varies from person to person. It is important to start slowly and build gradually with strength work to avoid injury. In general, two to three sessions per week are recommended. Each session should include at least one set of exercises for all major muscle groups, performing about 8 to 15 repetitions of each exercise. Once people have become accustomed to strength training, the exercises should be challenging enough to produce muscle fatigue but not injury. The benefits of strength exercise disappear rapidly if strength training is discontinued (Box 3-1).

Flexibility Training

Flexibility training refers to the performance of activities designed to increase flexibility, that is, the range of motion around joints. Because flexibility declines with age, sedentary lifestyle, injury, and immobilization, flexibility training helps reduce this loss, and preserve or increase range of motion. Flexibility training has been shown to increase joint range of motion in all age groups (Garber et al., 2011). Flexibility training is also an essential component of rehabilitation exercises, as it helps restore joint function. Adequate flexibility is required for most ADLs. Flexibility training can improve quality of life, especially for older adults and others with limited flexibility.

Research does not support the notion that flexibility training reduces risk of injury in otherwise healthy adults, nor does it reduce the delayed-onset muscle soreness that can follow physical activity. Flexibility exercise appears to reduce the muscles' ability to generate strength and power immediately after stretching, so people are advised to avoid stretching prior to sport performance, especially for activities requiring strength and power (McHugh & Cosgrave, 2010).

Many types of stretching exercises have been shown to increase flexibility (Garber et al., 2011). Passive static stretching involves holding a stretching position for 10 seconds or more, gradually increasing the stretch placed on the muscle group. Active static stretching adds contraction of the opposing muscle group to perform the stretching exercise. Ballistic stretching uses a bouncing movement of the body to rapidly place intermittent force on the muscle group

Box 3-1. Does Muscle Turn Into Fat When People Stop Exercising?

Muscle cells and fat cells bear little resemblance to one another physiologically, and muscle tissue cannot "turn into" fat tissue. When muscles hypertrophy, or increase in size, as a result of strength training, the increase in size occurs because muscle cells get larger. When training stops, the muscles atrophy, or become smaller, as the cells shrink. Fat cells can get larger and smaller as well. It is easy to see why people think that muscle turns to fat when training stops. Large athletes who train heavily often consume a higher-than-average amount of food to replenish calories burned during training and to provide protein for muscle building. If training stops but ex-athletes continue on their training diet, excess calories are stored as fat. Over time, muscles atrophy, and the ex-athletes grow fatter, so it looks like muscle has turned to fat.

Fat is stored in many locations, including in muscles. Intramuscular triglyceride stores refer to adipocytes located within muscles. Thus, although muscle tissue does not "turn into" fat tissue, fat tissue can accumulate in muscles. Think of a nice juicy steak with streaks of fat. Endurance athletes like intramuscular triglyceride, since the muscle mitochondria break down these triglycerides to make energy. But intramuscular triglyceride stores also have a dark side. Inactivity, aging, and higher levels of the stress hormone cortisol lead to higher levels of intramuscular triglyceride (Cree et al., 2010). Muscle fibers are lost with aging and inactivity, a condition called sarcopenia. As fiber number and size decline and intramuscular triglyceride stores grow, muscles get softer and weaker.

The good news is that strength training and muscle hypertrophy help delay sarcopenia. Strength training improves insulin sensitivity and counteracts the aging process. Building larger, stronger muscles in youth and midlife helps delay the processes that seem to "turn muscle into fat," rather than setting the stage for a fatter body later in life.

being stretched. Dynamic stretching involves slow movement from one stretching position to another. Proprioceptive neuromuscular facilitation (PNF), sometimes called contract-relax stretching, has many variations, most of which involve first isometrically contracting the muscle group to be stretched, and then following the contraction with a static stretch for the same muscle group. Force is applied to enhance the stretch either by the person stretching or another person trained in this method (Garber et al., 2011).

Flexibility training recommendations vary with each person's exercise program goals. For general health, flexibility training should be performed 2 to 3 days per week, and include stretches for all basic muscle groups. Each muscle group should be stretched for at least 60 seconds, either as a long static stretch, or a combination of shorter stretches using a variety of flexibility training techniques (Garber et al., 2011).

Functional Fitness Training

Functional fitness training employs motor skills such as agility, balance, and coordination in exercises designed to improve daily functional ability. Functional fitness training employs a wide range of activities that often include strength and flexibility training. Activities such as tai chi, martial arts, group exercise classes, and many sports provide functional fitness training. For older adults and those with limited fitness levels, activities designed specifically to improve functional fitness for ADLs have become popular. Functional fitness training may reduce fear of falling and fall risk in older adults by improving coordination and balance (Garber et al., 2011). Function fitness training is also called neuromotor exercise training or neuromuscular exercise training. Guidelines for functional fitness training generally recommend that people perform this type of training two to three times per week for 20 to 30 minutes per session (Garber et al., 2011).

Sedentary Lifestyle: A Pathological Condition

Some researchers suggest that instead of (or in addition to) extolling the health benefits of regular physical activity, scientists should also view the sedentary lifestyle as an unnatural and pathological condition. Regular exercise "normalizes" human physiology. Because inactivity leads to so many negative health consequences, many believe that physical inactivity is similar to a disease state (Lees & Booth, 2005). Researchers Thomas Buford and Todd Manini (2010) point out that when sedentary humans are used as a control group for comparison with a group with chronic disease, which may be caused in part by a sedentary lifestyle, results may be confounded by the inactivity of the control group. Just as one would want to eliminate cigarette smoking as a variable in the control group, so would one want to control for the effect of a sedentary lifestyle (Booth & Lees, 2006).

An interesting study on the effects of sedentary behavior asked a group of healthy young men (average age 27 years) to decrease daily activity from their normal level to less than 3,500 steps per day, as measured by a pedometer (Olsen, Krogh-Madsen, Thomsen, Booth, & Pedersen, 2008). The subjects began with an average of 10,501 daily steps and decreased to an average of 1,344 over the 2 weeks of the experiment. Subjects were instructed to stop exercising, to take the elevator instead of the stairs, and to take transportation rather than walking. A number of metabolic variables were measured at the beginning and end of the 2 weeks. In just 2 weeks of sedentary living, the men showed abnormal changes in insulin response and blood lipid regulation and a small but significant increase in visceral adipose stores. The results of this study confirm the pathological health effects of a sedentary lifestyle, even in healthy young men. Subsequent studies have also shown that prolonged periods of sitting are associated with increased risk of cardiovascular and all-cause mortality, even for nonobese, physically active people (Dunstan et al., 2010; Patel et al., 2010). Interrupting sitting time with short periods of low- to moderate-intensity physical activity helps reduce risky blood chemistry variables, including blood glucose and insulin levels (Dunstan et al., 2012).

EXERCISE AND PSYCHOLOGICAL HEALTH

How is exercise related to psychological health? To answer this question, one must first consider the definition of psychological health. Like physical health, some people view psychological health as an absence of mental illness. According to this limited view, if people are not depressed, anxious, delusional, or exhibiting any other major symptom, they are healthy. But researchers and writers in the wellness camp would argue that one should consider the World Health Organization's definition of health, presented in Chapter 1. Health was defined as "a state of complete physical, mental, and social well-being." Just as physical health is not merely the absence of disease, psychological health is more than just not feeling bad.

The World Health Organization describes mental health as "a state of well-being in which an individual realizes his or her own abilities, can cope with the normal stresses of life, can work productively, and is able to make a contribution to his or her community. In this positive sense, mental health is the foundation for individual well-being and the effective functioning of a community" (WHO, 2010). Psychological health might be visualized as a continuum that runs from very ill on one end, through a neutral point of no illness, and to the other end of high-level psychological well-being (Fig. 3-7). Optimal psychological well-being, like high-level physical wellness, does not mean people reach a state of perfection. Rather, wellness is a dynamic, ever-changing process, where people strive to maximize their well-being given the circumstances of their daily lives. People with high-level psychological well-being are not necessarily always happy, enlightened, and well adjusted; this is rarely the human condition. Stress and negative emotions such as anger, sadness, and worry happen to everyone. People with optimal psychological health understand that negative emotions are important and often help one figure out

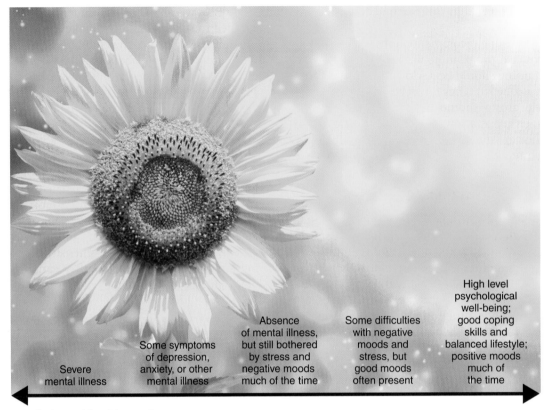

High level
psychological
well-being;
good coping
skills and
balanced lifestyle;
positive moods
much of
the time

Some difficulties
with negative
moods and
stress, but
good moods
often present

Absence
of mental illness,
but still bothered
by stress and
negative moods
much of the time

Some symptoms
of depression,
anxiety, or other
mental illness

Severe
mental illness

Figure 3-7. **Psychological health continuum.** Photograph © Thinkstock

what needs attention. But psychologically healthy people deal as effectively and efficiently with sources of stress as their situation permits, and they know how to manage their emotions and lead a balanced lifestyle in ways that help them avoid chronic stress overload most of the time.

Research shows that exercise has something to offer at each point on this spectrum. Physical activity may help people feel great and serve as a tool that people use to promote states of well-being and happiness. Physical activity has been shown to improve several measures of mood, increasing feelings of vigor and reducing feelings of fatigue, irritability, and anger. Many studies suggest that regular physical exercise improves people's response to psychological stress, with subjects showing less of an overreaction and fight-or-flight response in laboratory stress situations. Participating in exercise training has the potential to improve self-confidence and body image in some people. Cognitive improvements have been measured in subjects performing regular exercise training, including improvements in reaction time, memory, and information processing. Exciting research investigating the effects of physical activity on mild-to-moderate anxiety and depression suggests that physical activity can be part of a therapeutic approach to treatment of these common disorders.

Exploring the Psychophysiology of Exercise

Exercise psychologists have long been intrigued by people's descriptions of feelings of euphoria during and following exercise. Euphoria refers to feelings of intense happiness or well-being. Research on these reports of euphoria led to interesting research in exercise psychology and the neurobiology that accompanies the psychological effects of exercise.

The first people to describe exercise-induced euphoria in the sports medicine field were runners, as running was one of the most popular forms of exercise back in the 1970s. Early accounts of exercise-induced euphoria sounded very similar to descriptions of drug-induced euphoria, which led researchers to coin the term "runner's high." Psychiatrist and psychopharmacologist Arnold J. Mandell was one of the first to popularize the concept of the runner's high. His description provides a vivid portrayal of the term:

The first half hour . . . is pure agony, exaggerated body pain and philosophical crisis . . . . Thirty minutes out and something lifts . . . . The fatigue goes away and feelings of power begin. I think I'll run 25 miles today. I'll double the size of the research grant request. I'll have that talk with the dean . . . . Then, sometime into the second hour comes the spooky time. Colors are bright and beautiful, water sparkles, clouds breathe, and my body, swimming, detaches from the earth. A loving contentment invades the basement of my mind, and thoughts bubble up without trails. I find the place I need to live if I'm going to live (Mandell, 1979).

Since that time, people participating in other forms of intense exercise have also described experiences like the runner's high.

The Endorphin Theory

Interest in the runner's high led to a search for biological explanations for changes in mental state. This search led to formation of the hypothesis that intense physical activity may stimulate the body to produce chemicals similar to those in the opiate family. Opiates are drugs that come from the poppy flower, including opium, heroin, morphine, and cocaine. As psychologists explored this hypothesis, neuroscientists such as Candace Pert, discussed in Chapter 2, discovered neurochemicals they dubbed endorphins, for "endogenous morphine." Endogenous means produced by the body. In the human body, endorphins reduce pain, but they have other roles in the brain and body as well, including important roles in memory, learning, and registering emotions. The Endorphin Theory proposed that the psychological changes experienced with exercise, such as the runner's high, are due to increased levels of endorphins in the brain. Many people jumped to the conclusion that endorphins explained *everything* about the psychological effects of exercise.

Research on endorphins in humans is limited by the fact that endorphins are large molecules that do not cross the blood-brain barrier, thus remaining either in the brain, if produced there, or in the rest of the body, if that is their origin. Therefore, sampling endorphins in the peripheral circulation does not give researchers information about what is happening in the brain. Animal research has shown that endorphins are produced in the CNS with exercise that is prolonged or intense. However, extrapolation of this research to humans is limited. Some exercise psychologists have criticized the way both the public and exercise scientists have assumed that endorphins are the primary explanation for the psychological effects of physical activity, when the reality of this relationship is much more complex (Dishman & O'Connor, 2009). Endorphins interact with a number of other neurotransmitters, such as dopamine, a neurotransmitter known for its role in establishing sensations of pleasure in the brain. In fact, dopamine can be converted into endorphins. Animal research has shown that endorphins also interact with the NO production pathways (Esch & Stefano, 2010a) and are involved in the formation of new brain cells (Koehl et al., 2008). Thus, the big picture of the neurobiology of exercise is much larger than the original endorphin hypothesis.

Even though endorphins are not the total picture, they appear to at least play an important role in the runner's high and other positive emotions associated with exercise. Evidence suggests that this is most likely for exercise bouts of high volume. One intriguing study performed by Boecker et al., (2008) used positron emission tomography (PET) scans to examine the brains of runners before and after 2 hours of running. PET scans use a radioactive tracer and record activity involving the tracer substance. Boecker and colleagues found that after running, fewer endorphin receptor sites were available for binding, suggesting that endorphins that had been manufactured and released during exercise were bound to the receptor sites. The higher the levels of euphoria in the runners, the lower the receptor availability and, presumably, the higher the levels of endorphins in the brains of the runners after exercise.

Endocannabinoids and Exercise

Cannabis refers to a group of plants. One of these is the marijuana plant, which contains a psychoactive compound known to reduce pain and enhance enjoyment. In the 1990s, a chemical similar in structure to the active ingredient in marijuana was discovered to be produced by humans and laboratory animals. The molecule was named anandamide, after the Sanskrit word *ananda*, which means bliss or delight. Anandamide is one of a family of compounds called endocannabinoids, meaning cannabinoids produced endogenously. The endocannabinoids are neurotransmitters, binding to postsynaptic receptors on neurons. They reduce pain, enhance mood, and participate in many other important psychophysiological pathways. They appear to be involved in exercise behavior. Endocannabinoids motivate mice to run on their running wheels for longer periods of time, an activity that they find enjoyable (Fuss & Gass, 2010). In mice, the cannabinoid receptors in the CNS become "remarkably potentiated" or activated following exercise (DeChiara, et al., 2010). In humans, exercise is associated with increased levels of endocannabinoids in the bloodstream (Dietrich & McDaniel, 2004). Because endocannabinoid molecules are smaller than the endorphins, they are able to cross the blood-brain barrier, so serum levels are indicative of both peripheral and CNS production. Are endocannabinoids linked with euphoria? Neuroscientists speculate that these chemicals are not the only players, but they probably participate in the complex picture of mood production in humans (Esch & Stefano, 2010b).

The Complex Picture of the Psychological Effects of Exercise

Exploration of the runner's high, endorphins, and the endocannabinoids is just a small part of a very large area of research. Many exercisers experience positive psychological effects during and after an exercise session and find that they generally "feel better" when they are participating in regular physical activity. While they may not report feeling euphoric or high, they experience many other positive states. For over 40 years, psychologists have explored the associations between exercise and various psychological effects (Game Changers 3-1), including the following:

- Changes in mood
- Reduced feelings of stress and psychophysiological responses to sources of stress
- Changes in self-esteem
- Altered perception of body image
- Changes in sleep quality

- Better memory and other markers of cognitive function
- Reduction in symptoms of anxiety
- Reduction in symptoms of depression

These topics are explored in following sections. Research on all such topics has included investigations into the psychophysiology of the exercise experience. Some of the research has been prompted by an intellectual curiosity to simply explain the mind-body relationship. Other research studies have attempted to elucidate what types and volumes of activity could best be used in humans for therapeutic purposes,

---

Game Changers 3-1. William P. Morgan Expands the Big Picture of Exercise Science

Throughout his long and productive career, William P. Morgan has often changed the way that exercise scientists view important concepts. He is known for his ability to see the "big picture" of sport and exercise psychology and exercise science. He has combined impeccable research methods with acute observation and critical thinking to devise theoretical models to explain and predict a variety of interesting phenomena.

One of Morgan's first contributions to sport psychology was the identification of the "iceberg profile" for the mood states of male and female elite athletes (Morgan & Costill, 1972; Morgan, O'Connor, Sparling, & Pate, 1987). The iceberg profile describes the results typically seen in these athletes' scores on the Profile of Mood States (POMS) questionnaire. The elite runners in Morgan's study sample scored below general populations on the traits of tension, depression, anger, fatigue, and confusion. However, they scored higher than average on the trait of vigor, which forms the tip of the iceberg. A later study in 15 older, elite, male marathon runners compared their POMS profiles from the 1990s with data gathered from the same runners about 20 years earlier. The older runners (average age of 50 years) showed the same iceberg profile on the POMS that they showed in their younger years (Morgan & Costill, 1996).

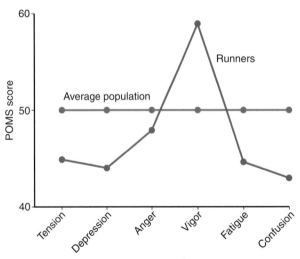

Iceberg profile. *(Adapted from Morgan, W. P. (1980). Test of champions: the Iceberg Profile. Psychology Today, 14(2): 92-108, with permission.)*

William Morgan was one of the first to suggest that some people with depression experience a significant reduction in symptoms of depression after starting a regular exercise program (Morgan, Roberts, Brand, & Feinerman, 1970). Subsequent research has since explored and supported his hypothesis.

Morgan is known as an inspiriting teacher and mentor. He has enjoyed explaining the psychological aspects of physical activity to exercise physiologists as well as the interactions of physical activity and psychology to exercise psychologists. In 1985, Morgan published the lead paper for a symposium on exercise psychology for the American College of Sports Medicine (ACSM), called "Affective Beneficence of Vigorous Physical Activity," highlighting the important psychological effects of exercise (Morgan, 1985). It was just like Morgan to use a lovely phrase like "affective beneficence" in reference to exercise effects. Affective describes the beneficence as relating to affect, or mood. Beneficence means kind, charitable, and beneficial. One can imagine exercise generously bestowing its benefits on the exerciser.

Morgan was one of the first psychologists to convince mainstream psychologists that the field of sport and exercise psychology was a distinct and growing area of research, and he founded the division of Exercise and Sport Psychology of the prestigious American Psychological Association in 1986 and served as its first president.

Game Changers 3-1. William P. Morgan Expands the Big Picture of Exercise Science—cont'd

In 2001, Morgan again suggested a paradigm shift in the way exercise scientists prescribe physical activity (Morgan, 2001). He studied people with long-term adherence to physical activity and found that they tended to (1) engage in purposeful activity, such as walking or bicycling for transportation, chopping wood for fuel, and gardening; and (2) ignore recommendations regarding exercise intensity, instead working at their preferred level of exertion. His observations, especially regarding exertion and exercise adherence, have been confirmed in subsequent studies.

Sources: Morgan, W. P. (1985). Affective beneficence of vigorous physical activity. *Medicine and Science in Sports and Exercise, 17*(1): 94-100; Morgan, W. P. (2001). Prescription of physical activity: a paradigm shift? *Quest, 53*(3): 366-382; Morgan, W. P., & Costill, D. L. (1972). Psychological characteristics of the marathon runner. *Journal of Sports Medicine and Physical Fitness, 12*(1): 42-46; Morgan, W. P., & Costill, D. L. (1996). Selected psychological characteristics and health behaviors of aging marathon runners: a longitudinal study. *International Journal of Sports Medicine, 17*(4): 305-312; Morgan, W. P., O'Connor, P. J., Sparling, B. P., & Pate, R. R. (1987). Psychological characterization of the elite female distance runner. *International Journal of Sports Medicine. 8*(Suppl 2), 124-131; Morgan, W. P., Roberts, J. A., Brand, F. R., & Feinerman, A. D. (1970). Psychological effect of chronic physical activity. *Medicine & Science in Sports, 2*(4): 213-217.

such as in the treatment of anxiety and depressive disorders.

Exercise and Mood

Researchers have studied the influence of exercise on mood in many different settings and with a variety of activities. Psychologists use the word mood to refer to how a person feels. Some researchers distinguish mood from emotion, using emotion to refer to shorter, often more-intense feelings experienced in response to a specific stimulus, such as something perceived to be disgusting, frightening, and so forth. Mood is generally used to refer to more-diffuse and longer-lasting feelings that may not be triggered by anything in particular. Another term, affect, refers to the nature of moods and emotions in terms of whether a person evaluates them as positive or negative. The three terms—mood, emotion, and affect—tend to be used interchangeably (Pressman & Cohen, 2005).

Evaluating Mood

Several tools are available to evaluate mood. One of the most commonly used questionnaires in this area of research is the Profile of Mood States (POMS). The POMS scores individuals on several scales for common moods, including levels of anxiety and tension, anger and hostility, depression, fatigue, confusion, and vigor. The POMS is used for many different purposes, not just to measure mood associations with physical activity.

Exercise psychologists have developed an interesting research tool to evaluate mood changes with physical activity (Ekkekakis & Petruzzello, 2002). Moods are categorized along two dimensions known as valence and activation. Valence refers to how positive an emotional state feels to a person, and it runs from unpleasant to pleasant. Activation is the second dimension, and it refers to energy level, with deactivated meaning low energy level and activated meaning high energy level. Moods are categorized as follows:

- Pleasant, activated—enthusiastic, excited, happy, alert
- Pleasant, deactivated—calm, peaceful, relaxed, content
- Unpleasant, activated—nervous, tense, upset, stressed
- Unpleasant, deactivated—sluggish, bored, sad, depressed

The Exercise-Induced Feeling Inventory (EFI) was designed by researchers Gauvin and Rejeski (1993) as a quick and easy questionnaire to measure mood changes most commonly associated with physical activity (Fig. 3-8). The EFI has subscales for feelings of positive engagement, revitalization, tranquility, and physical exhaustion—the mood descriptors that most commonly change in association with exercise. The EFI has been used to compare mood before and after exercise and also to compare general mood before and after weeks or months of regular exercise participation. Health and fitness professionals may find it useful in their work, as it helps clients consider a wide range of mood benefits commonly experienced with physical activity.

Another scale useful in studies of physical activity is the Feeling Scale (FS) (Hardy & Rejeski, 1989), which is a one-item scale that is a sort of emotional RPE scale. People rate how they are feeling on a scale of –5 (very bad, unpleasant feeling) to +5 (very good, pleasant feeling), with 0 as a neutral midpoint. This simple scale is useful during an exercise session when people do not have the time or energy to focus on anything longer.

Changes in Mood With Exercise

What have researchers found? Changes in mood have been measured before and after a single exercise session as well as before and after initiating a regular exercise program. Results regarding changes in mood have been similar for both acute and

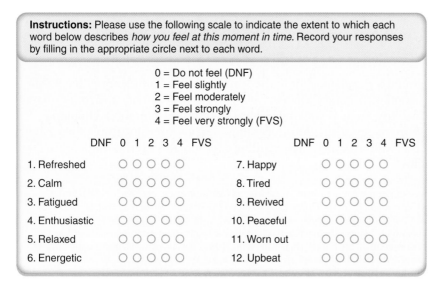

Figure 3-8. **The exercise-induced feeling inventory** *(From Gauvin, L., & Rejeski, W. J. (1993). The exercise-induced feeling inventory: development and initial validation. Journal of Sport and Exercise Psychology, 15(4): 403-423, with permission.)*

chronic exercise. The most frequently observed changes in mood include the following:

- **Energy level:** People often report feeling more energetic following a session of mild- to moderate-intensity exercise. They score higher on the POMS category of vigor and describe themselves as feeling more refreshed and invigorated. (Students can take advantage of this phenomenon with exercise study breaks (Health Psychology in Your Life 3-1).) At higher levels of exercise intensity, subjects with lower fitness levels may be less likely to experience improvements in energy level, whereas highly fit subjects tend to respond positively to and report feeling energized by even vigorous exercise. Interestingly, although people report feeling more energy after exercise, many also report feeling calm and peaceful at the same time. People enjoy this state of "calm energy." In fact, many psychologists believe that levels of energy and stress strongly influence people's moods (Box 3-2).
- **Fatigue level:** Not surprisingly, along with feeling more energy, people report feeling less fatigue. However, following high-intensity exercise, subjects with lower fitness levels may be more likely than highly fit subjects to report more, rather than less, fatigue.
- **Negative mood:** People report reductions in feelings of depression, anxiety, anger, tension, and irritability after a single exercise session as well as after participation in a regular exercise program.

One study found that college students with higher levels of physical activity reported higher levels of pleasant-activated moods than their less-active peers (Hyde, Conroy, Pincus, & Ram, 2011). In addition, all subjects reported more pleasant-activated moods on days when they had more physical activity. Subjects recorded their activity levels and moods at the end of

HEALTH PSYCHOLOGY IN YOUR LIFE 3-1: Can Exercise Energize Your Studying?

Can a 10-minute exercise break invigorate a college student's studying? After you have been sitting and doing schoolwork for a period of time, rate your energy level on a scale of 1 (very low energy) to 10 (very high energy). Then take a break and perform 10 minutes of moderately vigorous exercise. You could walk or run up and down the stairs, take a brisk walk, or whatever is convenient for you. At the end of the exercise period, use the same scale to rate your energy level again. Did you find a change? What are some of the variables that may have influenced your energy level? For example, if you are sleep deprived, exercise may not have a significant effect on deep fatigue. If you were already feeling energetic at the beginning of the exercise break, you may not have had room for improvement with exercise. If you spent 10 minutes jumping around to your favorite music, perhaps the music also helped to lift your spirits.

each day during this study, so it is unknown whether a better mood caused people to engage in more activity, whether the activity itself was responsible for the good moods, or perhaps some of each. It is likely that physical activity and mood interact, with physical activity causing improvements in mood and positive mood in turn prompting people to engage in more activity.

Variables and Mechanisms Associated With Exercise-Induced Mood Changes

The nature of a person's affective response to exercise likely depends on a number of variables (Fig. 3-9). Mood is affected by many factors, and all these factors interact with and influence a person's exercise experience. Some

Box 3-2. Calm Energy

Psychologists have commented on the interesting paradoxical effect of exercise on energy level. One might think (and many people do) that physical activity would be more likely to lead to feelings of fatigue and, consequently, negative mood rather than feelings of energy and relatively positive moods. Robert Thayer has proposed that people can learn to use exercise (along with eating habits, adequate sleep, and a balanced lifestyle) to regulate their moods to feel more energetic, engaged, and productive (Thayer, 2001). Thayer's research led him to categorize moods on two dimensions. One is where mood sits on a continuum running from calmness to tension; the other dimension runs from tiredness to energy.

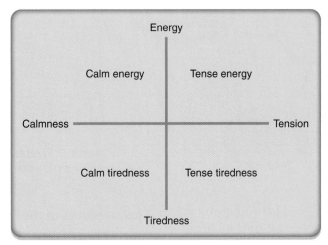

Calm energy. *(Adapted from Thayer, R. E. (2001). The Origin of Everyday Moods. New York: Oxford University Press, with permission.)*

Exercise can contribute to a pleasurable affective state that Thayer refers to as "calm energy," the title of his book summarizing his years of research on mood (Thayer, 2001). Calm energy is synonymous with feelings of enthusiasm, interest, and engagement. Sometimes people experience a sort of agitated tense energy, which can stimulate productivity but is often felt as anxiety and tension. Calm energy refers to more of a flow state of engagement without the nervous energy attached. Exercise is beneficial in reducing the anxious edge many people feel.

Similarly, feeling tired is not necessarily bad, if people are finished with their work and ready to relax. Thayer distinguishes between calm tiredness, which is experienced as relaxation and calmness, and tense tiredness. Feelings of depression are often experienced as tense tiredness, where one feels tense but lacking energy. Tense tiredness is also associated with feelings of boredom and fatigue. In fact, Thayer found that people dislike feelings of tense tiredness the most of the four quadrants.

Thayer believes people consciously manage and unconsciously respond to their moods with many health behaviors, especially eating and exercise. People often overeat in response to tense tiredness, a mood induced or worsened by stress and/or insufficient sleep. Cultivating states of calm energy with exercise, enough sleep, good stress-management strategies, and a healthful diet helps people feel better more of the time. It also helps prevent mindless munching in response to tense tiredness and, consequently, obesity.

Source

Thayer, R. E. (2001). *Calm Energy: How People Regulate Mood With Food and Exercise.* Oxford: Oxford University Press.

---

of the most widely recognized variables are discussed in the following subsections.

Neurobiological Changes

The research on endorphins, endocannabinoids, and other neurotransmitters such as dopamine and serotonin has established a model in which numerous neurochemicals interact with each other and in response to physical activity. Neurobiological changes that accompany exercise may help explain mood effects. This is most likely to be true at higher exercise intensities, where greater changes have been found. While, in general, exercise becomes less pleasurable at higher intensities, some people still report positive feelings following such exercise.

Changes in brain electrical activity suggest that increased activity occurs in several areas of the brain, including the limbic system (one of the locations involved with the processing of emotion) and in the ventral prefrontal cortex (also associated with mood states). Researchers have hypothesized that changes in

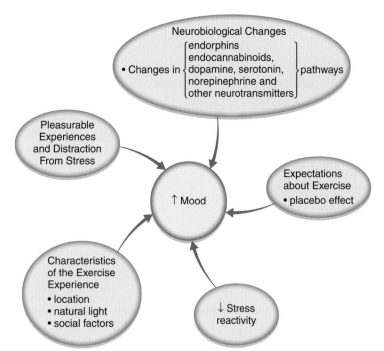

Figure 3-9. Factors that may mediate the effect of exercise on mood.

brain activity may reflect changes in neurotransmitter systems, such as changes in the release and binding of serotonin (Fumoto et al., 2010).

Expectations and Cognitions Regarding the Exercise Experience

Just as people who expect to experience inebriation from a laboratory beverage get drunk on a placebo, so might people who expect exercise to feel good experience mood improvements with exercise. People learn from others how to think about exercise. When family and friends have continually told a story of how unpleasant exercise is, a person may come to believe this. Consequently, a person may focus on the unpleasant sensations that accompany exercise and ignore any positive effects. Similarly, prior negative exercise experiences may color current impressions and lead to negative feelings during and after physical activities. The same goes for positive expectations. People who expect to feel good during and/or after exercise are more likely to do so.

Other thoughts influence people's experiences during exercise as well. Concerns about one's ability to perform the exercise, perceptions of control over the exercise situation, and other positive and negative thoughts about the exercise experience color a person's affective response to an exercise session (Rose & Parfitt, 2010).

Lower Stress Reactivity

Over time, exercise training is associated with reduced arousal in response to psychosocial stressors. This phenomenon is discussed in more detail in the next section on exercise and reduced feelings of stress. When people have less sympathetic nervous system overactivation in response to daily stressors, they generally have a more-positive mood.

Characteristics of the Exercise Experience

Not all exercise experiences are alike. An interesting study compared the response of women to a 10-minute walk at a self-selected intensity both in the laboratory and in an outdoor environment (Focht, 2009). Researchers measured affective state, enjoyment, and intention for future participation in walking exercise before, during, and after the 10-minute walks. Both indoor and outdoor walking sessions were associated with improvement in affective state. However, scores for the outdoor walking condition showed greater affective improvements, enjoyment, and intention to participate in future walking exercise (Focht, 2009).

Other variables related to exercise enjoyment might include socialization, exercise difficulty, and activity preference. Exercising with a friend may be perceived as more pleasant than exercising alone or with a group one does not like. Exercise that is not too hard or too long is probably also perceived to be more enjoyable and has a more-beneficial effect on mood. A given individual might enjoy and feel motivated by some activities but not others.

MOTIVATING CHANGE: Selecting Activities

Effective health and fitness professionals help clients select the best activities possible for their exercise programs. This may involve trading in faster improvements in measurable fitness for enjoyment. Professionals who work in fitness centers often keep their recommendations focused on the equipment and activities available in the fitness center. Clients have often paid to join the center and want to get their money's worth by coming as often as possible. But, for some people, the fitness center gets boring pretty quickly as they walk on the "treadmill to nowhere." These clients may do better coming to the fitness center 2 or 3 days a week and performing other activities outside the center on other days. For example, they might enjoy walking, golfing, cross-country skiing, or other opportunities outdoors. Ask about these and see if clients would like a little variety, without overwhelming them with suggestions.

In order to match exercise recommendations to client preferences, ask about previous experiences with exercise. What worked best in the past and why? What were the elements that helped your client stick to his or her program? What led to the client dropping out? Some clients are very forthcoming about their preferences, whereas others may not have strong opinions. Listen carefully to the stories that clients tell about their lives and to their responses to your suggestions. Consider clients' preferences as much as possible rather than giving them a standard workout.

Pleasurable Experiences and Distraction From Stress

Psychologists have often suggested that participation in physical activities may lead to improvements in psychological states because they serve as a distraction from the daily grind. This observation is especially useful in explaining why people experience positive changes in mood with activities provoking very little physiological change. For example, people report improvement in mood with playing darts or pool or going bowling, none of which tend to cause enough pain to activate the endorphin or endocannabinoid pathways (unless one is stabbed by a dart or drops the bowling ball on one's foot). Researchers suggest these distractions nevertheless change the channel on stress by redirecting a person's focus, perhaps interrupting ruminations on unpleasant tasks at hand.

Pressman et al. (2009) performed an interesting study examining the relationship between enjoyable leisure activities and measures of psychological and physical health. Leisure activities were defined as "pleasurable activities that individuals engage in voluntarily when they are free from demands of work or other responsibilities" (Pressman et al., 2009). These activities thus included both physical activities and other hobbies, such as reading, socializing, and so forth. In their study, 1,399 subjects completed questionnaires regarding their participation in leisure activities and the level of enjoyment experienced during these activities. Researchers also measured a number of physical variables, including blood pressure, body mass index, waist circumference (a measure of obesity), and salivary cortisol levels (an estimate of stress level). Pressman and colleagues found that higher scores on the enjoyable leisure activities questionnaire were associated with lower resting blood pressure, cortisol levels, waist circumference, and body mass index. A higher enjoyable leisure activities score was associated with better measures of psychosocial states and lower levels of depression and negative affect. The effect on psychosocial measures held across all demographic groups, irrespective of age, sex, and ethnicity.

It is likely that enjoyable activities, including but not limited to physical activities, provide a break and pleasant diversion from daily obligations. In addition, positive emotions reduce feelings of stress and dampen negative emotions. Positive emotions themselves enhance psychological and physical health (Pressman & Cohen, 2005). As the famous Dr. Seuss character, the Cat in the Hat, once said, "These things are fun, and fun is good."

Melissa tries to sneak quietly into the back row of the line-dancing class, but the instructor, Victor, gives her a big smile and comes over to say hello and to make sure Melissa is in the right class. Two other women are trying out the class for the first time, so Victor introduces them to each other. Victor turns on the music and begins the show. He is a born performer and obviously loves to dance. His energy is contagious, and Melissa throws herself into the combinations. Before she knows it, the hour has passed, and people are filing slowly out the door, laughing and chatting with each other. Victor says good-bye to everyone by name. He tells Melissa she is a fabulous dancer, and he hopes she will register for the class. Melissa realizes she feels great— energized and happy.

Melissa tells Victor she would love to take the class, but often at the end of the day she feels stressed and tired. Victor gives her a look, and says, "Don't you realize yet that you have to change the way you think? Instead of saying, 'I am too stressed and tired for exercise,' you have to say, 'I am feeling stressed and tired; therefore, I MUST get some exercise right away to feel better!'" He gives Melissa a big smile and hands her an article about the energizing, mood-improving effects of exercise. ∎

Flow and Exercise: The Ultimate Pleasure and Distraction From Stress

Exercise psychologists have explored the psychophysiology of a state of consciousness commonly experienced during sport and exercise known as "flow" (Nakamura & Csikszentmihalyi, 2007). Flow refers to an enjoyable state of consciousness where people feel totally engaged and at one with the activity with which they are involved. People experiencing flow are alert, tuned into the present moment, and responding to an intense challenge, such as skiing, kayaking, playing a musical instrument, dancing, or playing chess. Flow states closely resemble other descriptions of positive moods associated with physical activity. Csikszentmihalyi studied a wide range of subjects who reported feeling states of flow, including athletes (Box 3-3). He noted that high-caliber athletes engrossed in sport performance have reported enjoyable states of consciousness they call "being in the zone," synonymous with the definition of flow. Csikszentmihalyi believes that flow experiences are common and that it is possible to cultivate flow states of consciousness. While the runner's high tends to be associated with prolonged, fairly intense exercise, flow is more about feeling challenged and engaged. Flow is often experienced as euphoric, as in the runner's high, but is described in other words as well.

Box 3-3. Mihalyi Csikszentmihalyi and the Experience of Flow

Csikszentmihalyi (pronounced cheek-sent-muh-high) has described his research on states of consciousness as beginning in his young adulthood in Hungary following the horror of World War II upon observing the adults around him. All were devastated as a result of the war, having lost social status, financial support, friends, family members, and especially hope. Csikszentmihalyi began a search to understand what makes life worth living. He interviewed people who seemed to find satisfaction in life—artists, musicians, and athletes—asking them to describe their lives, work, thoughts, and feelings. Later, he developed a data-collection procedure that he called the Experience Sampling Method. He and his colleagues fitted volunteers with pagers that beeped at random times within every 2-hour period during the day. When the pager beeped, subjects completed a short questionnaire about what they were doing and how they were feeling. Data were collected on thousands of subjects.

Csikszentmihalyi found that people report flow experiences most often when facing a challenge that elicits peak performance in some area. In other words, flow most commonly results from a good match between a task's level of challenge and the skill set of a given individual to perform that task. When the level of challenge is too high compared with people's perceptions of their skills, they feel anxious. If a task is too easy in an area where people's skills are high (an accomplished tennis athlete playing with a group of amateurs), people are bored. The skills-challenge balance is always task specific.

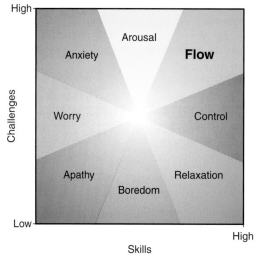

Flow. *(Adapted from Csikszentmihalyi, M. (1997). Finding Flow: The Psychology of Engagement with Everyday Life. New York: Basic Books, with permission.)*

Csikszentmihalyi described seven characteristics of the flow experience (Csikszentmihalyi, 1997) as follows:
- Complete engagement in the activity; engagement requires total concentration
- State of ecstasy, where one temporarily is so focused on the activity that one is not thinking about everyday life
- Sense of inner clarity; one knows what to do and does it
- Confidence, feeling that one's skills are adequate for the challenge at hand and that the challenge is doable
- Serenity, perhaps because one's focus excludes the opportunity to worry
- Sense of timelessness, not noticing the clock or being aware of time passing
- Intrinsic motivation, which means feeling motivated to perform the task because of the inherent benefits of the task, not for gaining secondary benefits such as money, prestige, and so on.

Source
Csikszentmihalyi, M. (1997). *Finding Flow: The Psychology of Engagement With Everyday Life*. New York: Basic Books.

Flow is not centrally about the effect of exercise, but sport and exercise experiences can offer conditions for total engagement that set the scene for the flow experience. Flow theory proposes that people feel most satisfied when they are both challenged and successful. Sport and exercise experiences that require total concentration are most frequently associated with flow experiences. While flow is more about states of consciousness, it does underscore the "feel-good" potential of sport and exercise experiences.

Mood and Exercise Adherence

Research on affective response to exercise has important implications for exercise behavior. It seems sensible that if people find exercise aversive, they are less likely to stick to an exercise program than people who find exercise pleasant. Research seems to support this commonsense notion. One study asked a group of volunteers to rate a number of variables during an exercise session in the laboratory. Subjects reported levels of positive affect, negative affect, tranquility, and fatigue. They also reported their intentions to exercise in the future and their current levels of physical activity. Three months later, subjects were contacted once again and asked to report how much they were exercising. The researchers found that subjects who responded more positively to the exercise session had stronger intentions to exercise and higher levels of exercise participation 3 months after the laboratory testing (Kwan & Bryan, 2009). Other researchers have found similar results (Williams et al., 2008). Successful health and fitness professionals work diligently to create positive exercise experiences for their clients as well as exercise programs that deliver both physical and psychological benefits (Health Psychology at Work 3-1).

Exercise Recommendations for Mood Improvement

What amounts, intensities, and types of exercise are best for improving energy level and mood? Researchers have studied the effect of exercise on mood in many different populations and for many different types and amounts of exercise to understand when and how exercise has a positive effect on mood. Most studies have examined aerobic activity, although strength exercise also leads to mood improvements. A meta-analysis on aerobic exercise reached the following conclusions (Reed & Buck, 2009). In general, the optimal dose of

---

HEALTH PSYCHOLOGY AT WORK 3-1: Addressing Health Issues and Improving Quality of Life

Rosalie Peri, R.N., Yoga and Pilates Instructor, and a National Strength and Conditioning Association Certified Personal Trainer

Rosalie Peri teaches yoga and Pilates privately in her own studio, Fluid Motion Pilates and Yoga Studio, and at the Northampton (MA) Athletic Club. She is also an adjunct instructor at Smith College, where she teaches a variety of group exercise classes. Rosalie began her health and fitness career in nursing, starting as a nurse's aide in a nursing home at the age of 15, because she has always liked older people. After nursing school at Massachusetts General Hospital, she worked in coronary care, the hospital unit that treats serious heart problems, for many years. Rosalie began teaching group exercise classes and working as a personal trainer when she decided that she would rather help people prevent heart attacks than treat them. She continued to do both for many years, recently transitioning out of coronary care and into fitness full time.

"Over half of my personal training clients are coping with previous and current injuries and chronic health problems. People appreciate my 20 years of experience in fitness and my training and experience as a nurse; it's a great combination. Many clients are worried about getting injured by exercise; they are motivated to try harder when they feel safe.

"The biggest motivators for my clients are health problems. They have risk factors for chronic illness or pain, and they are motivated to do something about this. Health problems can be extremely motivational. As we work together, they begin to feel more in control of their health situation, and this helps to keep them exercising.

"My clients are also motivated when they realize that they feel better when they are active. Sometimes they don't even realize exercise is helping until they stop—then they feel worse. I try to get them to pay attention to what they are feeling as they work out and to note how exercise helps them move more easily, have less pain and more energy. With Pilates and yoga, we work a lot with alignment and body mechanics, and clients often find relief for pain that they have been carrying around for years.

"My goal working with people is to find out what's important to them and help them use exercise to reach their goals. People have to do what they love. It takes time to discover what clients' goals are; and goals change over time. You have to develop good relationships with your clients and listen carefully. Clients may come in wanting to lose weight but then change their focus to working on their back issues or feeling less depressed. Muscle aches and pains are often intertwined with emotional health issues, and the right kind of exercise training can help both."

aerobic exercise for mood improvement is about 30 to 35 minutes of activity, performed 3 to 5 days per week at a low-to-moderate intensity regularly for a period of at least 10 to 12 weeks. Of course, regular participation in physical activity must continue, or benefits cease. While this amount of exercise will not work the best for everyone, it can be a good place to start. Highly fit, active people often prefer higher intensities and amounts of exercise, whereas previously sedentary people need to start more slowly.

People are more likely to enjoy physical activities that they choose voluntarily and perform for positive reasons (Cerin, Leslie, Sugiyama, & Owen, 2009). For some people, walking after work with a friend might be perceived as enjoyable, whereas housework or yard work may not. Other people might perceive the opposite and enjoy accomplishing a necessary task with their activity. People also generally prefer exercising at a self-selected pace, rather than a pace prescribed for them. Even when the prescribed pace is only slightly higher than the self-selected pace, people report a decline in the pleasure experienced with physical activity (Ekkekakis, 2009). Individualization of exercise recommendations is important for capturing exercise preferences and tailoring exercise programs to meet individual expectations.

Exercise, Stress Response, and Stress Reactivity

The stress response described in Chapter 2 is activated when people perceive themselves to be facing a challenge or threatening situation. The stress response mobilizes a person's mental and physical resources to cope with the situation. An appropriately strong stress response comes in handy when psychophysiological arousal is helpful for dealing with a source of stress. The nature and strength of a person's stress response is known as stress reactivity. An appropriate level of arousal can improve an athletic performance, the quality of a presentation, or a job performance. Once the challenge or threat has passed, the body returns to normal, and no harm is done.

So why does stress feel so bad sometimes? The stress response is harmful when people feel they are constantly under threat. Stress is especially harmful when it feels uncontrollable, unrelenting, and likely to have a negative outcome. Many people (including college students) can develop a "high-stress lifestyle," where deadlines and pressures loom continually on the horizon, and there never seems to be enough time to recover between challenges.

Yet, in a given situation of deadlines and pressures, some people are able to maintain a balanced perspective (at least some of the time) and feel challenged by the work, whereas others feel tormented by the sense of stress and are unable to unwind. Researchers have investigated the many factors that may help explain why some people are more stress resistant than others.

Scientists have examined both the role of physical fitness as well as the effect of regular physical activity. Many people report that they feel "less stressed" after an exercise session and when they are regularly active.

Physical Fitness and Stress Reactivity

Researchers have suggested that people with higher *fitness* levels have a lower physiological response to laboratory stressors, a phenomenon known as the cross-stressor adaptation hypothesis. The basic idea is that people who become accustomed to the stress of exercise may become less reactive to other stressors, such as having to give a speech or perform a frustrating task. While some research has supported this connection, other studies have found no relationship between fitness and stress reactivity. A meta-analysis performed by Forcier et al. (2006) found that in general, fit subjects tended to show about a 15% to 25% lower HR and blood pressure response to a laboratory stressor than unfit subjects. Another analysis, however, concluded that fit subjects had a slightly *higher* cardiovascular stress response but recovered slightly faster than unfit subjects (Jackson & Dishman, 2006). These contradictions indicate that the relationship between fitness level and cardiovascular reactivity to stress is highly variable from person to person and that the relationship may not be very robust. Most of the studies have relied on cross-sectional data, in which groups of fit people are compared with groups of unfit people. Often, the fit and unfit groups differ on other variables as well as fitness. For example, fit people may have more time to exercise, have higher incomes that support their exercise habit, or may just be genetically different from the unfit group. If a fit group has higher levels of self-esteem, for example, this could contribute to their lower responses to stress (O'Donnell, Brydon, Wright, & Steptoe, 2008).

It is important to note that the stress response includes not only the cardiovascular system but other systems as well. An interesting study by Hamer and Steptoe (2007) looked at the relationship between fitness and a number of stress-response variables in 207 adult men and women. While the researchers did not find a relationship between fitness (predicted from a submaximal exercise test) and cardiovascular reactivity, they did find that higher fitness levels were significantly associated with lower levels of stress-related proinflammatory cytokines (Hamer & Steptoe, 2007). Because proinflammatory cytokines are thought to speed the development of artery disease and other chronic illnesses, this study may illustrate an important mechanism by which exercise reduces risk of these chronic illnesses.

As the sympathetic nervous system charges up the body for fight or flight, heart rate variability (HRV) declines. Hamer and Steptoe found lower reductions in HRV in response to stress in the fit subjects, suggesting a greater parasympathetic response in fit individuals.

Physical Activity and Stress Reactivity

Some research has examined the effect of a single session of exercise on subsequent reactivity to a laboratory stressor. A meta-analysis of these studies concluded that prior exercise reduced the rise in systolic blood pressure in response to subsequent laboratory stressors (Hamer, Taylor, & Steptoe, 2006). The stressors were generally administered both before and soon after the exercise session, usually within the first hour post-exercise. One study in children found reduced HR and a reduction in systolic and diastolic blood pressure response to stress following a session of interval exercise (Roemmich, Lambaise, Salvy, & Horvath, 2009).

Studies on laboratory animals suggest that those who perform regular physical activity show several differences in brain structure compared with those deprived of the opportunity to be active. For example, studies on rats have found differences in the neural pathways of the limbic system (Greenwood, et al., 2011). Whether comparisons can be made between caged rats and humans is open to discussion. Nevertheless, such results suggest that regular activity may have neurological effects, which might explain the observed relationships among physical activity, stress reactivity, and feelings of stress in humans.

Variables and Mechanisms Associated With Reduced Stress Reactivity

Numerous variables seem to interact to provide the mechanisms by which physical activity may reduce stress reactivity (Fig. 3-10).

- **Neurobiological changes:** Described in the section above, animal research suggests that exercise may be associated with the way the brain responds to stress and the way that the brain tells the body to respond to stress (Greenwood et al., 2011.
- **Changes in sympathetic and parasympathetic nervous system response to stress:** Lower HR

variability and lower blood pressures in response to laboratory stressors suggest increases in parasympathetic tone in those accustomed to regular activity and possibly less sympathetic arousal. Animal models have shown a reduced norepinephrine response to stress following exercise (Hamer, Taylor, & Steptoe, 2006). (Norepinephrine rises with activation of the sympathetic nervous system.)

- **Relaxed muscles:** Relaxation and stress-reduction techniques often focus on the induction of muscular relaxation, which in turn contributes to feelings of psychological relaxation as well. Athletes often note a feeling of muscular relaxation following a good workout. It is possible that this muscle relaxation contributes to lower self-reported stress levels.
- **Improved mood:** In everyday conversation, people use the term "feeling stressed" to refer to various negative mood states. If exercise increases positive affect and reduces negative mood states, as suggested in the preceding section, exercise would be associated with reduced feelings of stress.

Exercise Recommendations for the Reduction of Stress and Stress Reactivity

The exercise recommendations for stress reduction in humans echo those for mood improvement. Stress reactivity is often reduced with only a single session of exercise. Regular exercise sessions of at least 30 minutes duration at least 5 days a week, as recommended by public health organizations, are likely to help reduce stress reactivity.

MOTIVATING CHANGE: Helping Clients Use Exercise to Reduce Feelings of Stress and Fatigue

People commonly give fatigue and feelings of stress as their reasons for dropping out of their exercise programs. Exercising takes time and energy and, when both are in short supply, it is easy to rationalize skipping a workout. In addition, both stress and fatigue feel bad. Psychologists who study health behavior have found that when people are experiencing negative emotions such as stress, depression, anxiety, anger, or sadness, the need to cope with the negative emotion becomes a top priority. The need to feel better now overrides the drive to do something that may lead to future benefits. In other words, if people think a big slice of chocolate cake helps get rid of the depression they are feeling right now, they are likely to eat it, even if they had previously been avoiding desserts to improve their health. If people feel bad and they think skipping their workout would make them feel better, they will skip the workout, even though they would like to get back in shape. Stress is the most common reason that people resume an addiction they had given up, such as smoking or drinking.

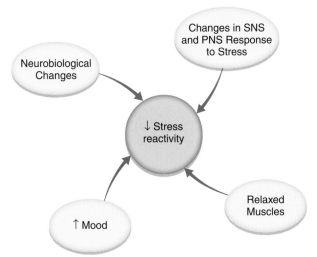

Figure 3-10. Factors that may mediate the effect of exercise on stress reactivity.

You can help your clients stick to their exercise programs by talking to them about the importance of using exercise to manage stress and negative emotions. If they can make the connection that exercise helps them feel good, perhaps they can learn to turn to exercise as a positive way to manage stress and fight fatigue (Behavior Change in Action 3-1).

Physical Activity, Self-Esteem, and Body Image

Most successful athletes will attest to the observation that sports and physical activity can have profound effects on self-concept and self-esteem. Self-concept refers to the way people perceive or define themselves. Self-concept includes the various roles people play in their family, community, and work lives. It includes people's ideas about their strengths and weaknesses, abilities, character, and all the stories built around what they have done in life. Related to self-concept is the notion of self-esteem. Self-esteem refers to people's evaluation and judgment about their self-concept. Self-esteem is a general sense of people's evaluations of their self-worth. While self-concept is the way that people might describe themselves, self-esteem reflects their evaluation of this description. For example, a person might believe he is a poor dancer, but this part of his self-concept may

have little or no influence on his self-esteem, unless he places a high value on dancing skill. An elite athlete who values athletic performance incorporates her role as an athlete into her self-concept. Her self-esteem is enhanced by her athletic success. The development of self-concept and self-esteem begin in infancy and is based on feedback received from caretakers. Later, the circle of influence grows to include friends, teachers, media, and the world at large. Experiences with recreational activities, schoolwork, sports, hobbies, work, and significant others all influence self-concept and self-esteem.

People with high self-esteem tend to have a lower risk of developing depression and anxiety and to be less likely to develop self-destructive addictive behaviors such as smoking, alcohol and drug abuse, or practicing pathogenic weight-control methods such as overly restrictive dieting or purging behaviors. Self-esteem may improve resistance to stress and be associated with a number of positive health variables, such as better cardiovascular and immune responses to acute stress (O'Donnell, Brydon, Wright, & Steptoe, 2008).

Sport and physical activity can have both positive and negative effects on self-esteem. Obviously, success feels better than failure, and people's self-esteem is most likely to improve when they feel competent in their participation in any valued realm, including physical activity. People who are shamed and bullied when participating in

BEHAVIOR CHANGE IN ACTION 3-1

Using Exercise to Decrease Stress and Fatigue

■ **CHALLENGE**

When clients list stress and fatigue as factors contributing to nonadherence to exercise programs, how do I motivate them to exercise?

■ **PLAN**

Motivate your clients to use exercise to fight fatigue and stress by suggesting the following:

Include emotional health goals in exercise program design. When you work with clients to set goals on which to base their exercise program design, ask about stress. Ask, "Are you ever bothered by feelings of stress or fatigue?" If your client says yes or sometimes, ask, "Did you know that exercise can help you feel invigorated and less stressed?" If they seem interested, explain briefly how exercise has been shown to improve mood and reduce stress.

Encourage clients to tune into the psychological effects of physical activity. From time to time, suggest that exercise should be having positive psychological effects. If clients are keeping some kind of exercise log, provide a place for recording mood and stress level after each workout. Ask clients how they are feeling after exercise sessions. Are your suggestions causing the placebo effect? It doesn't matter, since this is not a research project. If you are helping a client stick to an exercise program, the placebo effect is your ally and your client's ally as well. The power of suggestion can help your client find very real stress relief and mood improvement from regular physical activity.

Adjust exercise recommendations if clients are experiencing fatigue or a decline in mood following exercise. If exercise is not pleasurable, your client is more likely to quit. It's better to keep your client involved in a less-than-perfect exercise program than to push for a perfect program that they do not perform. Suggest lower exercise intensities, enjoyable activities, working out with a friend, or other ideas likely to make exercise more enjoyable.

Model positive thinking about exercise. Suggest that clients change their thinking from "I'm too tired to exercise" to "I feel tired; I think I will exercise so that I'll feel better."

physical activities (think about the clumsy or overweight kids in physical education classes) probably experience negative effects on self-concept and self-esteem.

Self-confidence refers to how much people feel likely to perform well in a given situation. Self-confidence is situation specific, although a general confidence in one's abilities contributes to a positive self-esteem. One of the interesting concepts that contributes to self-confidence, especially in the physical activity arena, is self-efficacy. **Self-efficacy** is the belief in one's ability to successfully accomplish a given task. Self-efficacy is situation specific. The stronger a person's self-efficacy, the more he or she persists at trying to succeed at a task in that area despite obstacles. For example, people with strong self-efficacy regarding their ability to walk regularly will be likely to stick to their walking programs despite bad weather or other factors that make walking more problematic. Self-efficacy contributes to self-concept as one piece of how people picture themselves.

Exercise and Body Image

The way that people feel about their appearance contributes to their self-concept and self-esteem (Lau, Cheung, & Ransdell, 2008). Self-esteem and body image are also related to risk of depression (Ryan, 2008). Participation in athletics and other forms of physical activity is often associated with improvements in the way people feel about their bodies and their appearance. But sometimes exercise can have the opposite effect, making people more aware of their physical shortcomings and creating anxiety about appearance. Such anxiety may cause people to avoid exercise and drop out of exercise programs.

Body image is all about perception. **Body image** refers to the way people see their bodies and to their subjective evaluations of their physical appearance. People's ideas and judgments about their bodies are influenced by many factors. For example, basic self-esteem affects the way people perceive their physical

attractiveness, as do cultural ideals of attractiveness and how much people buy into these ideals. Values regarding physical appearance are absorbed from family and friends. Just as self-esteem influences body image, the reverse is also true: body image affects people's self-esteem, especially if they value physical appearance.

Exercise is most likely to improve body image when people notice and value the changes that occur as a result of an exercise program. People often report feeling better about their bodies when they perceive improvements in health, fitness, or emotional well-being. People coping with health problems are especially responsive to exercise benefits when exercise helps them feel better and more energetic. Those who have more-realistic expectations about how their bodies should look are generally more satisfied with, or at least less concerned about, their appearance. They are more likely to experience positive feelings about their physical selves with improvements in fitness.

Exercise is most likely to have a negative effect on body image when it reinforces or increases existing disparities between people's ideals of physical attractiveness and their perceptions of their appearance. This occurs most often in adolescents and young adults who value an unrealistically thin (often the case for women) or muscular physique. While young people are especially at risk, problems with body image can develop at any age.

Variables and Mechanisms Associated With Improvements in Self-Esteem and Body Image

Many researchers have studied the effect of physical activity participation on self-esteem (Spence, 2005). Many variables affect the relationship between physical activity and self-esteem (Fig. 3-11). Three of the most important appear to be improvement in physical fitness, type of exercise program, and improvements in physical activity self-efficacy. As might be expected,

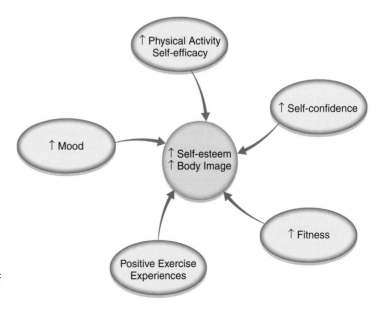

Figure 3-11. Factors that may mediate the effect of exercise on self-esteem and body image.

fitness improvement increases self-esteem. In terms of program type, exercise and lifestyle change programs typically show greater improvement in self-esteem than classes simply teaching skills (Spence, 2005). Improvements in physical activity self-efficacy likely contribute to improvements in self-esteem (White, Kendrick, & Yardley, 2009).

Both self-esteem and body image may be affected by the neurobiological changes and mood improvements discussed in previous sections. As people feel better in general, that good feeling may extend to feelings about themselves and their bodies. A longitudinal study by White, Kendrick, and Yardley (2009) found improvements in positive affect after as little as 1 to 3 weeks of participation in an exercise program. Increased positive affect and decreases in negative affect, along with increases in physical activity self-efficacy, preceded and thus may have contributed to improvements in self-esteem.

Participation in sport and physical activity can change the way people evaluate their bodies and thus affect their body image. In some cases, people learn to appreciate what their bodies can do, rather than just what their bodies look like. On the other hand, appearance-focused activities can worsen body image, as participants spend too much time in front of the mirror or obsessing about how they look.

The social elements of exercise and sport participation can exert strong effects on body image and self-esteem, in both positive and negative directions, depending on the quality of the group interactions. In the best cases, being around others who enjoy exercise and accept their less-than-perfect bodies can lead to improved self-esteem and body image. Supportive instructors, coaches, and friends are also important.

Exercise Recommendations for Improving Self-Esteem and Body Image

Researchers have not found a relationship between amount of exercise and self-esteem or body image improvements, although some studies have suggested that higher frequencies of participation (participating more days per week) may have a stronger effect than less-frequent participation (Spence, 2005). No particular intensities or amounts have been demonstrated to be particularly significant in improving self-esteem or body image or in changing self-concept. It is likely that the perceived quality of the exercise experience itself is more important than the amount or intensity of exercise (Behavior Change in Action 3-2). Perceived

BEHAVIOR CHANGE IN ACTION 3-2

Improving Body Image

CHALLENGE
Most clients ask for my advice because they are dissatisfied with their bodies. How do I help?

PLAN
A negative body image can motivate people to begin an exercise program, so it is common for health and fitness professionals to see people with negative body images. Sometimes, the exercise program you recommend consequently helps improve body image, but other times exercise and the fitness environment make body image worse. Sometimes, clients feel they fall short of the fitness ideals modeled by the instructors and clients at the fitness center. Such feelings may lead to exercise dropout, as people avoid exercise because it makes them feel bad. In some cases, people with a negative body image compulsively overexercise to the point of injury. Sometimes people with a negative body image also have eating disorders. If you are worried about a particular client, you should speak to your supervisor and follow guidelines for referral.

Health and fitness instructors can do many things to help clients develop a positive body image that promotes increased participation in regular physical activity, including the following:

Provide a friendly atmosphere that welcomes a variety of body types. As a health and fitness professional, you must set an example. Be friendly to everyone and encourage them to accept themselves they way they are, even as they strive to improve or maintain fitness.

Focus on positive reasons for exercising. Positive reasons for exercising, such as wanting to manage stress, have more energy, have fun, or improve health, are associated with a better body image. Negative reasons, such as wanting to achieve a very low weight or improve appearance, are more commonly associated with a negative body image and poorer exercise adherence. Suggest positive reasons for exercise as much as possible.

Help clients see progress. Look for valuable changes, such as better mood, more energy, and less stress. Point out how clients are lifting more weight or working at a higher intensity. Help them set short-term, reachable goals.

Encourage positive thinking, but don't promise unrealistic results. How much can appearance really change? Yes, people can lose a little fat, but usually not very much. They may get stronger and develop better muscle tone. But, except for a few unusual cases as featured in the media, changes in appearance are often not that significant. Yet healthful effects, such as improved blood pressure and blood sugar regulation, are still occurring.

improvements in physical fitness appear to be important, along with feeling successful regarding one's participation, however that may be defined.

Exercise and Sleep

Sleep needs and sleeping behavior vary from person to person. In general, adults need about 7 to 8 hours of sleep per night, and adolescents need an hour more. Sleep problems are common in all age groups and in many countries around the world. Sleep deficits have deleterious effects on many cognitive functions, including memory, reasoning, and decision-making. Many accidents result from fatigue associated with lack of sleep. Sleeping problems also have a negative effect on emotional health because fatigue increases feelings of stress, irritability, depression, and other negative emotional states. Lack of sleep is associated with higher levels of the hormone ghrelin, which increases feelings of hunger, and may lead to overeating and risk of obesity.

Insomnia refers to the inability to get an adequate amount of good-quality sleep. Insomnia is usually marked by difficulty falling asleep or waking during the night and being unable to get back to sleep. Insomnia is not the same thing as running a sleep deficit because of not allowing oneself to get adequate sleep (students pulling all-nighters take note), although many of the negative physical and psychological health effects are the same. Common symptoms of insomnia include the following:

- Trouble falling asleep
- Waking frequently during the night
- Difficulty getting back to sleep once awake
- Waking too early in the morning
- Daytime fatigue

Insomnia may occur for many reasons. It is often the side effect of medications, caffeine, nicotine, and other stimulants. Feelings of stress are frequently responsible for sleep problems. People suffering from chronic insomnia (insomnia lasting more than a few nights) should see their health-care providers if insomnia does not respond to the usual lifestyle change measures. Sometimes insomnia is a symptom of a larger problem that should receive medical attention.

Effects of Exercise on Sleep Quality

Epidemiological studies generally find an association between regular physical activity and sleep quality (Youngstedt & Kline, 2006). Teasing out causative relationships in such studies is difficult, of course, and such studies provide a great example of how many variables interact to affect each other. Does exercise cause psychophysiological changes that enable good sleep? Or do people who sleep well feel rested enough to exercise the next day? Researchers have suggested that if exercise occurs outdoors, natural light may help normalize circadian rhythm and thus promote better sleep. It is also possible that people who exercise may have other healthy behaviors that enhance sleep quality, perhaps drinking less coffee or alcohol, not smoking, and not overeating before bed, which can disrupt sleep quality.

Cross-sectional studies also show that in general, people who exercise tend to sleep better (Brand et al., 2010). Of course, the same variables that may be at work in the epidemiological studies may exert an influence in cross-sectional studies.

Experimental studies that have administered exercise treatments to subjects and examined changes in sleep produce few results if the subjects are young and healthy, with a low incidence of sleep problems (Gerber, Brand, Holsboer-Trachsler, & Puhse, 2010). People without sleep problems appear unlikely to benefit further with the addition of regular physical activity to their days. The largest effects of exercise on improvements in sleep quality have been seen in studies of older adults with mild-to-moderate sleep problems. For example, one well-controlled study found that subjects in the exercise group reported improvement on subjective and objective measures of sleep quality (Buman, Helker, Bliwise, & King, 2011). The greatest area of improvement noted in this study was that individuals reported less variation in their ability to fall asleep, although the average time to fall asleep for people did not change. This observation suggests that regular exercise may have reduced the number of "bad nights" in which people took a long time to fall asleep. Sometimes a bad night or two is followed by an easy time falling asleep the next night. So smoothing out this variation can lead to better sleep quality. Other studies suggest that reducing this variation is associated with higher levels of positive affect the following day (McCrae, 2008).

Exercise is probably most helpful as part of a comprehensive sleep-hygiene program. An interesting study by Kathryn Reid (2010) found that exercise treatment combined with sleep-hygiene education improved sleep duration, the ability to fall asleep, and subjective satisfaction with sleep in older adults with chronic insomnia. Subjects who exercised (compared with controls who attended museums, cooking classes, and other interesting activities three to five times a week) also experienced greater reductions in symptoms of depression and reduced daytime sleepiness, along with increased scores for vitality.

Variables and Mechanisms Associated With Exercise Effects on Sleep Quality

Regular physical activity seems to improve sleep the most for those with mild-to-moderate sleep problems. Older adults often appear as subjects in exercise and sleep studies because they frequently experience problems with sleep, but exercise may help reduce symptoms of insomnia in other age groups as well. Exercise probably exerts an effect through several mechanisms, depending on the exercise situation (Fig. 3-12).

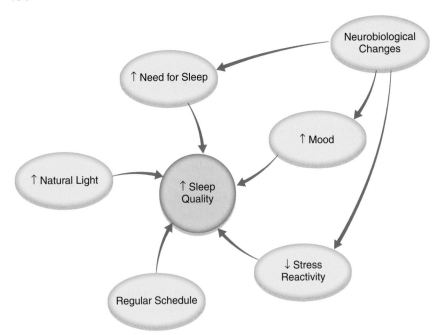

Figure 3-12. Factors that may mediate the effect of exercise on sleep quality.

- Increasing the body's need for restorative sleep. Sleep provides an opportunity for healing and restoration. Exercise increases the need to repair damaged muscles and replenish energy stores.
- Improving mood and reducing feelings of stress. Improvements in psychophysiological state may be the most important contribution of exercise to sleep quality. Many of the neurobiological mechanisms discussed in previous sections on mood and stress, such as changes in neurotransmitter pathways, may contribute to better sleep.
- Establishing a regular schedule. While research evidence is lacking for this variable, researchers in this area often mention the possibility that getting exercise during the day may help establish a regular routine, especially for older adults. A regular routine is an important component of sleep hygiene.
- Increasing exposure to natural light. Exposure to natural light during the day strengthens circadian rhythm and thus the sleep cycle.

Exercise Recommendations for Improving Sleep Quality

Sleep quality improvement with exercise was observed in studies that administered exercise programs in line with current public health recommendations of at least 30 minutes of moderately vigorous exercise most days of the week, although some studies have used lower doses and still observed significant effects. Both strength training and aerobic exercise have been associated with improvements in sleep. Because one of the mechanisms for improving sleep may involve stress reduction, health and fitness professionals should follow the previous exercise recommendations for reducing stress. Health and fitness professionals should suggest to clients with sleep issues that they may see improved sleep quality as they

begin exercising. Exercise dosage should be adjusted depending on a person's fitness level, time availability, activity preferences, and health concerns.

■ *Oh my, what a week! Melissa's coworker has left her job, and Melissa is trying to pick up the slack. She leaves work late, feels very stressed, and decides to go grocery shopping instead of attending the line-dancing class that she has been enjoying for several weeks. Melissa rushes through her shopping and arrives home. The kitchen is a mess, and she snaps at her son when he comes to ask her a question about his homework. "You must have skipped your exercise class!" he says. "Usually you come home singing, rather than yelling."*

Melissa takes a deep breath and prepares a quick meal. But, while she is cooking, she feels agitated and irritable. She realizes that her son is right: things like the messy kitchen do not get to her so much after her exercise class. That is interesting. She does not sleep very well that night. In the morning, she resolves to leave work on time and take a walk before dinner . . . and not to miss any more line-dancing classes. What was it Victor told her to say? "I am feeling stressed and tired; therefore, I must get some exercise right away to feel better!" ■

Exercise, Memory, and Cognitive Function

The adult brain contains about 100 billion nerve cells, or neurons, and 1,000 billion neuroglia, which are cells of the nervous system that perform a number of supportive functions. The cells of the brain communicate with each other and with the rest of the body by neurotransmitters sent from cell to cell and by hormones sent and received through the bloodstream and the cerebrospinal fluid.

With aging, the number of neurons in the brain declines, as does the number of synapses formed between cells. A gradual decline in short-term memory and a slowing of cognitive function begins in mid-adulthood. Adults have slower reflexes and information processing than children and teens. The evidence of cognitive defects is more striking in the elderly, who generally take much longer to learn a new task or understand new information than younger adults. Research suggests that many of the changes in brain structure and function observed with the aging process are mediated by a number of lifestyle variables, including level of physical activity.

Physical Activity and Brain Structure and Function

Several epidemiological and cross-sectional studies have found associations between physical activity and brain functions such as memory and learning. A recent meta-analysis found modest relationships between aerobic exercise training and improvements in attention, processing speed, executive function, and memory in humans (Smith et al., 2010). Executive function refers to processes that are involved in future-oriented behavior, such as planning, multitasking, setting priorities, and coping with distractions.

A study by Andel and colleagues examined the association between physical-activity level in midlife with the risk of dementia 30 years later (Andel et al., 2008). This study was particularly valuable because the investigators controlled for the effects of other variables known to affect risk for dementia, such as alcohol intake, smoking, diet, body mass index, age, and education. The researchers found that people who were exercising in midlife had a lower risk of developing dementia 30 years later.

An interesting study of college students found that a single bout of aerobic exercise (30 minutes of running) improved working memory 30 minutes after the exercise session (Pontifex, Hillman, Fernhall, Thompson, & Valentini, 2009). The experiment subjected students to three conditions on three separate days: sitting quietly, 30 minutes of running, and 30 minutes of weight training. The students performed a working memory test before and then 30 minutes after the end of the treatment conditions. The test consisted of memorizing a string of letters and then selecting the correct sequence from a list flashed at them. The students performed significantly better after the running condition but not after the other two conditions.

Variables and Mechanisms Associated With Exercise Effects on Memory and Cognitive Function

Scientists have identified many variables that may help explain the effect of exercise on memory and cognitive function (Fig. 3-13). One of these is the health of the circulatory system feeding the brain. Physical activity

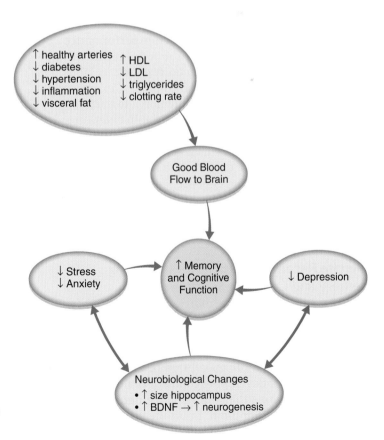

Figure 3-13. Factors that may mediate the effect of exercise on memory and cognitive function.

may help preserve the health of the arteries supplying the brain.

Exercise may also prevent memory loss by reducing feelings of stress. Animal studies have shown that high levels of severe chronic stress are associated with significant reduction in the size of the hippocampus, an important area for memory. The reduction in size may be due to cell death and/or reduction in neuron size (Lucassen et al., 2010). Exercise appears to increase the size of the hippocampus in both humans and laboratory animals. An interesting study in 120 older adults (aged 55 to 80) assigned subjects to year-long exercise programs (Erickson, 2011). One group participated in aerobic exercise, building up to walking 40 minutes a day, 3 days a week. The second group performed nonaerobic calisthenics and yoga. Subjects received functional magnetic resonance imaging (fMRI) brain scans, memory tests, blood tests, and fitness tests at the beginning, middle, and end of the study.

Subjects in the aerobic exercise group demonstrated slight increases (about 2%) in their hippocampal areas, whereas the same areas of the other group declined slightly (almost 1.5%), a significant difference. The researchers also found an association between improvements in aerobic fitness and an increase in hippocampal volume. In the aerobic exercise group, the blood levels of an important protein called brain-derived neurotrophic factor (BDNF) were correlated with larger increases in hippocampal volume. BDNF plays a role in stimulating the formation of new brain cells, a process called neurogenesis, from stem cells or precursor cells in the brain. In the aerobic exercise group, increased hippocampal volume was also associated with better performance on the memory tests. Although the numbers in this study were fairly small, they echo research in laboratory animals on the relationships among exercise, BDNF, hippocampal volume, and memory. Research on mice has shown that exercise changes brain chemistry, even in middle-aged animals, producing conditions that promote stem and precursor cell proliferation and maturation into new neurons in the brain (Wu et al., 2008). Exercise appears to enhance signaling molecules promoting new cell production and blocking other factors that inhibit neuron production and maturation (Gobeske et al., 2009).

Exercise Recommendations for Improving Memory and Cognitive Function

Animal studies suggest that more exercise is better for generating new brain cells. Studies in humans have tended to focus on moderate amounts of aerobic exercise. It is likely that general public health guidelines are sufficient to promote good brain health by reducing inflammation, developing good artery health, and providing conditions that can enhance neurogenesis in the brain. For optimal brain health, exercise throughout life is important. Because exercise exerts acute as well as chronic effects on memory, people can benefit from regular physical exercise at all ages.

Exercise and Anxiety

Anxiety refers to feelings of worry, self-doubt, and fearful uncertainty about the future. Anxiety is a useful feeling when it motivates people to deal with problems causing anxiety. For example, anxiety about a physical symptom may motivate people to seek medical attention and receive treatment for medical conditions. Anxiety about an upcoming exam may motivate students to study. In many cases, addressing the problem reduces the feelings of anxiety. Anxiety is a close cousin of stress. Many people experience anxiety as a symptom of stress. The word anxiety is often used to describe feelings of worry and stress.

When is anxiety a problem? Like feelings of stress, feelings of anxiety are a normal part of life for most people. Anxiety can be viewed as occurring along a continuum from occasional, mild feelings of anxiety to full-blown clinical anxiety disorders. Anxiety becomes a problem when it occurs frequently, arises without a real reason for fear, becomes a chronic state of mind, contributes to health problems such as high blood pressure, or interferes with ADLs. Clinical anxiety disorders are diagnosed when anxiety becomes excessive and uncontrollable, arises without a specific reason, and results in problematic changes in behavior and thinking. For example, fear of a panic attack may cause people to never leave their homes. Or excessive feelings of fear can interfere with a student's ability to perform well on an exam. Box 3-4 summarizes the most common types of anxiety disorders. According to the National Institute of Mental Health (2010), in 2005–2008 approximately 18% of U.S. adults were diagnosed with an anxiety disorder every year (12-month prevalence), and about 29% of U.S. adults will be diagnosed with an anxiety disorder at some point during their lives (lifetime prevalence). Women are 60% more likely than men to be diagnosed with an anxiety disorder.

Psychologists differentiate mental health symptoms into chronic and acute categories. When anxiety is a part of a person's personality profile and is a fairly common and enduring characteristic, psychologists refer to this as trait anxiety. People with trait anxiety generally respond to challenges with feelings of anxiety and typical fight-or-flight symptoms such an increased HR, sweating, and muscle tension. In response to diagnostic questionnaires about how they generally feel, they would be more likely to say that they tend to worry rather than they tend to feel relaxed. When anxiety arises for a short period of time but then resolves, psychologists refer to this as state anxiety. Everyone experiences state anxiety from time to time. Health and fitness instructors often see clients who are anxious about exercise and can ease this anxiety with education, clear explanations, and programs that build success. However, health and fitness instructors must learn

Box 3-4. Characteristics of Common
Anxiety Disorders

Generalized Anxiety Disorder
- Frequent experiences of fear most days, for at least 3 months
- Excessive anxiety about a variety of situations
- Feeling unable to control feelings of anxiety, which creates more anxiety
- Physical and behavioral symptoms such as insomnia, muscle tension, and fatigue

Phobias
- Excessive fear of something not regarded by most people as worthy of excessive fear, such as spiders, exams, or snakes
- Changes in behavior, as people attempt to avoid encountering the object of their phobia
- Distress because of worrying about the phobia or because behavior to avoid the phobia interferes with performance or quality of life
- A phobia of exams or public speaking can occur in college students and block performance on these important tasks

Panic Disorder
- Experience of panic attacks. A panic attack is a short, intense period of fear. People often feel they are dying. A panic attack is marked by a strong fight-or-flight response, with a rapid, pounding HR, sweating, trembling, and nausea. During a panic attack, people often feel the need for "flight" to escape a situation.
- Preoccupation with worrying about having a panic attack, especially in public.
- Changes in behavior because of worrying about panic attacks. People with panic disorder often develop agoraphobia.
- Panic disorder occurs in college student populations. Feelings of anxiety can lead to a fight-or-flight response, which leads to more anxiety and full-blown panic attacks. Feelings of fear snowball, as fear of fear feeds on itself to produce panic.

Agoraphobia
- Fear of being in situations from which one cannot escape if a panic attack strikes, such as in public situations or in transportation situations (on airplanes, trains, buses, etc.). Students with agoraphobia may fear going to class and not being able to leave.
- Changes in behavior as a result of anxiety, such as being unable to leave one's home. Students may stop attending class.

Source
American Psychiatric Association. (2013). *The Diagnostic and Statistical Manual of Mental Disorders*, 5th ed. Washington, DC: American Psychiatric Association.

to recognize when clients have mental health disorders that require referral to a mental health specialist (Box 3-5).

The Effect of Exercise on Anxiety

Interpreting research on the effects of physical activity on anxiety symptoms should be done with caution because there are so many types of anxiety disorders. Most of the research has focused on generalized anxiety disorder and panic disorder, although the effect of exercise on the other anxiety disorders has been studied as well. In addition, the effect of exercise on feelings of anxiety in people not diagnosed with anxiety disorders has yielded interesting results. Overall, exercise is generally helpful for reducing feelings of anxiety in most population groups.

Box 3-5. Mental Health Disorders and Your Scope of Practice

Although it is appropriate for health and fitness professionals to promote the positive emotional health benefits of physical activity, make sure that you do not slip into the role of therapist. Personal trainers are especially likely to be invited into their clients' personal lives, as conversation develops during workouts. But always maintain your professional distance and monitor your level of involvement, never diagnosing illness or recommending treatment.

When clients complain about stress and their problems, you can certainly listen with a sympathetic ear. Clients may even share the fact that they are exercising with you because they hope to reduce symptoms of depression. That is fine. You may discuss with them how studies have found that exercise may help reduce feelings of stress, anxiety, and depression for many people, keeping the focus on general research findings, rather than framing your remarks as your recommendations for their health problems. If clients convey the idea that depression or other emotional health problems are a significant force in their lives, or are interfering with their ability to function, suggest that they seek professional psychological guidance.

Many health and fitness professionals have had the sense that certain clients were beginning to lean too heavily on them. Some have even fallen gradually into a "helping" relationship where clients were calling them at all hours when feeling stressed or lonely. It is natural to want to be helpful, but realize you are not helping if you keep clients from getting professional help. Talk the situation over with your supervisor. And don't be afraid to discontinue your relationship with a troubled client if you are getting in over your head.

Just as a single bout of exercise tends to improve mood, it also tends to reduce anxiety levels. Reviews of the literature suggest that in most studies, people generally report lower levels of anxiety following exercise, as compared with pre-exercise levels (Strohle, 2009). These studies tend to overlap with studies of the effect of acute exercise on positive and negative affect, and they verify the tendency of acute exercise to increase positive affect and reduce negative affect, including feelings of anxiety. These effects, previously found in the population at large, have also been demonstrated in patients with anxiety disorders (e.g., Knapen et al., 2009).

A meta-analysis of randomized trials investigating the effects of exercise on anxiety concluded that exercise is as effective as psychotherapy and almost as effective as medication in reducing anxiety symptoms (Wipfli, Rethorst, & Landers, 2008). The results of this analysis suggest that anxiety symptoms can decline even without a significant increase in measures of physical fitness. Similarly, no particular amount or type of exercise stood out as the most strongly related to anxiety symptom reduction (Wipfli, et al., 2008). Another analysis examining the effect of exercise training on anxiety symptoms in patients with chronic illness also found a significant association (Herring, O'Connor, & Dishman, 2010). This is good news, as many patients with chronic illness develop symptoms of anxiety due to worry about their illnesses. Exercise is often recommended for chronic illness and may reduce anxiety symptoms even as it helps treat illness. Although exercise appears to reduce anxiety symptoms in all age groups, some studies suggest that physical activity is especially effective in older people (Youngstedt, 2010).

Variables and Mechanisms Associated With Exercise Effects on Anxiety

The same variables associated with improvements in stress response following exercise probably apply to anxiety reduction. In humans, anxiety is associated with many variables that also mediate the effect of exercise (Fig. 3-14), including the following.

- Improvements in self-esteem, self-confidence, and self-efficacy. When people feel more capable of coping with sources of stress, they sometimes feel less generalized anxiety.
- Changes in neurobiological pathways. The endorphin, endocannabinoid, and other neurotransmitter pathways discussed earlier in this chapter may be part of the explanation for the anxiolytic (anxiety-reducing) effects of physical activity.
- Increased levels of BDNF. Studies in humans have found that BDNF levels are lower in those with anxiety and depressive disorders. One very interesting study compared BDNF levels in people who have panic disorder with levels in normal controls both before and after 30 minutes of exercise (Strohle et al., 2010). BDNF levels were lower in people with panic disorder before exercise. Happily, following exercise their BDNF levels reached those of the normal controls.
- Changes in epigenetic regulation of gene expression. Studies in rats suggest regular physical activity causes epigenetic changes that alter gene expression (Gomez-Pinilla, Zhuang, Feng, Ying, & Fan, 2011). Some of these may be responsible for changes in neurotransmitter pathways and regulation of BDNF, for example.

Exercise Recommendations for Reducing Anxiety

No strong dose-response effect has been reported for exercise and anxiety reduction. While most studies have examined aerobic activity of moderate duration and intensity in line with public health recommendations, strength training and activities such as yoga and tai chi

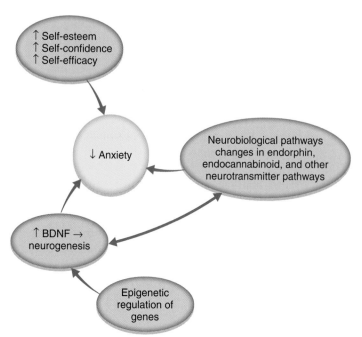

Figure 3-14. Factors that may mediate the effect of exercise on anxiety.

also appear to be effective in reducing anxiety. Because exercise performed at an individual's preferred pace may be best for improving positive affect, it makes sense for health and fitness professionals to work with individuals to establish the most effective exercise recommendations that not only work best to reduce feelings of anxiety but also improve exercise adherence (Box 3-6).

It has been another long day at work and, as Melissa gets into her car, she is thinking, "I am too busy to do the line-dancing class. No, that is not what I am supposed to say. I am supposed to say, 'I am feeling stressed and tired; therefore, I must get some exercise right away to feel better!' Okay, I will go." Her heart is not in it, but she remembers snapping at her son the other day.

Victor is smiling and seems so happy to see her. Melissa cannot resist smiling back. Just smiling makes her feel better! Another member of the class tells her she missed Melissa earlier in the week and wonders if she is okay. Melissa explains about work but that she knows she needs the class more than ever when she is feeling stressed out. Music, movement, Victor laughing and telling jokes. Where does he get the energy? Melissa feels the anxiety leave her body as her spirits lift. As she says good-bye to Victor after the class, she thanks him for helping her change the way she thinks. She adds, "I really feel so much better after this class!"

Box 3-6. When Exercise Feels Like Panic

Occasionally, clients may report feeling anxious in response to exercise symptoms, such as elevations in HR. This is especially likely in patients who experience anxiety, panic disorder, or less-severe problems involving occasional feelings of panic. When examined closely, exercise does bear a resemblance to panic: higher HR and faster breathing rate, higher systolic blood pressure, increased muscle tension, and sweating. With panic, such symptoms are perceived to be problematic, which leads to fear and an even higher HR and other symptoms as clients struggle to maintain control. Clients who are sensitive to elevations in HR or other exercise symptoms may need to begin exercise programs using activities with a fairly low level of intensity until they can tolerate, and hopefully enjoy, activities with a higher intensity. Such clients may be fine with low-intensity strength training and low-intensity aerobic activities. They may enjoy walking, biking, or swimming at slower paces that do not result in high HRs or other problematic symptoms.

Exercise and Depression

Depression is a mental health disorder marked by both mental and physical symptoms (Box 3-7). Symptoms of depression vary from person to person. In general, depression is diagnosed when people experience a number of symptoms, including prolonged feelings of sadness or anxiety, hopelessness, guilt, or worthlessness; or loss of interest or pleasure in activities once enjoyed. Depression may be severe or mild and last for weeks or years. Many people suffer from a combination of both depression and anxiety.

According to the National Institute of Mental Health (2010), in 2005–2008, over 6% of adults in

Box 3-7. Characteristics of Common Depressive Disorders and Bipolar Disorder

Major Depressive Disorder
Major depressive disorder is diagnosed when a person shows five symptoms in the list below, symptoms have continued for at least 2 weeks, and he or she has experienced a change in ability to function in daily life. Symptoms include the following:
- Depressed mood much of the time and/or inability to enjoy and loss of interest in activities previously perceived as interesting or pleasurable. This is the primary symptom of depressive disorders.
- Changes in appetite and weight
- Difficulty sleeping, or sleeping more
- Fatigue, lack of energy
- Feelings of guilt, worthlessness
- Feelings of hopelessness
- Difficulty concentrating
- Recurrent thoughts of death or suicide

Dysthymic Disorder (Dysthymia)
Dysthymia is a chronic, less-intense form of depression. Although less disabling than major depression, dysthymia causes the person to feel unwell or to function at less-than-optimal levels. Symptoms include a depressed mood a majority of the time and two or more of the symptoms listed above, with symptoms having continued for at least 2 years.

Bipolar Disorder (Manic-Depressive Disorder)
Bipolar disorder is diagnosed when depressive symptoms alternate with periods of extremely elevated mood (mania).

Source
American Psychiatric Association. (2013). *The Diagnostic and Statistical Manual of Mental Disorders*, 5th ed. Washington, DC: American Psychiatric Association.

the United States were diagnosed with major depressive disorder every year (12-month prevalence). An estimated 9.5% of U.S. adults were diagnosed with all forms of depression, which include major depressive disorder (also 12-month prevalence). Approximately 20% of adults in the United States will be diagnosed with a depressive disorder at some point during their lives. Depression rates are about 70% higher in women than men (NIMH, 2010). The prevalence of depressive disorders has doubled since the 1990s (Compton, Conway, Stinson, & Grant, 2006). This increase has occurred across all demographic groups, including whites, blacks, and Hispanics, and for almost all age groups, including children and adolescents.

Depression is a debilitating disorder that interferes with every aspect of a person's life. The combination of fatigue, negative mood, and inability to feel pleasure result in a downward spiral of doing less and feeling worse. The best thing for people who are depressed is to get out and do things, but people with depression often have difficulty summoning the desire or energy to do the things that might help them feel better (like exercise). Although regular physical activity helps reduce symptoms of depression, people with depression face huge emotional hurdles when attempting to stick to an exercise program.

The Effect of Exercise on Depression

Many people have wondered whether the mood-elevation effects of exercise might help people with depression. The answer appears to be a cautious maybe for some people, some of the time. Large-scale analyses of research evaluating the effects of exercise on depressive symptoms in normal and clinically depressed people suggest that exercise is about as effective as psychotherapy or medication (Blumenthal & Ong, 2009; Mead et al., 2009; Rethorst, Wipfli, & Landers, 2009). Then why the cautious qualifications above? Depression is notoriously difficult to treat and has high rates of recurrence. Researchers do not yet understand the causes of depression; thus, treatment recommendations are limited by this incomplete understanding. Although one might cheer that exercise is as effective as other treatments, it is important to note that many people do not respond adequately to any available treatment.

Studies show that sedentary behavior is associated with increased risk for depression, whereas regular physical activity is associated with reduced risk (Teychenne, Ball, & Salmon, 2010). Because depression is characterized by a lack of motivation to engage in activities, one might speculate that depression might be causing the sedentary behavior, and this may be true in many cases. However, it is also likely that people who are physically active are more resistant to developing depression than people who stay home and resort to sedentary activities such as watching a lot of television.

A number of interesting studies have examined the effect of increasing the physical-activity level for people with symptoms of depression. Because depression is such a complex illness, results for exercise effects have been mixed. A meta-analysis of randomized trials did find that subjects in the exercise treatment groups experienced on average a greater decline in depressive symptoms than subjects in the control groups (Rethorst et al., 2009). The result held for studies looking at both people diagnosed with depressive disorders as well as for people without diagnosed disorders. The most clinically significant studies were focused on people diagnosed with mild-to-moderate depression. Rethorst and colleagues examined 16 high-quality research studies that compared exercise versus control treatment groups of subjects diagnosed with depression. Of the 16 studies, average depression scores for the exercise treatment groups in nine of the studies were classified as "recovered," and the scores for the exercise treatment groups in three of the studies were "improved" (Rethorst et al., 2009). This means that although not every subject in the exercise treatment group recovered or improved, on average the group scores indicated recovery or improvement. Such improvements suggest that it is worth recommending exercise for people with depression. Even though many practitioners worry that patients with depression do not have the energy or drive to exercise, Rethorst and colleagues noted that the dropout rates for subjects in the exercise groups were observed to be similar to dropout rates for patients in the medication or psychotherapy treatment programs.

Although the results of the previous meta-analysis as well as other meta-analyses are fairly positive, it is important to recognize the limitations of studies on exercise for depression. One of the most significant limitations is that all subjects used in every study were volunteers (Blumenthal & Ong, 2009). Research has shown that volunteers differ significantly from the rest of the population. This holds true for every study ever conducted, not just studies of depression. But, in the field of depression research, this difference exerts an even stronger effect on the application of results. Depression is characterized by low energy and a lack of ability to get involved in activities. Volunteers probably have at least the beginning of a desire to get better as well as the energy and wherewithal to get to the researchers' laboratory or office. People who adhere to their treatment plans, especially a plan such as an exercise program that requires a significant commitment of time and energy, are more likely to experience at least a spark of hope that can be fanned into the flames of recovery. This is likely not true for everyone suffering from depressive disorders.

The effect of exercise on depressive symptoms in humans may be mediated in part by genetics. Certain combinations of genes may help predict which people are most likely to respond to depression treatments. For example, certain genes involved in the regulation of serotonin kinetics in the CNS appear to be related to depressed subjects' response to both medications and physical activity (Rethorst, Landers, Nagoshi, & Ross, 2010). The link between genetics and response to a variety of treatments is being investigated for a large range of illnesses. It is likely that in the future genetic profiles will help health-care providers better match treatments to individual patients.

The consensus among researchers in the area of depression and exercise is that regular physical activity is certainly worth a try. Many people with depression experience significant improvement in their symptoms with exercise. And, because exercise generally improves physical health (which can itself make people feel better), advising people with depression to increase physical activity level makes sense. Exercise is often recommended as part of a comprehensive depression treatment program that may also include psychotherapy and possibly medication.

Variables and Mechanisms Associated With Exercise Effects on Depression

Many variables and mechanisms may help explain the effect of exercise on symptoms of depression (Fig. 3-15). These include the following.

- Changes in activity patterns. One of the most problematic symptoms of depression is the tendency to disengage from people and to stop participating in activities. People with severe depressive disorders sometimes rarely leave their homes and have extreme difficulty just getting out of bed. When feeling bad leads to disengagement and lack of activity, bad feelings worsen, and the downward spiral of depression becomes even harder to reverse. If people are able to get

out and engage in activities, including physical activities, just getting out begins to reverse this problematic symptom of holing up alone at home.
- Reductions in anxiety symptoms. Many people with depression also suffer from anxiety. They may feel both nervous and worried as well as unmotivated and exhausted—not a pleasant combination. If exercise reduces feelings of anxiety, symptoms of depression may improve.
- Improved self-esteem, self-confidence, and body image. Another problematic symptom of depression is the feeling of worthlessness. Depression often manifests as low self-confidence and low self-esteem. Poor body image often accompanies these feelings. Exercise participation helps improve self-esteem, self-confidence, and body image, and research suggests that symptoms of depression may improve as a result of these changes (Ryan, 2008).
- Improvement in mood. Feeling good helps in elevating a person's mood. Improvements in energy level and a reduction in feelings of fatigue can be especially beneficial for people with depression, since depression is usually marked by fatigue.
- Better sleep quality. A disruption in sleep behavior is a common symptom of depression. People with depression often have difficulty falling and staying asleep. If exercise improves sleep quality, then this symptom of depression may become less severe.
- Changes in endorphin and endocannabinoid pathways. Endorphin pathways appear to play

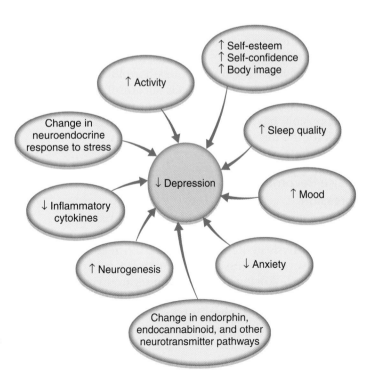

Figure 3-15. Factors that may mediate the effect of exercise on depression.

important roles in stress response and other regulatory systems involved in depression (Hegadoren, O'Donnell, Lanius, Coupland, & Lacaze-Masmonteil, 2009). Research in both humans and animals continues to reinforce the importance of endorphins and endocannabinoids in the psychophysiology of mood and mood disorders. Exercise appears to affect the production of these molecules as well as receptor response.

- Changes in other neurotransmitter pathways. Several neurotransmitter systems seem to be impaired by depressive illnesses. Exercise may exert salutary effects on depression by improving serotonin, dopamine, norepinephrine, and other neurotransmitter systems.
- Increased neurogenesis. Some types of antidepressants seem to exert their effects by stimulating neurogenesis. Since exercise has also been shown to increase neurogenesis, this mechanism may be one of the ways in which exercise helps relieve symptoms of depression (Lucassen et al., 2010).
- Reductions in inflammatory cytokines. An increase in inflammatory cytokine levels has been observed in people with depression. Some researchers have hypothesized that these proinflammatory substances may play a role in the onset and development of depressive symptoms (Hallberg et al., 2010). Studies have found that exercise reduces blood levels of these cytokines in people with depression (Hallberg et al., 2010).
- Changes in endocrine response to stress. People with depression have a number of physiological differences in their responses to stress compared with people not suffering from depression. Some evidence suggests that regular physical activity may improve endocrine response to stress for people with depression, increasing levels of norepinephrine (indicating a less-harmful stress response) and decreasing levels of cortisol. Elevated levels of cortisol, seen in some people with depression, have been associated with increased risk for the negative health effects associated with stress.

Exercise Recommendations for Reducing Depression

Exercise seems to have the greatest depression-reducing effects in people with mild-to-moderate depression. The meta-analysis by Rethorst et al. (2009) regarding the response of depression symptoms to exercise examined the following variables with regard to exercise recommendations. No particular type of exercise emerged as the clear winner, although a combination of aerobic and strength exercise appeared slightly more effective than aerobic exercise alone. Exercise sessions lasting 20 to 29 minutes were more effective than

longer sessions at reducing depression symptoms for nonclinical populations. (Nonclinical populations include people experiencing some depression symptoms but not at a level required for diagnosis with full-blown depressive disorders.) On the other hand, for people already diagnosed with depression, more exercise was better. Sessions lasting 45 to 59 minutes were more effective than shorter sessions. Health and fitness professionals should interpret this result with care, however. Motivation for exercise is a significant problem for people with depression and, although long exercise durations may be the most effective, they may be unapproachable for many, especially those beginning an exercise program.

Among nonclinical subjects, exercise intensities representing 61% to 74% of maximal HR were more effective than lower or higher intensities. However, for clinical populations, exercise intensity did not appear to be significantly related to symptoms of depression. Although only one study reviewed in this meta-analysis used an exercise treatment with a frequency of 5 days a week, clinically depressed subjects improved more in this study than in studies using lower exercise frequencies. In summary, the results above support general public health guidelines for exercise when recommending exercise for people with depressive symptoms and for people already diagnosed with clinical depression.

Negative Psychological Consequences of Physical Activity

This chapter would not be complete without noting that in addition to the exercise benefits presented above, exercise can become part of a compulsive behavior pattern for some people. Physical activity can become a way for people with eating disorders to purge calories. Compulsive exercise behavior and eating disorders are discussed in more detail in Chapter 11 in the context of addictions. Psychologists have noted that exercise, per se, is not really the problem. Rather, people struggling with stress and other difficult psychological issues may turn to exercise for a sense of stability and control.

EXERCISE RECOMMENDATIONS AND GUIDELINES

The discussion included in this chapter underlines the importance of regular physical activity for the promotion of optimal physical and psychological health and well-being. How much exercise is necessary for achieving all these benefits? The answer to this question, of course, depends on many variables. The right amount of exercise for an athlete training for the Olympics is different from the amount of exercise recommended for a person recovering from a heart attack.

Public health and professional organizations have reviewed thousands of research studies examining the effects of a wide range of types and amounts of exercise on fitness and health in various population groups. Over the past several decades, guidelines aimed at the general public have been written and extensively reviewed and revised (Pratt, Epping, & Dietz, 2009). Exercise physiologists and exercise psychologists have also worked to devise guidelines for health and fitness professionals working with individual clients, to guide exercise prescription for healthy people of all ages as well as for people diagnosed with physical or psychological illnesses.

The Public Health Perspective

Public health scientists have had endless discussions reviewing studies on the relationship of physical activity to health and have attempted to balance their recommendations, based on the best possible exercise programs, with what real people actually do. The goal of public health recommendations is to get the greatest return for a given recommendation. Public health officials are more concerned with getting more people to do a moderate amount of exercise, which result in the greatest overall gains in health for the population, than in getting active people to diversify their programs or to better use their time to meet individual fitness goals.

Public Health Recommendations for Physical Activity

Early exercise recommendations from the 1970s were somewhat complicated, in that they spelled out exercise intensity recommendations in terms of target HRs and included several categories of physical activity that should be performed. People reading these recommendations often lost interest halfway through, reluctant to spend time calculating target HR or following complicated instructions. In response, public health exercise recommendations no longer contain target HR calculations and advice has been simplified (Fig. 3-16). Leading exercise-promotion organizations have also worked together to reach consensus on their recommendations to reduce public confusion. These recommendations do a good job of laying out guidelines that are encouraging and easy to understand, and evidence suggests that people who adhere to these guidelines are significantly healthier than their sedentary peers (What's the Evidence? 3-1).

These guidelines for adults aged 18 to 64 can be found at the CDC's website.

- 2 hours and 30 minutes of moderate-intensity aerobic activity (e.g., brisk walking) every week, and
- Muscle strengthening exercises at least 2 days a week that use all the major muscle groups (legs, hips, back, abdomen, chest, shoulders, and arms)

------ OR ------

- 1 hour and 15 minutes of vigorous-intensity aerobic activity (e.g., jogging or running) every week, and
- Muscle strengthening (as described above)

------ OR ------

- An equivalent mix of moderate and vigorous aerobic activity, and
- Muscle strengthening

Moderate intensity is described as being hard enough so that you are breathing harder and breaking a sweat. You can talk but not sing. Vigorous intensity is described as breathing hard and fast, with your HR up quite a bit, and unable to say more than a few words without pausing to catch your breath.

Figure 3-16. Physical activity guidelines. *(From Centers for Disease Control and Prevention, with permission.)*

WHAT'S THE EVIDENCE? 3-1

Physical Activity Level and Health Outcomes

Haskell, W. L., Blair, S. N., & Hill, J. O. (2009). Physical activity: health outcomes and importance for public health policy. *Preventive Medicine, 49*(4): 280-282.

■ **PURPOSE**

The researchers sought to summarize the relationship between activity level and mortality and to explore whether public health recommendations regarding exercise are effective in practice.

■ **STUDY**

This is a review article, which means that the authors have reviewed many studies and drawn conclusions based on the combined data. These data derived from prospective studies of 252,925 men and women aged 50 to 71. Using standard biostatistical procedures, the data analyses performed attempted to isolate the relationship of physical activity level and mortality rates, removing the important effects of other variables such as age, education, gender, and fruit and vegetable intake. Subjects were divided into groups according to whether and how they were meeting the public health guidelines for exercise, according to self-reported answers on a questionnaire. One group of subjects was somewhat active but failed to meet public health recommendations. Some were meeting

Continued

WHAT'S THE EVIDENCE? 3-1–cont'd

or exceeding the guidelines by performing only moderate-intensity exercise, some by meeting the recommendations for vigorous exercise, and some by meeting the recommendation for combined moderate and vigorous exercise. The exercise groups were then compared with people who were completely sedentary. The group performing both moderate- and vigorous-intensity exercise had a relative risk for all-cause mortality of about 0.5. This means their risk of death at a given point in time was about half that of the inactive group.

■ **IMPLICATIONS**

This analysis illustrates the striking effect on mortality rate of doing even a little activity. Even the group failing to meet public health guidelines but doing a little exercise had a much lower mortality rate than the inactive group. The data suggested that meeting the public health guidelines for physical activity significantly reduced risk of death.

Public Health Messages and Motivation

Motivating people to become more active is the goal of public health information. A review of public health guidelines reveals many attempts to make physical activity palatable for the general public. Most urge people to select activities that they enjoy and offer other good advice on making physical activity more fun. Some remind readers they can "count" as exercise the more-vigorous ADLs, such as yard work, gardening, and cleaning tasks. They also encourage people who have difficulty exercising for 30 continuous minutes to try several bouts of 10-minute activity instead. Readers may note that these recommendations help build feelings of self-efficacy by making exercise seem doable. Images on the websites about the guidelines usually feature people of all shapes, sizes, ages, and ethnic backgrounds, to help viewers see themselves in the exercise picture. Sites suggest social support (exercising with a friend, either in pictures or as advice), ideas on making a plan, and education on the importance of exercise for good health and weight loss. Positive images of people exercising make exercise look interesting and fun.

MOTIVATING CHANGE: Explain Why Individualized Exercise Recommendations May Not Match Public Health Guidelines

Public health exercise recommendations are confusing to some clients who do not know much about exercise but are doing much more than the recommended minimum. It is common for a client to have worked up to exercising an hour a day several days a week to help address a health issue such as obesity or diabetes. Then a well-intentioned health-care provider comes along and recommends only 30 minutes. Clients come to their personal trainer or other advisor and wonder why they cannot just do 30 minutes a day.

Such situations provide an opportunity for health and fitness professionals to point out the importance of tailoring the exercise recommendations to the individual client's health problems and fitness goals. A one-size-fits-all exercise recommendation is bound to be unfit for many. Explain to your clients that the public health guidelines are meant to get people off the couch and doing something but that clients will gain far greater benefits by sticking to the more-comprehensive recommendations they have been following.

The Health and Fitness Professional's Perspective

Public health guidelines help raise awareness of the importance of physical activity and provide a starting place for picking up the pace, but people often need more education and support than public health guidelines alone can deliver. Individualized exercise recommendations help tailor both the exercise program activities and the motivational approach to the specific needs of individuals and groups and, thus, can more effectively help people increase physical activity levels.

Importance of Individualized Recommendations for Effective Exercise Program Design

The public health recommendations for physical activity described in the previous section apply explicitly to healthy individuals. Individuals with health concerns may need to modify these recommendations. In addition, even healthy individuals vary greatly in their health concerns, fitness goals, and exercise preferences. Individualized exercise programs help people more closely match where they are with where they want to be in terms of health and fitness. Individualized fitness recommendations can help people make the best use of their exercise time. Health and fitness professionals who have studied exercise program design learn how to modify these basic public health recommendations for individual clients.

Individualized exercise recommendations are especially important for people with health limitations or specialized sport performance goals. Although public health guidelines help people achieve overall health, athletes need to follow more specific training protocols to improve power, quickness, agility, or other skills. People training for an endurance event such as a marathon or triathlon need sprint training to improve their metabolic capacities and pace and certainly more than 30 minutes of exercise per day. In addition to individualizing exercise recommendations, health and fitness professionals can tailor their advice to improve the likelihood that clients stick to their exercise programs by helping them design effective action plans and giving them the information and support they need to make their health and fitness top priorities.

Importance of Individualized Recommendations for Motivation and Exercise Adherence

Health and fitness professionals can work with individuals and groups to support exercise behavior change. Although some people successfully increase physical activity by themselves, many respond to interaction with health and fitness professionals. Such professionals can improve people's likelihood of successful behavior change in many ways. They can help clients see the significant personal benefits of participating in regular physical activity, and they can design exercise programs that best meet individual needs and preferences. Health and fitness professionals can help clients understand the factors that hinder and promote exercise behavior, and they can work with clients to design effective strategies to support behavior-change intentions.

Health and fitness professionals can also advise clients regarding injury prevention and help them recognize overuse injuries in their early stages. Because injury is a leading cause of exercise dropout, health and fitness professionals must do everything possible to help clients prevent and cope effectively with exercise injuries.

Three months have passed, and a new session of line dancing is beginning. Two new people are in the class, checking it out before signing up. Melissa smiles, remembering her first day and how much fun the class turned out to be. She talks to some of the other "regulars" before the music begins. "This music is great," she thinks. "The music and the dance combinations take up all my brain power. There is no room for worrying."

After the class, Victor is talking to the newbies. One of them is telling Victor how very busy and stressed she is. Victor calls Melissa over. "Tell her what to say to herself when she is feeling stressed and tired!" Melissa smiles and repeats the mantra Victor taught her 3 months ago: "'I am feeling stressed and tired; therefore, I must get some exercise right away to feel better!' It sure has worked for me!" Melissa tells her.

KEY TERMS

accelerometer

activation

active static stretching

adiposopathy

aerobic exercise

affect

agoraphobia

anaerobic

anaerobic exercise

anandamide

anxiety

anxiolytic

atrophy

ballistic stretching

bipolar disorder

body image

brain-derived neurotrophic factor (BDNF)

cardiovascular exercise

chromosomes

cross-stressor adaptation hypothesis

depression

dynamic stretching

dysthymic disorder

emotion

endocannabinoids

endogenous

endorphins

ergometer

euphoria

executive function

exercise

exercise duration

exercise frequency

exercise intensity

exercise mode

exercise volume

flexibility

flexibility training

flow

functional fitness training

generalized anxiety disorder

hypertrophy

insomnia

intramuscular triglyceride

interval training

major depressive disorder

maximal heart rate

mood

motor unit

neurogenesis

neuromotor exercise training

neuromuscular exercise training

nitric oxide (NO)

nitric oxide synthase

opiates

panic disorder

passive static stretching

pedometer

phobia

physical activity

proprioceptive neuromuscular facilitation (PNF)

rating of perceived exertion (RPE)

repetitions (reps)

self-concept

self-confidence

self-efficacy

self-esteem

set

sport

state anxiety

strength

strength training

stress reactivity

stretching

telomerase

telomeres

trait anxiety

valence

volume of oxygen consumed ($\dot{V}O_2$)

CRITICAL THINKING QUESTIONS

1. Your grandmother hears that you are taking a course about exercise and health. She asks, "I have heard exercise is good for improving bone density. Is this true?" How do you reply?

2. You are a professional exercise psychologist reviewing a research paper that has been submitted to your journal. The study compares adolescents who participate on athletic teams with those who do not. The results from this study show that the athletes have higher self-esteem than the nonathletes. The authors conclude that high levels of exercise training improve self-esteem in adolescents. Do you think their conclusion is valid? Why or why not? What could be some other reasons that athletes differ from nonathletes? What would you say to the authors?

3. Using the public health guidelines in Figure 3-16 design an exercise program for yourself or a friend. Describe what types of exercise you would include and specify frequency, duration, and intensity of these activities.

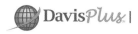 For additional resources log in to DavisPlus (davisplus.fadavis.com/ keyword "Brehm") and click on the Premium tab. (Don't have a PlusCode to access Premium Resources? Just click the Purchase Access button on the book's DavisPlus page.)

REFERENCES

Allen, J. D., Miller, E. M., Schwark, E., Robbins, J. L., Duscha, B. D., Annex, B. H. (2009). Plasma nitrite response and arteria l reactivity differentiate vascular health and performance. *Nitric Oxide, 20*(4), 231-237.

American Psychiatric Association. (2013). *The Diagnostic and Statistical Manual of Mental Disorders*, 5th ed. Washington, DC: American Psychiatric Association.

Andel, R., Crowe, M., Pedersen, N. L., Fratiglioni, L., Johansson, B., & Gatz, M. (2008). Physical exercise at midlife and risk of dementia three decades later: a population-based study of Swedish twins. *Journal of Gerontology: Medical Sciences, 63*(1), 62-66.

Bays, H. E., Gonzalez-Campoy, J. M., Henry, R. R., Bergman, D. A., Kitabchi, A. E., Schorr, A. B., . . . Adiposopathy Working Group (2008). Is adiposopathy (sick fat) an endocrine disease? *International Journal of Clinical Practice, 62*(10), 1474-1483.

Blumenthal, J. A., & Ong, L. (2009). A commentary on 'Exercise and depression,' (Mead et al., 2009): and the verdict is . . . . *Mental Health and Physical Activity, 2*(2), 97-99.

Boecker, H., Sprenger, T., Spilker, M. E., Henriksen, G., Koppenhoefer, M., Wagner, K. J., . . . Tolle, T. R. (2008). The runner's high: opioidergic mechanisms in the human brain. *Cerebral Cortex, 18*(11), 2523-2531.

Booth, F. W., & Lees, S. J. (2006). Physically active subjects should be the control group. *Medicine and Science in Sports and Exercise, 38*(3), 405-406.

Borg, E., Borg, G., Larsson, K., Letzter, M., & Sundblad, B. M. (2010). An index for breathlessness and leg fatigue. *Scandinavian Journal of Medicine and Science in Sports, 20*(4), 644-650.

Borg, G. A. (1982). Psychophysical bases of perceived exertion. *Medicine and Science in Sports and Exercise, 14*(5), 377-381.

Brand, S., Gerber, M., Beck, J., Hatzinger, M., Pühse, U., & Holsboer-Trachsler, E. (2010). High exercise levels are related to favorable sleep patterns and psychological functioning in adolescents. *Journal of Adolescent Health, 46*(2), 133-141.

Buford, T. W., & Manini, T. M. (2010). Sedentary individuals as "controls" in human studies: the correct approach? *Proceedings of the National Academy of Sciences, 107*(34), E134.

Buman, M. P., Helker, E. B., Bliwise, D. L., & King, A. C. (2011). Exercise effects on night-to-night fluctuations in self-rated sleep among older adults with sleep complaints. *Journal of Sleep Research, 20*(1 Pt 1), 28-37.

Centers for Disease Control and Prevention. *Physical activity for everyone: how much physical activity do you need?* : www.cdc.gov/physicalactivity/everyone/guidelines/index.html. Updated 3/11/11. Accessed 12/4/12.

Cerin, E., Leslie, E., Sugiyama, T., & Owen, N. (2009). Associations of multiple physical activity domains with mental well-being. *Mental Health and Physical Activity, 2*(2), 55-64.

Compton, W. M., Conway, K. P., Stinson, F. S., & Grant, B. F. (2006). Changes in the prevalence of major depression and comorbid substance use disorders in the United States between 1991-1992 and 2001-2002. *American Journal of Psychiatry, 163*(12), 2141-2147.

Cree, M. G., Paddon-Jones, D., Newcomer, B. R., Ronsen, O., Aarsland, A., Wolfe, R. R., & Ferrando, A. (2010). Twenty-eight day bed rest with hypercortisolemia induces peripheral insulin resistance and increases intramuscular triglycerides. *Metabolism, 59*(5), 703-710.

Csikszentmihalyi, M. (1997). *Finding Flow: The Psychology of Engagement with Everyday Life*. New York: Basic Books.

DeChiara, V., Errico, F., Musella, A., Rossi, S., Mataluni, G., Sacchetti, L., . . . Centonze, D. (2010). Voluntary exercise and sucrose consumption enhance cannabinoid CB1 receptor sensitivity in the striatum. *Neuropsychopharmacology*, 35(2), 374-387.

Denvir, M. A., & Gray, G. A. (2009). Run for your life: exercise, oxidative stress, and the ageing of the endothelium. *Journal of Physiology*, 587(17), 4137-4138.

Devos-Comby, L., Cronan, T., & Roesch, S. C. (2006). Do exercise and self-management interventions benefit patients with osteoarthritis of the knee? A meta-analytic review. The *Journal of Rheumatology*, 33(4), 744-756.

Dietrich, A., & McDaniel, W. F. (2004). Endocannabinoids and exercise. *British Journal of Sports Medicine*, 38(5), 536-541.

Dishman, R. K., & O'Connor, P. J. (2009). Lessons in exercise neurobiology: the case of endorphins. *Mental Health & Physical Activity*, 2(1), 4-9.

Dreifus, C. (2007). Finding clues to aging in the fraying tips of chromosomes: a conversation with Elizabeth H. Blackburn. *New York Times*, July 3. www.nytimes.com/2007/07/03/science/03conv.html. Accessed 12/4/12.

Dunstan, D. W., Barr, E. L., Healy, G. N., Salmon, J., Shaw, J. E., Balkau, B., . . . Owen, N. (2010). Television viewing time and mortality: the Australian Diabetes, Obesity, and Lifestyle Study (AusDiab). *Circulation*, 121(3), 384-391.

Dunstan, D. W., Kingwell, B. A., Larsen, R., Healy, G. N., Cerin, E., Hamilton, M. T., . . . Owen, N. (2012). Breaking up prolonged sitting reduces postprandial glucose and insulin responses. *Diabetes Care*, 35(5), 976-983.

Durrant, J. R., Seals, D. R., Connell, M. L., Russell, M. J., Lawson, B. R., Folian, B. J., . . . Lesniewski, L. A. (2009). Voluntary wheel running restores endothelial function in conduit arteries of old mice: direct evidence for reduced oxidative stress, increased superoxide dismutase activity and down-regulation of NADPH oxidase. *Journal of Physiology*, 587(13), 3271-3285.

Ekkekakis, P. (2009). Let them roam free? Physiological and psychological evidence for the potential of self-selected exercise intensity in public health. *Sports Medicine*, 39(10), 857-888.

Ekkekakis, P., & Petruzzello, S. J. (2004). Affective, but hardly effective: a reply to Gauvin and Rejeski (2001). *Psychology of Sport and Exercise*, 5(2), 135-152.

Ekkekakis, P., & Petruzzello, S. J. (2002). Analysis of the affect measurement conundrum in exercise psychology: IV: a conceptual case for the affect circumplex. *Psychology of Sport and Exercise*, 3, 35-63.

Erickson, K. I., Voss, M. W., Shaurya Prakash, R., Basak, C., Szabo, A., Chaddock, L., . . . Kramer, A. F. (2011). Exercise training increases size of hippocampus and improves memory. *Proceedings of the National Academy of Science*, 108(7), 3017-3022.

Esch, T., & Stefano, G. B. (2010a). Endogenous reward mechanisms and their importance in stress reduction, exercise, and the brain. *Archives of Medical Science*, 6(3), 447-455.

Esch, T., & Stefano, G. B. (2010b). The neurobiology of stress management. *Neuroendocrinology Letters*, 31(1), 19-39.

Focht, B. C. (2009). Brief walks in outdoor and laboratory environments: effects on affective responses, enjoyment, and intentions to walk for exercise. *Research Quarterly for Exercise and Sport*, 80(3), 611-620.

Forcier, K., Stroud, L. R., Papandonatos, G. D., Hitsman, B., Reiches, M., Krishnamoorthy, J., & Niaura, R. (2006). Links between physical fitness and cardiovascular reactivity and recovery to psychological stressors: a meta-analysis. *Health Psychology*, 25(6), 723-739.

Freedson, P., Pober, D., & Janz, K. F. (2005). Calibration of accelerometer output for children. *Medicine and Science in Sports and Exercise*, 37(11), S523-S530.

Fumoto, M., Oshima, T., Kamiya, K., Kikuchi, H., Seki, Y., Nakatani, Y., & Arita, H. (2010). Ventral prefrontal cortex and serotonergic system activation during pedaling exercise induces negative mood improvement and increased alpha band in EEG. *Behavioural Brain Research*, 213(1), 1-9.

Garber, C. E., Blissmer, B., Deschenes, M. R., Franklin, B. A., Lamonte, M. J., Lee, I. M., . . . American College of Sports Medicine. (2011). American College of Sports Medicine position stand. Quantity and quality of exercise for developing and maintaining cardiorespiratory, musculoskeletal, and neuromotor fitness in apparently healthy adults: guidance for prescribing exercise. *Medicine and Science in Sports and Exercise*, 43(7), 1334-1359.

Gauvin, L., & Rejeski, W. J. (1993). The exercise-induced feeling inventory: development and initial validation. *Journal of Sport and Exercise Psychology*, 15(4), 403-423.

Gerber, M., Brand, S., Holsboer-Trachsler, E., & Puhse, U. (2010). Fitness and exercise as correlates of sleep complaints: is it all in our minds? *Medicine and Science in Sports and Exercise*, 42(5), 893-901.

Gobeske, K. T., Das, S., Bonaguidi, M. A., Weiss, C., Radulovic, J., Disterhoft, J. F., & Kessler, J. A. (2009). BMP signaling mediates effects of exercise on hippocampal neurogenesis and cognition in mice, *PLoS ONE*. 4(10), e7506.

Goldberg, A. S., Moroz, L., Smith, A., & Ganley, T. (2007). Injury surveillance in young athletes: a clinician's guide to sports injury literature. *Sports Medicine*, 37(3), 265-278.

Gomez-Pinilla, G., Zhuang, Y., Feng, J., Ying, Z., & Fan, G. (2011). Exercise impacts brain-derived neurotrophic factor plasticity by engaging mechanisms of epigenetic regulation. *European Journal of Neuroscience*, 33(3), 383-390.

Greenwood, B. N., Foley, T. E., Le, T. V., Strong, P. V., Loughridge, A. B., Day, H. E., & Fleshner, M. (2011). Long-term voluntary wheel running is rewarding and produces plasticity in the mesolimbic reward pathway. *Behavioural Brain Research*, 217 (2), 354-362.

Hallberg, L., Janelidze, S., Engstrom, G., Wisén, A. G., Westrin, A., & Brundin, L. (2010). Exercise-induced release of cytokines in patients with major depressive disorder. *Journal of Affective Disorders*, 126(1-2), 262-267.

Hamer, M., & Steptoe, A. (2007). Association between physical fitness, parasympathetic control, and proinflammatory responses to mental stress. *Psychosomatic Medicine*, 69(7), 660-666.

Hamer, M., Taylor, A., & Steptoe, A. (2006). The effect of acute aerobic exercise on stress related blood pressure responses: a systematic review and meta-analysis. *Biological Psychology*, 71(2), 183-190.

Hardy, C. J., & Rejeski, W. J. (1989). Not what, but how one feels: the measurement of affect during exercise. *Journal of Sport and Exercise Psychology*, 11(3), 304-317.

Harris, T., Owen, C. G., Victor, C., Adams, R., Ekelund, U., & Cook, D. G. (2009). A comparison of questionnaire, zaccelerometer, and pedometer: measures in older people. *Medicine and Science in Sports and Exercise*, 41(7), 1392-1402.

Haskell, W. L., Blair, S. N., & Hill, J. O. (2009). Physical activity: health outcomes and importance for public health policy. *Preventive Medicine*, 49(4), 280-282.

Hays, N. P., Galassetti, P. R., & Coker, R. H. (2008). Prevention and treatment of type 2 diabetes: current role of lifestyle, natural product and pharmacological interventions. *Pharmacology & Therapeutics*, 118 (2), 181-191.

Healy, G. N., Matthews, C. E., Dustan, D. W., Winkler, E. A., & Owen, N. (2011). Sedentary time and cardio-metabolic biomarkers in U.S. adults: NHANES 2003-06. *European Heart Journal*, 32(5), 590-597.

Hegadoren, K. M., O'Donnell, T., Lanius, R., Coupland, N. J., & Lacaze-Masmonteil, N. (2009). The role of beta-endorphin in the pathophysiology of major depression. *Neuropeptides*, 43(5), 341-353.

Herring, M. P., O'Connor, P. J., & Dishman, R. K. (2010). The effect of exercise training in anxiety symptoms among patients: a systematic review. *Archives of Internal Medicine, 170*(4), 321-331.

Hyde, A. L., Conroy, D. E., Pincus, A. L., & Ram, N. (2011). Unpacking the feel-good effect of free-time physical activity: between- and within-person associations with pleasant-activated feeling states. *Journal of Sport and Exercise Psychology, 33*(6), 884-902.

Jackson, E. M., & Dishman, R. K. (2006). Cardiorespiratory fitness and laboratory stress: a meta-regression analysis. *Psychophysiology, 43*(1), 57-72.

Knapen, J., Somerijns, E., Vancampfort, D., Sienaert, P., Pieters, G., Haake, P., . . . Peuskens, J. (2009). State anxiety and subjective well-being responses to acute bouts of aerobic exercise in patients with depressive and anxiety disorders. *British Journal of Sports Medicine, 43*(10), 756-759.

Koehl, M., Meerlo, P., Gonzales, D., Rontal, A., Turek, F. W., & Abrous, D. N. (2008). Exercise-induced promotion of hippocampal cell proliferation requires beta-endorphin. *The FASEB Journal, 22*(7), 2253-2262.

Krauss, J., Farzaneh-Far, R., Puterman, E., Na, B., Lin, J., Epel, E., . . . Whooley, M. A. (2011). Physical fitness and telomere length in patients with coronary heart disease: findings from the Heart and Soul Study. *PLoS One, 6*(11), e26983.

Kwan, B. M., & Bryan, A. (2010). In-task and post-task affective response to exercise: translating exercise intentions into behaviour. *British Journal of Health Psychology, 15*(Pt. 1), 115-131.

Lau, P. W. C., Cheung, M. W. L., & Ransdell, L. B. (2008). A structural equation model of the relationship between body perception and self-esteem: global physical self-concept as the mediator. *Psychology of Sport and Exercise, 9*(4), 493-509.

Lees, S. J., & Booth, F. W. (2005). Physical inactivity is a disease. *World Review of Nutrition & Dietetics, 95*, 73-79.

Leitzmann, M. F., Park, Y., Blaire, A., Ballard-Barbash, R., Mouw, T., Hollenbeck, A. R., & Schatzkin, A. (2007). Physical activity recommendations and decreased risk of mortality. *Archives of Internal Medicine, 167*(22), 2453-2460.

Lucassen, P. J., Meerlo, P., Naylor, A. S., van Dam, A. M., Dayer, A. G., Fuchs, E., . . . Czéh, B. (2010). Regulation of adult neurogenesis by stress, sleep disruption, exercise, and inflammation: implications for depression and anti-depressant action. *European Neuropsychopharmacology, 20*(1), 1-17.

Mandell, A. J. (1979). The *second* second wind. *Psychiatric Annals 9*: 57-68; cited in Morgan, W. P. (1985). Affective beneficence of vigorous physical activity. *Medicine and Science in Sports and Exercise, 17*(1), 94-100.

Marcora, S. (2009). Perception of effort during exercise is independent of afferent feedback from skeletal muscles, heart, and lungs. *Journal of Applied Physiology, 106*(6), 2060-2062.

McCrae, C. S., McNamara, J. P. H., Rowe, M. A., Dzierzewski, J. M., Dirk, J., Marsiske, M., & Craggs, J. G. (2008). Sleep and affect in older adults: using multilevel modeling to examine daily associations. *Journal of Sleep Research, 17*(1), 42-53.

McHugh, M. P., & Cosgrave, C. H. (2010). To stretch or not to stretch: the role of stretching in injury prevention and performance. *Scandinavian Journal of Medicine and Science in Sports, 20*(2), 169-181.

Mead, G. E., Morley W., Campbell, P., Greig, C. A., McMurdo, M., & Lawlor, D. A. (2009). Exercise for depression. *Mental Health and Physical Activity, 2*(2), 95-96.

Mendelson, A. D., McCullough, C., & Chan, A. (2011). Integrating self-management and exercise for people living with arthritis. *Health Education Research, 26*(1), 167-177.

Milton, D., Porcari, J. P., Foster, C., Gibson, M., Udermann, B., & Greany, J. (2008). The effect of functional exercise training on functional fitness levels of older adults. *Gundersen Lutheran Medical Journal, 5*, 4-8.

Morgan, W. P. (1980). Test of champions: the iceberg profile. *Psychology Today, 14*(2): 92-108.

Morgan, W. P. (1985). Affective beneficence of vigorous physical activity. *Medicine and Science in Sports and Exercise, 17*(1), 94-100.

Morgan, W. P. (2001). Prescription of physical activity: a paradigm shift? *Quest, 53*(3), 366-382.

Morgan, W. P., & Costill, D. L. (1972). Psychological characteristics of the marathon runner. *Journal of Sports Medicine and Physical Fitness, 12*(1), 42-46.

Morgan, W. P., & Costill, D. L. (1996). Selected psychological characteristics and health behaviors of aging marathon runners: a longitudinal study. *International Journal of Sports Medicine, 17*(4), 305-312.

Morgan, W. P., O'Connor, P. J., Sparling, B. P., & Pate, R. R. (1987). Psychological characterization of the elite female distance runner. *International Journal of Sports Medicine, 8*(Suppl 2), 124-131.

Morgan, W. P., Roberts, J. A., Brand, F. R., & Feinerman, A. D. (1970). Psychological effect of chronic physical activity. *Medicine & Science in Sports, 2*(4), 213-217.

Nakamura, J., & Csikszentmihalyi, M. (2007). Flow theory and research. In: Ong, A. D. & Van Dulmen, M. H. M., eds. *Oxford Handbook of Methods in Positive Psychology,* vol. 13. Oxford and New York: Oxford University Press, pp 195-207.

National Institute of Mental Health (2010). Statistics. www. nimh.nih.gov/statistics/index.shtml. Accessed 12/4/12.

O'Donnell, K., Brydon, L., Wright, C. E., & Steptoe, A. (2008). Self-esteem levels and cardiovascular and inflammatory responses to acute stress. *Brain, Behavior, and Immunity, 22*(8), 1241-1247.

Olsen, R. H., Krogh-Madsen, R., Thomsen, C., Booth, F. W., & Pedersen, B. K. (2008). Metabolic responses to reduced daily steps in healthy nonexercising men (letter). *Journal of the American Medical Association, 299*(11), 1261-1263.

Patel, A. V., Bernstein, L., Deka, A., Feigelson, H. S., Campbell, P. T., Gapstur, S. M., . . . Thun, M. J. (2010). Leisure time spent sitting in relation to total mortality in a prospective cohort of US adults. *American Journal of Epidemiology, 172*(4), 419-429.

Pedersen, B. K. (2011). Muscles and their myokines. *Journal of Experimental Biology, 214*(2), 337-346.

Pontifex, M. B., Hillman, C. H., Fernhall, B., Thompson, K. M., & Valentini, T. A. (2009). The effect of acute aerobic exercise and resistance exercise on working memory. *Medicine and Science in Sports and Exercise, 41*(4), 927-934.

Pratt, M., Epping, J. N., & Dietz, W. H. (2009). Putting physical activity into public health: a historical perspective from the CDC. *Preventive Medicine, 49*(4), 301-302.

Pressman, S. D., & Cohen, S. (2005). Does positive affect influence health? *Psychological Bulletin, 131*(6), 925-971.

Pressman, S. D., Matthews, K. A., Cohen, S., Martire, L. M., Scheier, M., Baum, A., & Schulz, R. (2009). Association of enjoyable leisure activities with psychological and physical well-being. *Psychosomatic Medicine, 71*(7), 725-732.

Puterman, E., Lin, J., Blackburn, E., O'Donovan, A., Adler, N., & Epel, E. (2010). The power of exercise: buffering the effect of chronic stress on telomere length. *PLoS One, 5*(5), e10837.

Reed, J., & Buck, S. (2009). The effect of regular aerobic exercise on positive-activated affect: a meta-analysis. *Journal of Sport and Exercise Psychology*, *10*(6), 581-594.

Reid, K. J. (2010). Aerobic exercise improves self-reported sleep and quality of life in older adults with insomnia. *Sleep Medicine*, *11*(9), 934-940.

Rethorst, C. D., Landers, D. M., Nagoshi, C. T., & Ross, J. T. (2010). Efficacy of exercise in reducing depressive symptoms across 5-HTTLPR genotypes. *Medicine and Science in Sports and Exercise*, *42*(11), 2141-2147.

Rethorst, C. D., Wipfli, B. M., & Landers, D. M. (2009). The antidepressive effects of exercise: a meta-analysis of randomized trials. *Sports Medicine*, *39*(6), 491-511.

Roemmich, J. N., Lambaise, M., Salvy, S. J., & Horvath, P. J. (2009). Protective effect of interval exercise on psychophysiological stress reactivity in children. *Psychophysiology*, *46*(4), 852-861.

Rose, E. A., & Parfitt, G. (2010). Pleasant for some and unpleasant for others: a protocol analysis of the cognitive factors that influence affective responses to exercise. *International Journal of Behavioral Nutrition and Physical Activity*, *7*(7), 15.

Ryan, M. (2008). The antidepressant effects of physical activity: mediating self-esteem and self-efficacy mechanisms. *Psychology and Health*, *23*(3), 279-307.

Smith, P. J., Blumenthal, J. A., Hoffman, B. M., Cooper, H., Strauman, T. A., Welsh-Bohmer, K., . . . Sherwood, A. (2010). Aerobic exercise and neurocognitive performance: a meta-analytic review of randomized controlled trials. *Psychosomatic Medicine*, *72*(3), 239-252.

Spence, J. S. (2005). The effect of exercise on global self-esteem: a quantitative review. *Journal of Exercise and Sport Psychology*, *27*(3), 311-334.

Strohle, A. (2009). Physical activity, exercise, depression and anxiety disorders. *Journal of Neural Transmission*, *116*(6), 777-784.

Strohle, A., Stoy, M., Graetz, B., Scheel, M., Wittmann, A., Gallinat, J., . . . Hellweg, R. (2010). Acute exercise ameliorates reduced brain-derived neurotrophic factor in patients with panic disorder. *Psychoneuroimmunology*, *35*(3), 364-368.

Teychenne, M., Ball, K., & Salmon, J. (2010). Sedentary behavior and depression among adults: a review. *International Journal of Behavioral Medicine*, *17*(4), 246-254.

Thayer, R. E. (2001). *Calm energy: how people regulate mood with food and exercise*. Oxford: Oxford University Press.

White, K., Kendrick, T., & Yardley, L. (2009). Change in self-esteem, self-efficacy and the mood dimensions of depression as potential mediators of the physical activity and depression relationship: exploring the temporal relation of change. *Mental Health and Physical Activity*, *2*(1), 44-52.

Williams, D. M., Dunsiger, S., Ciccolo, J. T., Lewis, B. A., Albrecht, A. E., & Marcus, B. H. (2008). Acute affective response to a moderate intensity exercise stimulus predicts physical activity participation 6 and 12 months later. *Psychology of Sport and Exercise*, *9*(3), 231-245.

Wipfli, B. M., Rethorst, C. D., & Landers, D. M. (2008). The anxiolytic effects of exercise: a meta-analysis of randomized trials and dose-response analysis. *Journal of Sport and Exercise Psychology*, *30*(4), 392-410.

World Health Organization (WHO). (2010). Mental health: strengthening our response. Fact Sheet Number 220. www.who.int/mediacentre/factsheets/fs220/en. Accessed 12/4/12.

Wu, C.-W., Chang, Y.-T., Yu, L., Chen, H. I., Jen, C. J., Wu, S. Y., . . . Kuo, Y. M. (2008). Exercise enhances the proliferation of neural stem cells and neurite growth and survival of neuronal progenitor cells in dentate gyrus of middle-aged mice. *Journal of Applied Physiology*, *105*(5), 1585-1594.

Youngstedt, S. D. (2010). Comparison of anxiolytic effects of acute exercise in older versus younger adults. *Journal of Applied Gerontology*, *29*(2), 251-260.

Youngstedt, S. D., & Kline, C. E. (2006). Epidemiology of exercise and sleep. *Sleep and Biological Rhythms*, *4*(3), 215-221.

CHAPTER OUTLINE

LEARNING OBJECTIVES

After reading this chapter, you will be able to:

1. Describe ecological perspectives on health behavior and how health and fitness professionals use these perspectives to design health-promotion programs.

2. List the six stages of change in the Transtheoretical Model and illustrate these stages with an example.

3. Discuss the Health Belief Model and the Theory of Planned Behavior and describe how the components of these two models explain the process of forming decisions to change a target behavior.

4. Explain the concept of self-efficacy.

5. Describe the types of motivation that are part of Self-determination Theory.

6. Explain the concept of locus of control and its behavior-change applications.

7. Discuss several behavioral-learning and cognitive-behavioral strategies for helping people change health behaviors.

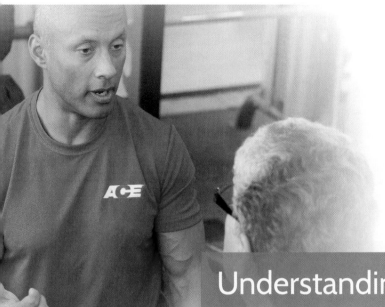

Sharon R. Sears, Barbara A.
Brehm, and Kristina Bell

CHAPTER 4

Understanding Behavior Change: Theoretical Models

UNDERSTANDING BEHAVIOR CHANGE: Theoretical Models

■ *Kristen has just begun a new job as wellness director for a large insurance company. She works in the human resources (HR) department and reports to Janice, the head of HR. A major part of Kristen's job is overseeing the on-site fitness center, which employs several part-time people as exercise instructors and personal trainers. Kristen spends part of each day as a lifestyle coach, working one on one with clients who need to make lifestyle changes for medical reasons. Alarmed at the rising obesity rates she sees in the company's employees, Janice has recently introduced a variety of initiatives to encourage employees to lose weight. She has asked Kristen to use her lifestyle-coaching skills to work with employees individually and in small groups to motivate them to improve their eating and exercise habits. Janice has also asked Kristen if she has any other recommendations for helping overweight employees improve their lifestyles.*

Kristen knows that the statistics on successful weight loss are pretty discouraging and wonders where to start. She decides to begin with a needs assessment to determine employees' perceptions of what they need to support more-healthful lifestyles. She gets Janice's permission to e-mail each employee a short questionnaire and to conduct several focus groups to obtain feedback from a variety of employees. Kristen spends quite a bit of time her first month there introducing herself to people in various departments and watching people in the cafeteria. ■

Psychologists have been studying health behavior and behavior change for many years. Numerous factors influence how a person develops health habits. Psychologists have created theoretical models to help conceptualize the behavior-change process. As explained in Chapter 1, a theoretical model is a set of ideas to help people understand and predict the way that things work. Psychologists develop models using many sources of evidence, including observation and scientific research. Understanding where health behaviors originate can help people to develop strategies for effective interventions. Psychologists acknowledge that human behavior is complex. No single model is sufficient for explaining all behaviors for all people. Models are simply a starting point for conceptualizing why people do what they do.

This chapter introduces some important concepts in behavior change, including a description of the many areas in which behavior-change theory is applied. The chapter then presents some well-known behavior-change models and theories. The focus is on models and theories supported by scientific research and that are useful to health and fitness professionals. As described in Chapter 1, the overarching model that health and exercise psychologists use is the biopsychosocial model. Considering factors in the biological, psychological, and social domains gives psychologists the most complete view of human behavior and the best understanding of behavior change.

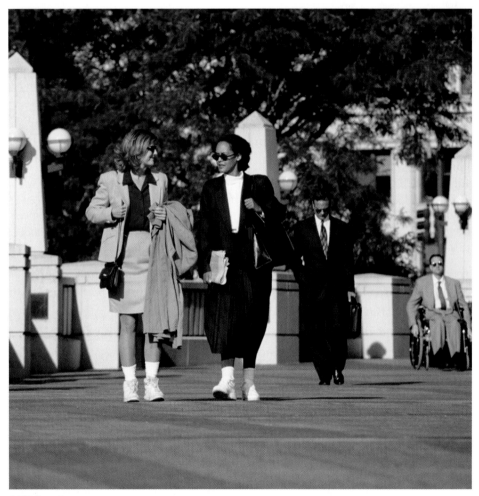

© Thinkstock

INFLUENCES ON HEALTH BEHAVIOR:
Ecological Models

People's behavior is strongly influenced by the environments in which they live. Understanding the many factors that influence behavior can help health and fitness professionals understand clients and design effective behavior-change interventions. Changing individual behavior may be an obvious and common approach to improving health; yet individuals exist in social systems.

Thus, health promotion can occur through a variety of paths and networks.

Ecological Perspectives

Researchers have proposed using an ecological perspective for understanding health behavior and for structuring effective behavior-change programs (Kok, Gottlieb, Commers, & Smerecnik, 2008; Richard, Potvin, Kishchuk, Prlic, & Green, 1996). An ecological perspective views health as a function of individuals and the environments in which they live, including the people around them. The ecological approach focuses on interrelationships between individuals and various environmental levels and helps health and fitness professionals understand how people interact with their environments. Figure 4-1 depicts an ecological model with several layers of environmental influences (Fig. 4-1). Ecological models help health and fitness professionals understand both supportive influences as well as barriers for behavior change. Generally, they include some variation of the following layers (terminology for the layers varies among research groups, depending on the behavior of interest and a target population's situation) (Fisher, 2008):

- Intrapersonal Level, including a person's knowledge, values, beliefs, and preferences
- Interpersonal Level, including close interpersonal relationships, such as family members and close friends, and social network
- Organizational Level, including influences such as a person's workplace, health-care systems, and community groups
- Community Level, including the built environment as well as neighbors
- Societal and Cultural Level, including larger social and cultural influences, such as government structures, public health policies and programs, and economic structures

Experts have shown that an ecological perspective facilitates the understanding of many types of lifestyle behaviors, including exercise behavior. Although a great deal of behavior-change research focuses on the way that people make decisions about changing how they behave, behavior is the result of more than their individual decisions. For example, cultural factors and social networks exert a great deal of influence on the behavior of individuals. Ecological perspectives help bring these factors to the attention of people designing behavior-change programs. For example, a study of physical activity levels in 318 Greek older adults found that an ecological perspective helped to explain why subjects were active (Thøgersen-Ntoumani, 2009). One of the most predictive factors was number of friends exercising. This study is interesting in that it reminds psychologists that behavior-change models usually focus on individual decision-making. These models have been developed and tested primarily on English-speaking and northern European populations, which tend to value autonomy and individuality. It is possible that these models are less predictive for cultures, like those in southern Europe, that place higher value on collective behavior (valuing one's role as part of a group).

The ecological approach is important to health and fitness professionals because it offers a broad view of how to understand behavior and promote health. Working with individual clients may be a direct and satisfying way to influence health behavior. However, health and fitness professionals can also serve as visionaries and advocates for broader social change by doing research to design programs that target communities, organizations, and public policy.

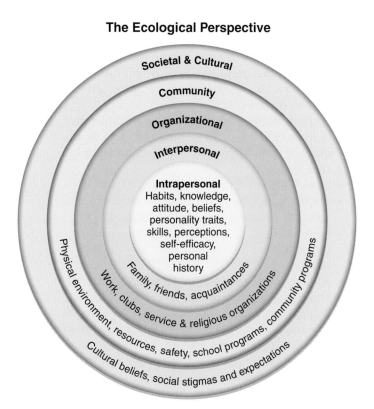

Figure 4-1. Ecological model.

Kristen examines the food choices as she waits in the cafeteria line. "Not too bad," she thinks, "but the salad bar could use a little more diversity in the vegetable department." She wonders if there really needs to be five dessert choices, each more tempting than the last. Where is the fresh fruit? The entrée is fried and the vegetable is overcooked. The prices are low, which may account for the limited vegetable selections. Kristen wonders if people would be willing to pay a little more for better food. The cafeteria is full, and people seem to enjoy eating together and taking a break from work.

The needs-assessment questionnaires have been coming back. Many people mentioned the donut culture that pervades the company. Donuts seem to make an appearance at every meeting, and several respondents mentioned that they have a hard time saying no. Vending machines feature sodas, candy, and salty snacks. Kristen decides to include some recommendations for healthier food options in her next meeting with Janice. ■

Health Promotion

Ecological perspectives can help inform and guide health-promotion efforts. Health promotion refers to activities and programs designed to change behaviors in ways that are likely to lead to better health outcomes. Health promotion is based on a philosophy that health and wellness are both individual and collective endeavors.

Promotion Across the Layers

Health-promotion efforts occur at all ecological perspective layers and in many settings. Examples follow:

- An individual decides to improve his health by taking a walk every day or by reducing screen time in the evening.
- A family member suggests eating healthier and the family group gathers more regularly for the evening meal to improve nutrition and family cohesion.
- Close friends attend an exercise class together.
- A community bookstore organizes and promotes a display of books about eating locally grown produce, inviting guest speakers and encouraging patrons to think about their food-buying habits.
- A town builds recreational facilities or improves school lunch offerings.
- Public service announcements on television promote health-minded behaviors with messages such as "Do not drink and drive."
- Laws requiring public places and businesses to be smoke-free reduce people's exposure to second-hand smoke.

Health and fitness professionals often find themselves working at all these levels. The theme that connects all health-promotion efforts is behavior change. In every case, health promotion targets one or more behaviors that people could change in ways that produce better health outcomes. Health and exercise psychology research helps to inform these health-promotion efforts.

Health-promotion efforts typically target behaviors that will most effectively promote good health and prevent disease. Because health-promotion work at every level requires resources in terms of time and money, it makes sense to put resources into those efforts that will produce the greatest return.

Health-related behaviors such as physical activity, smoking cessation, stress management, and healthy eating all influence one another. Whereas behavior-change discussions typically focus on a single target behavior, the real-life picture of behavior change is much more complex. Often changes in one area influence other behaviors. For example, finding healthful ways to limit feelings of stress may, in turn, reduce the drive to smoke or overeat. Health and fitness professionals will often find themselves working with clients who are trying to change more than one behavior.

Types of Intervention

People can change their behavior to promote good health in a variety of ways. The goal of health-promotion efforts may be to prevent health problems or to cope more effectively once problems arise and to reduce the harm that results from these problems. Health psychologists refer to three types of intervention for health promotion: primary prevention, secondary screening, and tertiary treatment.

Primary prevention is a way of addressing health behaviors before people become ill. Primary prevention has two strategies. One strategy is to keep people from ever developing poor health habits. For example, teaching effective hand washing in child-care centers is a way to help people prevent the spread of illness early in life. A second strategy is to help people change existing poor health habits before they become a physical problem. Helping people change from eating highly processed sugary foods to eating more fresh fruits and vegetables before they develop diabetes is an example of this strategy. Primary prevention efforts are often broad in scope and target population.

Like primary prevention, secondary screening is a way of addressing health behaviors before people become ill or early in an illness when the problem is most treatable. Whereas primary prevention is often broad in scope, secondary-screening strategies try to identify people who are most at risk for having specific diseases or conditions. This more-focused strategy can guide an efficient use of resources and help people who need health-care intervention the most. For example, increased age is a risk factor for developing breast cancer.

Thus, government organizations such as the National Cancer Institute and National Institutes of Health recommend that women over a certain age get mammograms to detect breast cancer at its earliest stages when it is most treatable. Routine measurements of blood pressure, blood sugar, and blood lipids aim to detect early changes in these variables. If early changes are detected, lifestyle modifications may help prevent the development of more-serious problems. For example, many people are able to avoid, or at least delay for several years, taking medication for hypertension by making changes in diet and increasing their physical activity. Such measures are most likely to be effective with borderline hypertension when problems are first developing.

Tertiary-treatment interventions address health behaviors after people become ill or injured. Some people think of this approach as harm reduction. Even after people are ill, promoting health-behavior change may reduce the effect or slow the progression of disease (Fig. 4-2). An example of this strategy is getting people with diabetes to take their insulin medication regularly and control blood sugars. This approach may prevent further harm from diabetes complications, such as vision and kidney problems. Similarly, cardiac-rehabilitation programs often encourage aggressive lifestyle changes to slow the progression of artery disease in people who have already experienced a heart attack. In some cases, tertiary treatment can even reverse the disease process, as when lifestyle measures stop the formation of arterial plaque or normalize blood glucose regulation.

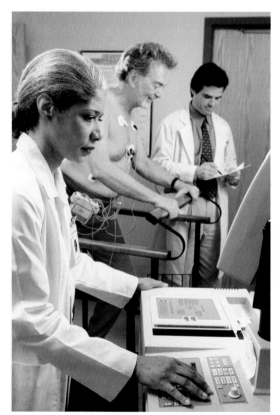

Figure 4-2. Exercise as tertiary treatment for heart disease.
© Thinkstock

THE PROCESS OF BEHAVIOR CHANGE: The Transtheoretical Model

The process of behavior change is complex, and, when people attempt to change lifestyle behaviors to improve health and prevent illness, they typically go through several stages. For example, individuals usually do not go from being sedentary one day to engaging in physical activity several times a week the next day. Rather, they may begin by simply thinking about changing their behavior. They may form intentions to change that they then ignore. Or they may try several times to initiate a new behavior, such as walking 3 days a week. Most people do not succeed in staying active for several months the first time they try. Similarly, quitting smoking often takes many attempts. People may sustain new behaviors for days, weeks, or even months, and then relapse and go back to their old ways. The best-known model of the process of behavior change is the Transtheoretical Model (TTM). James O. Prochaska and colleagues proposed this model to describe the idea that behavior change is a process that goes through stages (Game changers 4-1) (Norcross, Krebs, & Prochaska, 2011; Prochaska & DiClemente, 1982; Prochaska & DiClemente, 1983). Transtheoretical refers to "across theories," or drawing from many theories, and incorporates concepts, such as self-efficacy, from other theories.

Learning about the TTM can help health and fitness professionals have a better understanding of the mental processes that each client goes through. A client stands a better chance of making a significant change when a program is personalized based on his or her readiness to change (Levesque, Cummins, Prochaska, & Prochaska, 2006). Readiness to change has become a key concept in behavior-change programs. Readiness simply refers to how willing and prepared a person is to change a given behavior.

The TTM has two dimensions: stages of change and processes of change. Stages of change involve the temporal, motivational, and adherence (Does the person stick to his intentions to change?) aspects of change. Processes of change involve activities and events that contribute to successful behavior modification (DiClemente et al., 1991).

The Stages of Change

There are six different stages of change, and people can cycle through them both backwards and forwards (Fig. 4-3).

- Precontemplation. At this stage, the client is not ready to change and is not even thinking about making any kind of change in the near future. Sometimes people in this stage are subdivided into nonbelievers and believers. Nonbelievers do not see the value of behavior change. Believers recognize the value of change but are not confident in their ability to make the change at any time in the near future.

Game Changers 4-1. James Prochaska and the Stages of Change

Historically, researchers tended to view behavior change as an all-or-nothing phenomenon. Either people changed or they did not: people stopped smoking or kept smoking, stopped drinking or kept drinking, lost weight or did not lose weight. Over time, researchers and clinicians began to realize that the process of behavior change is very complex. One of the key players to shift the paradigm for understanding how people change behavior is James O. Prochaska.

Based on research data and clinical observations, Prochaska and colleagues (i.e., Prochaska & DiClemente, 1982) noted that behaviors such as smoking, weight loss, and alcohol use are not one-time endeavors with a dichotomous (yes or no) outcome. Instead, they argued:

> In order to do justice to data on changes in smoking, weight control, or alcohol abuse, the stages of change need to be represented as cyclical rather than linear in sequence. For addictive problems, such as smoking, a revolving-door schema is a more accurate representation of the sequence that smokers pass through in their efforts to become nonsmokers (*Prochaska & DiClemente, 1982, p. 283*).

Prochaska and his colleagues thus proposed the Transtheoretical Model to include the stages and processes of change that people go through on the path of behavior change. A study by DiClemente et al. (1991) provided early support for the Stages of Change Model for smoking cessation. The researchers found that classifying smokers into precontemplation, contemplation, and preparation stages of change predicted 1-month and 6-month smoking cessation. Thus, the researchers suggested that asking people whether they planned to quit smoking does not provide enough information. Instead, the researchers found that intentions to quit in the near versus distant future as well as recent quit attempts can be the gateway to future quitting success. Since that time, countless other researchers and clinicians have implemented and evaluated the Transtheoretical Model as a component of behavior-change programs.

James Prochaska earned his Ph.D. in clinical psychology and has published over 300 journal articles, book chapters, and books on behavior change for health promotion and disease prevention. He has been the principal investigator on millions of dollars' worth of research grants for the prevention of chronic diseases. He was named one of the five most influential authors in psychology by both the Institute for Scientific Information and the American Psychological Society.

Sources: DiClemente, C. C., Prochaska, J. O., Fairhurst, S. K., Velicer, W. F., Velasquez, M. M., & Rossi, J. S. (1991). The process of smoking cessation: an analysis of precontemplation, contemplation, and preparation stages of change. *Journal of Consulting and Clinical Psychology*, 59(2): 295-304; Pro-Change Behavior Systems, Inc. (2011). James A. Prochaska, PhD: founder. www.prochange.com/staff/james_prochaska. Accessed 11/30/12; Prochaska, J. O., & DiClemente, C. C. (1982). Transtheoretical therapy: toward a more integrative model of change. *Psychotherapy: Theory, Research & Practice*, 19(3): 276-288.

- **Contemplation.** The client is beginning to think about possibly making a change within the next 6 months.
- **Preparation.** The client is making small attempts at behavior change and plans to make a full change within the next 30 days.
- **Action.** The behavior change is in progress; however, the new behavior has not yet lasted 6 months.
- **Maintenance.** The client is actively engaged in the continuation of the behavior change; the new behavior has lasted longer than 6 months.
- **Relapse.** The client has reverted back to the previous behavior.

The stages of change can be illustrated by considering people who are not yet thinking about changing a certain behavior. For instance, some smokers are not considering quitting. Although they have read the literature and seen the pictures of scarred lung tissue, they do not think about stopping. They remain in the precontemplation stage. But, once they begin to think about changing the behavior, they enter the contemplation stage. For example, Sarah, a client who smokes, begins to consider the need to quit. If Sarah decides to quit within the next 6 months, she is then in the contemplation stage. As Sarah begins to investigate quitting and decides that the time has come, she then progresses into the preparation stage. When Sarah does finally throw the pack away and stops smoking completely, she has successfully entered into the action phase. Once she has given up cigarettes for at least 6 months, she is in the maintenance phase. It is possible that Sarah will continue with her behavior change and never smoke again. However, it is also possible that she may relapse, going back to her old smoking habit.

Many people make multiple attempts at behavior change before experiencing long-term success. Rather than viewing these relapses as failures, it is helpful to view them as learning opportunities for future change. Relapse prevention may be particularly helpful during the action and maintenance phases to help clients anticipate pitfalls and pinpoint problem-solving strategies.

Some models of the stages of change include a final stage called termination. Termination refers to a stage

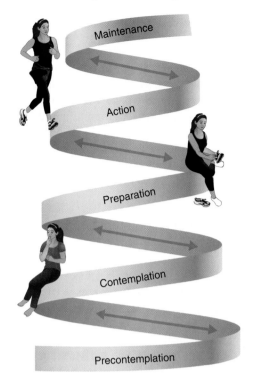

Figure 4-3. Stages of behavior change.

in which the individual continues the behavior change indefinitely. If the client discussed above never has another cigarette for the rest of her life, she would be in the termination stage of smoking cessation. The termination stage is helpful for models of addiction treatment because many people do succeed in eliminating addictive substances and behaviors from their lives. Other behaviors, such as eating and exercise behaviors, generally continue to change throughout people's lives. Researchers rarely use the termination stage to describe the adoption of regular physical activity. Instead, they usually describe regular exercisers as "long-term maintainers."

The Stages of Change Model grew out of research about smoking cessation (i.e., DiClemente et al., 1991), but it has been applied to numerous health behaviors, from making dietary changes (i.e., Di Noia & Prochaska, 2010), to drinking behavior in college students (i.e., Vik, Culbertson, & Sellers, 2000) to making decisions about health-care plans such as Medicare (i.e., Levesque et al., 2006). Chapters 8 through 10 will examine the Stages of Change Model as applied to common health behaviors with which health and fitness professionals work, including physical activity, eating, and weight-control behaviors.

MOTIVATING CHANGE: Adjusting the Role of the Health and Fitness Professional According to the Client's Stage

Just as the client's tasks and behaviors evolve over time, so too does the role of the health and fitness professional. Norcross, Krebs, and Prochaska (2011) describe these changing roles as follows. With clients in precontemplation, the role may be

one of a nurturing parent. The parent joins with a resistant and defensive youngster who is both drawn to and repelled by the prospect of becoming more independent. The health and fitness professional is supportive and understanding with clients in precontemplation. With clients in contemplation, the role is like that of a Socratic teacher, who encourages clients to achieve their own insights into their condition through skillful questioning. With clients in the preparation stage, the stance is like that of an experienced coach who has been through crucial matches and can provide a game plan or review the participant's own plan. With clients who are progressing into action and maintenance, the professional becomes more of a consultant who is available to provide expert advice and support when action is not progressing smoothly. As termination approaches, clients consult the professional less and less as they experience greater autonomy to live free from previous problems. The professional may be available on an as-needed basis if a client's situation changes such that he or she needs additional support to prevent relapse.

Although the use of the Stages of Change Model is promising, it is important to remember that not all clients will be ready for change. It is also important to remember that, although the stages seem to be fairly black and white, there is actually a lot of gray area between each individual stage. These models and treatment programs are based on work with individual clients whose needs differ. A program that works for one person may not work for the next. If a program seems to work initially, that does not mean the client will not relapse into an earlier stage. Each client is looking for something different in his or her work with the health and fitness professional. It is up to the professional to determine what the client is looking for, what the client is ready for, and the best possible recommendations that will help that client become as healthy as possible.

Decisional Balance

Decisional balance is an important concept in the TTM and other models of behavior change. Decisional balance is the idea that, as people move through the stages, the way they feel about the behavior will change. The balance of positive and negative thoughts associated with the behavior may shift in ways that lead to a decision to change. Professionals can use this to help clients make a decision to change. For example, as Sarah begins to contemplate quitting smoking, she may devise a pros and cons list reflecting her thoughts about the behavior. At this stage, Sarah's list may have pros for smoking such as stress reducer and appetite suppressor. Sarah may have difficulty recognizing cons other than those she hears about in the media. As she moves into the action and maintenance stages, her con list may begin to surpass the pros list. Her thoughts surrounding the behavior have changed.

In the precontemplation stage, people typically feel that the benefits of their current behavior outweigh the costs. People in this stage can usually give a long list of reasons for not changing and spell out the many barriers they would face were they to try to change. As people enter the contemplation stage and actually consider changing, they are drawn to at least a few of the benefits of changing. As they think about barriers, they may begin exploring ways to cope with these. The decisional balance may shift frequently throughout the contemplation stage, as people go back and forth about whether to change.

The Processes of Change

People use a variety of strategies to work through the different stages of change. These strategies are known as the processes of change. Whereas stages of change represent *when* people change, the processes represent *how* people change. There are 10 processes of change described by the TTM, many of which are drawn from other theories and models. Five of these are cognitive processes that result in new ways of thinking that reinforce motivation to change. Five are behavioral processes that support the new behavior. Processes of change include the following (Norcross, Krebs, & Prochaska, 2011; Prochaska, DiClemente, & Norcross, 1992).

Cognitive Processes
- **Consciousness raising:** A person experiences increasing awareness of the advantages of changing.
- **Dramatic relief:** A person feels emotional relief upon experiencing and expressing feelings about his or her problems and solutions. Relief occurs when people decide to change, and this decision eases the discomfort caused by the realization that the current behavior is problematic.
- **Environmental reevaluation:** A person assesses how his or her problem affects the environment, especially the social environment.
- **Self-reevaluation:** A person sees himself or herself in a new way that is incompatible with the old behavior.
- **Self-liberation:** A person chooses or commits to behavior change and has a new belief in his or her ability to change.

Behavioral Processes
- **Helping relationships:** Social support from friends, family, helping professionals, and others can inspire or support change.
- **Reinforcement management:** A person rewards himself or herself or is rewarded by others for making changes.
- **Stimulus control:** A person avoids stimuli that elicit problem behaviors by restructuring the environment (e.g., removing alcohol or unhealthy foods) or avoiding high-risk cues.

- **Counterconditioning:** A person uses response substitution, replacing problem behaviors with alternative healthier behaviors (e.g., taking a short walk rather than smoking in response to feelings of stress, drinking tea rather than coffee after dinner to reduce caffeine intake).
- **Social liberation:** A person takes advantage of increased social opportunities to be with people who model the new behavior, noticing and using these opportunities to reinforce behavior change.

Box 4-1 uses the example of Sarah to illustrate these processes.

These processes of change help clients focus on activities that will help strengthen their commitment to behavior change (DiClemente et al., 1991). As with the stages of change, the use of processes varies from person to person. Researchers and clinicians have observed clients using these processes of change both when getting professional help to change an unwanted behavior and when making behavior changes without any help. In general, the cognitive processes tend to be more commonly used in the earlier stages of change, whereas the behavioral processes appear to be more useful in the preparation, action, and maintenance stages (Norcross, Krebs, & Prochaska, 2011).

MOTIVATING CHANGE: Applying the Processes of Change

Health and fitness professionals may see several of the cognitive processes of change from time to time, especially if they work with clients in the precontemplation and contemplation stages of change. Health and fitness professionals often participate in the consciousness-raising process as they educate clients about risks and benefits of behaviors. As they explore with clients the importance of health risks and health behaviors, sometimes the conversation goes in directions where clients express thoughts reflecting the other four cognitive processes, especially if they are making a decision to change.

Health and fitness professionals often work with the five behavioral processes of change. These are specific skills the professional should be able to teach clients. More information about using these processes to help clients change exercise, diet, weight control, and other behaviors will be explored in Chapters 8 through 11. The Transtheoretical Model drew these from behavioral-learning theory (discussed in more detail below), and these processes have been shown to be very helpful in behavior change.

FACTORS INFLUENCING THE PROCESS OF BEHAVIOR CHANGE

Much of the research on behavior change has focused on the factors that influence an individual's thinking and decision-making about changing behavior.

Box 4-1. Processes of Change

The example smoker Sarah can provide an illustration of the 10 processes of change. The terms for these processes can be difficult to remember, but the processes themselves are very common; and most readers have had many of these experiences in their own lives.

Consciousness raising. Sarah begins to think about changing because something has occurred to raise her consciousness, or awareness, about the risks of her smoking behavior. Although she probably has always known smoking was risky, she learns something new that changes or raises her awareness regarding the behavior. Perhaps someone close to her develops lung cancer from smoking. Or she becomes angry as she reads an article about the chemicals secretly added to the brand of cigarette she smokes. Something changes the way she sees smoking.

Dramatic relief. As Sarah becomes worried or angry about her smoking habit, her discomfort increases. She no longer smokes a cigarette mindlessly, without remembering the consciousness raising she has experienced. The discomfort grows as Sarah explores her need to smoke and her need to quit. When Sarah decides to think about quitting, she experiences dramatic relief.

Environmental reevaluation. Environmental reevaluation involves clients considering how the health behavior affects the environment around them, including their social networks. How does Sarah's smoking affect the people with whom she associates? Sarah has decided to one day have children and realizes that she must quit smoking to have a healthy family. Environmental reevaluation may also help Sarah realize that she wants to be known as healthy and a good role model for younger friends and family.

Self-reevaluation. Sarah sees herself and her smoking habit in new ways that encourage quitting. She has fallen in love with a man who hates smoking and finds that smoking no longer belongs in her lifestyle.

Self-liberation. As Sarah feels moved to quit smoking, she feels freed from the constraints of being a smoker. Self-liberation resulting from committing to behavior change feels good and reinforces her motivation, at least temporarily.

Once Sarah has taken action to quit smoking, she uses the behavioral processes to reinforce her decision to change. These include the following:

Helping relationships. Sarah accepts help from the friends and family members who support her desire to quit. She spends time with these friends to stay busy and keep her mind away from smoking. Their emotional support helps motivate Sarah to stick to her plans to quit.

Reinforcement management. Sarah decides to reward herself periodically for not smoking. For example, she decides to use the money saved from not buying cigarettes to get a massage.

Stimulus control. Sarah needs to avoid certain situations that are strong triggers of her smoking behavior. For example, she avoids certain parties where almost everyone smokes. On the other hand, she goes more frequently to environments that reinforce not smoking, such as movie theaters, fitness centers, and restaurants that do not permit smoking.

Counterconditioning. Because Sarah cannot avoid all smoking triggers, she plans new responses to those triggers. For example, Sarah used to smoke when speaking to a friend on the phone; now she paces or doodles on a piece of paper instead. She is conditioning herself to make a new response to a stimulus.

Social liberation. Sometimes behavior change opens up new opportunities. Sarah is motivated by opportunities to participate in new activities now, so needing to smoke frequently is not an issue. She lives in an area where smoking is frowned on and difficult to engage in, so she experiences social liberation by no longer being weighed down by her smoking habit. She enjoys going out with the new nonsmoking guy she has met. She enjoys exercise more since she becomes less out of breath as her lungs function better.

Researchers have developed several models to help explain the important factors that motivate health-behavior change on an individual level and predict whether an individual will decide to change and then carry out that change. These models vary in their usefulness, depending on the target behavior. Some behaviors are relatively simple, and the decision to change often leads to actual change. For example, going to the dentist for a checkup or getting an annual physical examination takes little preparation—only the wherewithal to get to a single appointment.

Attending some physical therapy sessions and performing a set of therapeutic exercises several times a day takes more organization and energy. An individual may decide to receive physical therapy for an injury but then fail to follow through. Even more complex is maintaining a program of physical activity for several months. The decision to change may not play a large role in how successful change efforts are. Nevertheless, these models are important for understanding certain steps in the behavior-change process.

The Health Belief Model

According to the Health Belief Model (Rosenstock, 1966), people's ideas and underlying emotions about illnesses, prevention, and treatments may influence health behaviors and decisions about health behaviors.

Variables

The Health Belief Model has at least four variables: perceived susceptibility to illness, perceived seriousness of illness, perceived benefits of a health behavior, and perceived barriers to a health behavior (Fig. 4-4). The first two variables involve the individual's beliefs about a health threat. The second two variables reflect the individual's beliefs about the health behavior that could reduce the threat.

The belief in a health threat has two components. These are perceived susceptibility to an illness and perceived seriousness of the illness. Perceived susceptibility refers to people's perceptions as to how likely they are to acquire or develop the illness. Perceived seriousness refers to people's perceptions regarding the short- and long-term severity of the illness. For example, this theory could apply to whether people will get a flu vaccine. Perceived susceptibility to an illness such as the flu may include people's beliefs about how contagious the illness is, how likely they are to be in situations where they might catch the flu, and how strong their immune system is in fighting the flu. Perceived seriousness of the disorder might include people's beliefs about how bad they would feel if they got the flu, how long they would have the flu, how much work or school they would miss, and how much it would cost to treat the disorder. Overall, the theory would suggest that the more people believe they are vulnerable and perceive the disorder to be severe, the more likely they would be to engage in a specific beneficial health behavior.

Secondary screenings sometimes motivate behavior change because they may alter people's perceptions of susceptibility when screenings indicate a potential problem. For example, people who have not thought much about what they eat may become more aware of their eating habits if they hear their blood pressure is high. They may suddenly feel more susceptible to hypertension and hopefully feel motivated to prevent its development through beneficial lifestyle behavior change.

The second set of variables relates to perceptions of the health behavior. People may perceive both benefits and barriers to taking action with a specific health behavior. Beliefs about benefits may include how effective the person thinks a health behavior and its alternatives would be in preventing an illness. Using the flu vaccine example, the more a person believed that a flu shot could reduce the chances of getting the flu, the more likely the person would be to get it. A final component to the Health Belief Model is people's ideas about the barriers or drawbacks of a health behavior. For example, people might have an excessive fear of pain and needles. They also might have a busy school schedule and little extra money to pay for vaccines. Even if people know it is flu season and think the flu shot would reduce their chances of getting the flu, the emotional and practical barriers may get in the way of them getting flu shots.

MOTIVATING CHANGE: Helping Clients Evaluate and Correct Perceptions

An important role for health and fitness professionals is to help people become aware of scientific evidence about their vulnerability to illness, the severity of disorders, and the effectiveness of health behaviors in preventing or treating disorders. Left to their own devices, people may use unreliable sources of evidence to make health decisions. A powerful but often incomplete source of information is limited personal experience, anecdote, or testimonial. An informal name for this phenomenon is the "Aunt Edna effect." For example, if someone had an Aunt Edna who smoked all her life, ate greasy food, and never exercised, yet lived to be 90, the person might be tempted to engage in similar poor health behaviors. Health and fitness professionals can kindly acknowledge that this outcome may have been true for this one individual but that most people should follow recommendations to quit smoking, eat more fresh fruits and vegetables, and exercise.

Clients may also have read unreliable information on Internet sites or in other media. The health and fitness professional should help them question the source and explore the site's motivations for posting the information (Box 4-2). Many websites sell products based on testimonials. One person's story is not enough to prove that a particular observation is true or will work for everyone. By sharing readable, accurate articles and websites with clients, the professional can steer them in the direction of useful and scientifically supported information.

Scientific Research Using the Health Belief Model

One meta-analysis by Carpenter (2010) of 18 longitudinal studies using the Health Belief Model to predict health behavior suggested that the variables of perceived benefits and barriers might be particularly strong predictors of actual behavior over time. They also

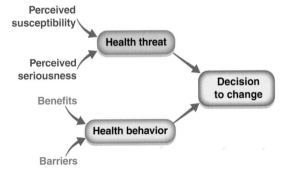

Figure 4-4. The Health Belief Model.

Box 4-2. Helping Clients Evaluate Health Information on the Internet

Many consumers rely on the World Wide Web for health, fitness, and nutrition information because they can find a wealth of information there, from advertisements to scientific articles. Some clients may use the Web to seek information on a health topic that concerns them or a family member. They may find information sites or even discussion groups that provide personal accounts of experiences with the health topic.

Although a number of clients are quite savvy about evaluating the quality of the information that they find on the Web, some clients may accept product advertisements as scientific fact. When clients mention questionable information that they have found on the Web, you can help correct their misunderstandings, perhaps examining the website together. Furthermore, you should screen the health and fitness information that you share with clients prior to sharing it. In addition, understanding the factors that characterize quality websites can help health and fitness professionals design a site that has a positive effect on visitors. To gain the best-quality information, keep the following in mind.

Differentiate advertisements from scientific information.

Most people who use the Web know when they have wandered into a website that is advertising a product. They may have clicked on an ad that appeared on their screen, or they may have been seeking information on related products. Some ads masquerade as "infomercials," and unwary readers may be taken in by the scientific appearance of the website. Web users must use the same discrimination that they use with print media to evaluate marketing materials and understand that marketing is, well, marketing. Claims about product efficacy may or may not be valid, and the surfer must beware.

Compare information on several websites.

Users often compare material listed on various sites, which is an intelligent strategy. Contradiction abounds in health research, whether in print or nonprint media. When users find material in several places on the Web, it is more likely to be generally accepted as truthful, even though their understanding of "truth" may change with the next research study published.

Find out who is responsible for the website.

Note the website's address, because it may give the name of the institution or organization that has posted the information. If not, go to the site's home page and explore. Some organizations, such as the American Heart Association or the Food and Drug Administration, may be familiar to you. If you have never heard of the organization, find out more. Links such as "About Us" or "Contact Us" often lead to a page that tells you about the organization. Some sites give quite a bit of information about the organization's purpose, history, policies, and even funding sources. Some disclose relationships between the organization and special interests that might bias their views. It is also important to determine who screens the information posted on that website. Is there an editorial board or some sort of review panel? If the website was created by an individual, what can you find out about him or her?

Explore the website's reasons for posting the information.

Many websites will state their purpose in posting information on the Web. Government and educational institutions often provide facts of interest to consumers as part of their organization's mission. The organizations sometimes earmark some of their resources for these educational purposes.

Sometimes information is posted to help sell products. If this is the case, you will see advertisements for products related to the topic that you are researching. This does not necessarily invalidate the article you have found, but you must ask yourself whether selling products might affect the website managers' choice of information that they make available to consumers.

Identify who wrote the material on your topic of interest.

Many websites offer a variety of information written by diverse authors. Who wrote the material? Are authors listed? Can you find any information about the authors? Do they have an educational degree and are they affiliated with a respected institution, such as a college or governmental agency? In other words, are they qualified to provide the posted information?

---

found that other variables interacted with the ones in the Health Belief Model to predict behavior. For example, it mattered whether a health behavior was a preventive measure or a treatment. Specifically, perceived benefits and barriers were stronger predictors of behavior for preventing a negative health condition compared with treating an existing negative health condition. For instance, perceived benefits and barriers may be good predictors of behaviors such as getting vaccines to prevent the flu or getting mammograms to detect breast cancer. Perceived benefits and barriers may not be as good at predicting treatment behaviors such as dental care or taking prescription drugs.

Another meta-analysis by DiMatteo, Haskard, and Williams (2007) found that how people perceived disease severity significantly and positively related to their adherence to health behaviors. In other words, the higher the perceived severity, the more likely people are to adhere to medical recommendations. However, they also found that people who already have serious illnesses such as cancer or HIV may be at greatest risk of not engaging in health-promoting behaviors. People facing such challenges may become psychologically and physically worn down by their disease, medical regimens, financial costs, and legal issues. They may lose hope, become socially isolated, and be less likely to engage in health behaviors. The "lived experience of illness" over time can alter perceptions of the benefits and barriers for health behavior. Thus, the process of making decisions about health behaviors is dynamic and complex.

■ *Janice agrees with Kristen's suggestions for making more fruits and vegetables available and reducing the availability of empty-calorie and high-fat foods, and they set up some meetings with the cafeteria director to discuss possible changes. They both agree it will be harder to change the "donut culture." Kristen emphasizes the importance of department heads signing on to promote a more-positive eating culture. Kristen cautions Janice to phase the donuts out very slowly, or they might face a rebellion from the donut-deprived workers. She suggests beginning with donuts and fresh fruit and muffins and then maybe progressing to donut holes instead of large donuts.*

Kristen suggests an educational campaign for the entire workforce to help them rethink certain eating behaviors, including the donuts provided at meetings. She explains the Health Belief Model to Janice and suggests they use the model to help frame the educational campaign. Kristen explains that people tend to underestimate their susceptibility to diet-related illness because the physiological effects of poor nutrition do not manifest immediately. Because no single food or meal causes much damage, people also underestimate the seriousness of poor eating habits. Similarly, improving eating habits is not usually perceived to have many benefits or a large effect on health. In addition, many people feel that there are many barriers to improving their nutrition and that eating habits are difficult to change.

Kristen and Janice agree to educate employees about the risks associated with poor eating habits and the health benefits of improving eating behaviors. Kristen agrees to give fun and engaging workshops for various departments on the benefits of good nutrition and simple and easy changes that

can be made to one's eating habits. She and Janice hope that giving people more information will strengthen their health beliefs supporting the importance of improving their eating habits. ■

Self-Efficacy

Self-efficacy (SE) is the degree to which an individual believes he or she can successfully perform a behavior. Albert Bandura defined an efficacy expectation as "the conviction that one can successfully execute the behavior required to produce the outcomes" (Bandura, 1977, p. 193). According to Bandura, these thoughts about oneself may influence motivation, action, and emotional arousal (Bandura, 1982). Events that people believe they can cope with successfully become less fearsome. People are more likely to want to approach things they believe they are capable of doing and avoid things they do not think they can do.

SE can be general or specific. General SE is an individual's belief that he or she can accomplish or cope with a wide range of demands. Domain-specific SE is an individual's confidence in his or her ability to carry out a specific action (What's the Evidence? 4-1). Researchers have examined general and specific SE as predictors of a wide range of behaviors, from exercise to smoking cessation to condom use (e.g., Casey, Timmermann, Allen, Krahn, & Turkiewicz, 2009; Gwaltney, Metrik, Kahler, & Shiffman, 2009; Luszczynska, Scholz, & Schwarzer, 2005; Sears & Stanton, 2001; Yarcheski, Mahon, Yarcheski, & Cannella, 2004). Overall, SE itself is a fairly good predictor of future behavior change. Although interventions to increase SE directly have been mixed in their ability to change behavior, there may be indirect ways that health and fitness professionals can work with clients to increase their SE.

■ **MOTIVATING CHANGE:** Understanding How Client Self-Efficacy Influences Motivation for Behavior Change

The concept of self-efficacy is important to health and fitness professionals in understanding how confident clients may feel about making health-behavior changes. Health and fitness professionals may or may not be able to directly change an individual's SE for a specific behavior; however, understanding the client's existing beliefs can give professionals a sense of where the client is starting. The health and fitness professional can offer social support, empathy, and in some cases specific strategies and success experiences that may empower the client to make behavior changes. Perhaps a client had a bad experience in the past that leads him to believe he is not capable of a particular behavior. It may be helpful to ask clients to describe their past experiences. Perhaps there were unfavorable conditions that affected the client's likelihood of success. These questions can help clients disentangle beliefs about themselves from

WHAT'S THE EVIDENCE? 4-1

The Specificity of Exercise Self-Efficacy

Rodgers, W. M., Murray, T. C., Courneya, K. S., Bell, G. J., & Harber, V. J. (2009). The specificity of self-efficacy over the course of a progressive exercise programme. *Applied Psychology: Health and Well-Being, 1*(2): 211-232.

■ PURPOSE

The purpose of this study was to examine changes in exercise self-efficacy (SE) over 6 months of participation in either a walking or traditional fitness center–based exercise program. The researchers wanted to see whether exercise self-efficacy was specific to the type of exercise performed, or whether if SE improved for one form of exercise, such as walking, it would improve for the other form, even though subjects were not performing that type regularly. In addition, the researchers examined specific types of exercise self-efficacy thought to be important for successful behavior change and how these measures changed over time.

■ STUDY

A total of 115 volunteers, including 83 women and 32 men, completed the study. The average age of participants was about 49 years old, and average body mass index (BMI) was about 30. (A BMI of 25 to 30 is considered over-weight.) Subjects were randomly assigned to three groups: walking, traditional exercise, and a control group. The walking activity group wore pedometers and tried to achieve a target number of steps per day, gradually working up to 10,000 steps per day. The traditional exercise group performed exercise on machines (e.g., treadmill, elliptical trainer, etc.) in a fitness center. They began with 20 minutes of exercise 3 days a week, progressing to longer durations (about 40 minutes) and 4 days a week to meet public health guidelines for exercise participation. The third group served as a "lifestyle maintenance" control group and had the opportunity to begin exercise programs at the end of the study.

All participants completed questionnaires about feelings of SE for walking activity and for traditional exercise. Researchers measured three types of exercise SE:

- Task exercise SE (how confident people were that they could perform the specific exercise tasks, such as using proper technique)
- Scheduling exercise SE (how confident people were that they could perform the exercise regularly)
- Coping exercise SE (how confident people felt about overcoming general barriers to exercise participation)

The experiment showed that improvements in exercise SE were specific to exercise mode; for example, subjects who walked had greater improvements in SE for walking than for traditional exercise. This held true for all three types of exercise SE. The study supported the notion that successful experiences in exercise settings have the power to increase exercise SE.

Interesting patterns for all three types of SE emerged over time. The researchers had hypothesized that exercise-specific SE would increase over the 6 months of the study. Task SE typically increased, specific to exercise mode, over the first 3 months of the exercise program, but then declined. Especially concerning was a decline noted in coping SE for the traditional exercise group. All participants evaluated coping self-efficacy for both walking and traditional exercise. Coping SE scores for the walking group declined over the first 12 weeks of the program, as initial optimism may have faded, but then increased over the second half of the program. SE scores for the traditional exercise group rose for the first half of the program but then declined sharply in the second half. This decline may have been due to increased program demands.

■ IMPLICATIONS

Health and fitness professionals can help clients increase all forms of exercise SE by ensuring they are successful in meeting the demands of their exercise programs. However, the decline in coping SE between 3 and 6 months as the traditional exercise program became more demanding is a concern. This decline did not occur for walking exercise. Health and fitness professionals typically recommend exercise in a fitness center environment, with a target of reaching public health guidelines. It may be important for health and fitness professionals to examine this practice, working closely with individual clients, if possible, to be sure that the demands of the exercise program do not exceed client coping SE.

situations that may have impeded their potential. The health and fitness professional may be able to offer new and more-favorable conditions for early success. Even small achievements can change the client's emotional landscape, improve SE, and increase motivation for future action.

The Theory of Planned Behavior

The Theory of Planned Behavior (Ajzen, 1991) suggests that attitudes, subjective norms, and perceived behavioral control influence behavioral intentions (Fig. 4-5). Those intentions, in turn, influence actual

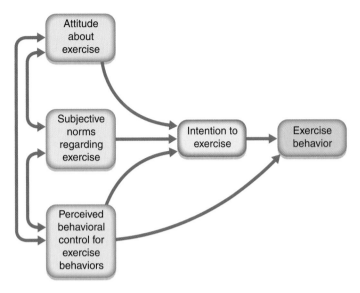

Figure 4-5. Theory of Planned Behavior: application to exercise.

behavior. Attitudes include people's thoughts and feelings about the positive and negative aspects of a behavior. Subjective norms are people's beliefs about what they think others typically do, as well as what they think others want them to do. Perceived behavioral control is the same idea as self-efficacy—people's beliefs about their own ability to engage in a behavior.

For example, consider wearing a bicycle helmet. The theory would suggest that the more positively people view wearing a helmet, the more they believe others wear helmets and want them to wear a helmet; additionally, the more they think that they could be successful at wearing a helmet, then the more likely they will be to intend to wear a helmet. Finally, the more they intend to wear a helmet, the more likely it is that they actually will wear a helmet.

Numerous research studies offer scientific support for each piece of the Theory of Planned Behavior. However, few studies examine tests of the full model simultaneously. In other words, to really support the model, a study should ideally examine how all the components unfold over time. Likewise, few studies have examined whether interventions to change attitudes, norms, and perceived control subsequently affect intentions and behavior.

Armitage and Talibudeen (2010) designed a safer-sex experiment. Their intervention about condom carrying led to increases in participants' subjective norms about condom carrying, which in turn predicted behavioral intentions to carry condoms. The subjective norms mediated, or explained, the relationships between the intervention and intentions to carry condoms. However, these researchers did not measure actual future condom-carrying behavior or condom-use behavior.

Wyszynski, Bricker, and Comstock (2011) found that a parent quitting smoking cigarettes by the time a child was in third grade led to the child having more-negative attitudes about smoking in ninth grade, which in turn led to that child being less likely to smoke in

12th grade. Indeed, the negative attitudes about smoking mediated the relationship between parental smoking cessation and future smoking behavior by children.

◼ *Kristen has enjoyed giving several healthy eating workshops. Janice has allowed these to be offered during work hours, which ensured good attendance. Kristen is now organizing a physical activity incentive program–the Century Club. Employees who log 100 miles of walking, or the equivalent, win a free t-shirt and a book of coupons to local businesses.*

Several employees have signed up for individual lifestyle counseling sessions with Kristen and her personal trainers. Kristen usually meets with sedentary clients herself because she has the most training in working with this group. Her goal is to help them make a decision to enroll in the Century Club. She hopes that once they enroll, they will be motivated to walk several times a week. Her strategy in her counseling sessions is to explore a client's motivations for coming to see her and then build on the motivations to help people form the intention to exercise regularly. Based on what clients tell her, she then asks questions concerning their attitudes toward exercise. Her theme with many clients is informing them that even small increases in physical activity reap benefits because many clients seem to think only high volumes and intensities of exercise count. By focusing on amounts of exercise matched to clients' abilities, she hopes to strengthen their self-efficacy, or perceived behavioral control. She helps them make specific plans for when, where, and how they will walk and encourages them to walk with a friend or family member when possible. Kristen knows that whereas social norms are not strongly predictive of exercise behavior, social support is very helpful. ◼

MOTIVATION FOR BEHAVIOR CHANGE

The word "motivation" comes from the Latin root, *movere*, which means to move. Motivation is the internal force that moves clients to action. Motivation is central to every stage of behavior change. Psychologists have studied the many factors that affect motivation for behavior change and how health and fitness professionals can best work with people to increase their motivation for positive behavior change.

Self-Determination Theory: The Nature of Motivation

Researchers Edward Deci and Richard Ryan (2008a) have studied motivation and psychological well-being. They believe that people are naturally active and motivated to pursue activities and goals in which they are interested or from which they believe they will obtain some benefit. They have observed that people also act in response to external forces that put pressure on them to behave in certain ways. Deci and Ryan propose that there are different types of motivation that drive behavior and that some types of motivation are more likely to result in successful behavior change than others. They talk specifically about two basic types of motivation: autonomous motivation and controlled motivation. Autonomous motivation means that people feel like they are behaving of their own free will, in accordance with their own wishes. They are doing something because they want to do it. Controlled motivation means people do something because they feel pressured by demands from external forces. These types of motivation feel very different to people. The theory of motivation developed by Deci and Ryan is called Self-determination Theory (SDT).

Factors That Affect Motivation

SDT holds that the three most important factors that influence motivation include autonomy, competence, and connection.

Autonomy

People generally do not like to be told what to do, unless they have actively sought and asked for advice. People like to feel that they have choices and can make choices about behavior according to their own wishes, in accordance with their own values and goals. Autonomous motivation is stronger than controlled motivation for this reason: people like autonomy.

Competence

People like to feel competent at the activities in which they engage. They like to feel good about their performance and are pleased when their work goes well, when they receive good grades, or when they become proficient at skills that they are working to develop. Competence is similar to self-efficacy. Both are specific to behavior. A person may feel competent and have high self-efficacy for work situations but low competence in the fitness center—and thus low self-efficacy for following an exercise program. When people feel incompetent, they generally do not feel good, and they may lose motivation to continue in the area of incompetence. Feelings of competence are motivational and strengthen people's efforts in the area of competence.

Connection

People are social creatures and tend to seek relationships with other people. They like to feel understood, have the approval of others they respect, talk to one another, and reach out to others who need help. Connection means that people feel they belong in a particular group or place. Positive connections make people feel good and reinforce motivation.

Types of Motivation

Deci and Ryan have proposed that in addition to classifying motivation as autonomous or controlled, motivation can be further divided into six broad categories that vary in the degree to which people feel they are autonomously motivated (Fig. 4-6). Most people exhibit health behaviors for all these motivations at various times throughout their lives (Health Psychology in Your Life 4-1). Intrinsic motivation occurs when people pursue an activity because it is inherently interesting or enjoyable. People who play basketball with a group of friends during their lunch hour just for fun are intrinsically motivated. They are not driving themselves to do something unpleasant just to get some exercise or joining the group because they do not want to disappoint a friend who is expecting them to come. They play because they enjoy playing. Intrinsic motivation is the strongest form of motivation because it feels the best.

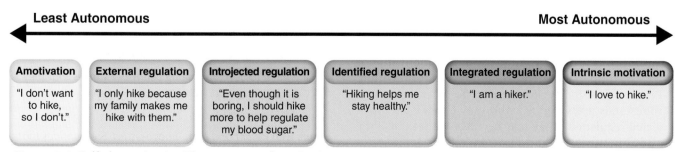

Least Autonomous ← → Most Autonomous

Amotivation	External regulation	Introjected regulation	Identified regulation	Integrated regulation	Intrinsic motivation
"I don't want to hike, so I don't."	"I only hike because my family makes me hike with them."	"Even though it is boring, I should hike more to help regulate my blood sugar."	"Hiking helps me stay healthy."	"I am a hiker."	"I love to hike."

Figure 4-6. Self-determination Theory: types of motivation.

HEALTH PSYCHOLOGY IN YOUR LIFE 4-1.
Motivation for Health Behaviors

List five behaviors you perform regularly that help you to stay healthy or improve your health. Examples might include eating a salad every day, taking the stairs instead of the elevator, playing a sport or engaging in another form of physical activity, going to bed by a certain time on weeknights, or scheduling (and attending) regular dental hygiene appointments. For each behavior, consider whether your motivation is intrinsic, integrated regulation, identified regulation, introjected regulation, or external regulation.

The opposite of intrinsic motivation is extrinsic motivation. Extrinsic motivation occurs when a person behaves a certain way to achieve a desired outcome, not because the behavior is inherently interesting or enjoyable. When people exercise because they will get a free t-shirt, obtain the approval of a friend, or feel less stressed later in the day, they are extrinsically motivated. Deci and Ryan propose that people can feel autonomous with extrinsic motivation, especially when the goals achieved by the behavior in question are valued. They call this type of motivation identified regulation. People identify with the goal or value of the behavior, so they use (regulate) a behavior to pursue the goal, thus feeling a form of autonomous motivation. The motivation comes from within. Motivation for health behaviors often comes from identified regulation. Many people have strong motivation for exercise, even though they do not particularly enjoy working out, because they like the way exercise makes them feel after the session has ended, or they believe that exercise helps them look better or sleep better, or they perceive other benefits from exercise. Identified regulation feels good, as people feel autonomous with this type of motivation. Deci and Ryan describe a similar but even more-autonomous form of motivation, integrated regulation. People with integrated regulation believe the behavior is consistent with their personal values, and they have integrated the behavior into their self-concept. For example, people may bicycle regularly because they see themselves as cyclists. Although the motivation for the behavior is not yet purely intrinsic, it is highly autonomous.

Introjected regulation refers to behavior that occurs because people feel they "should" perform the behavior but do not really want to do it. The motivation is coming from external forces, rather than from within. People who sign up for an exercise class because a spouse has pressured them to may experience introjected regulation. They may say they want to take the class, but in reality they do so to please or appease another person. Because introjected regulation interferes

with feelings of autonomy, it does not feel good and is a fairly weak form of motivation for behavior change.

External regulation occurs when people act solely from external pressure. Children who must sit and not talk in class often do so because they must, not because they want to or see any benefit to this behavior, other than avoiding punishment. When people perform a behavior because they "have to" as a result of rules they must follow, their motivation is poor, and the behavior usually ceases once the person leaves that situation. An example of external regulation might be an unwilling child in physical education class running a mile because he must complete a fitness test. Amotivation is the last category of motivation and refers to no motivation whatsoever.

SDT has application for behavior in all realms of life. It is especially applicable to health-behavior change, since motivation is so important for changing lifestyle behaviors. Research suggests that people who pursue autonomous goals are more likely to report feelings of well-being and better coping strategies that reduce feelings of stress and strengthen feelings of self-control (Miquelon & Vallerand, 2008). Researchers have also examined SDT in relationship to exercise and physical activity behaviors. A review focusing on SDT proposes that it can help both researchers and practitioners understand decisions to begin exercising as well as adhere to an exercise regimen (Wilson, Mack, & Grattan, 2008). Researchers have also applied SDT in studies of close relationships, parenting, education, and work (Deci & Ryan, 2008b).

■ *Over 15% of the employees have signed up for the Century Club program, and Kristen is very pleased. She understands that the incentives offered for participation are a form of extrinsic motivation and hopes that as employees become active, they will enjoy their activities and develop a more-integrated regulation of their exercise behavior. To this end, her workshops, bulletin boards, and e-mails to employees help them focus on the psychological benefits of physical activity. Kristen has urged Janice not to focus on a company-wide weight-loss program because weight loss can be a discouraging goal for many people. Instead, the focus has been on feeling more energetic, and she is hoping that these positive feelings will better support employees' behavior-change efforts.*

Of course, many of the employees making appointments to meet with Kristen want to lose weight. Kristin discusses their ideas for improving their diet and exercise behaviors, urging them to develop lifelong behavior changes that they can live with. She also explores their motivations for weight loss. One client, Carrie, tells Kristin she has struggled for years with weight and body-image issues. She confides that she has been in and out of therapy. "I used to want to lose weight so people would like me better. I would feel ashamed and like a bad person when my crazy starvation diet failed. I thought I had failed. I now know that these crazy diets were the biggest problem. Plus feeling ashamed and depressed made me eat even more than usual." She tells Kristen she has made steady progress in learning to manage stress without overeating and is ready to exercise. Kristen is pleased to hear that Carrie is on the right track and finding better motivations for weight control. Carrie does not want to exercise at work. Kristen tells Carrie about a water exercise class for beginners held at a nearby facility. Carrie likes this idea and decides to try it. Kristen also suggests walking in a nearby park. Carrie feels self-conscious about walking in public. Kristen suggests that Carrie get a dog to walk. Carrie laughs but then gets a surprised expression on her face. "You know, my neighbor is elderly and has difficulty getting out to walk her dog. Maybe I could help her out." ■

Motivational Interviewing

Today the health-care field is different from the past. No longer is the professional–client relationship based on the doctor telling the patient what to do and the patient simply accepting the information. Today, a person can search the Internet for answers before ever speaking with a health and fitness professional. Clients are looking for more than just instructions to follow. They want to be actively involved with their self-care and treatment decisions.

How do health and fitness professionals promote behavior change with clients without simply giving advice or reciting information from a book? After all, many clients already know what they should be doing. They have the information they need but may lack the motivation and social support to apply this knowledge. Motivational interviewing might be the key (Miller & Rollnick, 2013). **Motivational interviewing is both a treatment philosophy and a set of strategies to help people increase their own internal drive to change.** It is a way for the trained professional to lead clients into forming their own decisions about the changes they need to make regarding their health behaviors. Professionals work with clients to explore and resolve ambivalence about behavior change. The professional and the client are collaborators (Lundahl & Burke, 2009). Ideally, motivational interviewing helps clients develop intrinsic motivation, or at least integrated regulation of the target behavior. The purpose of motivational interviewing is to help clients feel autonomous, competent, and connected.

Much research has been devoted to motivational interviewing in recent years. Motivational interviewing grew out of treatments for substance-use disorders in the 1980s. Since then, researchers have applied it to many behaviors such as diet, exercise, and risky activities related to HIV and other sexually transmitted infections. Motivational interviewing has been found to be a consistently better treatment than none at all and has also been found to work just as well and in some cases even better than other established treatments ranging from cognitive-behavioral approaches (discussed in the next section) to 12-step programs (Lundahl & Burke, 2009). Motivational interviewing also has been found to be an effective intervention in the health care of chronically ill cohorts (e.g., Linden, Butterworth, & Prochaska, 2010), as well as increasing attempts to quit smoking in college students (e.g., Harris, Catley, & Good, 2010).

For professionals interested in learning motivational-interviewing techniques, Lundahl and Burke (2009) recommend starting by participating in a two-day interactive workshop, followed by ongoing supervision and coaching. Their research suggests that practitioners with a variety of professional and educational backgrounds (e.g., bachelors-, masters-, and doctoral-level training) can be successful at learning motivational-interviewing strategies (Health Psychology at Work 4-1).

Motivational interviewing is especially helpful for people in the early stages of change. Professionals need great skill when using motivational-interviewing techniques with people resistant to change or coping with complicated psychological issues and situations. Some of the components of motivational interviewing, such as effective communication skills, will be discussed in Chapter 5. All health and fitness professionals can practice the good communication skills that are the foundation of motivational interviewing to enhance understanding of their clients and to help them feel respected and valued.

MOTIVATING CHANGE: In the Early Stages of Change, Let Clients Do the Talking

Motivational interviewing is especially helpful when working with clients in the precontemplation or contemplation stages of change. These clients have not yet made a decision to change, so jumping into writing exercise recommendations or giving advice on changing eating behaviors may be a waste of time—and may even make clients feel overwhelmed and less confident than ever about changing. For professionals who see many clients in this stage, learning motivational-interviewing techniques is helpful. The best way to work with clients not yet ready to change is to help them explore their ideas about the behavior and its importance and relevance to them. It is also important to explore clients' feelings of self-efficacy and the barriers that they see preventing them from changing. When clients have some ambivalence about changing, a good listener can help them explore this ambivalence in productive ways and provide helpful information that might move clients closer to changing.

HEALTH PSYCHOLOGY AT WORK 4-1. Motivational Interviewing on College Campuses

Brian L. Burke, Ph.D.

Brian L. Burke (Ph.D., University of Arizona, 2003) is an Associate Professor of Psychology at Fort Lewis College, a public liberal arts college in Durango, Colorado. Dr. Burke is a licensed clinical psychologist whose principal academic interests include terror management, motivational interviewing, and college teaching. Dr. Burke won the New Faculty Teaching Award at Fort Lewis College in 2005 and the Featured Scholar Award at Fort Lewis College in 2010. He originally hails from Montreal, Canada (yes, he does play ice hockey). Dr. Burke has published several scholarly articles on motivational interviewing, including five meta-analyses (or quantitative summaries) of outcome studies. Dr. Burke published a seminal meta-analysis on outcome studies of motivational interviewing in 2003 [Burke, B. L., Arkowitz, H., & Menchola, M. (2003). The efficacy of motivational interviewing: a meta-analysis of controlled clinical trials. *Journal of Consulting and Clinical Psychology, 71*(5): 843-861], which remains one of the most highly cited papers in Essential Science Indicators. Dr. Burke offers a unique practicum course at Fort Lewis College to give students the opportunity to learn and apply motivational interviewing on campus. He trains students in the course to be peer consultants for fellow students who are in need of help after violating the college's drug and alcohol policies, who are experiencing academic difficulties in their math classes, or who are thinking about quitting smoking.

"Motivational interviewing (MI) is an evidence-based treatment for substance abuse and other problems, which integrates the relationship-building skills of client-centered therapy with active strategies for change. In my MI practicum course, undergraduate psychology and public health students learn how to do motivational interviewing by practicing the component skills and then using them in 'live' one-on-one interviews with other students sanctioned for substance-related campus policy violations or who are on the cusp of failing their math class. This course thus gives students an opportunity to learn about and deliver interventions designed to reduce substance use and improve academic success on campus.

"A large and expanding number of controlled research studies have shown that MI is more effective (10% to 20% more) than no treatment and at least as effective as other viable treatments for many problems. These problems range from improving diet and exercise behaviors to reducing substance abuse and other risky behaviors and increasing client engagement in treatment.

"The MI practicum class is very small and reserved for students who are academically capable and socially mature. I put my psychologist license on the line when I send my students out there to do peer consulting. They get close supervision from me and the Coordinator for Student Wellness Initiatives.

"The work the practicum students are doing benefits the college. It's also a different way for them to learn. They look beyond the college classroom and think about their future careers. The following comments from my students illustrate this point.

"'It's very rewarding knowing that you could have made a difference with somebody. It's all about them,' said one of my students. 'You're not telling them what to do, but you're helping them realize what and how they might decide to change to make their own lives better.'"

"'I was attracted to this class because I knew I was going to get skills for being a social worker in the future, and I have,' said another MI student. 'I have gained some skills that I know I'm going to be able to use in my career.'"

Attribution Theory and Locus of Control

Attributions are explanations that people have for why things happen. Most people have a tendency to attribute their own behavior to the situation while attributing others' behavior to personality. After all, individuals see themselves in many contexts and see other people in only one or a few contexts. People have more data about themselves, so it makes sense that they can generate more reasons for why they do things. This phenomenon is important to health and fitness professionals because a fitness professional's ideas about why clients are doing (or not doing) what they are supposed to may be very different from a client's view. For example, a health and fitness professional might recommend walking first thing every morning for 30 minutes. When the client fails to stick to this plan, the health and fitness professional might attribute his failure to personality traits like laziness or lack of self-discipline. On the other hand, the client may feel that he simply has no spare time in the morning, perhaps needing to dress and feed children for school and get to work early himself. Thus, health and fitness professionals need to be careful about making only personality or internal attributions about their client's behavior. It is important to work with the client to also assess and address external or situational factors that might be barriers to following behavior-change recommendations.

Individual clients also may have a tendency to emphasize internal or external causes for their own health and behavior. Another name for this tendency is locus of control. Locus of control is the extent to which people think things happen for internal versus external reasons (Rotter, 1975). For example, two students in the same course might get a "D" on an exam. They both have the same low grade on the same test. However, one student might think, "That exam was so unfair. That professor is such a witch!" This student is making an external attribution and may have more of an external locus of control. Another student might think, "I am so dumb. I can't do this." This person is making an internal attribution and may have a more-internal locus of control. Some events truly are outside of individual control. Natural disasters such as earthquakes are one example. Other events may be more within individual control. Most events have a combination of causes, and regardless of the nature of initial cause, people often have control over how they respond to events.

A concept called health locus of control (HLOC) has helped researchers study the role that locus of control might play in health-behavior applications (Wallston, Wallston, & Devellis, 1976). Scales that measure HLOC determine how strongly people believe that their health is determined by factors under their personal control. People with a strong internal HLOC believe that they have a great deal of control over their personal health. People with a strong external HLOC believe that their health is more likely to be determined by powerful others (such as health-care providers) or chance. It makes sense that people with a strong internal HLOC might be more likely to follow through with behavior-change programs designed to reduce health risks, but the research has not always supported this common-sense notion (Baumeister & Bengel, 2007; Grotz, Hapke, Lampert, & Baumeister, 2011). Some researchers have argued that HLOC is an indication of perceived behavioral control (from the Theory of Planned Behavior Model) or self-efficacy, and that measuring HLOC separately does not add much predictive value in studies examining behavior change (Armitage, 2003).

The attributions that people make are all relative to the individual. Perception is key. Without delving too deeply into philosophy about the nature of reality, finding one's own truth is a unique interplay between the individual's ideas, emotions, and interactions with the environment. Two different people may respond to the exact same event in very different ways depending on their genetic makeup, prior experiences, and culture.

MOTIVATING CHANGE: Help Clients Explore Locus of Control

The issue of locus of control is important to health and fitness professionals because too many external or internal attributions can create problems. Too much of an external locus of control can create a sense of anger and blame directed at others or of helplessness and dependency directed at oneself. Too much of an internal locus of control can create a sense of self-blame, guilt, and depression. For example, many women in mainstream U.S. culture internalize media ideals about tall, underweight models. If some women believe that they can control and change everything about their bodies—that is, too much internal locus of control— they may be more apt to become frustrated and depressed when their diet and exercise efforts do not let them become the media ideal. The challenge for health and fitness professionals is to help clients realistically evaluate what they can and cannot control. By doing this, professionals can help clients find a balance between acceptance and change.

BEHAVIOR-CHANGE STRATEGIES

Psychologists have always been interested in how people learn new behaviors. Because learning new behaviors is the basis for behavior change, this research has applications for health and fitness professionals. Behavioral-learning theory research typically studies the rewards and punishments that people (and animals) learn to associate with certain behaviors and how these associations shape future behavior. Cognitive-behavioral approaches examine how people's thinking and emotional states are linked to their behavior.

Behavioral-Learning Theory

Behavioral-learning approaches focus on how people and other animals learn through associations. Strict behaviorists emphasize externally observable, measurable actions. Other theorists believe that internal events such as thoughts and feelings may develop through behavioral-conditioning principles.

Classical Conditioning
Classical-conditioning principles may be useful in understanding how people have developed associations in their lives. The basic idea is that people learn to associate previously neutral stimuli with naturally occurring connections between stimuli and responses. Figures 4-7 and 4-8 offer some examples. Figure 4-7 illustrates a famous experiment performed by Ivan Pavlov (1849-1936), a Russian physician and neurophysiologist who initially studied digestive secretions in dogs (Fig. 4-7). He became famous for a serendipitous discovery that dogs begin to salivate in anticipation of food. When dogs taste or smell meat (unconditioned stimulus or UCS), they naturally salivate (unconditioned response or UCR). Pavlov called these associations "unconditioned" because they occur without having to teach them. When a previously neutral stimulus such as a metronome ticking is repeatedly paired with the unconditioned stimulus of meat, over time the ticking alone (conditioned stimulus or CS) will itself elicit salivation (conditioned response or CR). The

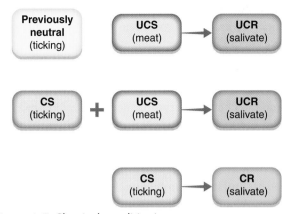

Figure 4-7. Classical conditioning.

associations that are learned are called conditioned. The responses that occur with classical conditioning are often called reflexive, meaning they are unconscious and automatic.

Many people have stories of foods that they no longer eat because they became associated with unpleasant sensations. For example, if a person eats a hot dog and then experiences motion sickness from a car ride, which results in vomiting the hot dog, the person may forever after find the taste of hot dogs aversive. The previously neutral stimulus (hot dog) becomes associated with the aversive experience of vomiting (Fig. 4-8).

Many anxiety disorders such as post-traumatic stress disorder and some phobias have classically conditioned aspects to their development and treatment. For example, very loud noises naturally elicit a startle reflex. A child who is startled by a balloon popping may become intensely afraid of balloons. Balloons themselves are not inherently frightening, but by association they become so. Paradoxically, the treatment for many phobias is to train the client in a relaxation response and then expose him or her to the feared object. The idea is that relaxation is incompatible with anxiety and fear. If the person can learn a new association between the feared object and relaxation, then counterconditioning occurs. Psychologists use counterconditioning as one component of treatment programs for some psychological disorders.

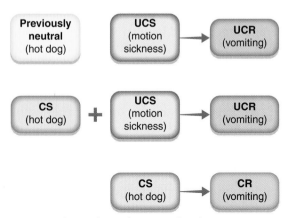

Figure 4-8. Classical conditioning: food aversion.

For health and fitness professionals, classical conditioning may be useful in a broad sense. Offering a positive, relaxing environment and professional relationship could counteract previous negative associations that people may have regarding working with health and fitness professionals. In addition, clients interested in changing eating behaviors may find that many overeating responses have evolved in a classical-conditioning manner. For example, some people have a conditioned response that stimulates them to eat when watching a movie. A formerly neutral stimulus (the movie) becomes associated with the pleasurable activity of eating. Just as Pavlov's dog learned to salivate in response to a ticking metronome, so do some eaters reach for food when watching movies, even though they may not be hungry. Chapter 9 discusses eating behavior in more detail and how health and fitness professionals can use behavioral strategies to help clients address eating behavior.

Operant Conditioning

Operant conditioning is about rewards and punishment. As in classical conditioning, learning occurs based on associations between behaviors and stimuli. However, there are some important differences between classical and operant conditioning (Fig. 4-9). The most important differences are that operant conditioning views a person's behavior as voluntary and believes that behavior occurs (or resists occurring) in anticipation of a reward or punishment. Operant conditioning refers to the idea of organisms "operating" on their environment. The fact that behavior is voluntary opens up a world of options for the health and fitness professional and client.

The person most often credited with developing the ideas of operant conditioning is B.F. Skinner (1904-1990). For example, Skinner trained pigeons to engage in all kinds of behaviors (e.g., "dancing" in circles, pecking certain colored disks) in anticipation of a food reward. Skinner and other behaviorists use terms such as positive reinforcement, negative reinforcement, positive punishment, and negative punishment.

These concepts can be tricky to master because some of these words do not mean the same thing as in everyday language. Reinforcement refers to behaviors that you want to increase in frequency. Punishment refers to behaviors that you want to decrease in frequency. Positive refers to applying a stimulus. Negative refers to removing a stimulus. Here, positive and negative do not signify whether the target behavior or stimulus is good or bad. Positive and negative refer only to whether you are introducing or taking away a stimulus.

An example of positive reinforcement is giving a dog a treat for sitting. The dog trainer applies a pleasant stimulus (treat) to increase behavior (sitting).

An example of negative reinforcement is a car "dinging" until passengers fasten their seat belts. They remove an aversive stimulus (dinging sound) to increase behavior (fastening their seat belts).

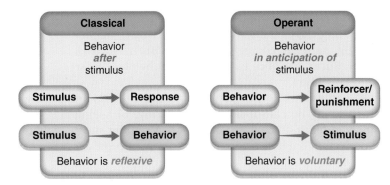

Figure 4-9. Differences between classical and operant conditioning.

An example of positive punishment is getting a ticket for speeding. The police officer applies an aversive stimulus (expensive ticket) to decrease behavior (speeding). Note that the term "positive" refers to applying the stimulus. Neither getting a ticket nor speeding is good!

An example of negative punishment is revoking one's driver's license for driving under the influence of alcohol. The justice system removes a pleasant stimulus (the privilege of driving) to decrease behavior (driving when intoxicated).

Most adults, children, and animals respond best to positive reinforcement as a learning strategy whenever possible. Punishment may be necessary in some circumstances to protect people. However, punishment has many drawbacks, including inducing fear, avoidance, and concealment.

For health and fitness professionals, positive reinforcement will likely be the most useful behavioral-learning tool. The kinds of behaviors and rewards that clients can experience are infinite. Strict behaviorists would focus on behaviors that are observable to others and rewards that come externally from the environment. For example, people might get paid a certain amount of money for every time they exercise. Some employee workplace programs operate on this principle.

Other theorists would say that rewards can be internal, such as good thoughts and feelings that come from engaging in healthy behaviors. An important role for the health and fitness professional is to help clients notice the benefits of their efforts. SDT suggests that behaviors performed in response to intrinsic motivations will be more likely to continue than those performed for external rewards. External rewards, however, can enhance people's motivation to make a decision to change. External rewards may motivate people to start exercising or make other changes in their health behaviors. Hopefully, over time clients will develop intrinsic motivation or integrated regulation to continue these positive behaviors.

Cognitive-Behavioral Approaches

Whereas behavioral approaches emphasize externally observable behavior, cognitive-behavioral approaches recognize the interrelationships between thoughts,

feelings, and behaviors. If people can change their thoughts, then perhaps they can change how they feel and act. Indeed, some theorists view thoughts as "internal mental events" that can be reinforced over time.

Cognitive-behavioral approaches comprise one of the most scientifically researched areas of psychological intervention for a wide range of experiences and disorders including behavior change, major depression, generalized anxiety disorder, panic disorder, anger management, and stress. Recently researchers have examined the usefulness of cognitive-behavioral approaches for irritable bowel syndrome (Jones, Koloski, Boyce, & Talley, 2011), chronic pain (Turner, Holtzman, & Manel, 2007), insomnia (Espie, 2009), and bereavement (Currier, Holland, & Neimeyer, 2010).

Cognitive-behavior theory initially developed out of work by psychologists who research, diagnose, and treat clinical depression. Aaron Beck (Beck, Rush, Shaw, & Emery, 1979) discovered that people with depression tend to have patterns of thinking that are internal, stable, and global. People who make internal attributions have an excessive tendency to blame themselves. People who make stable attributions assume that things will never get better. People who make global attributions assume that, if something is going wrong in one area of life, then it means that everything is bad. Beck called this constellation the "depressogenic cognitive triad," meaning that these three tendencies together are a recipe for developing depression. Taken to an extreme, these thoughts can create feelings of profound sadness and hopelessness that are characteristic of clinical depression.

For example, imagine that Greg has recently experienced the breakup of a romantic relationship with his girlfriend. He might think, "It's all my fault (internal). I am never going to get another date (stable). My friends are all going to think I am a loser, so I can't go to school (global)." This line of thinking may suggest an excessive tendency to blame oneself and to assume that things will never get better and that this single unpleasant event negatively affects multiple areas of life such as friendships and school.

The effects of our thoughts are not just psychological. Research suggests that thinking about the unwanted breakup of a romantic relationship can affect the brain in ways similar to the pain from a physical stimulus (Kross, Berman, Mischel, Smith, & Wagner, 2011).

Another classic framework for identifying unhelpful thought patterns comes from David Burns (Burns, 1999). Burns describes 12 patterns of unhelpful thinking (Box 4-3).

A common thought pattern in health-behavior change may be "all-or-nothing" thinking, or seeing things in black-and-white categories. Anything short of perfection is a failure. For example, some people as-sume that they have to look like a fashion model to be physically attractive, train like a professional athlete to exercise, or eat an exclusively vegan diet (i.e., consume no animal products whatsoever) to gain health benefits from fruits and vegetables. In reality, most people will wear regular clothes, exercise recreationally, and would benefit from small and consistent changes in their eating behavior. Although this description is less glamorous than the first one, it is probably more attainable and sustainable for most people.

MOTIVATING CHANGE: Tactfully Challenging Unhelpful Thought Patterns

So what does all this mean for health and fitness professionals? The goal here is not for every health and fitness professional to become a psychotherapist. Like any career choice, becoming a psychotherapist requires extensive education and training to practice ethically and effectively. The goal for health and fitness professionals is to have a sense of psychological phenomena that may arise in the context of a working relationship with clients. If health professionals can identify psychological patterns, they may be able to use some general concepts and strategies suggested here, collaborate with a trained psychologist on a health-care team, or make a referral to a psychologist working independently.

If health and fitness professionals note that clients might be engaged in unhelpful thought patterns, there are some simple ways to respond. The basic goal of cognitive-behavior therapy is to help the client identify and challenge his or her own automatic thoughts. For example, if a 30-year-old client says she needs to train for a marathon next month but she has not run since high school, the fitness professional might say something like, "That is great you are so excited about running again. However, increasing your exercise volume too quickly could lead to injury. What would it be like to start by training for a 5K run over the next 3 months?" This strategy affirms the client's desires and enthusiasm. At the same time, it gently invites the client to examine her own thinking. Raising the question, "What would it be like to..." is a nice way to introduce new ideas without being overly prescriptive or dashing the client's hopes. The health and fitness professional can offer some realistic options and also ask the client to brainstorm alternative suggestions.

Box 4-3. Twelve Patterns of Distorted or Unhelpful Thinking

1. All-or-nothing thinking: Seeing things in black-or-white categories; if a situation falls short of perfect, seeing it as a total failure
2. Jumping to conclusions: Interpreting things negatively without examining the evidence
3. Mind reading: Without checking it out, arbitrarily concluding that someone is reacting negatively
4. Fortune-telling: Predicting that things will turn out badly
5. Emotional reasoning: Assuming that negative emotions reflect the way things really are (e.g., "I feel terrified about going on airplanes; therefore, it must be dangerous to fly.")
6. Personalization and blame: Holding oneself or others personally responsible for an event beyond one's own or another's control
7. Overgeneralization: Seeing a single negative event, such as a romantic rejection or a career reversal, as a never-ending pattern of defeat; using words such as "always" or "never" when thinking about it
8. Mental filter: Picking out a single negative detail and dwelling on it to the exclusion of other information
9. Discounting the positive: Rejecting positive experiences by insisting that they do not count
10. Magnification: Exaggerating the importance of problems or shortcomings or minimizing the importance of desirable qualities
11. Should statements: Telling oneself that things should be a certain way
12. Labeling: An extreme form of all-or-nothing thinking where someone interprets behavior as an attribute (e.g., instead of saying "I/he/she made a mistake," the person also attaches a label such as "I am a failure.")

(Adapted from Burns, D. D. (1999). *The Feeling Good Handbook.* New York: Plume: 8-11.)

Behavior-Change Skills

Behavior-change skills are techniques that research shows are useful in helping people change behavior. Many of these skills are based on the behavioral-learning models and theories presented above. Health and fitness professionals can easily teach these skills to clients changing health behavior. Although the skills are easy to teach, they are not always easy to practice, as behavior change can be a difficult undertaking. The most helpful behavior-change skills include the following:

- **Setting goals and making specific plans:** Health and fitness professionals should be well versed in goal setting and planning. Goals must be clear and achievable. Plans must be specific. Clients must drive the planning process and professionals help clients make plans realistic.
- **Self-monitoring:** Self-monitoring systems are ways for clients to keep records of their activities and progress, as related to behavior change. Examples of self-monitoring systems include exercise logs, diet records, and smoking logs. Self-monitoring systems can be handwritten or electronic—whatever works best for clients. Systems can be used to record behaviors, as well as descriptions of events that triggered behaviors and thoughts related to the behaviors.
- **Problem solving:** Information gathered from self-monitoring systems can provide information for problem solving. Clients can learn to identify triggers that initiate both wanted and unwanted behaviors and think of ways to work around or with these. The processes of stimulus control and counterconditioning, discussed above, can be used to cope with common things that trigger behavior.
- **Cognitive restructuring:** Because people are thinking creatures, even programs focused primarily on observable behavior usually teach clients how to examine thinking that influences their behavior, as described in cognitive-behavioral approaches above (Fabricatore, 2007). Clients can learn to identify the thinking that leads to excuses to overeat or not exercise or have one more cigarette. With practice, clients can also learn to replace automatic thought patterns that lead to unwanted behaviors with more-productive thinking (Behavior Change in Action 4-1). This is all cognitive restructuring.

BEHAVIOR CHANGE IN ACTION 4-1

Cognitive Restructuring Supports Behavior-Change Efforts

■ **Challenge**
Some clients have negative thought patterns that lead to too many excuses for not exercising. How can health and fitness professionals help clients examine and change unhelpful thought patterns?

■ **Plan**
Psychologists have found that cognitive-restructuring strategies can help people change negative thinking patterns. Cognitive restructuring is the practice of examining and changing one's conscious thoughts. Cognitive restructuring means learning to perceive and think about a situation in a new way. Health and fitness professionals can help clients notice and challenge unhelpful thought patterns in several ways. The following suggestions focus on exercise behavior, but they can also apply to overeating, smoking cigarettes, and other health behaviors.

Encourage clients to keep a record of negative thoughts and self-talk that "cause" or almost cause them to skip an exercise session. Give clients 1 to 2 weeks to observe and record these thoughts. If clients have trouble becoming aware of their thoughts, instruct them to pay special attention to what is going through their minds when they are feeling stressed or conflicted about exercising or what thoughts prompt them to decide to not exercise. Thoughts may take the form of words, phrases, and even sentences, or they may be images or pictures combined with emotions.

Spend part of a session looking at these thoughts together. Which statements reflect real problems that you can address with the client? Let the client suggest ways that he or she could deal with these problems. Which tend to be "excuses"?

Suspend your judgment and allow clients to evaluate their self-talk. If clients feel that their problems are valid, and not excuses, be sympathetic. If clients feel that you are belittling their problems, they may become defensive and no longer be open to your guidance or cognitive-restructuring efforts.

Examine misconceptions that may underlie negative thoughts. Clients may exhibit some of the unhelpful thought patterns from Box 4-3. When exposed to the light of day, these patterns often seem less powerful, and clients can begin to observe and correct problematic misconceptions. For example, some clients are perfectionists with "all-or-nothing" thinking. If they can't exercise for 2 hours a day, they decide they may as well not exercise at all. Some clients may think exercise is adding to their stress. Perhaps they can see exercise as helping to reduce stress, if they feel more relaxed after an exercise session.

Help clients rephrase negative self-talk. This is harder than it sounds. The new self-talk should be less negative but also something that does not strike the client as unrealistic or silly. Here are two examples:
Unhelpful thinking: "I'm too tired to exercise today."

Continued

BEHAVIOR CHANGE IN ACTION 4-1–cont'd

New thinking: "I am going to exercise even though I feel tired. I know I'll feel better and have more energy after my workout."

Unhelpful thinking: "This exercise program is a waste of time. I've got more-important things to do."

New thinking: "I need exercise to stay healthy. What's more important than my health? Staying healthy is just as important as my work, and I must make time each day to exercise so that I can stay healthy and work as effectively as possible."

Help clients anticipate and cope with common negative thoughts. Once clients have uncovered and rephrased unhelpful thoughts, ask them to imagine getting ready to exercise with the negative thoughts springing up in their minds. Ask them to imagine restructuring the negative thoughts and exercising anyway. Clients should finish this visualization by imagining how good they feel during or after the exercise session.

■ *Kristen beams as she hands out t-shirts at the Century Club awards ceremony. Although some of the employees who have earned their awards are already regular exercisers, several are new to exercise or have not exercised regularly in several years.*

Kristen is pleased with the changes that the cafeteria director has made in lunch offerings. There are now two desserts, instead of five, and the menu has expanded to include a better selection of fruits and vegetables and fewer fried foods. Even though donuts still make their appearance at meetings from time to time, several employees have told Kristen that they appreciate the fruit platters as well.

Carrie enjoys walking her neighbor's dog so much that she takes it out every morning before work. This gives her a "reason" to walk. She has even met another dog owner who is on the same schedule, and some days they enjoy walking together. Her neighbor is grateful, and Carrie feels good about helping her.

At Kristen's weekly meeting with Janice, Janice observes that although weight loss may be slow in coming, several department heads have mentioned improved morale in their departments, as people compared their Century Club logs and bragged about their progress. ■

KEY TERMS

action (stage of change)
amotivation
attitudes
attributions
autonomous motivation
autonomy
behavior-change skills
behavioral-learning theory
classical conditioning
cognitive-behavioral approaches
cognitive restructuring
competence
connection
contemplation (stage of change)
controlled motivation
decisional balance
ecological perspectives
external regulation
extrinsic motivation
Health Belief Model
health locus of control
health promotion
identified regulation
integrated regulation
intrinsic motivation
introjected regulation
locus of control
maintenance (stage of change)
motivational interviewing
operant conditioning
perceived behavioral control
precontemplation (stage of change)
preparation (stage of change)
primary prevention
processes of change
punishment
readiness
reflexive
reinforcement
relapse
secondary screening
Self-Determination Theory
self-efficacy
self-monitoring
stages of change
subjective norms
termination (stage of change)
tertiary treatment
Theory of Planned Behavior
Transtheoretical Model

CRITICAL THINKING QUESTIONS

1. Consider the factors that affect your consumption (or nonconsumption) of alcohol. Draw a diagram similar to Figure 4-1 and apply an ecological perspective to your drinking behavior. Which factors at each level encourage you to drink alcohol? Which factors discourage this behavior?

2. Imagine you are working with a client who was diagnosed with high blood sugar several years ago but has not been back to a doctor since that time and is not sure whether he has diabetes. Use the Health Belief Model to list points that you might bring up in a conversation with him to help him form the decision to make a medical appointment to see if he has diabetes.

3. Use the Theory of Planned Behavior to compare the attitudes, subjective norms, and perceived behavioral control of a student who has just joined a sports team with a student who has never exercised and whose social group is not physically active. How might these three variables differ? How might they influence the amount of activity in which the two students engage?

4. Think about a habit you have tried to change. This could be any habit, from procrastinating less or keeping your desk clean, to eating more fruits and vegetables or quitting smoking. Use the Stages of Change Model from the TTM to describe your progress from precontemplation through whatever other stages you reached.

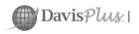 | For additional resources log in to Davis*Plus* (**http://davisplus.fadavis.com**/ keyword "Brehm") and click on the Premium tab. (Don't have a *Plus*Code to access Premium Resources? Just click the Purchase Access button on the book's Davis*Plus* page.)

REFERENCES

Ajzen, I. (1991). The theory of planned behavior. *Organizational Behavior and Human Decision Processes, 50*(2): 179-211.

Armitage, C. J. (2003). The relationship between multidimensional health locus of control and perceived behavioural control: how are distal perceptions of control related to proximal perceptions of control? *Psychology and Health, 18*(6): 723-738.

Armitage, C. J., & Talibudeen, L. (2010). Test of a brief theory of planned behaviour-based intervention to promote adolescent safe sex intentions. *British Journal of Psychology, 101*(1): 155-172.

Bandura, A. (1982). Self-efficacy mechanism in human agency. *American Psychologist, 37*(2): 122-147.

Bandura, A. (1977). Self-efficacy: toward a unifying theory of behavioral change. *Psychological Review, 84*(2): 191-215.

Baumeister, H., & Bengel, J. (2007). Psycho-social correlates of health and health behaviours: challenges and methodological pitfalls. *International Journal of Public Health, 52*(1): 6-7.

Beck, A. T., Rush, A. J., Shaw, B. F., & Emery, G. (1979). *Cognitive Therapy of Depression.* New York: Guilford Press.

Becker, M. H., ed. (1974). The Health Belief Model and personal health behavior. *Health Education Monographs, 2*: 324-473.

Burns, D. D. (1999). *The Feeling Good Handbook.* New York: Plume.

Carpenter, C. J. (2010). A meta-analysis of the effectiveness of health belief model variables in predicting behavior. *Health Communication, 25*: 661-669.

Casey, M. K., Timmermann, L., Allen, M., Krahn, S., & Turkiewicz, K. (2009). Response and self-efficacy of condom use: a meta-analysis of this important element of AIDS education and prevention. *Southern Communication Journal, 74*(1): 57-78.

Currier, J. M., Holland, J. M., & Neimeyer, R. A. (2010). Do CBT-based interventions alleviate distress following

bereavement? A review of the current evidence. *International Journal of Cognitive Therapy, 3*(1): 77-93.

Deci, E. L., & Ryan, R. M. (2008a). Facilitating optimal motivation and psychological well-being across life's domains. *Canadian Psychology, 49*(1): 14-23.

Deci, E. L., & Ryan, R. M. (2008b). Self-determination theory: a macrotheory of human motivation, development, and health. *Canadian Psychology, 49*(3): 182-185.

DiClemente, C. C., Prochaska, J. O., Fairhurst, S. K., Velicer, W. F., Velasquez, M. M., & Rossi, J. S. (1991). The process of smoking cessation: an analysis of precontemplation, contemplation, and preparation stages of change. *Journal of Consulting and Clinical Psychology, 59*(2): 295-304.

DiMatteo, M. R., Haskard, K. B., & Williams, S. L. (2007). Health beliefs, disease severity, and patient adherence: A meta-analysis. *Medical Care, 45*(6): 521-528.

Di Noia, J., & Prochaska, J. O. (2010). Mediating variables in a transtheoretical model dietary intervention program. *Health Education & Behavior, 37*(5): 753-762.

Espie, C. A. (2009). "Stepped care": a health technology solution for delivering Cognitive Behavioral Therapy as a first-line insomnia treatment. *Sleep, 32*(12): 1549-1558.

Fabricatore, A. N. (2007). Behavior therapy and cognitive-behavioral therapy of obesity: is there a difference? *Journal of the American Dietetic Association, 107*: 92-99.

Fisher, E. B. (2008). The importance of context in understanding behavior and promoting health. *Annals of Behavioral Medicine, 35*: 3-18.

Grotz, M., Hapke, U., Lampert, T., & Baumeister, H. (2011). Health locus of control and health behaviour: results from a national representative survey. *Psychology, Health & Medicine, 16*(2): 129-140.

Gwaltney, C. J., Metrik, J., Kahler, C. W., & Shiffman, S. (2009). Self-efficacy and smoking cessation: a meta-analysis. *Psychology of Addictive Behaviors, 23*(1): 56-66.

Harris, K. J., Catley, D., Good, G. E., Cronk, N., Harrar, S., & Williams, K. B. (2010). Motivational interviewing for smoking cessation in college students: a group randomized controlled trial. *Preventive Medicine, 51*(5): 387-393.

Jones, M., Koloski, N., Boyce, P., & Talley, N. J. (2011). Pathways connecting cognitive behavioral therapy and change in bowel symptoms of IBS. *Journal of Psychosomatic Research, 70*(3): 278-285.

Kok, G., Gottlieb, N. H., Commers, M., & Smerecnik, C. (2008). The ecological approach in health promotion programs: a decade later. *American Journal of Health Promotion, 22*(6): 437-442.

Kross, E., Berman, M. G., Mischel, W., Smith, E. E., & Wagner, T. D. (2011). Social rejection shares somatosensory representations with physical pain. *Proceedings of the National Academy of Sciences, 108*(15): 6270-6275.

Levesque, D. A., Cummins, C. O., Prochaska, J. M., & Prochaska, J. O. (2006). Stage of change for making an informed decision about Medicare health plans. *Health Services Research, 41*(4): 1372-1391.

Linden, A., Butterworth, S. W., & Prochaska, J. O. (2010). Motivational interviewing-based health coaching as a chronic care intervention. *Journal of Evaluation in Clinical Practice, 16*(1): 166-174.

Lundahl, B., & Burke, B. L. (2009). The effectiveness and applicability of motivational interviewing: a practice-friendly review of four meta-analyses. *Journal of Clinical Psychology, 65*(11): 1232-1245.

Luszczynska, A., Scholz, U., & Schwarzer, R. (2005). The general self-efficacy scale: multicultural validation studies. *Journal of Psychology, 139*(5): 439-457.

Miller, W. R., & Rollnick, S. (2013). *Motivational Interviewing: Preparing People for Change*, 3rd ed. New York: Guilford Press.

Miquelon, P., & Vallerand, R. J. (2008). Goal motives, well-being, and physical health: an integrative mode. *Canadian Psychology, 49*: 241-249.

Norcross, J. C., Krebs, P. M., & Prochaska, J. O. (2011). Stages of change. *Journal of Clinical Psychology, 67*(2): 143-154.

Pro-Change Behavior Systems, Inc. (2011). James A. Prochaska, PhD: founder. www.prochange.com/staff/james_prochaska. Accessed 11/30/12.

Prochaska, J. O., & DiClemente, C. C. (1982). Transtheoretical therapy: toward a more integrative model of change. *Psychotherapy: Theory, Research & Practice, 19*(3): 276-288.

Prochaska, J. O., & DiClemente, C. C. (1983). Stages and processes of self-change of smoking: toward an integrative model of change. *Journal of Consulting and Clinical Psychology, 51*(3): 390-395.

Prochaska, J. O., DiClemente, C. C., & Norcross, J. C. (1992). In search of how people change: applications to addictive behaviors. *American Psychologist, 47*(9): 1102-1114.

Richard, L., Potvin, L., Kishchuk, N., Prlic, H., & Green, L. W. (1996). Assessment of the integration of the ecological approach in health promotion programs. *American Journal of Health Promotion, 10*(4): 318-328.

Rosenstock, I. M. (1966). Why people use health services. *Milbank Memorial Fund Quarterly, 44*: 94-127.

Rotter, J. B. (1975). Some problems and misconceptions related to the construct of internal versus external control of reinforcement. *Journal of Consulting and Clinical Psychology, 43*(1): 55-66.

Sears, S., & Stanton, A. (2001). Expectancy-value constructs and expectancy violation as predictors of exercise adherence in previously sedentary women. *Health Psychology, 20*(5): 326-333.

Thøgersen-Ntoumani, C. (2009). An ecological model of predictors of stages of change for physical activity in Greek older adults. *Scandinavian Journal of Medicine and Science in Sports, 19*: 286-296.

Turner, J. A., Holtzman, S., & Mancl, L. (2007). Mediators, moderators, and predictors of therapeutic change in cognitive-behavioral therapy for chronic pain. *Pain, 127*(3): 276-286.

Vik, P. W., Culbertson, K. A., & Sellers, K. (2000). Readiness to change drinking among heavy-drinking college students. *Journal of Studies on Alcohol, 61*(5): 674-680.

Wallston, K. A., Wallston, B. S., & Devellis, R. (1978). Development of Multidimensional Health Locus of Control (MHLC) Scales. *Health Education Monographs, 6*(2):160-170.

Wilson, P. M., Mack, D. E., & Grattan, K. P. (2008). Understanding motivation for exercise: a self-determination theory perspective. *Canadian Psychology, 49*: 250-256.

Wyszynski, C. M., Bricker, J. B., & Comstock, B. A. (2011). Parental smoking cessation and child daily smoking: a 9-year longitudinal study of mediation by child cognitions about smoking. *Health Psychology, 30*(2): 171-176.

Yarcheski, A., Mahon, N. E., Yarcheski, T. J., & Cannella, B. L. (2004). A meta-analysis of predictors of positive health practices. *Journal of Nursing Scholarship, 36*(2): 102-108.

CHAPTER OUTLINE

LEARNING OBJECTIVES

After reading this chapter, you will be able to:

1. Discuss how health and fitness professionals can strengthen important factors in behavior-change models to help clients change health behaviors.

2. Describe the communication skills that are most helpful to health and fitness professionals when working with clients.

3. Assess a client's readiness to change.

4. Suggest possible approaches to discussing behavior change with clients who are resistant to or ambivalent about changing.

5. Create effective behavior-change goals and action plans.

6. Teach behavior-change skills.

7. Discuss common ethical challenges that arise when working with clients who are trying to change their health behaviors.

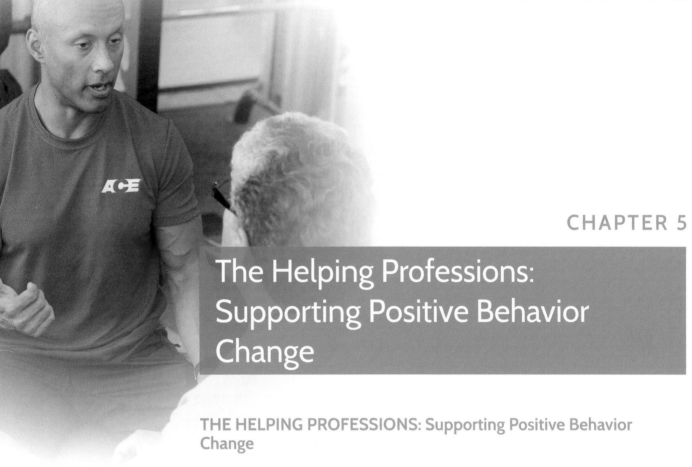

CHAPTER 5

The Helping Professions: Supporting Positive Behavior Change

THE HELPING PROFESSIONS: Supporting Positive Behavior Change

■ *Erica works in a cardiac-rehabilitation department at a busy hospital. Most of her patients are recovering from either a recent heart attack or revascularization surgeries, such as angioplasty or bypass graft surgery. Erica is an exercise physiologist by training, but in addition to prescribing exercise for patients, she also talks with them about how their other behavior-change efforts are going while they walk on the treadmill or indoor track or use other exercise equipment. Most of Erica's patients have met at least once with the dietitian and with a psychotherapist. Erica gets reports and recommendations from those professionals and then works with patients as they strive to implement new lifestyle behaviors.*

Erica's department head has recently hired a consultant to work with all staff members to improve their communication skills so that they can work more effectively with patients. "This must be mostly for the doctors," Erica thinks. The surgeons are especially notorious for having no people skills. She feels that she communicates well with her patients already and presumes the mandatory workshops will be a waste of her valuable time. "What is there to learn? The recommendations for patients recovering from heart attacks and surgeries are pretty cut and dried," she says to herself. "Sure, changing diet, exercise, and maybe quitting smoking and managing stress are a lot for most of these patients, but what choice do they have? Lifestyle change works, and patients need the information to get with the program." ■

Chapter 1 presented information on the most common health problems found in North America and around the world, emphasizing that a majority of these relate to health behaviors. Behaviors often cause the problem, as when smoking causes carcinogenic changes in lung cells or the destruction of the alveoli seen in emphysema. Sometimes a number of behaviors contribute to a disorder, as with type 2 diabetes. Health professionals often recommend lifestyle changes to reduce the negative effects of chronic health problems, such as heart disease, and to improve longevity and quality of life. Health researchers and policy makers alike agree that people must develop healthful lifestyles to prevent, delay, and treat the major threats to health and well-being (Freudenberg & Olden, 2011).

It is impossible to ignore the urgent need for all health professionals, including health and fitness professionals, to be more effective agents for behavior change as they work with their clients and patients. As researchers have come to understand the importance of health behaviors, a cry for more effective health-care delivery that includes support for more healthful lifestyles has gone out to every type of health professional (Klein et al., 2004). Some physicians, nurses, and other medical personnel are changing their focus from simply delivering advice to helping motivate patients to follow advice and, in many cases, are encouraging patients to help shape the advice and inform treatment decisions (Vickers, Kircher, Smith, Petersen, & Rasmussen, 2007). Allied health professionals such as dietitians, athletic trainers, exercise physiologists, physical therapists, health and lifestyle coaches, personal trainers, occupational therapists, and counselors have a keen interest in providing more effective support to patients and clients who need to improve health behaviors. This chapter presents information on how health and fitness professionals can be most effective in their work with clients trying to develop more healthful lifestyles.

The first step in providing effective behavior-change services is to learn about the psychology of health and fitness, behavior-change theories and models, and the many factors that influence behavior—the topics covered in this book. The next step is to understand the role that health and fitness professionals can play in the behavior-change process and how helping professionals can best apply behavior-change theory and models in their work. That is the purpose of this chapter. Effective health and fitness professionals discover early in their career that excellent communication skills are central to their role as agents of behavior change. This chapter discusses how they use these skills to establish productive working relationships, to assess clients' readiness to change, and then to help clients decide to change. If clients are ready to change, health and fitness professionals can help them create goals and action plans and teach behavior-change skills. This chapter concludes with a section on a few of the ethical challenges that most often arise when working with clients to change behavior.

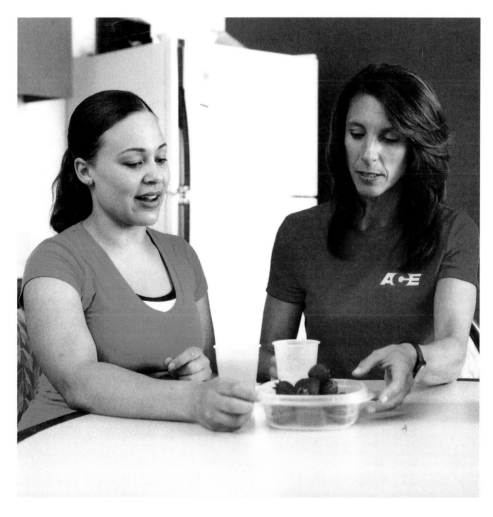

BEHAVIOR CHANGE AND THE HEALTH AND FITNESS PROFESSIONAL

The behavior-change theories and models presented in Chapter 4 apply to behavior change in general, whether individuals are working to change on their own or are working with one or more health and fitness professionals. A primary goal of health and fitness professionals is to take advantage of the knowledge provided by behavior-change research to help clients strengthen the factors that lead to a decision to change and to support the behavior-change process.

Client-Centered Behavior Change

What is the best way to help clients decide to change and to support the behavior-change process? The answer depends on the context and the people involved. Traditionally, health and fitness professionals, along with other allied health professionals and health-care providers, have seen their role as that of advice giver. This role is still an important one, and giving advice is still a critical part of the professional's job in these fields. An effective professional is able to give directive advice when that is the best way to deal with a client's situation. Research on health provider–patient relationships suggests that patients often just want a diagnosis and a treatment recommendation, especially if they have a new physical complaint or want a prescription (Taylor, 2009). Similarly, clients at a fitness center interested in beginning a weight-training program are often eager to get started and do not want to spend a great deal of time in discussion. An effective professional listens enough to know how to best move forward with a given client or patient.

Sometimes patients and clients have more complicated situations or have trouble implementing treatment recommendations. When the patient must be more involved in the treatment process, it becomes more important for providers to gain patient buy-in. When professionals recommend lifestyle treatments, a more patient-centered approach appears to lead to more effective behavior change, better health outcomes, and higher patient satisfaction (Berwick, 2009). Patient-centered generally refers to a treatment philosophy and procedures that put the patient first, explaining things clearly, listening carefully to understand a patient's questions and concerns, and, when appropriate, giving patients a choice in treatment plans (Berwick, 2009). The term client-centered refers to the same approach in settings where the person is a client rather than a patient.

Self-determination Theory Guides Client-Centered Approaches

Patient- and client-centered approaches are often based on Self-determination Theory (SDT; Chapter 4). These approaches strive to strengthen the client's perceptions of autonomy, competence, and connection in provider settings and in the client's behavior-change programs (Fig. 5-1). Whether behavior change involves taking daily medication or full-fledged lifestyle change, a motivated client is more likely to stick to treatment recommendations. Client-centered approaches try to connect with clients' intrinsic motivations for change (or treatment, depending on the situation) in order to maximize client willingness to address problems that occasionally arise. Health and fitness professionals can learn to communicate in ways that enhance clients' feelings of autonomy, competence, and connection (Hunter, 2008). Professionals can also learn to listen to clients' stories to uncover what is meaningful and motivational and then connect behavior-change recommendations to clients' meaningful goals. Research has shown that the quality of support provided by the helping professional can enhance clients' adherence to behavior-change programs (Ryan, Lynch, Vansteenkiste, Deci, 2011).

The Health Belief Model and the Theory of Planned Behavior Help Focus Discussion

Factors in the Health Belief Model can provide good "talking points" for health and fitness professionals in their behavior-change discussions with clients. However, professionals must first listen carefully to learn what clients think about health threats in terms of the importance of the threat and their perceived vulnerability. The health and fitness professional can uncover this information by asking good questions, listening carefully, and gaining the client's trust. Similarly, good communication can help professionals understand how clients perceive behavior-change interventions in terms of their effectiveness and the clients' self-efficacy, or ability to perform the intervention (Fig. 5-2). Health

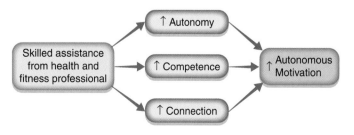

Client's perceptions of:

Figure 5-1. Client-centered approaches.

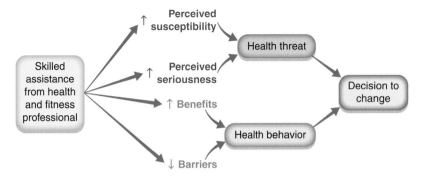

Figure 5-2. **Using the Health Belief Model.**

and fitness professionals can help change clients' understandings of health problems and behaviors, but only if they first listen carefully and lead clients to productive conclusions rather than simply telling them what to do.

Similarly, the Theory of Planned Behavior offers factors that help move people to form the intention to change. The factors of attitude toward the behavior change and perceived behavioral control (similar to self-efficacy regarding the performance of that behavior) are the factors most strongly related to forming the intention to change in behavior-change programs, with social norms exerting a somewhat weaker effect (Jacobs, Hagger, Streukens, De Bourdeaudhuij, & Claes, 2011; Fig. 5-3). An interesting study by Nele Jacobs and colleagues paired SDT with the Theory of Planned Behavior in programs designed to change diet or exercise behaviors (Jacobs et al., 2011). The researchers found that guiding clients to strengthen intrinsic motivation regarding behavior change affected their attitudes and self-efficacy, which in turn strengthened intentions to change both diet and exercise behavior. Approaches like this, which integrate applicable models and theories to guide intervention approaches, help make professionals more effective in their behavior-change work.

MOTIVATING CHANGE: Behavior-Change Models Inform Work With Clients

Although behavior-change theories and models can seem overwhelmingly complex, when working

with clients you can begin by focusing on four important goals, including:

1. Use good communication skills to establish a productive working relationship, building a client's sense of autonomy, competence, and connection and understanding the client's motivations for change.
2. Evaluate how the client feels about health threats, if any.
3. Evaluate how the client feels about the behaviors in question. How important is it to change?
4. Evaluate the client's self-efficacy for changing.

Does Professional Support Help?

Does working with a health and fitness professional to change behavior have a positive effect or are most people better off changing on their own? Fjeldsoe and colleagues (Fjeldsoe, Neuhaus, Winkler, & Eakin, 2011) looked at research studies that reported on whether subjects maintained behavior change following exercise or dietary interventions. The highest levels of behavior-change maintenance were associated with face-to-face contact with a health and fitness professional during the program and periodic contact with a professional after the end of the program, suggesting that work with a professional is more likely to lead to successful behavior change. In addition, longer interventions (over 24 weeks) tended to be more successful than shorter ones, again supporting the idea that professional support can be helpful.

COMMUNICATION SKILLS SUPPORT BEHAVIOR-CHANGE MOTIVATION

Patient- and client-centered approaches require the ability to interact with people in ways that further progress toward mutually agreed-upon goals. Although this sounds simple, human interactions are fraught with difficulty. Professionals may accidentally say things that insult clients. Clients may misunderstand the professional's recommendations. Professionals may overestimate the time and energy clients are willing to spend on behavior change. Unless they have actively

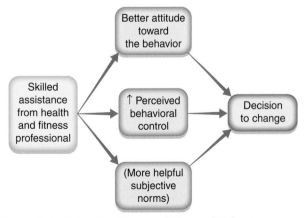

Figure 5-3. **Using the Theory of Planned Behavior.**

sought out advice, people generally do not like to be told what to do, and clients may push back against professional advice. When things do not work well, people become judgmental and defensive and stop trying to communicate with each other. Behavior–change plans stall and good intentions fade away.

Many professional groups have extensively studied provider–patient and provider–client communication to understand ways to improve it and to teach professionals how to communicate more effectively. Researchers have found that participation in programs designed to improve communication skills significantly increases health-provider effectiveness in delivering patient-centered care by, for example, primary care providers (Helitzer, LaNoue, Wilson, de Hernandez, Warner, Roter, 2011; Neumann et al., 2010), nurses (Pfister-Minogue & Salveson, 2010), and dietitians (Whitehead, Langley-Evans, Tischler, & Swift, 2009). Experts in the education of allied health professionals, fitness professionals, and educators agree that excellent communication skills are essential for professionals in these fields (Hunter, 2008; Rink & Hall, 2008).

Communication Goals

The overarching goal of health and fitness professionals is to help clients decide to improve health behaviors and stick to their behavior-change plans. Underlying this important goal are several other objectives that lay the groundwork for a productive working relationship with clients (Fig. 5-4).

Creating Positive Emotions and Optimism for Change

Health and fitness professionals should try to set a positive tone from their first contact with clients. Clients must begin their behavior-change journeys feeling as energetic and optimistic as possible. Positive emotions such as hope and anticipation of success give clients the energy they will need to stick to their programs. Positive emotions also help create a more productive bond between the professional and the client. Clients who do not enjoy working with a health and fitness professional are likely to leave, either abandoning behavior-change efforts or looking for other professionals with whom to work.

Establishing Feelings of Connection and Trust

Clients must feel that health and fitness professionals are trustworthy, since behavior change often involves very personal issues. Clients often feel vulnerable discussing health issues, past behavior-change failures, and other information important in the behavior-change counseling process. Health and fitness professionals will elicit the most trust and client buy-in if they convey a professional, unconditional positive regard for clients. Clients feel valued and ready to proceed with behavior-change programs when they feel that the professional is interested in them and cares about the outcome of their work together. The positive regard and involvement must feel authentic. This creates a climate that allows clients to be more open and honest, giving the professional a greater ability to design individualized behavior-change recommendations. A professional, trusting relationship contributes to feelings of connection that motivate people (Ryan et al., 2011).

Gathering Information and Setting the Agenda

Good communication skills and a caring demeanor allow the health and fitness professional to gather information from clients that helps set a productive direction. This information gives professionals a sense of clients' motivations for change, ideas about health and behavior change, and past experiences with behavior change. Using that information, the professional can design the most effective behavior-change program for each client.

Communicating Behavior-Change Recommendations

Effective health and fitness professionals give sound behavior-change advice but try to do so when clients are most receptive and motivated to change behaviors. Good communication skills help professionals find those moments when clients are open to advice. Good communication skills also help professionals deliver advice in ways that are most likely to resonate with clients. Effective professionals make behavior-change recommendations that build each client's sense of autonomous motivation in a way that matches his or her personal sense of self-efficacy for behavior change.

Establishing a Positive and Professional Relationship

The first few meetings between a client and the health and fitness professional should establish good rapport.

The Communication Process

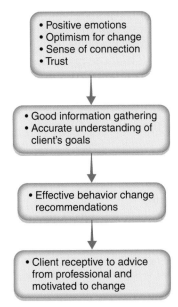

Figure 5-4. The communication process.

Rapport refers to a relationship marked by mutual understanding and trust. Because rapport begins with first impressions, health and fitness professionals should do everything possible to present themselves as approachable. Rapport continues to build over time, and the longer professionals and clients work together, the more they come to understand one another. An early foundation of trust and respect increases the likelihood that a positive and productive relationship will develop.

First Impressions

Most people have a first impression, consisting of an initial judgment or emotional response, when meeting another person for the first time. People's first impressions of others are often fairly accurate (Biesanz et al., 2011). Many factors influence clients' first impressions of a health and fitness professional. Some of these factors are under the professional's control, such as attire and screening procedures. Health and fitness professionals have interacted, as clients or patients themselves, with health professionals and can likely recall both positive and negative first impressions. When people are asked to recall both negative and positive experiences with health and fitness professionals, many common themes emerge (Brehm, 2010).

Negative experiences are marked by rudeness, indifference, ineptitude, neglect, and even malpractice. In describing negative experiences, people often report being left waiting a long time in environments that were dirty, disorganized, or dull. They describe professionals as appearing bored, uninterested in the client, uncaring, or distracted. They perceive communications with the professional as unclear, with clients saying they did not understand the information or the reasons for the treatments or recommendations. Questions were not encouraged or answered clearly.

Positive experiences are characterized by a sense of caring, respect, clear communication, and professionalism. Clients perceive that the professional takes their concerns seriously and that he or she is highly qualified, knowledgeable, and helpful. Questions are carefully considered and clearly answered, and the environment is clean and organized. Box 5-1 lists characteristics that contribute to positive first impressions and positive professional relationships.

Positive first impressions provide a great start for the rapport-building process. Because first impressions are so important, health and fitness professionals must remember that they may be contributing to a potential client's first impression before they have even met the client. For example, fitness professionals may work out in the fitness facility where they work. This means that they are always in the public eye. Their behavior in these settings may influence whether clients form a favorable impression of them. Similarly, health and fitness professionals often run into clients in public places such as grocery stores, shopping malls, theaters, and so forth. Conduct in

Box 5-1. Creating Professional First Impressions

Many factors contribute to people's first impressions of a health and fitness professional. Some relate to the professional's appearance and behavior and others to the appearance of the facility in which a meeting takes place. Factors that health and fitness professionals should consider when meeting clients for the first time include the following.

Appearance of the Health and Fitness Professional

- Professional wears appropriate and professional attire
- Professional cultivates an appearance that looks fit, neat, and clean
- Professional avoids wearing strong scents (e.g., musk, patchouli), controversial apparel, and anything that might irritate or offend clients
- Professional gives clients full attention to show professional interest
- Professional treats clients with respect and a warm, positive attitude

Interactions With the Health and Fitness Professional

- Clients have confidence in the professional's qualifications, training, experience, and skills
- Clients have enough time to express their concerns
- The professional listens carefully and tries to understand clients' concerns
- Clients believe that the professional is giving full attention and is interested in what they have to say
- Clients perceive an unconditional positive regard from the professional
- Clients believe that the professional respects them and their opinions
- Clients trust that the professional will maintain their confidentiality and will work on behalf of their best interests
- Instructions are clearly explained, and clients' questions are answered

Environment

- Facility is neat, clean, and pleasant
- Offices and staff have a well-organized appearance
- Meeting location is relatively quiet and without too many distractions

Adapted with permission from Brehm, B. A. (2004). *Successful Fitness Motivation Strategies.* Champaign, IL: Human Kinetics, 11.

these environments can contribute to the impression that the professional makes on others and also to the professional's reputation.

First impressions are also created by technologies such as telephone messages, Web pages, blogs, and other social networking tools. Health and fitness professionals should consider what sort of professional image they project when they employ these tools. New professionals and young people must be especially careful to avoid offensive images and text that could turn off potential employers and clients.

In emerging professions, such as personal training and lifestyle coaching, where credentialing is not always required or well understood by the public, it is especially important for professionals to establish credibility (George, 2008). Health and fitness professionals should be sure that clients know about their education, training, certifications, other qualifications, and work experience. These can be highlighted on websites, business cards, and materials given to clients. Professionals should describe their experience and their scope of practice when orienting new clients at the first meeting.

Health and fitness professionals who have had little difficulty developing rapport with clients similar to themselves may find that it takes a little longer to build trust with people who differ in age, gender, ethnicity, size, socioeconomic status, educational background, ability, or fitness level (Brehm, 2009). Building rapport may take more effort when clients are reluctant to change their behavior, afraid of injury, or depressed and anxious about health issues. Some clients have had bad experiences that led them to develop prejudices against athletes, physical educators, dietitians, physical therapists, and other health and fitness professionals. They may have less trust of young people, old people, women, men, people who appear to be overweight, or people of a different ethnic background. Nevertheless, health and fitness professionals who consistently behave professionally and employ good communication skills often win the hearts and trust of even the most reluctant clients.

Nonverbal Communication

People's verbal communications are only a small part of the messages they send. People pay attention to much more than words in their effort to decipher messages and understand social situations, including interactions with health and fitness professionals (Mast, 2007). When listening to each other's words, people seek to verify verbal content by evaluating the speaker's appearance, facial expressions, body language, and tone of voice. If someone's words ("I am glad to meet you") and body language (lack of eye contact, disinterested facial expression, body turned away, low energy) do not match, people generally trust body language over verbal content (Ambady & Weisbuch, 2010).

When talking with clients, the health and fitness professional should speak clearly and use language that clients can easily understand, without speaking down to them. It is certainly appropriate to use exercise science and medical vocabulary, but professionals should be sure to define terms that may be unfamiliar to clients. They can enhance verbal content with visual information, such as pictures, diagrams, and charts that illustrate concepts. Exercise demonstrations may accompany verbal explanations.

People often develop distracting habits that interfere with effective verbal communication. Peppering explanations with frequent fillers such as "um," "you know," and "like" gives a first impression that clients may perceive as uneducated and unprofessional. Older clients often complain that young people speak too quickly. To exacerbate matters, new professionals may have a tendency to speak even more quickly and add more fillers when nervous. Students who are new to professional–client interactions can benefit from conducting and then viewing and evaluating mock sessions that are filmed.

Nonverbal communication occurs in many ways, including:

- **Voice quality:** A weak, hesitant, or soft voice does not inspire client confidence. On the other hand, a loud, tense voice tends to make people nervous. Health and fitness professionals should try to develop a voice that is firm and confident to communicate professionalism. Some people end their sentences with a higher pitch, as though asking a question. This communicates indecisiveness and can detract from the confident impression the health and fitness professional should make.

- **Eye contact:** Direct, friendly eye contact shows clients that they are the focus of attention. When a listener looks away when a person is speaking, the speaker does not feel heard. Similarly, when a speaker looks away, the listener does not feel important and thinks the speaker does not care about his or her reaction.

- **Facial expression:** Facial expressions convey emotion but work best when the emotion is sincere. Most clients can sense an artificial smile, so health and fitness professionals must reach deep to portray a genuine display of positive regard for clients. As professionals work with clients, their faces should display the concern, thoughtfulness, and/or enjoyment they are feeling.

- **Hand gestures:** Use of hand gestures varies from culture to culture. In general, people are most comfortable when a speaker uses relaxed, fluid hand gestures while explaining things. When listening, health and fitness professionals should refrain from hand gestures. Fidgeting hands, clenched fists, abrupt gestures, and finger pointing are distracting to many clients.

- **Body position:** An open, well-balanced, erect body position communicates confidence. Good posture is especially important for health and fitness professionals, whose bodies serve as symbols of their professional expertise (Maguire, 2008). A body posture that is leaning or stooped suggests fatigue and boredom (not to mention poor health and physical fitness), whereas a rigid, hand-on-hips stance may be interpreted as aggressive. When the professional and client sit together talking, the professional should look attentive by leaning slightly forward and keeping arms uncrossed. He or she should eliminate distracting nervous activity such as foot or finger tapping or constantly shifting position.

- **Behavior:** Many behaviors serve as forms of communication. For example, when the health and fitness professional is late for an appointment or frequently reschedules appointments, this communicates a lack of respect for the client. Professionals communicate a lack of involvement when they interrupt an appointment to make a phone call or perform other tasks. A cell phone ringing in the middle of a discussion can throw conversation off track. Unless the meeting is explicitly taking place during a meal, eating when meeting with a client is distracting.

Gathering Information and Setting the Agenda

The early sessions between the health and fitness professional and the client depend on the nature of the work and the client's commitment and motivation. Health and fitness professionals often see clients in the preparation stage of change, ready to take on a behavior-change program to improve health and fitness. Good communication skills are essential in these situations so that health and fitness professionals can clearly understand client goals and use the information gathered to craft effective recommendations. Many health professionals see clients or patients who are not even thinking of changing but want a quick fix for a health problem. In these cases, professionals must become skilled in techniques such as motivational interviewing (discussed in Chapter 4), to help clients become open to thinking about behavior change. Some professionals have time for only a brief conversation with a new client, whereas others will work with individuals for months or even years. Even when contact with clients is limited, it is still important for the health and fitness professional to gather information on what clients are looking for and to individualize advice as much as possible.

The best way to gather information in any setting is to ask good questions and listen mindfully to the answers. These answers reveal how clients view behavior change in terms of its importance to them as well as their feelings of self-efficacy for changing. Answers will reveal clients' readiness to change and

factors that will enhance the likelihood of behavior-change success. Effective communication tools for structuring information-gathering sessions come from motivational interviewing (Rollnick, Miller, & Butler, 2008). Chapter 4 emphasized that using motivational interviewing techniques requires training and practice. However, learning to listen mindfully and reflectively, the basis of the information-gathering practice described in the following, is an important skill useful to everyone in everyday life. Many health professionals use modified motivational interviewing procedures to engage with clients about behavior change (Pfister-Minogue & Salveson, 2010). Modified procedures capture the collaborative, supportive spirit of motivational interviewing. Learning to ask good questions and listen in an effective and mindful fashion is appropriate and helpful for health and fitness professionals discussing lifestyle change with clients to gather information from the client on their behavior-change goals and to design effective and motivational interventions.

Client-centered communication includes four important techniques: open-ended questions, affirmations, reflective listening, and summarizing. Health and fitness professionals often remember these techniques as a group using the acronym OARS (Miller & Rollnick, 2013) (Fig. 5-5).

Open Questions

Closed questions elicit brief answers and are useful for gathering information on specific topics. Examples of closed questions include "Are you hoping to lose weight?" "Do you have time to exercise before work?" "Does that exercise feel too difficult?" Closed questions may often be answered with "yes" or "no" or a short sentence.

Open questions, or open-ended questions, invite clients to give the professional more information, tell their stories, and paint a broader picture. Whereas closed questions take the conversation in directions important for the health and fitness professional's agenda, open questions allow information important to clients to surface. Examples of open questions include, "How can I help you?" "What does your typical weekday schedule look like?" "What kinds of situations lead to overeating?" Closed questions can be turned into open questions very simply by following up the answers with another question or request, such as "Can you tell me more about that?"

*O*pen questions

*A*ffirmations

*R*eflective listening

*S*ummarizing

Figure 5-5. OARS: Components of effective communication for health and fitness professionals.

Skilled use of open questions accomplishes several goals at once:

- **Breaks the ice of early meetings:** Open questions asked during the first meeting get the conversation started in a client-centered fashion. Open questions direct thinking in productive ways that get work off to a good start.
- **Builds rapport:** As clients sense that the professional is interested in their situation, they feel more trusting.
- **Provides useful information:** Open questions allow clients to provide information on their reasons for consulting the health and fitness professional and factors that may affect adherence to a behavior-change plan. Health and fitness professionals learn about clients' strengths and positive characteristics to highlight in the future for building self-efficacy and motivation.
- **Nurtures autonomous motivation in clients:** Asking open questions hands the direction of the conversation to the client. It suggests that the client is the focus not only of the information-gathering procedures but also of the direction that the behavior-change program will take. Since the client is influencing recommendations, the result is more client buy-in and responsibility for results. Open questions can lead to the development of goals and plans most relevant to and realistic for individual clients.
- **Increases client satisfaction:** Open questions show clients that the health and fitness professional has their interests at heart. Clients feel valued and empowered.

After the first two communication skills training sessions, Erica is shocked to realize that she does most of the talking in her sessions with patients. She always figured that the more forceful and persuasive she was, the more likely patients would be to understand what she was asking them to do. It often seemed to Erica that patients just didn't realize the importance of behavior change, and this made her argue even more forcefully, hoping to ignite a motivational fire in her patients.

Today she is going to try using open questions with her patient Marilyn, a 68-year-old widow recovering from triple bypass surgery that was performed over a month ago. Erica has been frustrated by Marilyn's lack of progress and low level of adherence to the cardiac-rehabilitation program. Instead of lecturing Marilyn on the importance of her lifestyle change program as she ordinarily would, Erica asks open questions as they walk around the track together. Marilyn does not say much at first, but eventually she does talk to Erica about her struggles with depression and how difficult it is some days to get out of the house.

Erica listens sympathetically, stunned by how much Marilyn has shared with her. As Erica and Marilyn review how things are going, Erica feels overwhelmed with all of the issues Marilyn is dealing with. She talks with Marilyn about the emotional health benefits of regular physical activity. Marilyn is interested and asks for more information on this. Erica and Marilyn agree that using exercise to help improve Marilyn's energy level and outlook will be the focus of their next meeting. Instead of focusing solely on heart health, Erica realizes that addressing depression will probably do just as much for Marilyn's rehabilitation. In the meantime, Erica urges Marilyn to try and take a short walk every morning to reduce her symptoms of depression and lift her mood. Marilyn smiles and says she will give this a try.

Affirmations

Affirmations are statements that reinforce clients' strengths and accomplishments or indicate that they are making progress. Health and fitness professionals use affirmations to build a client's self-efficacy for behavior change. Affirmations must not be empty praise but should refer to specific situations and actions that showed character strengths and progress. Affirmations might be responses to a story the client tells. "That was a good strategy." Affirmations might be reminders to clients of past accomplishments that illustrate their ability to be successful. "You said last year you were able to continue walking several days a week by walking at the indoor track once it started getting dark early. That was a good idea."

Affirmations are designed to help clients build autonomous motivation, rather than changing in order to achieve praise from the health and fitness professional. Long-lasting lifestyle change is more likely to result from clients building the skills to make decisions and plan changes in their own lives, rather than changing to win recognition from health and fitness professionals. It is fine for the health and fitness professional to indicate approval, but affirmations should help clients create a positive story about their abilities to succeed. "Look at how many more repetitions you are doing this week compared to last week," is a way to praise a client's efforts, show evidence of improvement, and build exercise self-efficacy.

Reflective Listening

Reflective listening refers to active listening combined with verbal and nonverbal responses to indicate interest and understanding and to encourage the speaker to continue. Reflective means that listeners reflect back to the speakers what they (the listeners) have heard to confirm accurate understanding. Reflective listening shows the speaker that the listener has heard not only the speaker's words but is also trying to perceive and understand the feelings that the words convey. Reflective listening helps speakers feel understood and valued and thus helps build connection and rapport.

Professionals who work with people need to be good listeners. Unfortunately, many health and fitness professionals tend to believe that, because they get paid to give advice, the more they say, the better. They love to talk about exercise and health and equate information delivery with performance and giving clients their money's worth. Unfortunately, this focus on talking can interfere with good communication if the professional always dominates discussions with clients and interrupts clients before they are finished speaking.

Listening is important but difficult. Lives are busy and noisy, and it is not possible to listen mindfully to everything everyone says. Some of the time people pretend to listen but don't really pay attention. They may pretend to listen so that people will like them or not think them rude. People may hear only part of what the speaker is saying and tune out parts they find boring, offensive, or hard to understand. Instead of listening carefully to a speaker, listeners are often busy formulating arguments, forming judgments about the speaker, or thinking about what they will say next. They may simply be daydreaming about something else entirely. They might be preoccupied with themselves, perhaps distracted by their own problems.

Even if people try to listen, they may not hear what the speaker is saying. People often reconstruct messages to reflect their own beliefs and needs. They may have prejudices about the speaker and look for confirmation of these in the speaker's words. They may tend to hear what they expect to hear and neglect to take in other things the speaker is saying. Fortunately, listening skills can be learned, and reflective listening improves with practice (Health Psychology in Your Life 5-1).

Reflective listening occurs when the health and fitness professional listens carefully and empathetically to a client, with an open mind, trying to identify with the client's situation. When trying to listen, professionals should give clients their full attention. Effective communication occurs most easily in quiet, private spaces to limit distraction.

Health and fitness professionals should direct the conversation during early meetings by asking clients open questions. As clients answer, professionals should show that they are listening with appropriate eye contact and body language. Professionals can also demonstrate reflective listening by responding to clients' answers in several ways, including the following:

- **Encouraging:** The professional may use short words or phrases such as "I see," "Yes," and "That's interesting," that encourage the client to continue speaking when there is a natural pause in the client's speech. These phrases let the client know that the professional is listening carefully and following what is being said. Nodding and smiling can also indicate listening and encourage speakers to continue.

HEALTH PSYCHOLOGY IN YOUR LIFE 5-1.
Practice Your Skills

Practice reflective listening with a classmate, friend, or family member. Let them know you are working on a class project and ask them to describe a problem they have had or are having in changing a health behavior. This might be a problem getting enough exercise or a problem with their diet. Maybe they are having difficulty quitting smoking or doing their back exercises regularly. It is best if you can get the person talking about a real problem that he or she wants to discuss.

Once you have identified a helpful partner and a problem, your goal is simply to try to understand the problem, and the partner's situation, as clearly as possible. Do not try to solve the problem; simply try to listen and understand. Begin by asking open questions to get your partner to describe the problem. Try to focus totally on listening. Try to paraphrase what the person is telling you and use appropriate nonverbal communication cues.

Note how you felt during this exercise. Which paraphrasing attempts worked best? Which felt most awkward? How did the speaker respond? Did reflective listening feel different from how you usually interact with people? How could you further improve your reflective listening skills?

- **Paraphrasing:** The listener can demonstrate understanding by restating in a clear and concise way the essence of what the client has been saying. Paraphrasing may also extend the meaning of the client's answers. For example, the client may tell a story about how she maintained a lighter weight for several years. The health and fitness professional might paraphrase, "So that feels like it might be a realistic weight for you." If the paraphrase is not accurate, the speaker then has a chance to correct an erroneous impression.
- **Questioning:** Responding to a client's stories with more open questions demonstrates good listening and directs the conversation, encouraging the client to continue sharing relevant information. The professional might follow up a client's story with a comment such as, "You said you quit exercising last year. What made you stop?" Health and fitness professionals should ask questions at appropriate times to clarify points that they do not understand or to move the conversation in a more productive direction.
- **Reflecting emotional content:** The health and fitness professional should also find opportunities to confirm the emotional content of the

client's story if appropriate and important. "That must have been upsetting." "You seem discouraged." "That sounds like fun."

Summarizing

At appropriate points in the conversation, the health and fitness professional should try to summarize key points that have a bearing on meeting objectives. After summarizing, the professional should allow clients to comment on the summary to confirm its accuracy and correct misunderstandings. Summarizing not only demonstrates effective listening, but it gives the health and fitness professional an opportunity to guide a conversation that is wandering too far off topic or keep a meeting on track in terms of time. The summary also provides an opportunity for the professional to emphasize certain parts of the conversation that are especially helpful and useful. Summaries can serve as a way to wrap up a topic before moving on to another.

Is Effective Communication More Work for the Professional?

Health and fitness professionals who are accustomed to limiting client input and primarily giving advice may find that, like any form of behavior change, changing communication habits is not easy at first. In fact, developing good communication skills takes a great deal of practice for anyone. People generally enjoy talking more than listening, and health and fitness professionals are no exception. However, once professionals begin to practice reflective listening and a more mindful, present-moment awareness in their work, this approach can actually reduce work stress. Listening carefully is good for the listener. Listening with attention forces the health and fitness professional to slow down and focus on the present moment, which can help reduce the stress that people feel from trying to do too many things at the same time. In addition, by making conversations more productive, professionals feel better about their work. With practice, health and fitness professionals can gradually learn to improve their communication skills, avoiding behaviors that limit rapport building and information gathering as well as dealing with difficult conversations more easily (Box 5-2).

Technology and Communication

Technology has been harnessed in a number of promising ways in behavior-change interventions. In 2010, Krebs and colleagues conducted a meta-analysis of

---

Box 5-2. Conversation Stoppers

Too Much Self-Disclosure From the Professional
Self-disclosure refers to sharing personal thoughts and experiences, in the process revealing more about oneself. It is often appropriate for health and fitness professionals to use a limited amount of self-disclosure to demonstrate understanding and to forge bonds with a client. Self-disclosure should avoid boasting and showing off, which might make clients feel inadequate and inferior and stop the conversational flow. Instead, professionals may choose to reveal similar personal experiences to indicate that they understand a client's position. These self-disclosures should be limited to one or two sentences, keeping the focus on the client. For example, a personal trainer might say, "I think I know what you mean. When I moved to a new city last year, I didn't exercise for several weeks either. What did you do then?"

Difficult Disclosures From the Client
Health and fitness professionals are sometimes unsure of how to respond when clients share information that is very sad, such as a disclosure of a client's serious illness or the illness or death of someone close to the client. Often a short response is all that is required, such as, "I'm so sorry." "That must have been very hard." "I can't even imagine how difficult this must have been for you and your family." The personal trainer should follow the client's lead as to whether he or she wants to say anything more on this topic. If sad information affects exercise program design in any way, the professional can turn the conversation back to the practical details. For example, "Now that your mother has moved in with you and your family, what is the best time for you to do your food shopping?" If clients reveal new medical information that causes concern, the professional should refer them back to their health providers for medical clearance. If their new medical condition places them outside of the professional's scope of practice and expertise, he or she should refer them to someone with the necessary training and experience.

Professional's Judgmental Attitude
It is human nature to evaluate others. However, health and fitness professionals should be aware of judgmental feelings about clients and try to suspend judgment, approaching each client with a curious and open mind. Health and fitness professionals should strive to convey a professional, positive regard for clients, regardless of their personal characteristics. When people perceive negative judgment, they may feel defensive and angry. These negative emotions can interfere with rapport and reduce client self-efficacy.

88 studies that used computer-tailored interventions to promote health behavior change. They defined "computer-tailored" as methods that selected communication messages based on data provided by clients. The important point is that the messages were tailored, or individualized, to client response. For example, clients might be asked questions to assess self-efficacy. If they scored low on self-efficacy, they would receive messages different from those sent to clients who scored high on this variable. Those low in self-efficacy might receive suggestions for increasing their confidence for changing the target behavior. The computer-tailored interventions used various combinations of information delivery, including messages sent by computer or telephone or even delivered in print. The researchers found that tailored interventions were somewhat more effective than nontailored interventions (Krebs, Prochaska, & Rossi, 2010). As computer programs become more sophisticated at responding to client input, behavior-change interventions that use computer-tailored methods offer an opportunity to expand health behavior–change efforts.

An interesting example of a computer-tailored intervention is one designed to incorporate the principles of Self-determination Theory in its interface with clients (Patrick & Canevello, 2011). The researchers contrast the ability of the computer personal trainer to provide feedback that is need-supportive and empathetic versus standard programs that respond in a more controlling, evaluative, and judgmental fashion. Although this software is still in development, researchers hope that programs such as this will help public health efforts to reach people who are unable or unwilling to meet with health and fitness professionals. Professionals could use such programs to supplement their work with clients.

Technology such as Internet and telephone use has the capacity to expand communication options and opportunities. However, health and fitness professionals should use these communication channels with discretion, as too much contact becomes annoying. Both clients and personal trainers should give clear directions on how they prefer to be contacted. For example, many clients do not wish to receive e-mail every day reminding them to exercise, although they may not mind a reminder of an upcoming appointment. Health and fitness professionals may wish to let clients contact them at a work telephone number but not on their mobile or home telephone numbers.

Communication Skills for Clients and Patients

Because communication is always a two-way street, communication skills training has also been offered to patients to help them communicate more effectively with providers (Talen, Muller-Held, Eshleman, & Stephens, 2011). In a randomized control study conducted by Talen and colleagues, physicians rated patients receiving a short, one-session intervention as having better overall organization and communication skills and a more positive attitude during a subsequent office visit. Patients in the intervention group reported higher provider–patient communication quality and a greater feeling of being partners with their physicians in their treatments, compared with the control group. Health and fitness professionals may wish to consider helping clients understand their roles in the behavior-change process and teach communication skills for developing effective working relationships with helping professionals. The professionals in the study by Talen and colleagues described previously used a simple one-page information sheet that patients prepared before seeing their providers, so the patients were ready to provide helpful information and interact productively with providers.

READINESS TO CHANGE

As health and fitness professionals begin working relationships with new clients, one of their first objectives is to assess a client's readiness to engage in a behavior-change program. Chapter 4 presented the Stages of Change Model and the processes of change. One of the most important applications of the Stages of Change Model as well as other health behavior–change models is that a decision to change almost always precedes actual behavior change. Health and fitness professionals will be more effective if they can individualize their support based on how ready a client is to change.

Assessing Readiness to Change

Usually health and fitness professionals can get a sense of a client's stage of change by asking open questions and listening to the client's answers. During early conversations with clients, health and fitness professionals can ask why they have sought to meet with the professional, how they view their health/behavior–change situations, how they feel about their ability to change, and how ready they are to change. Clients who are resistant to change may be in precontemplation or contemplation stages. Clients who have actively sought to meet with a professional are likely at least contemplating or preparing for change. As discussed in Chapter 4, approaches for assisting clients would vary in these two situations.

When open questions have not helped the health and fitness professional decide whether a client is ready to change or not, simply asking clients how they feel about changing can help. Questions might be placed in context. For example, "It seems like you are concerned about your diagnosis of diabetes. Diabetes is managed best if you can add some physical activity to your day. You are already walking twice a week for 20 minutes during your lunch hour. Do you think you could add another session of this each week?" This closed question might lead to more discussion and a better idea of a client's willingness to change.

Sometimes professionals include readiness-to-change questions on the paperwork that clients complete before their first visit (Box 5-3). Answers to these questions can be helpful and may stimulate further discussion once professionals and clients begin working together.

Professionals can also use scaling to get a clearer idea of a client's readiness to change or any other variable of interest. Scaling refers to rating a variable on a numerical scale, for example, a scale from 1 to 10. "On a scale from 1 to 10, how confident are you that you will be able to exercise 3 days a week during your lunch hour?" The upper and lower limits of the scale should be defined. For example, "Let's say 1 represents no confidence, you think you will probably never do this, and 10 represents total confidence, you think you will have no problem doing this every week." If scaling suggests low confidence, the professional should work with the client to revise recommendations, so that they are more in line with client self-efficacy.

Ryan and colleagues (2011) emphasize that categorizing clients into an exact stage may not be helpful or necessary, as a person's stage can change from moment to moment. In the Stages of Change Model, clients often move forward or backward in their stage. Movement from preparation to action is especially difficult to predict. Clients must be not only ready to change but also have the skills and energy required to follow through on their decisions. Many health and fitness professionals have stories about clients who appear totally committed to a behavior-change program but drop out after a few sessions. Health and fitness professionals should still attempt to assess readiness but be somewhat flexible in their approach, listening carefully to clients' reasons for changing, and adapting their interventions to best meet clients' needs (Behavior Change in Action 5-1).

Change Talk: Helping Precontemplation and Contemplation Clients Decide to Change

When health and fitness professionals find themselves working with clients who are not yet willing to change their behavior, it is important to refrain from arguing or bullying the client into changing. Although it is tempting to forge ahead and tell clients what they should be doing, the professional's advice may be wasted if clients have not yet made a commitment to change. Arguing and pressuring tend to alienate clients and create defensive resistance. Clients may eventually seem to agree, and even say they will follow recommendations, but may ignore the advice once they leave the professional's office.

A more productive approach is to discuss with clients the reasons they feel unable or unwilling to change (Fig. 5-6). Using the OARS skills outlined above, professionals can talk to clients in ways that show supportive concern for them when challenging their current behavior. The health and fitness professional's goal in behavior-change counseling situations with people not ready to change is to guide them to see that their current lifestyle is likely contributing to current or future problems. Using effective questions, the health and fitness professional tries to help clients see that good health is important and a healthy lifestyle will help them reach goals and engage in activities important to them. Helpful strategies include the following:

- **Ask open questions:** The health and fitness professional may begin by asking clients open questions about their health concerns and relevant lifestyle factors. The professional should also ask clients questions about their families, work, and recreational pursuits. What do their days look like? What kinds of activities and hobbies do they enjoy?
- **Listen effectively:** The health and fitness professional should listen carefully to the client's answers. Listening effectively will help the professional understand the reasons a client feels, for example, unable to exercise, or does not feel the need to exercise. Listening carefully helps the professional uncover valuable information and shows clients that the professional respects them, even if he or she does not agree with them.

Box 5-3. Readiness-to-Change Questionnaire: Strength Training

Please check the description that best fits you.

____ 1. I do not participate in strength-training exercise, and I do not plan to begin a strength-training program in the next 6 months.

____ 2. I do not participate in strength-training exercise, but I am thinking about starting a strength-training program in the next 6 months.

____ 3. I do not participate in strength-training exercise, or participate only occasionally, but I am planning to begin a strength-training program in the next month.

____ 4. I am currently performing strength training regularly and have been training regularly for less than 6 months.

____ 5. I have been performing strength training regularly for 6 months or more.

Regular strength-training exercise means two or more sessions per week.

Note to health and fitness professionals: statements indicate stage of change. 1, precontemplation; 2, contemplation; 3, preparation; 4, action; 5, maintenance.

Adapted with permission from Brehm, B.A. (2004). *Successful Fitness Motivation Strategies.* Champaign, IL: Human Kinetics, 38.

BEHAVIOR CHANGE IN ACTION 5-1

Evaluating Stage of Change

■ **CHALLENGE**

Accurately evaluating a client's stage of change, especially whether the client has made the decision to change, and evaluating how committed the client is to following behavior-change recommendations

■ **PLAN**

Professionals will get a better idea of a client's commitment to change if they approach this subject in a variety of ways during their initial meetings.

Include a stage of change questionnaire on intake paperwork. Health and fitness professionals can make this question specific to their practice. The questionnaire in Box 5-3 applies to strength-training exercise. But you can adapt this questionnaire for any situation, such as eating a more healthful diet, managing blood sugar, consuming less salt, or walking 3 days a week. Answers to this questionnaire not only give you some indication of how the client is feeling about change but may also get clients to strengthen their commitment to the behavior-change program.

Include a readiness-to-change scale on intake paperwork. Include a scale from 1 to 10 and ask clients to circle how ready they feel to commit to a behavior-change program. Indicate on the scale that 1 means not at all willing to change and 10 extremely committed to changing.

Include scales for how important change is for the client, as well as client confidence in changing. Assessing both how clients view the importance of change and their confidence for changing gives health and fitness professionals good information for further discussions. Both factors are also important predictors of behavior-change success. Clients who feel that change is important and that they have the ability to change have probably made a stronger commitment to changing than clients who say they do not think change is important and/or who lack confidence in their ability to change.

There is no magic number on a 1-to-10 scale that ensures behavior-change success. The answers on these scales are simply an indication of how the client is thinking and feeling and can help guide future discussions and behavior-change recommendations. The professional might ask, "You say you are at a 5 for confidence about changing. What would it take to move you to a 6?"

Try to get a sense of a client's motivation for change. Ask clients why they are seeking professional advice. Questions like, "What brings you here today?" "What are you hoping to gain from this work?" or even, "How can I help you?" may get clients talking about their motivations for behavior change. As they are talking, try to assess motivation. Does it seem to be autonomous? Or are clients trying to please someone else?

Many clients are trying to do the right thing because their physician or someone else has recommended the change. That is perfectly normal and fine. This may develop into autonomous motivation for good health. Reinforce the importance of good health with clients. Most people do want to feel good and succeed in reaching their goals. Most life goals require decent health. A discussion with you can help clients make this connection.

Ask clients directly how ready they are to change. The professional might refer to clients' answers on the intake paperwork or simply ask them how committed they feel at some point during an early meeting. This question should be asked in a supportive, rather than a critical way. For example,

"Many people find that eating more fruits and vegetables takes some planning. I am looking forward to helping you with that. Are you ready to take this on?"

"People often find they have more energy and feel less stressed after only a few weeks of regular exercise. I suggest you begin with a 30-minute walk 3 or 4 days a week. Does that sound reasonable to you, with your schedule? Do you feel able to follow this recommendation?"

"I want to help you design a strength-training program that will enable you achieve your goals, but I also want the program to work in terms of your schedule. The program will only be successful if you can really do it. You will need to train at least 3 days a week here at the gym. Is that realistic for you? Do you think you will be able to get here 3 days a week for an hour each session to start? I think you will start to see results after just a few weeks if you can follow through with this."

Adjust recommendations as needed. If clients seem hesitant, ambivalent, or lacking confidence in their ability to change, keep recommendations fairly simply, in order to increase the likelihood that they will follow through and be successful, thus building their confidence. Clients may still be in contemplation or preparation stages of change and need to firm up their decision to engage wholeheartedly in a behavior-change program. Engage them in discussions, using reflective-listening techniques, to help them weigh the pros and cons of changing and make plans for dealing with their barriers to change.

Clients who seem fairly committed to changing and who seem to have autonomous motivation for changing may be ready to proceed with the professional's recommendations. Nevertheless, since people's commitment and motivation change from day to day, it is important to check in periodically to see how things are going and adjust behavior-change recommendations accordingly.

With clients in precontemplation and contemplation:

- Ask open questions.
- Listen effectively.
- Guide conversation → importance of health.
- Keep conversation friendly.
- Keep listening and monitoring client response.
- Explore ambivalence.
- Reinforce change talk.
- Build self-confidence/reinforce strengths.
- Encourage clients to generate ideas.
- Ask permission before giving advice.

Figure 5-6. Helping clients make a decision to change.

- **Guide clients to consider the importance of health:** Eventually, the professional should move to questions that will hopefully help clients conclude that good health is important, so they can continue to engage in those activities that are personally most meaningful and fulfilling. The professional can then turn the discussion to the behavior-change issues at hand, trying to connect behavior change with good health. For example, if clients have a family history of heart disease, the professional could follow up by asking, "Did you know that regular physical activity helps prevent heart disease?"

- **Keep the conversation friendly:** Although health and fitness professionals may challenge statements made by clients ("I don't have a weight problem, so I don't need to exercise"), they should avoid heated arguments, since negative feelings may make clients defensive. If clients start to seem angry, the professional should switch to a more neutral, information-gathering question. The professional may also express empathy and respect for the difficulties the client faces. Experts in motivational interviewing advise professionals to "avoid arguing" (Rollnick et al., 2008). This means to maintain an empathetic attitude toward the client, even if it means agreeing that change is too difficult right now. This prevents clients from shutting the professional out and may even convince clients that professionals are on their side and trying to help.

- **Keep listening and monitor client response:** The health and fitness professional should continually monitor clients' responses to questions. If the professional senses that the client has stopped listening, it's time to stop talking. Instead, the health and fitness professional can ask clients what they are thinking about or if they have any questions. These types of discussions can feel somewhat uncomfortable for professionals who tend to avoid conflict, but mild discomfort

may help clients feel the need to change. If all else fails, try "How can I help you?"

- **Explore ambivalence:** It is human nature to feel ambivalent. Ambivalence means having mixed or contradictory feelings about something. People often feel ambivalent about lifestyle change. On the one hand, a person might want to have more energy and might consider increasing physical activity to feel more energetic. On the other hand, that same person might find it difficult to summon the energy to actually get out and exercise. Although recognizing that exercise helps them feel better, people might also feel that exercise takes too much energy to perform. As they speak with clients, health and fitness professionals should listen carefully to statements and stories that indicate ambivalent feelings about behavior change. Sometimes it is helpful to bring ambivalent issues to light for discussion. As clients explore their contradictory thoughts and feelings about the topic, over time they may be able to strengthen their resolve to change and to recognize the factors standing in the way of behavior change. For example, they may learn to recognize a habit of starting to make excuses for why they cannot stick to the behavior-change recommendations at this moment and be able to move forward with change and ignore "the little voice" making excuses. They may be able to come up with strategies to deal with perceived barriers and to increase their perceptions of the importance and feasibility of behavior change.

- **Reinforce and support change talk:** Change talk refers to things clients say that favor positive behavior change. Health and fitness professionals try to ask questions that elicit change talk from the client. For example, the professional might ask, "Tell me more about the time 2 years ago when you enjoyed walking during your lunch hour." As the person describes his success, the professional nods and smiles and remembers the points that seem to have contributed to success. When clients make statements such as, "I know I would feel better if I started exercising again," or "I sleep better when I drink less coffee," the professional can agree with these statements and encourage clients to continue. When clients move into a more negative and resistant tone, the professional does not reinforce the negative talk but does not argue, either. Professionals must continually remind themselves that it is the client who must decide to change and to find positive, motivational reasons for changing. Ryan and colleagues (2011) suggest that "truly reflective and person-centered techniques are effective only insofar as they are fostering

HEALTH PSYCHOLOGY AT WORK 5-1. Reflective Listening Key to Fostering Change Talk
Sarah Keyes, M.S.W.

Sarah Keyes is a clinical social worker, meeting with individual clients in an outpatient facility in Cambridge, MA. Most of her patients are referred to her by health-care providers for treatment of a variety of psychological disorders. Sarah counsels clients to help them address issues in their lives and habits of thought that are causing distress. Although the issues addressed in clinical social work may differ from the lifestyle change focus of health and fitness professionals, the goal of professionals in both fields is helping clients make decisions to change and learning to approach life in more healthful ways. Sarah was a Division I swimmer at Clemson University and often recommends physical activity to her clients who have anxiety and depression.

"I often use motivational interviewing to help clients find a better direction in their lives. I help them call on past experiences to bring up discrepancies between how they want their life to look versus how it looks now. Active, mindful listening is critical for effectively motivating clients.

"In my master's degree program, we [the students] practiced reflective listening with each other. This practice was actually harder than working with clients, but it helps you develop the listening skills and questioning techniques, so, whatever content emerges with a client, you have practiced the structure. Mindfulness practice is also helpful for learning to keep your focus in the present moment when listening to others talk.

"When I first started as a counselor 2 years ago, I was surprised by how hard it is to just listen to someone, without cutting in or responding. It takes some practice to tune in and really listen, without thinking about the next thing you're going to say. When you listen mindfully, you can really soak up the person's story. You get a feel for who the person is by the way they choose their words and the way they convey their stories. Sometimes I wonder where the story is going, and I have a hard time focusing and being patient. But most of the time, the story makes a useful point. I don't take notes when I am listening to a client, since that can be distracting. But I catalogue the stories in my mind and write my notes once the session is over.

"The return on your listening investment is pretty high. You gather material to help motivate people. You can remind them later of things they have said that illustrate their strengths or their desire to change. You learn what is important to them and how they think about the changes they are working on. And people feel good about being heard, which builds your relationship with the client."

---

autonomous change talk." If health and fitness professionals continue working with a client for a while, they can continue to mention and reinforce statements that the client has made about positive, personally meaningful reasons for changing, guiding him or her to pay more attention to productive ways of thinking and behaving (Health Psychology at Work 5-1).

- **Build self-confidence:** Health and fitness professionals can help clients identify areas of success, no matter how small. For example, the professional might praise a client who currently walks the dog twice a day for 5 minutes and then ask whether the client might consider increasing the walk time by a minute or two each week. Health and fitness professionals can help clients identify personal strengths, based on stories clients have shared. "I admire the flexibility and persistence you showed when you were balancing your job and taking care of your children. Now that your children are older, I wonder if that same flexibility and persistence could be applied to fitting exercise into your day." Other strengths that health and fitness

professionals might observe include the ability to organize and plan, manage stress effectively, use a sense of humor to cope with difficulty, cultivate and sustain social support, conduct Web searches for helpful information, and solve problems creatively.

- **Encourage clients to generate ideas:** If clients seem willing to make even small changes, health and fitness professionals should let them take the lead in making suggestions that might work for them. Professionals should encourage clients to look for options that will work best in the context of their lives and abilities.

- **Ask permission before giving advice:** Clients only make use of advice to which they listen. Before launching into a lecture, health and fitness professionals should check to see whether clients are ready to listen. "Would you like more information on exercising to reduce high blood pressure?" If clients are ready to listen, professionals should be prepared to provide helpful information. Attractive, readable handouts may help explain relevant issues about which the client desires more information.

■ *Erica is getting the hang of this new communication style, and although it is hard giving up total control over her meetings with patients, she is finding that listening more helps her gather useful information. Her patients also seem to be livelier during the sessions, asking more questions and offering more suggestions.*

Her next patient, Mark, is a recovering alcoholic who smokes. After his recent heart attack, Mark cut down from two packs of cigarettes to one pack a day, but he has stalled at that level. Mark is exercising regularly and is pleased with his improvements in strength, endurance, and muscle definition. Erica knows that she is prejudiced against alcoholics and smokers, so she has always tried extra hard with Mark to suspend her judgment and be more supportive. Nevertheless, she can't restrain herself from launching into the dangers of smoking lecture every week or two, hoping Mark will finally make a commitment to quitting.

Mark arrives looking glum. When Erica asks him with a big smile how he is doing, his eyes well up with tears, and he tells her that yesterday his dog died suddenly; the vet suspects poisoning. Erica loves dogs herself and knows that losing a favorite pet can be a horrible blow. She offers her sympathy and then asks if the loss has affected his behavior-change program. Mark offers that he is working longer hours and trying not to be home as much, where he is more likely to miss the dog. As they review Mark's behavior-change records, she notices his smoking only increased slightly this week. She remarks on his efforts, especially during such a hard week. She asks what else he thinks would be helpful in getting through this tough period. He ponders her question and then mentions he has some vacation days to use up, and maybe he will go visit his sister, with whom he enjoys spending time. Erica is grateful she did not launch into her "you're a bad person for smoking" routine and instead took time to learn more about Mark's situation. ■

Weighing the Pros and Cons

Once clients seem to be seriously thinking about changing, the mark of the contemplation stage of change, it is important to keep the reasons for changing in sight. What is causing the client to consider changing? The motivating factors that initiated the thinking may help clients decide to make a change.

As clients talk about changing, it may be possible to hear them listing the pros and cons of changing or of the behavior in question. Sometimes, it is almost as if clients are arguing with themselves. These arguments are not only about logic but also about barriers to action, stress, emotions, and quality of life. It is tempting to jump in and cut down potential excuses with ideas for overcoming perceived barriers, but this type of arguing does not usually lead to real change. When clients' motivation is strong and their self-efficacy high, they can more easily deal with barriers. So weighing the pros and cons and helping clients decide to change is at heart about clients' motivations for change and their belief in their abilities to change.

Health and fitness professionals contribute best in these discussions by letting clients take the lead. Professionals should answer client questions and reinforce positive reasons for changing. They can help clients look at discrepancies that have arisen in discussions about behavior change. For example, when a client is bemoaning the fact that she has no time to exercise, the professional might gently remind her that at the last session she mentioned how bored she is in the evenings, when she tends to overeat. Perhaps the professional can guide the client to see that an evening exercise class might both relieve boredom and reduce emotional overeating.

It is easy when a client starts listing reasons for not changing to simply counter with a solution. Instead, prompt clients to come up with their own solutions. Clients who do their own problem solving come up with more realistic solutions and feel more invested in the process and then hopefully more committed to their behavior-change program.

Locus of Control and Learned Helplessness

People who have a stronger sense of control over their lives may be more likely to exhibit positive health-related behaviors, such as exercising regularly. People who tend to attribute events and outcomes to internal factors such as effort and ability have an internal locus of control, whereas those who generally attribute outcomes to external factors such as luck or the actions of others have an external locus of control, as discussed in Chapter 4 (Rotter, 1990). People with a stronger internal locus of control in terms of attributing health to personal behaviors may have more success in sticking to behavior-change programs. On the other hand, those with a more external locus of control, and particularly people who believe health is primarily a matter of luck, may be less likely to exercise or to seek health information (Grotz, Hapke, Lampert, & Baumeister, 2011).

Clients who seem to fail repeatedly are especially challenging for health and fitness professionals. Learned helplessness refers to a psychological state in which people have come to believe that they are helpless in, or have no power or control over, certain situations (Petersen, Maier, & Seligman, 1995; Game Changers 5-1). People who feel like they have little power or control over whether they are able to stick to a behavior-change program will probably need extra support to be successful.

Game Changers 5-1. Martin Seligman: From Learned Helplessness to Learned Optimism and Flourishing

Psychologist Martin Seligman is best known for his theory of learned helplessness and for his work as one of the originators of the positive psychology movement. Seligman's focus in higher education began with a major in philosophy at Princeton University and then transitioned to a Ph.D. in psychology at the University of Pennsylvania, where he continues his work.

Seligman's early work on learned helplessness grew out of the observation that animals placed in situations where they had no control over an aversive situation subsequently endured the aversive situation even though in later experimental conditions escape was possible. Seligman and colleagues were working with dogs that had been classically conditioned to expect an electrical shock from the cage floor after hearing a tone (Overmier & Seligman, 1967). The original purpose of the study actually was unrelated to the learned helplessness behavior, but like all good scientists, Seligman was also curious about serendipitous and interesting observations. The researchers observed that, even after these dogs were moved to a cage that allowed escape from floor shock, the dogs simply endured the shock, without trying to get to another part of the cage that did not deliver a shock. In a subsequent experiment, Seligman and colleague Steven F. Maier compared dogs exposed to uncontrollable foot shock with those who were able to stop the shock by pressing a panel (Seligman & Maier, 1967). When moved to the new cage allowing escape, the latter group of dogs quickly figured out how to get away from the part of the cage that delivered a shock, as did a control group of dogs not exposed to shock. However, the dogs exposed to uncontrollable shock did not attempt to escape. Seligman and others have explored the concept of learned helplessness in people and its relationship to explanatory style, that is, how people explain and interpret events.

Seligman's long and productive career took a new and interesting direction in the 1990s as he spearheaded what came to be known as the positive psychology movement. Elected president of the American Psychological Association in 1996, Seligman urged psychologists to expand their focus to study not only mental illness but also "what makes life worth living," in order to better understand and promote high-level psychological health. Seligman has continued to nurture the application of his and others' research in positive psychology. His books (Seligman 1998, 2002, 2011) and public appearances (Seligman, 2004) have brought the principles and practice of positive psychology to a wide audience. Collaborations with a variety of organizations have used methods developed in the field of positive psychology to reduce risks of depression, anxiety, and behavioral problems in schoolchildren and to promote resilience in military personnel (University of Pennsylvania, 2012). Seligman's work links psychological well-being to physical health and promotes the importance of physical activity and the prevention of chronic health problems (Seligman, 2008). Health and fitness professionals may enjoy exploring the assessment tools and material on positive psychology and behavior change on Seligman's website, www.authentichappiness.org, and sharing this information with their clients.

Sources: Overmier, J. B., & Seligman, M. E. (1967). Effects of inescapable shock upon subsequent escape and avoidance responding. *Journal of Comparative and Physiological Psychology, 63*(1): 28-33; Seligman, M. E. P. (1998). *Learned Optimism: How to Change Your Mind and Your Life.* New York: Simon & Schuster; Seligman, M. E. P. (2002). *Authentic Happiness: Using the New Positive Psychology to Realize Your Potential for Lasting Fulfillment.* New York: Simon & Schuster; Seligman, M. E. P. (2004). TED Talk: Martin Seligman: The new era of positive psychology. www.ted.com/talks/martin_seligman_on_the_state_of_psychology.html. Accessed 12/6/12; Seligman, M. E. P. (2008). Positive health. *Applied Psychology, 57*: 3-18; Seligman, M. E. P., & Maier, S. F. (1967). Failure to escape traumatic shock. *Journal of Experimental Psychology, 74*(1): 1-9; Seligman, M. E. P. (2011). *Flourish: A Visionary New Understanding of Happiness and Well-being.* New York: Simon & Schuster; University of Pennsylvania. Authentic happiness. www.authentichappiness.org. Accessed 11/28/12.

People with learned helplessness tend to see failure as inevitable and have learned to attribute their failures to internal, uncontrollable, and stable causes (Petersen et al., 1995). This means that they believe failure occurs because of unchangeable and uncontrollable personal qualities in themselves (Fig. 5-7). A client with learned helplessness might think, "I have never had enough energy or organization to stick to an exercise program. I can't take care of myself." Contrast this with successful exercisers who view failures as caused by external,

controllable, and changeable causes. "The last exercise program didn't work out because I moved to a new town, but I will try to find a new fitness center here."

In conversations with clients who seem to exhibit learned helplessness, health and fitness professionals can try to help clients view the behavior-change program as being achievable and under the client's control. When a client starts explaining why the program won't work, the professional can listen carefully and work with the client to design a program that is as simple and

Attribution Characteristics of Learned Helplessness
Explanations for Prior Failures

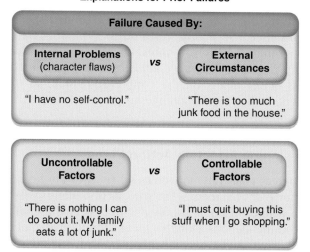

Figure 5-7. Attribution characteristics of learned helplessness.

convenient as possible. In addition, health and fitness professionals should help clients view challenges that arise as a function of controllable and changeable factors, rather than personal failings. This can be difficult, but emphasizing past successes (in any realm) and personal strengths can sometimes build client self-efficacy and internal locus of control.

CREATING GOALS AND ACTION PLANS

Many of the clients that health and fitness professionals see are in the preparation stage of change. They are seeking advice and are at least somewhat motivated to change. After a short period of questioning and listening, professionals may get a good sense of why clients have sought advice, their levels of self-efficacy for behavior change, and some of their motivations for change. Health and fitness professionals should help these clients establish behavior-change goals that will guide implementation plans.

Creating Motivational Goals

People usually begin behavior-change programs with some goals in mind. These initial goals may be connected to heartfelt hopes and dreams, and if so, they may help provide intrinsic motivation or at least help clients develop the integrated self-regulation that will sustain them through difficult times, giving them the energy they need to overcome barriers. Initial goals, even heartfelt ones, may be vague, however, or very unrealistic. Health and fitness professionals can help clients artfully transform vague and unrealistic goals into more measurable, reachable goals that still connect to clients' hopes and dreams.

Behavior-change practitioners often describe helpful goals as S.M.A.R.T. goals: specific, measurable, attainable,

relevant, and time-bound (Bryant & Green, 2010). This acronym can be helpful for health and fitness professionals working with clients to set motivational goals (Fig. 5-8).

Specific

Goals are more helpful when they are specific. Vague goals such as "get in shape," "manage stress," and "lose weight" are often the starting point for behavior-change programs. Since clients must translate goals into actions they can take, specific goals provide better information for creating a behavior-change program. For example, in order to make an action plan, clients must define terms such as "improve my diet." They need specific goals so that variables can be measured and progress toward goals can be evaluated occasionally to assure them the behavior-change program is effective. As health and fitness professionals work with clients, it is important to let clients clarify vague goals, aided by questions and suggestions from the professional.

A goal must be specific enough that clients can evaluate their progress toward it. Instead of "improve my diet," specific goals might be to consume four servings of vegetables a day, eat a salad with dinner every evening, or have dessert only three times a week. All of these goals help guide behavior-change recommendations and are specific enough that both the client and the professional know what they mean. Other examples of specific goals include climbing the stairs without getting winded or being able to fit into last year's jeans. Walking 4 days a week, eating fish twice a week, and

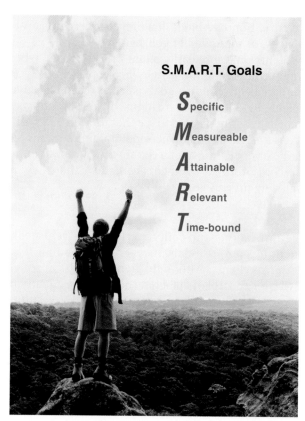

Figure 5-8. S.M.A.R.T. goals. Photograph © Thinkstock

drinking four glasses of water a day are other specific goals.

Measurable

Measurable goals allow clients to measure progress and assess whether they have reached their goals. Making progress and reaching goals are very motivational. Most health and fitness professionals know which fitness variables are easily measured; these will be discussed in more detail in Chapter 8. Servings of fruits or vegetables, number of cigarettes, number of alcoholic drinks, and minutes of strength training are measurable variables. Almost any subjective variable can be measured with scaling, described earlier in this chapter. For example, stress level can be subjectively assessed on a scale from 1 to 10, as can daily levels of fatigue, sleep quality, and other less objective variables.

Attainable

Some people find lofty goals motivating, but others find them intimidating. Even very motivated clients may run out of steam as time goes by and they feel that they have made little progress toward out-of-reach goals. Clients seem to be especially likely to set unobtainable goals in the areas of weight loss and body composition change. Large goals should be broken down into smaller goals, with all goals adjusted at periodic evaluations. Although studies have described the type of progress that health and fitness professionals are likely to see on different variables, each client is different. No one can predict with certainty how quickly (or even whether) an individual will lose weight, lower blood pressure, improve blood lipid levels, increase aerobic capacity, or improve her golf swing.

Clients can more easily attain process goals, where simply completing the activity accomplishes the goal, compared with product goals, such as reaching a given weight, blood pressure reading, or aerobic capacity. Many clients are pleased to see that they are exercising 4 days a week, attending personal training sessions regularly, or not eating after a certain time in the evening. A record of target behaviors can show that they are achieving process goals.

Relevant

Open questions and reflective listening help health and fitness professionals uncover the goals that really matter to clients. Although clients may have sought advice for control of diabetes, they may be equally interested in improving endurance enough to resume a hobby that they used to enjoy, such as square dancing or hiking. In this case, controlling blood sugar is one goal, and improving endurance with dancing or hiking might be another good goal. Clients can rate how much easier dancing or hiking is becoming as their behavior-change programs progress. Process goals such as hiking on the weekend may be extremely relevant to clients.

Time-bound

People want to know when they can expect to see improvements from their labor. Time-bound means spelling out the time it will take to reach specific goals. Because people respond to behavior-change programs at different rates, goals and predictions for progress usually need adjustment as time goes by. It is better to err on the conservative side, so that clients will see small changes as progress, rather than disappointments.

Designing Effective Action Plans

Whereas goals tell individuals where they are headed, action plans tell them what to do. Action plans spell out the where, when, and how details of behavior-change recommendations. Once health and fitness professionals and clients agree on goals, the next step is coming up with a good plan for reaching them (Fig. 5-9). Several studies have confirmed the common-sense observation that committing to a specific action plan or plans, also known as implementation intentions, increases the likelihood of successful behavior change (Andersson & Moss, 2011; de Vet, Oenema, & Grug, 2011; Wiedemann, Lippke, Reuter, Ziegelmann, & Schwarzer, 2011; Ziegelmann, Luszczynska, Lippke, & Schwarzer, 2007). For example, a study regarding the relationship between goal intentions (decisions to work toward a goal) and implementation intentions and adherence to a rehabilitation exercise program found that both types of intentions were significantly related to adherence during the first 6 months of the study, when patients were actively working with therapists. However, once patients were on their own, only implementation intentions predicted continued adherence to prescribed exercise programs 12 months after the beginning of the study (Ziegelmann et al., 2007). Similarly, action planning was associated with a successful increase in fruit and vegetable intake in a Swiss study conducted by Wiedemann and colleagues (Wiedemann et al., 2011).

Design of a behavior-change action plan should be based on client input, allowing clients to guide formation

Sample Action Plan

Goal: Eat more fruits and vegetables
ACTION PLAN
1. *Consume one fruit serving with breakfast.*
2. *Drink one cup of vegetable juice after work.*
3. *Add another serving of vegetables at dinner— make ½ plate vegetables.*

Figure 5-9. **Sample action plan.** Photograph © Thinkstock

of the action plan as much as possible. Professional input on the behavior-change plan should also be drawn from evidence-based studies, but client preference must help mold recommendations into a form that will fit the client's life, even if these forms are not "ideal" (Taylor, 2009). For example, clients who feel unable to reach public health guidelines for recommended amounts of physical activity should still be encouraged to do what they can, even if this results in suboptimal levels of physical activity. Some exercise is better than none and also better than a beautifully designed exercise program that causes anxiety and dropout. Health and fitness professionals can elicit clients' ideas for action plan design with open questions and reflective listening, guiding the development of a behavior-change plan that is feasible for that individual. Action plans should strive to be as realistic as possible, yet effective for addressing the client's goals.

The Planning Fallacy

Psychologists have observed that whether people plan to exercise, write a book, or build a space shuttle, they consistently underestimate the time, money, and energy required to accomplish their goals, a phenomenon called the planning fallacy (Thaler & Sunstein, 2008). Construction projects usually take longer and cost more than original estimates. New programs at work often take longer to design and implement than originally thought. Health and fitness professionals may note that a behavior-change program that looks great on paper turns out to require much more time and energy than clients actually have available.

Understanding this human tendency to think big can help people plan more realistically. Lack of time and energy are leading causes of behavior-change non-adherence. Good planning enhances the likelihood that people will reach their goals. Designing behavior-change programs that are realistic in their time and energy requirements can increase adherence.

The irony is that high expectations do help people make a decision to change. High expectations reinforce behavior-change benefits and help the benefits outweigh the costs in people's eyes. But what happens when these benefits are not immediately apparent? Studies suggest that, when high expectations are unmet, clients experience frustration and disappointment and are more likely to abandon their behavior-change programs than clients with more modest and more realistic expectations. These observations have led to the false hope theory (Trottier, Polivy, & Herman, 2009) and explain why overly optimistic and ambitious people are eager to start but are often the first to abandon their behavior-change programs. The false hope theory describes how people with unrealistically high expectations are motivated to make resolutions to change but are then likely to relapse once their expectations are unmet. Setting lofty goals actually makes people feel good, temporarily, and motivates people to try again, despite repeated failures in the past. Setting

goals improves self-image and induces feelings of optimism. But, as psychologists in this area of research have observed (Polivy & Herman, 2000), "Overconfidence breeds false hope, which engenders inflated expectations of success and eventually the misery of defeat."

MOTIVATING CHANGE: Balance Optimism and Realism

Balancing boundless optimism with realism can be tricky. People need hope. As you work to balance optimism with realism, use adjectives like "realistic," "sustainable," and "enjoyable." Instead of saying clients are taking on too much, praise their enthusiasm but reduce the expectations a little "to prevent injury," or "to be sure this recommendation works for you." Health and fitness professionals should always express confidence in their clients. "This is an ambitious program, but, since you have been successful in similar programs in the past, I think you will succeed in this one as well." If you work with clients over time, you will be able to adjust behavior-change programs if clients find them too discouraging.

Self-control

Changing a habit or routine takes self-control. Self-control refers to the control that people exert over their thoughts, feelings, and behavior. People use self-control when they walk by the bakery without going inside to buy a treat, limit alcohol intake, or say no when a friend offers a cigarette, if these are things that were previously customary behaviors.

Psychologists agree that self-control, also known as self-regulation, is a limited resource (Muraven, 2010). The less self-control energy a behavior-change program takes, the more likely people are to be successful. Coupled with underestimating time and energy, this lack of energy for self-control is a leading cause of nonadherence. People have a tendency to design overly ambitious programs that require much more daily self-control than they can summon. When they begin to translate their behavior-change plans into daily life, they often find that they cannot muster the willpower required to overcome old habits.

Psychologists have found that understanding and acknowledging that self-control is a limited resource can help people make more effective behavior-change plans. The following points help to clarify the nature of self-control:

- Intrinsic motivation and behavior-change self-efficacy increase self-control energy. Strong intrinsic motivation and integrated self-regulation that relate to a person's important goals increase self-control energy. In other words, motivation increases willpower.
- People vary in their levels of self-control. Some people have strong self-discipline for lifestyle changes, and others do not. People may have some idea of where they fall on the self-control

spectrum and be able to predict how much energy they can actually expend changing lifestyle behaviors. Making realistic plans enhances behavior-change adherence.

- Self-control improves with practice. Clients who practice self-control, starting with tasks that are not too difficult, may gradually improve their levels of self-control.
- Habits require less self-control than making decisions. Habits do not involve very much decision making, so they require little self-control energy. Once new behaviors are part of people's routines, they can operate on automatic pilot. Habits develop most quickly when behavior follows a "same-time, same-place" type of format.
- Social support reduces the need for self-control. People spend less energy deciding whether to perform a given behavior if the people they are with are also performing it (or not performing it in the case of behavior-cessation programs). For example, when people who have quit smoking are with nonsmoking friends, they are less likely to smoke. Helpful social support can reinforce new habits, increase motivation and self-efficacy, and reduce feelings of stress.
- Coping with stress depletes self-control energy. Stress is a leading cause of behavior-change program attrition. When people feel bad, doing something to feel better becomes more important than future health benefits (Vohs et al., 2008). Managing stress is a critical component of successful behavior-change programs. Fortunately, many people discover that exercise is a great way to reduce stress, and they learn to engage in physical activity to reduce feelings of stress.
- Self-control energy is strongest early in the day. People who exercise first thing in the morning have the best chance of sticking to their exercise programs because they are less likely to be derailed by other demands. Overeating tends to occur most frequently at the end of the day, perhaps partly because self-control is weakest at this time.

MOTIVATING CHANGE: The Force of Habit

Most people feel stressed by too much change. Unless people check into a spa or some sort of therapeutic training program, where meals are prepared for them and schedules dictate which activity comes next, it is hard to incorporate a lot of new behavior change into daily life. Although a spa or other health retreat can be a great way to jump-start a behavior-change program, changes must eventually be incorporated into daily life. People who are successful in changing health behaviors tend to make their new behaviors a habit. For example, people monitoring their blood glucose levels learn to do so at specific times each

day. Successful changers also do a great deal of planning to figure out how to make new behaviors fit as easily as possible into their lives. Instead of urging clients to rely on willpower, help them create as many supports as possible for their new behaviors.

TEACHING SELF-REGULATORY AND BEHAVIOR-CHANGE SKILLS

The successful adoption of new health behaviors relies heavily on people's self-regulatory ability. Thoughts, feelings, and behavior are connected, and self-regulation must reach into all three areas. Chapter 4 presented a brief overview of behavior-change and self-regulatory skills. This section will focus on these skills again and suggest ways that health and fitness professionals can best help clients acquire and improve these skills in behavior-change contexts.

Good Communication Is Essential for Teaching Skills

Good communication that includes the OARS skills described above continues to be at the heart of successful professional–client relationships. As clients embark on their behavior-change journeys, good professional support can help them build skills that will enhance the likelihood of success. As with creating effective goals and action plans, teaching self-regulation and behavior-change skills involves more than simply telling clients what to do. Good communication consists of a dialogue, where professionals ask open questions and clients explore what is and is not working. Professionals and clients then work as a team to revise goals and action plans, if necessary, and to refine strategies that will help clients stick to their programs.

Create Positive Affect

Teaching behavior-change skills is best done in a positive way that generates hope and builds self-efficacy. Health and fitness professionals should continue to tie suggestions and educational efforts to clients' hopes and dreams, in order to tap into clients' autonomous motivation for change. When possible, professionals should present behavior-change skills as producing positive emotions. For example, instead of focusing only on how much exercise clients should do, the professional should also focus on how regular exercise will begin to help reduce feelings of stress or on other emotional health benefits clients want. One study found that messages promoting positive affect (exercise will help you feel good) were associated with higher levels of physical activity in subjects than cognitive messages that simply conveyed information about exercise benefits (exercise is good for you) (Conner, Ryan, Morris,

McEachan, & Lawton, 2011). Good communication skills also create positive feelings because clients feel respected and valued as they work with the professional. If clients experience emotional health benefits with exercise, health and fitness professionals can encourage regular physical activity as part of behavior-change efforts.

Build Client Competence

People want to feel competent (Ryan et al., 2011). Health and fitness professionals should continually strive to be sure that the demands of behavior-change programs do not exceed clients' abilities, especially clients' perceptions of their abilities. Self-efficacy is strongly associated with people's abilities to employ self-regulation skills during a behavior-change program (Anderson, Winett, Wojcik, & Williams, 2010). Health and fitness professionals should realize that feelings of self-efficacy for behavior change can fluctuate widely from day to day and continue to check in with clients over time regarding how they are doing. Changes in other realms of life, such as difficulties at work, can change self-efficacy for behavior change, because clients feel busier or more stressed.

Implement Methods for Self-monitoring

Research has shown that self-monitoring is one of the most effective ways to support behavior change, including exercise-program adherence (Burke, Conroy, & Sereika, 2011; Helsel, Jakicic, & Otto, 2007). Self-monitoring systems, such as a log in which clients record their workouts or smokers record cigarette use, help in several ways (Fig. 5-10). First, they increase clients' self-awareness. Self-monitoring is especially useful in increasing self-awareness of unconscious behaviors such as eating and smoking. Self-monitoring

acts as a mirror to give clients a more objective view of their behavior.

Second, self-monitoring systems forge an important link between the health and fitness professional and the client. Clients come to expect careful surveillance of their records, which they present at each session with the professional. Knowing that someone will be checking on their adherence may prod clients into action and get them thinking about problems that they may wish to discuss at their next session with the professional (Brehm, 2009).

Third, self-monitoring systems can serve as important tools for evaluating behavior-change problems. Clients may note factors that helped or interfered with behavior-change plans. The health and fitness professional can analyze this information with clients and brainstorm solutions to problems that arise.

Lastly, self-monitoring records serve as a form of positive reinforcement and increase self-efficacy. For example, a completed exercise log shows clients that they are being successful in their exercise programs.

■ *This morning, Erica is looking forward to trying out her new communication skills with one of her biggest failures. Alice is 83, recovering from an angioplasty procedure, and has hypertension. Erica appreciates Alice's wry sense of humor and enjoys leading her through her workout. Alice doesn't mind the exercise program; that, at least, has worked well. But Alice seems to have made little progress in reducing her salt intake or in consuming more fruits and vegetables. She has always listened attentively and patiently to Erica's recommendations but then seems to ignore the dietary advice.*

After her workout, Alice sits down with Erica to go over her dietary record sheets from the past week. No progress:

...day	Tuesday	Wednesday	Thursday	Fri...
	2	**3**	**4**	**5**
...t fruit ...juice ...er veg	√ Bfast fruit √ Veg juice √ Dinner veg	√ Bfast fruit O Veg juice √ Dinner veg	√ Bfast fruit √ Veg juice O Dinner veg	√ Bfa... √ Veg... √ Din...
	9	**10**	**11**	**12**
...t fruit ...juice ...er veg	√ Bfast fruit √ Veg juice √ Dinner veg	√ Bfast fruit √ Veg juice √ Dinner veg	__ Bfast fruit __ Veg juice __ Dinner veg	__ Bfa... __ Veg... __ Din...
	16	**17**	**18**	**19**
...t fruit ...juice ...er veg	__ Bfast fruit __ Veg juice __ Dinner veg	__ Bfast fruit __ Veg juice __ Dinner veg	__ Bfast fruit __ Veg juice __ Dinner veg	__ Bfa... __ Veg... __ Din...

Figure 5-10. Self-monitoring example.

mostly take-out, prepared foods, and sugary snacks, but there is one fast-food salad. Over the past several sessions, Erica has heaped advice on Alice, regarding low-salt cooking, shopping for fresh fruits and vegetables, and food composition charts from fast-food restaurants. Today Erica is not going to give advice and instead prepares to listen. She asks Alice how she decides what to eat at a given meal. How is it she eats so much take-out and prepared foods? Alice seems surprised at the questions but then admits she doesn't really think about food very much and she hates vegetables. Erica is amazed to hear Alice doesn't like to cook; she thought women of that generation were all good in the kitchen. How silly. No wonder her earlier advice did not connect. Erica switches gears and discusses with Alice the simplest, easiest tips for fitting more fruits and vegetables into the diet. She asks Alice if she is comfortable making one small change. Alice says she will try to drink a glass of low-sodium vegetable juice with lunch every day. They create a box on Alice's self-monitoring sheet for vegetable juice, which she will try to check off each day. ■

Analyze Behavior Chains

Sometimes self-monitoring systems reveal behavior patterns that enhance or disrupt behavior-change efforts. A behavior chain refers to behaviors that are commonly linked together (Foster, Makris, & Bailer, 2005; Kumanyika et al., 2008). Behavior chains are usually analyzed in terms of antecedents, behaviors, and consequences. For example, smokers may light up a cigarette every time they make a telephone call to a friend. In this example, calling a friend triggers smoking behavior and is called an antecedent, in that the calling, or the decision to call, comes before and triggers the behavior—smoking. Consequences follow the behavior (Fig. 5-11). Smoking may cause the smoker to feel better, as the nicotine craving is satisfied. Additionally, talking to the friend may also be associated with positive feelings, so the smoking–telephone call link may be doubly reinforced.

When behavior chains that affect target behaviors are identified, clients and professionals can work

together to break the chain, with the client taking the lead. For example, consider a client who has worked with a health and fitness professional to design an exercise program to improve blood sugar regulation. The client has agreed to begin walking every day around his neighborhood for 30 minutes when he gets home after work. The client is successful for 2 days after his meeting with the professional but on the third day arrives home later than usual from work, feeling hungry and tired, and decides to skip walking. Unfortunately, the next few days are also late days, and the client returns to his next meeting with the health and fitness professional discouraged and frustrated.

As the professional and client examine this behavior chain, they can problem-solve ways to address the antecedents and consequences that led to a decision to not exercise. Would the client be more successful exercising before work if he is often fatigued at the end of the workday? Would stopping at a fitness center on his way home be an option, so that the temptations of dinner and rest would not be available to reinforce a decision to skip the walk? As the health and fitness professional and client "take apart" the links in the behavior chain, they can come up with a plan to reinforce the new, desired behavior (exercising). This process is called shaping, since the client is attempting to shape a new, more productive behavior chain. Shaping is an application of the stimulus control and counterconditioning processes of change, as described in Chapter 4.

Sometimes behavior chains point to environmental factors as triggers for undesirable behaviors. Environmental re-engineering means changing the environment in ways that promote (or at least do not inhibit) desirable behaviors. Environmental re-engineering includes simple changes, such as not keeping junk food in one's living or work area. It can also include large changes, such as building a fitness center at a workplace to make it easier for employees to exercise.

Encourage Coping Planning

Most clients have a fairly good idea of the factors that tend to interfere with their behavior-change efforts. Many have had previous experiences with relapse, where behavior-change efforts were temporarily or permanently abandoned and old behaviors resumed. These previous experiences are valuable when planning for future similar situations, where factors perceived as barriers to behavior change may arise. Research suggests that coping planning, or devising strategies for dealing with potential barriers to behavior change, is as important to the success of behavior-change programs as action planning (Wiedemann et al., 2011).

As always, clients should take the lead in suggesting factors likely to disrupt behavior-change plans. Common problems include anything that changes a client's schedule, since most health behaviors become routine habits. For example, travel, visitors, school holidays,

Behavior Chain

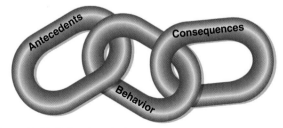

Figure 5-11. Behavior chain.

bad weather, and illness commonly upset a person's daily rhythm. Clients can anticipate and plan for these disruptions, so that behavior change continues. Clients can also make plans for coping with situations where behavior-change programs derail temporarily, so that they can resume their behavior-change efforts as soon as possible.

Discuss Stress-Management Options

Health and fitness professionals may notice that stress and negative emotions such as anger and worry are common components of behavior chains associated with relapse or difficulty sticking to a behavior-change program. Stress and negative emotions make clients feel tired, preoccupied with problems, and weaker in self-efficacy, and they stimulate people to search for ways to feel better. Chapter 6 details the effects of stress on behavior-change programs, along with common approaches for reducing feelings of stress. Cultivating a ready repertoire of stress-management strategies is especially important for clients who tend to respond to stress with harmful actions such as eating, substance abuse, or sedentary behaviors.

Explore Strategies for Increasing Social Support

People are social creatures, and the behavior of family, friends, and others exerts a strong influence. Social support refers to any behavior on the part of other people that helps someone achieve goals and objectives. Social support can be a supervisor at work who encourages employees to exercise during their lunch hour or a spouse who prepares a healthful meal. It can be a group of people focused on a similar goal, such as quitting smoking or addressing another addiction, or an exercise class. Health and fitness professionals provide social support for their clients by assisting them throughout behavior-change programs. One of the best forms of social support can be an exercise partner who exercises with the client. Social support enhances the likelihood that clients will succeed in behavior change (Anderson et al., 2010). It has the potential to influence many factors in behavior-change models, including the following (Fig. 5-12).

- **Clients' perceptions about health and behavior change:** People are swayed by the opinions of others. Close relationships can be especially influential in this regard (Sbarra & Hazan, 2008). Significant others help shape clients' beliefs about health threats, their personal vulnerability to health threats, behavior change, and whether behavior change alters personal vulnerability to health threats.
- **Social norms and a client's social network:** Smokers whose friends all smoke may have a harder time quitting than a smoker who has many nonsmoking friends and family members.

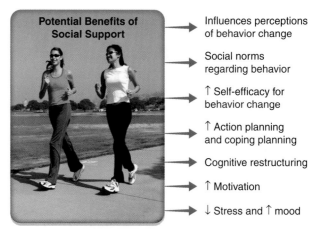

Figure 5-12. **Potential benefits of social support.** Photograph © Thinkstock

- **Self-efficacy and perceived behavioral control:** Both verbal persuasion from others and modeling seen in others enhance feelings of behavioral control (Molloy, Dixon, Hamer, & Sniehotta, 2010).
- **Action planning and coping planning:** Molloy and colleagues (Molloy et al., 2010) found that social support facilitated coping planning, especially for women (What's the Evidence? 5-1). The researchers proposed that planning can be socially interactive. Social support can reinforce a decision to change and then provide other helpful ideas and support as clients move forward in their behavior-change programs.
- **Cognitive restructuring:** Cognitive restructuring, explained in Chapter 4, refers to processes by which clients identify and attempt to change unproductive thought patterns that trigger negative emotions and behaviors. Family, friends, and others close to clients can reinforce more realistic and productive thoughts.
- **Motivation:** Although social support generally provides extrinsic motivation, which is not as effective at sustaining long-term behavior change as autonomous forms of motivation, extrinsic motivation sometimes can jump-start a behavior-change program and lead to subsequent development of more autonomous motivation. Chapter 4 presented the processes of change from the Transtheoretical Model. Relationships with others are involved in several of these, especially social liberation and helping relationships.
- **Reduced stress and improved mood:** Friends can help clients address problems and provide emotional support when feelings of stress threaten to interfere with behavior-change intentions. Friends can lighten the mood and reframe negative situations.

Health and fitness professionals can encourage clients to think about people (or animals; Fig. 5-13) who might provide helpful support. When clients do not seem to have much of a support network, they

WHAT'S THE EVIDENCE? 5-1

Social Support Facilitates Planning for Exercise

Molloy, G. J., Dixon, D., Hamer, M., & Sniehotta, F. F. (2010). Social support and regular physical activity: does planning mediate this link? *British Journal of Health Psychology, 15*(Pt 4): 859–870.

■ PURPOSE

The observation that social support for physical activity increases participation in exercise is well established. Molloy and colleagues wanted to learn more about the mechanisms by which social support influences physical activity patterns. The purpose of this study was to see if level of social support influenced the planning processes that help people translate goals into actual exercise behavior.

■ STUDY

All residential students (about 10,000) at Aberdeen University in Scotland received an e-mail at the beginning of the school year inviting them to participate in the study, and 903 students completed the study. Students answered questionnaires regarding their exercise frequency, level of intention to exercise regularly, and perceived behavioral control for regular exercise, as defined in the Theory of Planned Behavior. Subjects also answered questions about their action planning and coping planning and their level of social support for physical activity. Social support for physical activity was measured by scaled responses to three items: "In the last week, I . . . had somebody to encourage me to participate in physical activity on a regular basis . . . had somebody to participate in physical activity with me . . . felt supported in having a regular pattern of physical activity." Data were collected during the first 2 weeks of class. Seven weeks later, data on frequency of physical activity were collected again. The researchers looked at the associations between social support for physical activity and exercise frequency and other variables listed previously.

The researchers found somewhat different results for men and women. For men, greater social support for physical activity was significantly related to higher levels of perceived behavioral control. Higher levels of perceived behavioral control were related to higher levels of physical activity. Social support for physical activity was significantly related to action planning in men; however, planning was not associated with physical activity levels in this group. The researchers concluded that although social support for physical activity was related to a few variables, as described above, it did not have a significant overall effect on men's physical activity levels in this study.

The pattern for women was different. For women, more social support for physical activity was significantly related to both intention to exercise and to perceived behavioral control for physical activity. As with the men, higher levels of perceived behavioral control were related to frequency of exercise. Social support for physical activity for women was significantly related to action planning and coping planning. Coping planning, in turn, was significantly related to level of physical activity. The researchers concluded that social support for physical activity was a stronger predictor of exercise frequency for women than for men. The researchers also concluded that some of the effect of social support for physical activity is mediated through higher levels of planning.

■ IMPLICATIONS

Social support for physical activity can have important effects for both men and women and should be encouraged for clients of both genders. However, social support seems to have a stronger influence for women than men, at least for people under 30 years old, the age of this subject pool. Social support probably exerts its beneficial effects in several ways. One of the most important effects, especially for women, is to improve coping planning. The researchers suggest that behavior-change interventions should take advantage of the socially interactive nature of planning processes.

might find support in a group behavior-change environment, such as a weight-control program or exercise class.

Help Clients Visualize Success

Research suggests that simple visualization exercises can help clients build preconscious processes that will support behavior change (Andersson & Moss, 2011). Preconscious processes refer to memories and feelings people may not currently be aware of but that they can remember. Preconscious processes can influence people's thoughts and feelings about something, such as a behavior-change program. Many fitness professionals are familiar with the idea of using visualization to enhance sports performance, manage stress, and facilitate behavior change. Studies of athletes have found that mental performance of sports skills can enhance the improvement that comes with physical practice. Obviously, mental practice is not a substitute for physical training, but it can somehow sharpen an athlete's focus so that physical training produces faster results.

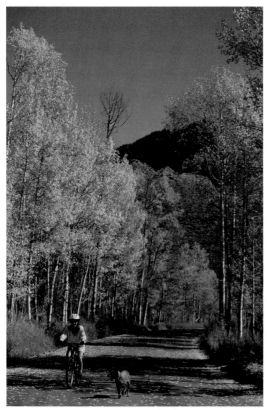

Figure 5-13. **Dogs can be social support.** © Thinkstock

must think about arranging childcare. The wheels start turning, and plans are put in motion. As people imagine the future, thoughts and feelings arise, and they often respond by devising solutions to possible problems.

As people visualize the future, they also practice coping with negative emotions. As they imagine events, they experience an emotional response to these events, albeit in a milder form than the actual event would elicit. But they still feel a full range of emotions, from joy and pleasure to anger, disappointment, and anxiety. For example, as the client imagines the chaos of school vacation, she may experience some anxiety about not having control of her time. Researchers suggest that when people anticipate upcoming emotions, they deal with them more effectively and are less likely to let negative emotions get in the way of their plans (Davis & Asliturk, 2011; Taylor, Pham, Rivkin, & Armor, 1998). This is very important, since negative emotions are a leading cause of relapse in behavior-change programs. Visualization may also work by giving people a sense that they will be successful in reaching their goals. Because their goals seem reachable, they are willing to work harder to achieve them and are less likely to give up in the face of negative emotions or the inevitable snafus that occur in real life.

Researchers have designed interesting applications for using visualization in changing behavior. Research suggests that visualization can aid planning and emotional self-regulation (Andersson & Moss, 2011). People who visualize the skills needed to accomplish a certain behavior-change goal appear to make better progress than those who simply visualize themselves as having already achieved their goals. So, for example, people trying to quit smoking seem to get more benefit from visualizing themselves deciding to sip tea after dinner instead of smoking rather than just being a non-smoker. People trying to lose weight may benefit more from imagining themselves getting up from their desks at lunchtime and going for a walk, rather than just visualizing themselves as thin.

Visualization seems to increase the engagement of people with the processes they are imagining and to increase the likelihood that they will behave in ways that help them succeed. By imagining the steps needed to achieve their goals, people may increase their problem-solving behavior. Health and fitness professionals can maximize the power of visualization by asking clients to imagine potentially difficult situations and to mentally rehearse skills for dealing successfully with these situations.

Take as an example a client who is worried that her children's upcoming school vacation will disrupt her exercise routine. As she imagines the vacation, she remembers that her schedule tends to fall to pieces whenever she takes days off from work to be home with the kids. To get to the fitness center, she

MOTIVATING CHANGE: Instructing Clients on Visualization

Health and fitness professionals can encourage clients to visualize successful behavior change. You can help your clients create visualization scenarios to practice on their own. For example, clients who have decided to walk first thing in the morning might envision themselves waking up, putting on their exercise clothes, and going out the door for a walk. You can coach clients to imagine how that experience might look and, while visualizing, make the scene as realistic as possible. Clients can also imagine what sounds they might hear and even smells or tastes associated with the experience they are visualizing. Clients should visualize what they hope for.

Visualization works best when people are in a relaxed state, such as before falling asleep or after a few minutes of deep breathing. But visualization can also be done anywhere when a client has a few moments, such as waiting in line at a store or waiting at a red light while driving.

Once clients get the hang of imagining their new behaviors under normal circumstances, they can extend visualization into the coping-planning realm. In the example above, the client might imagine that she wakes up, puts on her exercise clothes, but finds that it is raining hard. So instead, she gets on the exercise bike and does an interval workout for 30 minutes, watching the morning news.

SUPPORTING BEHAVIOR CHANGE: Ethical Considerations

Behavior change can be tricky and difficult work for many clients. Change can have unintended consequences influencing clients' family relationships, work situation, and social circles. Professionals can feel overwhelmed with the challenges faced by their clients. Human relationships often develop in complicated ways, and what began as a professional relationship can turn into codependency; for example, clients may contact professionals several times a day and demand far more attention than is reasonable. New professionals must be especially careful to become familiar with ethical guidelines that can prevent some of the most common problems that tend to arise in behavior-change work.

Respect Client Autonomy

Supporting client autonomy is an ethical priority (Ryan et al., 2011). The beauty of working in a client-centered fashion is that clients develop responsibility for the behavior-change goals and programs that are developed. Because client input guides behavior-change recommendations every step of the way, the professional is never solely "responsible" for behavior-change outcomes. Obviously, the health and fitness professional should always have clients' best interests at heart and should guide them in directions that are evidence-based for producing the desired health and fitness improvements clients seek. But clients must do the behavior-change work, such as exercising regularly, making better choices about food intake, quitting smoking, or learning to leave work at reasonable hours. Following the communication skills guidelines set forth in this chapter will help health and fitness professionals respect client autonomy.

Maintain Professional Boundaries

Effective health and fitness professionals strive to convey to clients an empathetic, positive regard. Thus, when professionals and clients work together for an extended period, it is normal for both to experience friendly feelings. However, the effectiveness of health and fitness professionals is undermined when they become too personally involved with their clients.

What is the difference between professional empathy and personal involvement? Empathy occurs when the professional demonstrates understanding and acceptance toward the client. Professionals can demonstrate empathy within their role in helping a client. Personal involvement occurs when the professional becomes friends with the client or enters into a sexual relationship. It is difficult to maintain a professional–client relationship once this has occurred.

Appropriate professional behavior for one health and fitness professional may not feel right to another. For example, should a personal trainer attend a party given by a client? Most personal trainers could participate professionally in such a situation, but others might feel uncomfortable or at least unable to really enjoy the party. Over time, health and fitness professionals develop certain boundaries that allow them to behave professionally and express empathy without becoming best friends with clients.

Stay Within Professional Scope of Practice

Every professional has a proscribed scope of practice spelled out by his or her certification or licensing organization. Health and fitness professionals must be very clear about their scope of practice and adhere strictly to their organization's guidelines in this area. Guidelines usually define the types of clients and concerns to which professionals should limit their practice.

Health and fitness professionals usually begin working with a client in good faith that the client's issues are within their scope of practice. However, other health or personal issues may arise that are beyond such scope. When these problems arise, it is appropriate for professionals to refer a client to someone whose scope of practice includes the issues that the client needs to address (Box 5-4).

Erica's department head, Adrian, asks everyone for feedback on their experience with communication skills training at the monthly department meeting. "Cute!" Erica thinks. "Even he is learning to listen!" Several people share stories, as well as frustrations. Most agree they

---

Box 5-4. Effective Referrals

Health and fitness professionals refer clients to other professionals for many reasons: to follow up on symptoms of illness or injury, to help them get dietary advice from nutrition professionals, or to encourage them to get professional help for psychological concerns such as substance abuse, depression, or eating disorders. They refer clients to other professionals when an issue exceeds their scope of practice and they feel that clients could benefit from good advice. They also refer when they feel their clients need to confront a serious issue they may be denying. Some clients are too needy. Some clients do not seem to be making progress and the work isn't working and the professional's help isn't helping. It is time for the client to try someone else.

Box 5-4. Effective Referrals–cont'd

Most health and fitness professionals are comfortable recommending that clients seek medical help for illness or injury, but they are less confident in their ability to confront a client about a possible psychological concern. Every client is different, so every referral situation is different. The following are some general suggestions on referring a client for professional help that can guide professionals in most situations.

Check in With the Work Team

Health and fitness professionals should discuss their concerns with their supervisor and work team. Colleagues can help professionals decide whether they are justified in their responses or overreacting to the situation. Colleagues may have faced similar situations themselves and have good suggestions.

The professional's employer may already have policies and guidelines in place for making referrals in various areas, including psychological concerns. The employer may also ask the professional to document the referral conversations and follow up in some way. If the health and fitness professional is uncomfortable confronting the client about the issue, perhaps someone with more experience can do this instead.

Prepare to Refer

Health and fitness professionals must be ready with a specific referral recommendation. They may wish to refer clients back to their health-care providers, or they may recommend another type of professional in their location. They should be prepared to give clients specific contact information for the dietitian, physical therapist, and so on who they plan to recommend. If clients need to complete a new medical clearance form, the professional should have that ready as well.

Professionals need to make a decision about the bottom line: what will they ask clients to do and how will they follow up? Will they continue to work with clients no matter what? Will they require new medical clearance or contact with the client's provider? Will the professional need to stop working with the client because the situation exceeds his or her scope of practice?

The professional gathers the evidence. Before speaking with the client, he or she makes a list of specific, observed behaviors and statements. Clients find it more difficult to dismiss the professional's point of view if presented with solid evidence. Rather than saying, "You seem too concerned about your body image," the professional will want to say, "Every time we meet, you make many derogatory comments about being fat. You say you never go out because you are worried about how you look. I am worried about you." For a client who is overexercising, the professional might use evidence as follows: "I have recommended that you reduce your exercise intensity, but your exercise log shows you are exercising longer and harder than you were last month."

Meet With the Client

Health and fitness professionals should schedule a time to speak with their clients in private about their concerns. If no private place is available, they should find a spot out of earshot of others. If the client is a minor, the professional should also speak to the parents on a separate occasion.

The professional should open the conversation by expressing concern. "I am worried about you because . . . ." For example, he or she might say something such as, "Here are the nutrient requirements for pregnant women. I am concerned that you are far short of these. I am worried about your health and your baby's development." Then the professional should cite the evidence that he or she has gathered.

Once professionals have voiced their concerns and evidence, they must give clients time to respond. They should not interrupt them when they talk and should listen with an open mind to their point of view. Professionals may wish to modify their recommendations or to tell clients that they need some time to formulate a response. They should express confidence in the client's ability to cope with the situation and to achieve a positive outcome.

Sources

Bartlett, S., Anderson, R., & Cotton, R. T. (2013). Chapter 11: Referral. In: Bryant, C. X., Green, D. J., & Merrill, S., eds. *ACE health coach manual.* San Diego, CA: American Council on Exercise.

Johnson, J. H., Haskvitz, E. M., & Brehm, B. A. (2009). *Applied Sports Medicine for Coaches.* Baltimore, MD: Lippincott, Williams, & Wilkins.

could use more training, because they sometimes find themselves in difficult conversations where they are not always sure what to say next. Adrian shares the recent results of a patient satisfaction survey, noting that patients

who report feeling satisfied or very satisfied with their experiences with professionals in the department has risen somewhat, compared with 6 months ago. Adrian is pleased, and he urges everyone to check their e-mail for their individual patient satisfaction reports this afternoon.

That afternoon, Erica is nervous as she opens the e-mail from Adrian. She breathes a sigh of relief when she sees that the feedback on her performance mirrors the improvements seen in the department as a whole. Although she still gets the usual disgruntled comment or two, there are more statements than usual from individuals praising her ability to try to understand them and to support their behavior-change efforts. Erica appreciates the irony that, even though she is giving less advice, her patients are following more of it. ■

KEY TERMS

action plan

affirmations

ambivalence

antecedent

behavior chain

change talk

client-centered

closed questions

consequences

coping planning

environmental re-engineering

false hope theory

goal intentions

implementation intentions

learned helplessness

open questions

patient-centered

planning fallacy

preconscious processes

process goals

product goals

rapport

reflective listening

scaling

self-control

self-disclosure

self-regulation

shaping

social support

CRITICAL THINKING QUESTIONS

1. The next time you visit a professional, such as a dentist, health-care provider, professor, counselor, or auto mechanic, be aware of the factors listed in Box 5-1. How did the professional rate on these factors? What aspects of your work together created a positive impression for you? What qualities, if any, detracted from the experience of working together?

2. Observe your thoughts as people talk to you throughout the next few days. Do you focus exclusively on what they are saying? Or do you notice yourself doing any of the following: thinking about what you will say next, forming judgments about the speaker, predicting what the speaker will say next, daydreaming about something else, or thinking about your own problems?

3. The following are closed questions. Create open questions that might elicit the same information but in a more expanded and contextual way.
   • Have you ever tried to exercise regularly?
   • Do you get enough sleep?
   • Do you have a good diet?

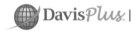 For additional resources log in to DavisPlus (davisplus.fadavis.com/ keyword "Brehm") and click on the Premium tab. (Don't have a *Plus*Code to access Premium Resources? Just click the Purchase Access button on the book's DavisPlus page.)

REFERENCES

Aikens, J. E., Bingham, R., & Piette, J. D. (2005). Patient-provider communication and self-care behavior among type 2 diabetes patients. *The Diabetes Educator, 31*(5): 681-690.

Ambady, N., & Weisbuch, M. (2010). Nonverbal behavior. In: Fiske, S. T., Gilbert, D. T. & Lindzey, G., eds. *Handbook of Social Psychology.* New York: McGraw-Hill: 464-497.

Anderson, E. S., Winett, R. A., Wojcik, J. R., & Williams, D. M. (2010). Social cognitive mediators of change in a group randomized nutrition and physical activity intervention: social support, self-efficacy, outcome expectations and self-regulation in the Guide-to-Health Trial. *Journal of Health Psychology, 15*(1): 21-32.

Andersson, E. K., & Moss, T. P. (2011). Imagery and implementation intention: a randomized controlled trial of interventions to increase exercise behaviour in the general population. *Psychology of Sport and Exercise, 12*(2): 63-70.

Bartlett, S., Anderson, R., & Cotton, R. T. (2008). Chapter 11: Referral. In: Bryant, C. X., & Green D. J., eds. *ACE Lifestyle & Weight Management Consultant Manual.* San Diego, CA: American Council on Exercise.

Berwick, D. M. (2009). What 'patient-centered' should mean: confessions of an extremist. *Health Affairs, 28*(4): w555-w565.

Biesanz, J. C., Human, L. J., Paquin, A., Chan, M., Parisotto, K. L., Sarracino, J., & Gillis, R. L. (2011). Do we know when our impressions of others are valid? Evidence for realistic accuracy awareness in first impressions of personality. *Social Psychological and Personality Science, 2*(5): 452-459.

Brehm, B. A. (2010). Communication and teaching techniques. In: Bryant, C. X., & Green, D. J., eds. *ACE Personal Trainer Manual.* San Diego, CA: American Council on Exercise: 39-61.

Brehm, B. A. (2009). Communication strategies and behavior change. In: Bryant, C. X., & Green, D. J., eds. *ACE Advanced Health & Fitness Specialist Manual.* San Diego, CA: American Council on Exercise: 57-77.

Brehm, B. A. (2013). Lifestyle modification and behavior change. In: Bryant, C. X., Green, D. J., & Merrill, S. eds. *ACE Health Coach Manual.* San Diego, CA: American Council on Exercise: 385-408.

Brehm, B. A. (2004). *Successful Fitness Motivation Strategies.* Champaign, IL: Human Kinetics.

Burke, L. E., Conroy, M. B., & Sereika, S. M. (2011). The effect of electronic self-monitoring on weight loss and dietary intake: a randomized behavioral weight loss trial. *Obesity, 19*(2): 338-344.

Conner, M., Ryan, R. E., Morris, B., McEachan, R., & Lawton, R. (2011). Changing exercise through targeting affective or cognitive attitudes. *Psychology and Health, 26*(2): 133-149.

Davis, C. G., & Asliturk, E. (2011). Toward a positive psychology of coping with anticipated events. *Canadian Psychology, 52*(2): 101-110.

de Vet, E., Oenema, A., & Grug, J. (2011). More or better: do the number and specificity of implementation intentions matter in increasing physical activity? *Psychology of Sport and Exercise, 12*(4): 471-477.

Fjeldsoe, B., Neuhaus, M., Winkler, E., & Eakin, E. (2011). Systematic review of maintenance of behavior change following physical activity and dietary interventions. *Health Psychology, 30*(1): 99-109.

Foster, G. D., Makris, A. P., & Bailer, B. A. (2005). Behavioral treatment of obesity. *American Journal of Clinical Nutrition, 82*(1): 2305-2355.

Freudenberg, N., & Olden, K. (2011). Getting serious about the prevention of chronic diseases. *Preventing Chronic Disease, 8*(4): A90. www.cdc.gov/pcd/issues/2011/jul/10_0243.htm. Accessed 11/25/12.

George, M. (2008). Interactions in expert service work: demonstrating professionalism in personal training. *Journal of Contemporary Ethnography, 37*(1): 108-131.

Grotz, M., Hapke, U., Lampert, T., & Baumeister, H. (2011). Health locus of control and health behavior: results from a nationally representative survey. *Psychology, Health, and Medicine, 16*(2): 129-140.

Helitzer, D. L., LaNoue, M., Wilson, B., de Hernandez, B. U., Warner, T., Roter, D. (2011). A randomized controlled trial of communication training with primary care providers to improve patient-centeredness and health risk communication. *Patient Education and Counseling, 82*(1): 21-29.

Helsel, D. L., Jakicic, J. M., & Otto, A. D. (2007). Comparison of techniques for self-monitoring eating and exercise behaviors on weight loss in a correspondence-based intervention. *Journal of the American Dietetic Association, 107*(10): 1807-1810.

Hunter, S. D. (2008). Promoting intrinsic motivation for clients. *Strength and Conditioning Journal, 30*(1): 52-54.

Jacobs, N., Hagger, M. S., Streukens, S., De Bourdeaudhuij, I., & Claes, N. (2011). Testing an integrated model of the theory of planned behavior and self-determination theory for different energy balance-related behaviours and intervention intensities. *British Journal of Health Psychology, 16*: 113-134.

Johnson, J. H., Haskvitz, E. M., & Brehm, B. A. (2009). *Applied Sports Medicine for Coaches.* Baltimore, MD: Lippincott, Williams, & Wilkins.

Klein, S., Sheard, N. F., Pi-Sunyer, X., Daly, A., Wylie-Rosett, J., Kulkarni, K., . . . American Society for Clinical Nutrition. (2004). Weight management through lifestyle modification for the prevention and management of type 2 diabetes: rationale and strategies. A statement of the American Diabetes Association, the North American Association for the Study of Obesity, and the American Society for Clinical Nutrition. *American Journal of Clinical Nutrition, 80*(2): 257-263.

Krebs, P., Prochaska, J. O., & Rossi, J. S. (2010). A meta-analysis of computer-tailored interventions for health behavior change. *Preventive Medicine, 51*: 214-221.

Kumanyika, S. K., Obarzanek, E., Stettler, N., Bell, R., Field, A. E., Fortmann, S. P., . . . American Heart Association Council on Epidemiology and Prevention, Interdisciplinary Committee for Prevention. (2008). Population-based prevention of obesity: the need for comprehensive promotion of healthful eating, physical activity, and energy balance. *Circulation, 118*(4): 428-464.

Larson, E. B., & Yao, X. (2005). Clinical empathy as emotional labor in the patient-physician relationship. *Journal of the American Medical Association, 293*(9): 1100-1106.

Maguire, J. S. (2008). The personal is professional: personal trainers as a case study of cultural intermediaries. *International Journal of Cultural Studies, 11*(2): 211-229.

Mast, M. S. (2007). On the importance of nonverbal communication in the physician-patient interaction. *Patient Education and Counseling, 67*(3): 315-318.

Miller, W. R. (1983). Motivational interviewing with problem drinkers. *Behavioural Psychotherapy, 11*: 147-172.

Miller, W. R., & Rollnick, S. (1991). *Motivational Interviewing: Preparing People to Change Addictive Behavior.* New York: Guilford Press.

Miller, W. R., & Rollnick, S. (2013). *Motivational Interviewing: Preparing People for Change,* 3rd ed. New York: Guilford Press.

Molloy, G. J., Dixon, D., Hamer, M., & Sniehotta, F. F. (2010). Social support and regular physical activity: does planning mediate this link? *British Journal of Health Psychology, 15*(Pt 4): 858-870.

Muraven, M. (2010). Building self-control strength: practicing self-control leads to improved self-control performance. *Journal of Experimental Social Psychology, 46*(2): 465-468.

Neumann, M., Edelhauser, R., Kreps, G. L., Scheffer, C., Lutz, G., Tauschel, D., & Visser, A. (2010). Can patient–provider interaction increase the effectiveness of medical treatment or even substitute it?—An exploration on why and how to study the specific effect of the provider. *Patient Education and Counseling, 80*: 307-314.

Norman, P., Bennett, P., Smith, C., & Murphy, S. (1998). Health locus of control and behavior. *Journal of Health Psychology, 3*(2): 171-180.

Overmier, J. B., & Seligman, M. E. (1967). Effects of in-escapable shock upon subsequent escape and avoidance responding. *Journal of Comparative and Physiological Psychology, 63*(1): 28-33.

Patrick, H., & Canevello, A. (2011). Methodological overview of a self-determination theory-based computerized intervention to promote leisure-time physical activity. *Psychology of Sport and Exercise, 12*: 13-19.

Petersen, C., Maier, S. F., & Seligman, M. E. P. (1995). *Learned Helplessness: A Theory for the Age of Personal Control.* New York: Oxford University Press.

Pfister-Minogue, K. A., & Salveson, C. (2010). Training and experience of public health nurses in using behavior change counseling. *Public Health Nursing, 27*(6): 544-551.

Polivy, J., & Herman, C. P. (2000). The false-hope syndrome: unfulfilled expectations of self-change. *Current Directions in Psychological Science, 9*(4): 128-131.

Rink, J. E., & Hall, T. J. (2008). Research on effective teaching in elementary school physical education. *The Elementary School Journal, 108*(3): 207-218.

Rollnick, S., Butler, C. C., Kinnersley, P., Gregory, J., & Mash, B. (2010). Motivational interviewing. *British Medical Journal, 340*:c1900. doi: 10.1136/bmj.c1900.

Rollnick, S., Miller, W. R., & Butler, C. C. (2008). *Motivational Interviewing in Health Care: Helping Patients Change Behavior.* New York: Guilford Press.

Roth, G., Assor, A., Niemiec, C. P., Ryan, R. M., & Deci, E. L. (2009). The emotional and academic consequences of parental conditional regard: comparing conditional positive regard, conditional negative regard, and autonomy support as parenting practices. *Developmental Psychology, 45*: 1119-1142.

Rotter, J. B. (1990). Internal versus external control of reinforcement: a case history of a variable. *American Psychologist, 45*(4): 489-493.

Ryan, R. M., Lynch, M. R., Vansteenkiste, M., & Deci, E. L. (2011). Motivation and autonomy in counseling, psychotherapy, and behavior change: a look at theory and practice. *The Counseling Psychologist, 39*(2): 193-260.

Sbarra, D. A., & Hazan, C. (2008). Coregulation, dysregulation, self-regulation: an integrative analysis and empirical agenda for understanding adult attachment, separation, loss, and recovery. *Personality and Social Psychology Review, 12*(2): 141-167.

Seligman, M. E. P. (1998). *Learned Optimism: How to Change Your Mind and Your Life.* New York: Simon & Schuster.

Seligman, M. E. P. (2002). *Authentic Happiness: Using the New Positive Psychology to Realize Your Potential for Lasting Fulfillment.* New York: Simon & Schuster.

Seligman, M. E. P. (2004). TED Talk: Martin Seligman: The New Era of Positive Psychology. www.ted.com/talks/martin_seligman_on_the_state_of_psychology.html. Accessed 12/6/12.

Seligman, M. E. P. (2008). Positive health. *Applied Psychology, 57*: 3-18.

Seligman, M. E. P. & Maier, S. F. (1967). Failure to escape traumatic shock. *Journal of Experimental Psychology, 74*(1): 1-9.

Seligman, M. E. P. (2011). *Flourish: A Visionary New Understanding of Happiness and Well-being.* New York: Simon & Schuster.

Talen, M. R., Muller-Held, C. F., Eshleman, K. G., & Stephens, L. (2011). Patients' communication with doctors: a randomized control study of a brief patient communication intervention. *Families, Systems, & Health, 29*(3): 171-183.

Taylor, K. (2009). Paternalism, participation and partnership—the evolution of patient centeredness in the consultation. *Patient Education and Counseling, 74*: 150-155.

Taylor, S. E., Pham, L. B., Rivkin, I. D., & Armor, D. A. (1998). Harnessing the imagination: mental stimulation, self-regulation, and coping. *American Psychologist, 53*(4): 429-439.

Thaler, R. H., & Sunstein, C. R. (2008). *Nudge: Improving Decisions About Health, Wealth, and Happiness.* New York: Penguin.

Trottier, K., Polivy, J., & Herman, C. P. (2009). Effects of resolving to change one's own behavior: expectations vs. experience. *Behavior Therapy, 40*(2): 164-170.

University of Pennsylvania. Authentic happiness. www.authentichappiness.org. Accessed 11/28/12.

Vickers, K. S., Kircher, K. J., Smith, M. D., Petersen, L. R., & Rasmussen, N. H. (2007). Health behavior counseling in primary care: provider-reported rate and confidence. *Family Medicine, 39*(10): 730-735.

Vohs, K. D., Baumeister, R. F., Schmeichel, B. J., Twenge, J. M., Nelson, N. M., & Tice, D. M. (2008). Making choices impairs subsequent self-control: a limited-resource account of decision making, self-regulation, and active initiative. *Journal of Personality and Social Psychology, 94*(5): 883-898.

Whitehead, K., Langley-Evans, S. C., Tischler, V., & Swift, J. A. (2009). Communication skills for behaviour change in dietetic consultations. *Journal of Human Nutrition and Dietetics, 22*: 493-500.

Wiedemann, A. U., Lippke, S., Reuter, T., Ziegelmann, J. P., & Schwarzer, R. (2011). How planning facilitates behaviour change: additive and interactive effects of a randomized controlled trial. *European Journal of Social Psychology, 41*: 42-51.

Ziegelmann, J. P., Luszczynska, A., Lippke, S., & Schwarzer, R. (2007). Are goal intentions or implementation intentions better predictors of health behavior? A longitudinal study in orthopedic rehabilitation. *Rehabilitation Psychology, 52*(1): 97-102.

CHAPTER OUTLINE

LEARNING OBJECTIVES

After reading this chapter, you will be able to:

1. Explain what is meant by the terms stressors, stress response, and coping and discuss how the three are related.

2. Discuss how feelings of stress often affect health behaviors.

3. Conceptualize the psychophysiology of the acute stress response, including the roles of the autonomic nervous system and the endocrine system.

4. Understand the psychophysiology of the chronic stress response and how chronic stress arousal affects physical and psychological health.

5. Discuss factors that influence the stress–health relationship, including factors that exert negative as well as positive effects on health.

6. Summarize what stress management means and describe some of the skills and techniques commonly thought to reduce feelings of stress and its negative health effects.

7. Teach a few simple relaxation exercises to others.

8. Describe several ways that health and fitness professionals can help clients reduce feelings of stress and increase resilience.

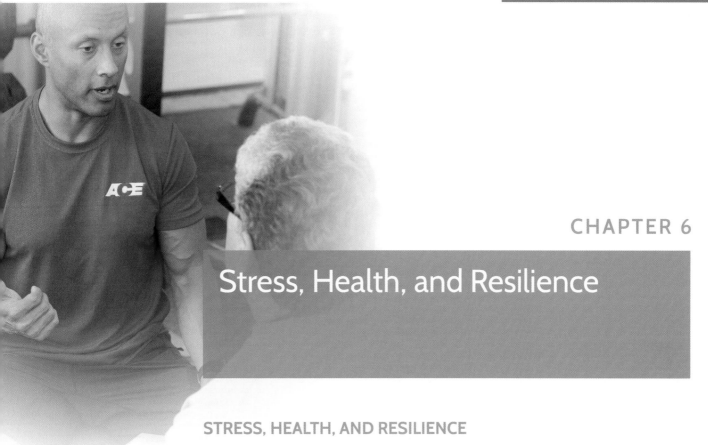

CHAPTER 6

Stress, Health, and Resilience

STRESS, HEALTH, AND RESILIENCE

Morgan is a personal trainer and fitness instructor at a large health club. He has worked as a health and fitness professional for over 10 years and is currently enrolled in a master's program in public health. This semester, he is taking a class on stress and health. Morgan is meeting with a new client, Sam, a 46-year-old mid-level manager who is married with two young children. When Morgan asks Sam why he wants to start exercising, Sam confides that he has been under increasing stress for the past few years, with no end in sight. Although he does not think he has much time to exercise, he has become motivated to make the time because he is experiencing some health problems, such as tightness in his chest. He also measured his blood pressure at a drugstore machine and found that it was 170/95, which disturbed him greatly since his father died from a stroke 15 years earlier. Morgan appreciates his initial conversation with Sam and assures him exercise could help reduce both feelings of stress and blood pressure. However, he gives Sam a medical clearance form and asks him to check in with his doctor before coming back. Morgan explains that the blood pressure monitoring machine may not have been accurate, and it is best to follow up on the chest discomfort and possible hypertension. Morgan hopes Sam obtains an appointment soon, receives medical clearance to exercise, and comes back to the fitness center before the motivation of his medical concerns passes.

The question, "What is stress?" elicits a variety of responses. Some people will talk about sources of stress: writing a paper, having too much work to do, or arguing with a friend. Others will describe emotions: anxiety, irritability, or feeling out of control and overwhelmed. Some will add physical symptoms to the list: tension headache, painful muscle spasms in the neck and shoulders, or difficulty sleeping. A few might mention behavioral symptoms: overeating, procrastinating, or drinking too much alcohol.

Responses to the "What is stress?" question usually carry a negative connotation, although some people will acknowledge that stress motivates them to get their work done and even to perform better. A few will actually admit to enjoying the "adrenaline rush" of impending deadlines or being in a high-pressure situation, such as a job interview or an athletic event. Many students swear that they work better when stressed by a looming deadline.

Stress is a part of life and can even provide the spice of life. But, when stress piles up and makes people feel overwhelmed and out of control, stress-related illnesses may develop. Stress can also interfere with behavior-change plans, as coping with stressful feelings now overrides future plans to quit smoking, start exercising, or eat fewer desserts. This chapter presents information on stress and health and the factors that affect that relationship. Because stress is a part of every client's life, health and fitness professionals must be able to discuss the impact of stress on health and on behavior change. This chapter concludes with some ways that professionals can help their clients build resilience and manage stress.

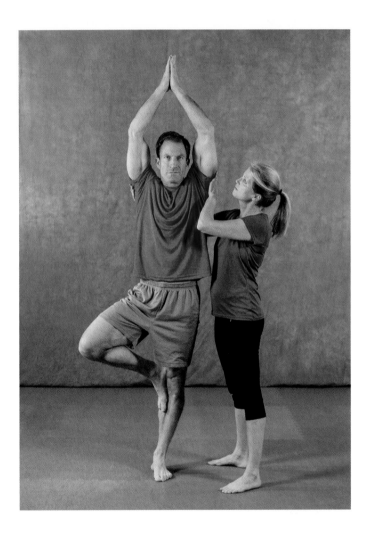

UNDERSTANDING STRESS

People generally use the term stress to describe a feeling of anxiety and tension that occurs when they feel that the demands they are experiencing exceed their abilities and resources for coping (Lazarus & Folkman, 1984; Fig. 6-1). Stress involves some sort of demand or challenge, a person's perception of and immediate response to that challenge, and the subsequent actions the person takes to deal with the challenge.

Demands, Resources, and Perception

The demand–resources relationship echoes Flow Theory. Demands are situations and events that are perceived by a person to require an adjustment or response. Resources

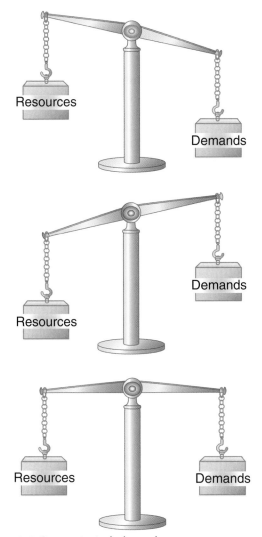

Figure 6-1. Stress: An imbalance between resources and demands.

can be material resources (such as money, housing, and food) as well as personal skills and attributes (such as intelligence, sport skill, and academic experience). When high demands match a person's high personal resources, including skills and abilities, the person is more likely to perceive the demand as a challenge that could be stimulating and even enjoyable. This happens when the challenge is in the area of a person's expertise and experience. When someone sees demands as beyond his or her ability to cope, feelings of stress arise, especially if the demand is important. However, if one has no challenges, this can lead to feelings of boredom. Although some relaxation feels good, a job that is repetitive, continues for a long time, and is not stimulating can be unpleasant.

Perception plays an important role in both people's interpretation of demands and their assessment of resources available to deal with events. Although people usually view cataclysmic events, such as natural disasters, armed conflict, and death of loved ones as stressful, many of the events of daily life are open to interpretation. Receiving a "B" on a paper may be disappointing to some students but cause for celebration for others. A list of assignments due during the semester may elicit feelings of panic for some or simply a desire to get organized for others.

Similarly, people's perceptions of their abilities and resources influence the stress content of a given demand. A required calculus course is not stressful to people who perceive their math abilities to be good, whereas math phobes may tremble at the thought. Of course, the math phobe may be motivated to try harder and study and may receive a better grade in the course. To complicate matters, perception often differs from reality. If people's perceptions of their abilities are too low, they feel overly stressed in the face of challenge and may unnecessarily avoid potentially fruitful opportunities for personal growth and development. For example, they may not ask for a raise they deserve at work or apply for a job for which they are qualified. On the other hand, overestimating one's abilities might also cause stress. For example, a student may not allot enough time to complete an assignment before it is due, thinking "Oh, this will be easy for me. I am a great writer, so this should not take more than an hour or two." When the paper actually takes about 5 or 6 hours, the student may feel stressed and exhausted from staying up late and handing in a low-quality project.

Sometimes people may have the skill to meet a challenge but not the time, energy, finances, or other necessary resources. For example, a math expert might not mind the idea of a required calculus class but be stressed when adding that class onto a full course load that he or she already perceives as challenging.

Stressors

Stress usually begins with a demand or challenge, called a stressor. A stressor is anything that causes stress. Stressors may be real (a vicious dog), distorted perceptions of something real (a friendly dog that someone perceives to be vicious), or purely imaginary (fear of walking into a new neighborhood because a vicious dog might appear).

Early research on stress suggested that people (and laboratory animals) exhibit components of the fight-or-flight response whether the source of stress is positive or negative (Game Changers 6-1). For example, heart rate and blood pressure increase whether people are getting ready for a party they are excited about or an exam they are dreading. Either way, people prepare to respond to an upcoming situation. Researchers coined the term eustress to describe sources of stress that people regard as positive. Of course, something regarded as eustress by one person may be a cause of distress for another. Although many of the immediate fight-or-flight symptoms are similar for eustress and distress, the long-term chronic health effects differ, with feelings of distress resulting in much more harm (Hatch & Dohrenwend, 2007). However, even eustress takes energy, and without sufficient recovery, sleep, and relaxation, even too much fun can be exhausting.

Game Changers 6-1. Stress Physiology Pioneers: Walter Cannon and Hans Selye

Walter Cannon is regarded as the first Western scientist to systematically study the physiology of emotion (Brown & Fee, 2002). Born in 1871, Cannon was a professor and chair of the Department of Physiology at the Harvard University Medical School. Cannon describes his early interest in the physiological effect of emotion. He was studying the gastrointestinal tract and the processes of digestion in animals. He noticed that when his animals were upset or frightened, the activity of their digestive systems stopped. He described these observations in his autobiography, *The Way of an Investigator* (1945):

> The whole purpose of my effort was to see the peristaltic waves and to learn their effects. Only after some time did I note that the absence of activity was accompanied by signs of perturbation, and when serenity was restored the waves promptly reappeared. This observation ... led to a long series of studies on the effects of strong emotions on the body. The idea flashed through my mind that [these changes] could be nicely integrated if conceived of as bodily preparations for supreme effort in flight or in fighting. The inhibition of digestive activity by emotional excitement was an interruption of a process which is not essential in a life-or-death emergency and which uses a supply of blood urgently needed elsewhere (Cannon, 1945).

As a result of these observations, Cannon coined the term "fight or flight" in 1915 to describe the physiological response to threat (Cannon, 1915). Cannon studied the role of the sympathetic nervous system and the adrenal glands in the fight-or-flight response and wrote about the effect of emotional states on health (Cannon, 1936).

Hans Selye, born in 1907 in Vienna, Austria-Hungary, greatly admired Cannon's work and picked up where Cannon left off. Selye first began researching stress physiology in 1936 at McGill University in Montreal, Canada. Nine years later, he moved to the University of Montreal where he supervised a large laboratory with dozens of assistants.

Selye created the first working physiological definition of stress, describing it as "the nonspecific response of the body to any demand made upon it" (Selye, 1956). He called the response nonspecific because he observed the same physical response in his laboratory animals to a wide variety of stimuli, including bacterial infection, trauma, heat, and cold (Selye, 1936). Selye believed that in humans, positive stressors, which he termed eustress, caused a physiological fight-or-flight response similar to that caused by more-disturbing change, which he called distress. He also noted that the same response occurred whether the threat was real or imagined (Selye, 1982).

Selye devised a theory about the health effects of chronic stress, which he called the General Adaptation Syndrome (GAS). When exposed to chronic stress, such as continuous loud noise, an animal exhibits three states of adaptation. Initially, the fight-or-flight response occurs, which Selye called the alarm reaction. Physiologists today link the alarm reaction to the autonomic nervous system's immediate response to stress. As exposure to the stressor continues, the animal develops some resistance to it. Selye referred to this as the stage of resistance. Physiologists note that during this stage, the various stress hormones that circulate throughout the period of stress sustain a long-term stress reaction. When the animal's resistance wears down, it enters what Selye called the stage of exhaustion. If the stressor continues, the animal eventually dies (Selye, 1982).

Selye's approach was typical of scientists working with laboratory animals in that its focus was on physiological response. Such a focus was important because it defined a stress stimulus in a controlled and clear way, and scientists could observe and measure results. This early research laid the groundwork for the expanded definitions of stress to follow and for the understanding of the more-complex primate stress response.

Sources: Brown, T. M., & Fee, E. (2002). Walter Bradford Cannon: pioneer physiologist of human emotions. *American Journal of Public Health, 92*(10): 1594-1595; Cannon, W. B. (1915). *Bodily Changes in Pain, Hunger, Fear, and Rage.* New York: D. Appleton & Co; Cannon, W. B. (1936). The role of emotions in disease. *Annals of Internal Medicine, 9*: 1453-1465; Cannon, W. B. (1945). *The Way of an Investigator: A Scientist's Experiences in Medical Research.* New York: W.W. Norton; Selye, H. (1936). A syndrome produced by diverse nocuous agents. *Nature, 138*:32; Selye, H. (1956). *The Stress of Life.* New York: McGraw-Hill; Selye, H. (1982). History and present status of the stress concept. In: Goldberg, L., & Breznitz, S., eds. *Handbook of Stress: Theoretical and Clinical Aspects.* New York: Free Press.

The Acute Stress Response: Preparing for Fight or Flight

One's immediate reaction to a stressor—the acute stress response—has both physical and psychological components. Physically, the body gets ready to fight or run away—the famous "fight-or-flight" response introduced in Chapter 2. The heart beats harder and faster, blood pressure rises, muscles brace for action, and breathing becomes shallower and more rapid. This physiology is important for understanding the relationship between stress and health.

The Physiology of the Acute Stress Response

When the brain perceives the need to deal with a source of stress, neurons in the hypothalamus activate the sympathetic nervous system (SNS) and set the fight-or-flight response in motion. As described in

Chapter 2, the sympathetic branch of the autonomic nervous systems activates those organs and systems most essential for action and suppresses functions such as digestion that can wait. The nervous system responds immediately, and the person instantly feels markers of the acute stress response, such as a pounding heart, tense muscles, and sweaty hands.

Because the stress response is so essential for survival, the endocrine system reinforces this response and helps maintain arousal for as long as necessary. Activation of the SNS stimulates the adrenal glands, made up of the outer adrenal cortex and inner adrenal medulla (Fig. 6-2).

The adrenal medulla secretes the hormones epinephrine and norepinephrine, collectively called the catecholamines. They are sympathomimetic, meaning that they mimic the action of the sympathetic nervous system. Like the SNS, they increase heart rate and the contractile force of the heart, which also increases blood pressure. They dilate the airways, increasing airflow to the lungs. The catecholamines increase blood sugar, giving the body fuel for muscle contraction. And, like the SNS, they slow the digestive processes, putting digestion on hold until the person deals with the immediate stressful situation.

As it orchestrates the autonomic nervous system response to stress and stimulates the response of the adrenal glands, the hypothalamus also secretes some hormones. The front portion of the hypothalamus secretes corticotropin-releasing hormone (CRH), which stimulates the pituitary gland, located at the base of the brain, to release adrenocorticotropic hormone (ACTH). ACTH moves through the bloodstream and soon reaches the adrenal glands. ACTH acts on the adrenal cortex, stimulating it to release two families of hormones called glucocorticoids and mineralocorticoids (Fig. 6-3). This pathway is called the hypothalamic-pituitary-adrenal (HPA) axis.

Cortisol, corticosterone, and cortisone are three glucocorticoids involved with the stress response. Glucocorticoids affect several metabolic processes by the following actions:

- Mobilizing energy sources by increasing the rate of protein breakdown in cells, especially muscles,

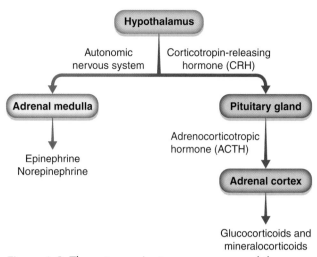

Figure 6-3. The autonomic stress response and the hypothalamic-pituitary-adrenal axis.

so the body can use these proteins for energy or to make enzymes. The glucocorticoids stimulate the liver to produce glucose from certain protein components when blood sugar is low.
- Making blood vessels more sensitive to agents promoting constriction, thus helping to increase blood pressure. This improves blood flow during physical activity, anticipating the need to fight or flee.
- Inhibiting the process of inflammation. Inflammation can make the inflamed area stiff. Limiting mobility helps in the short run but delays healing in the long term.
- Causing a decrease in the number of white blood cells released from the thymus gland. White blood cells are important components of the immune system defense against bacteria and other foreign invaders. This decrease in immune activity may be one of the "energy-conservation" processes of the glucocorticoids. White blood cells are not needed when facing an immediate emergency, and, with stress, the body's energy goes primarily to survival-promoting processes. Under conditions of chronic stress, elevated cortisol levels can negatively affect the immune system.

The adrenal cortex also secretes mineralocorticoids, which help control fluid and salt balance. The mineralocorticoid aldosterone is responsible for about 95% of the action in this hormone family. Aldosterone causes the kidneys to retain sodium and water—an action that increases blood volume and, consequently, blood pressure.

The thyroid gland also participates in the stress response by increasing the supply of fuel for the muscles (raising blood levels of fats and glucose) and speeding up metabolism. The hypothalamus releases a hormone called thyrotropic hormone-releasing factor (TRF), which stimulates the pituitary gland to secrete thyrotropic hormone (TTH). This hormone stimulates the thyroid gland to release thyroxin (Fig. 6-4). In addition to increasing blood fat and blood sugar levels,

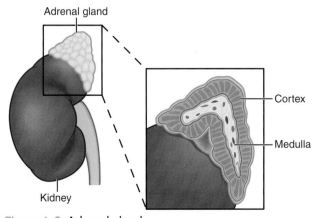

Figure 6-2. Adrenal gland.

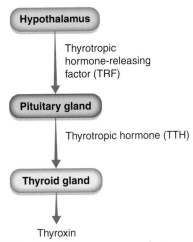

Figure 6-4. The thyroid hormones and stress.

thyroxin also increases breathing rate, heart rate, and blood pressure to reinforce the fight-or-flight response. Thyroxin also increases intestinal motility, which may cause diarrhea. Thyroxin decreases feelings of fatigue but can increase anxiety.

The hypothalamus stimulates the pituitary gland, through a direct nervous system pathway, to secrete the hormones oxytocin and vasopressin (also known as antidiuretic hormone, or ADH; Fig. 6-5). In addition to its work as the "tend-and-befriend" hormone, oxytocin raises blood pressure by contracting the small muscles lining the arteries; vasopressin does this too.

Psychological Components of the Acute Stress Response

The stress response is set in motion by a person's evaluation of a stressor, as the brain decides what is threatening and what is not. Several brain areas are involved in this evaluation. The prefrontal cortex helps guide decision making about a potential stressor by integrating remembered information (experiences as well as other forms of instruction) from various areas of learning and controlling impulsive behavior (McEwen & Gianaros, 2010). In other words, the prefrontal cortex helps people respond "reasonably" to a given stressor. It can respond to stress-management training and psychotherapy to help reduce unnecessary stress arousal.

The amygdala and hippocampus are parts of the limbic system involved with emotional perception and evaluation of stimuli. They are closely connected and work together. They are also connected to the prefrontal cortex, the hypothalamus, and other brain areas and can increase or decrease activation of the hypothalamus to initiate a stress response (McEwen & Gianaros, 2010). The amygdala remembers events associated with fear and threat and tells the hypothalamus to respond with a stress response if it senses that the new stimulus is a threat. The hippocampus helps put a new stimulus into the context of remembered events and can help inhibit the stress response by increasing understanding of the threat, so the amygdala is not as afraid.

Psychologically, people's thoughts and feelings interact with their physical arousal. Words, phrases, or images may pop into their heads. If these are negative (e.g., "Why me? I hate this job. I can't take it."), they may further intensify the physical stress response. More positive thoughts (e.g., "I've done this before; I can do it again. I can work through this.") may help reduce the fight-or-flight response. Sometimes during a stressful situation, people may not be aware of any thoughts but simply react as though "by instinct."

In some situations, emotions may be part of a person's stress response. People often report feeling anxious, frightened, helpless, and depressed when facing a stressor. Sometimes people report more positive feelings, such as feeling challenged, stimulated, excited, and even happy, if the stressor is something that they have some control over and if they expect the outcome to be positive. Thoughts and emotions interact with each other and with a person's physical response to a stressor (Fig. 6-6). Scary thoughts about a stressor (e.g., "My cousin died of rabies when he got bitten by a dog!") can increase fear and the physical stress response. Similarly, when a person feels her heart pounding, she may think, "I am in danger," or "This is really bad." Although models separate the stress response into physical, emotional, and cognitive components, in real life, all of these components occur simultaneously.

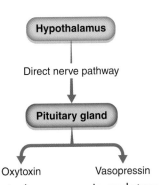

Figure 6-5. Oxytocin, vasopressin, and stress.

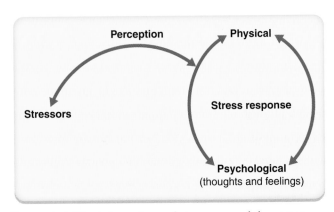

Figure 6-6. The interactions of stressors and the stress response.

Coping

Coping is what people do to deal with a source of stress or feelings of stress. It is helpful to conceptualize coping strategies as falling into two main categories: problem-focused coping and emotion-focused coping (Lazarus & Folkman, 1984). Problem-focused coping includes measures whose goal is to change or eliminate the source of stress or deal with a problem directly. As the deadline for a paper approaches, direct coping methods would include writing the paper or dropping the course. When a student chooses to write the paper, the source of stress is changed and eventually eliminated. Similarly, if the student drops the course, the paper is no longer a source of stress. Emotion-focused coping includes measures that do not directly change or eliminate the source of stress but instead change the way the person feels and reduce the stress response (Fig. 6-7). The problem still exists, but the person feels better. Emotion-focused coping for the problem of writing a paper includes going for a run to reduce anxiety, complaining to a friend about the professor, or deciding to work on the paper tomorrow instead of today.

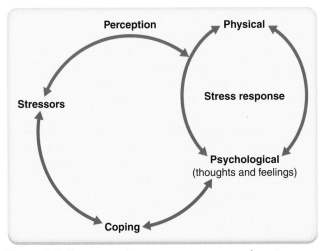

Figure 6-7. Stressors, the stress response, and coping.

Of course, some coping choices produce better long-term results than others. Adaptive coping responses are mostly helpful and generally do not contribute to long-term problems. They would include writing the paper that is due, changing a flat tire, or asking a noisy neighbor to turn down his music. Maladaptive coping responses might feel good in the short term but cause more stress or health problems later. Maladaptive coping responses would include buying a paper online (instead of writing it), driving the car with a flat tire, or punching the noisy neighbor in the nose. Emotion-focused coping can also be maladaptive. Getting drunk, overeating, or procrastinating on an important project in response to feelings of stress are examples of maladaptive coping.

These categories of coping are usually situational. Talking to a close friend when feeling stressed is generally considered adaptive, but some people complain so much that their friends run away to avoid listening. A good exercise session can reduce stress and calm one's nerves in preparation for completing an upcoming assignment; in this context, exercise is adaptive coping, since it helps the person reduce feelings of stress in a positive way. But what about people who train for hours a day and cannot find time to see friends or do homework? Exercise may make them feel good in the present moment, but it creates problems in the future as they lose their social networks and fail school. More examples of adaptive and maladaptive coping are in Table 6-1.

Coping includes both cognitive and behavioral responses to stress. When facing a stressor, people generally think about what their options are and then try to solve the problem or address the source of stress. Sometimes the stressor is difficult or impossible to change, and people cope by changing the way they see the stressor. This strategy, called positive reappraisal, involves thinking about the stressor in a new way that makes it appear less stressful. For example, a student who does not get into his first choice for graduate

Table 6-1. Illustrations of Adaptive and Maladaptive Coping Responses

This table gives examples of both problem-focused and emotion-focused coping responses that one might see students exhibit when feeling stressed about writing an upcoming assignment.

	ADAPTIVE	MALADAPTIVE
Problem-focused	Ask writing counselor or teacher for help	Send professor a threatening e-mail
	Talk to other students in the class to generate ideas	Plagiarize information to complete the assignment
Emotion-focused	Take a walk	Get drunk at a party and drive recklessly
	Go to a movie with friends	Go to the gym and get in a fight
	Go to the gym and work out	

school might think, "Oh well, I did not really want to live in that city anyway, and now I will be closer to my friends."

Another coping response is avoidance. Procrastination is one form of avoidance, where people put off dealing with an assignment, project, or something else they need to do. People usually use avoidance in areas of life that are difficult or distasteful or those in which they do not feel competent making decisions. For example, people successful in most areas of life may avoid going to the dentist or taking their car in for service. Sometimes avoidance works, in that a problem resolves itself. Other times, avoidance increases stress, if problems grow while being ignored. For example, a small cavity in one's tooth could get worse over time and require more-expensive and invasive treatment later.

Coping can also be proactive, both to avoid potential stressors and to improve well-being (Greenglass & Fiksenbaum, 2009). For example, when people engage in self-improvement activities such as anticipating potential health problems and changing diet and exercise to prevent such problems, they are coping proactively.

Health Behaviors and the Stress Response

Some health behaviors can intensify feelings of stress, whereas others can reduce them. People use some health behaviors to cope with stress. If these behaviors are healthy and reduce feelings of stress, they are considered a form of adaptive coping. But some coping behaviors can lead to future health problems and are considered maladaptive.

Caffeine Consumption

Caffeine and other drugs such as nicotine evoke the fight-or-flight response; they are sympathomimetic substances because they mimic the effect of the SNS. Caffeine and nicotine increase heart rate, blood pressure, and muscle tension and can make people feel edgy and irritable, especially when other stressors pile up.

One or two caffeinated beverages consumed judiciously at appropriate times during the day appear to do no harm for most people. Indeed, a little caffeine can increase alertness. The problem is that some people overuse caffeine when feeling tired and stressed. Caffeine cannot substitute for a good night's sleep. When people are truly fatigued, caffeine does not help them concentrate; it simply leaves them tired and wired—too jittery to sleep but too tired to do anything productive.

Caffeine tolerance varies. Some people can consume a great deal of caffeine with few negative results. Others find that any amount of caffeine causes undesirable symptoms, such as anxiety, an irregular heartbeat, or stomach irritation. Some people who forego caffeine find that they have a more even flow of energy throughout the day without caffeine's energy peaks and valleys.

Caffeine metabolizes very slowly, so it remains in the bloodstream for many hours. Thus, people who have trouble sleeping at night should not consume caffeine in the late afternoon and evening. Many beverages, energy drinks, and chocolate contain caffeine.

Tobacco Products

Since using tobacco products can lead to future health problems, tobacco use is considered a maladaptive coping mechanism. The nicotine in tobacco products is a highly addictive substance, and addictions can exacerbate feelings of stress. On top of a "normal" stress load, the need to smoke increases agitation. More detail about tobacco use and the nature of addiction is in Chapter 11.

The reason that people smoke to cope with stress is that once they satisfy their craving for nicotine, they feel better temporarily. This is why smoking is associated with relaxation. In addition, smoking is associated with breaks in the work routine, and this positive association helps people enjoy smoking. Add the social component of a cigarette break with a group of friends, and smoking becomes even more rewarding.

Reduced Sleep Quality and Quantity

Reduced sleep is a common response to stress overload. When there are not enough hours in a day to get everything done, people may decrease sleep time. In addition, many people have trouble sleeping well when feeling anxious and stressed. Sleep deprivation correlates with a more-negative emotional state and reduced productivity. The tense tiredness that results from a combination of stress and sleep deprivation makes stress feel worse. Small stressors appear much larger. On the other hand, a good night's sleep reduces feelings of stress and improves coping.

Physical Activity

When people feel stressed and overly busy, they tend to exercise less—especially if physical activity falls primarily into recreational hours. People who find that physical activity improves mood and relieves stress may notice that they feel more stressed when they are less active. As discussed in Chapter 3, regular physical activity often improves stress resistance and mood and reduces feelings of stress.

Eating Behavior

Eating behavior affects stress patterns in several ways. First, it can be a stressor itself, as when people worry about what to eat. Second, poor eating behavior can create feelings of fatigue and irritability that make minor stressors seem like major problems; and third, eating behaviors are often used as emotion-focused coping measures. In addition, many people find that periods of stress tend to worsen eating habits. On the other hand, positive eating behaviors, such as preparing and enjoying a healthy meal, can help reduce feelings of stress (Fig. 6-8).

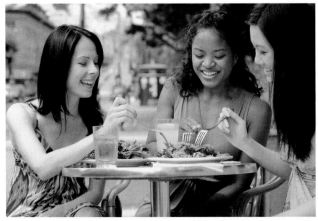

Figure 6-8. Eating behavior and stress reduction. © Thinkstock

Eating behavior is a source of stress when people worry about what to eat. Trying to eat less to lose weight or trying to eat more healthful foods can upset a person's routine and cause stress. Eating behaviors can become part of people's struggles with body image, self-concept, and self-esteem. Eating can be stressful for students who depend on dining halls whose hours do not coincide with their eating patterns or whose food is not appetizing. Feeding a family can be stressful for parents balancing finances and children's eating preferences with a desire to provide nutritious meals.

Poor eating habits make some people more vulnerable to feelings of stress. Many people work best with a regular eating schedule and healthful meals. For them, eating well reduces feelings of stress and increases their ability to deal with demands. Other people tolerate quite a bit of irregularity, and poor dietary habits do not generally worsen stress. Hunger, however, is associated with irritability and difficulty focusing, and searching for food while hungry often results in eating the foods most readily available—not necessarily what one feels like eating. On the other hand, some people find that big meals lead to sleepiness or fatigue.

Some people use food to cope with negative emotions and feelings of stress. Consuming comfort food feels soothing. Overeating in response to stress is common but can become a problem when it is one's coping method of choice and/or leads to substantial overeating.

Eating habits tend to get worse during periods of stress because consuming a healthful, balanced diet takes time, money, energy, and planning to keep nutritious foods on hand and prepare healthful meals. When people feel overwhelmed with stress, they may neglect grocery shopping and meal preparation, grabbing food that is easy and fast. This can result in a lower fruit and vegetable intake and a higher intake of empty calories and unhealthful fats. Irregular eating schedules and reduced satisfaction with meals can in turn increase feelings of stress.

■ *Morgan does not see Sam for over a month. Finally, Sam arrives with a smile on his face, medical clearance forms in hand. He is relieved that the stress test showed no signs of*

heart disease. The doctor did say his blood pressure was somewhat elevated and has counseled Sam to begin to address this problem with diet, exercise, and stress management. Sam is going to see his doctor again in 3 months to evaluate whether his borderline hypertension is responding to lifestyle change.

Morgan knows Sam's life could probably use a total overhaul, but he does not want to overwhelm Sam by asking him to address diet, exercise, and stress all at the same time. Instead, he decides to get Sam off to a good start with a simple exercise program. Because Sam has not exercised much beyond playing catch with his kids, Morgan begins with a low-intensity program combining 20 minutes of aerobic machines with seven strength-training exercises.

Morgan asks Sam about his caffeine consumption. He knows caffeine can cause chest tightness and contribute to temporary blood pressure elevation. Sam acknowledges that he tends to drink too much coffee and that his doctor recommended cutting back. Morgan asks Sam to simply keep track of his coffee consumption this week, observe whether it is related to feelings of stress and chest tightness, and report back next week. ■

Gender Differences in the Stress Response

Interesting research by Shelley Taylor and colleagues suggests that men and women may not respond to stressful situations in the same way. Observing that males were the subjects of most stress research, both in animals and humans, the researchers decided to study the fight-or-flight response to stressors in females. Taylor and colleagues mused on the evolutionary demands faced by women, who were often raising young and caring for the elderly. They reasoned that in many cases, weighed down by these responsibilities, females may not have been likely to respond to stress by fighting or running away, which would leave the vulnerable behind.

As predicted, the researchers found that in women, the fight-or-flight response did occur, but the intensity was tempered by a stronger tendency to build social support, which the researchers called "tend and befriend" (Taylor et al., 2000). In laboratory animals, stressed females increased their tending or caring for the young. In humans, stress led to actions of befriending others to form a stronger social network. Taylor and colleagues speculated that the likely causes of these gender differences in stress response were biological and social learning differences. Subsequent research confirmed this hypothesis. Women tend to produce more of the hormone oxytocin in response to stress. Oxytocin promotes caregiving behavior and relaxation and inhibits aggression. Girls and women also imitate other females around them, acquiring gender-role behavior as they mature.

Many other studies have found gender differences for various aspects of the stress response (McLean & Anderson, 2009; Smeets, Dziobek, & Wolf, 2009). Does this mean that women have fewer problems with stress? Women actually tend to report more stress than men and experience more stress-related emotional health disorders such as anxiety and depression (Kelly, Tyrka, & Anderson, 2008). It is important, however, to not generalize or make too many assumptions about any given individual's response to stress or his or her coping strategies.

The Time Bind: Self-care and Work–Life Balance

One of the most common sources of stress is not a single bad thing but simply too much to do in too little time. In fact, a majority of college students and working adults express concern about achieving a balanced,

healthy lifestyle in the face of a perceived lack of time. This concern is widespread among both men and women in all age groups, from teens to seniors. Men and women with young children seem to experience the most acute time crunch, coupled with feelings of guilt and frustration about not being able to "do it all" perfectly. Occupations that require a high level of social contact and long hours often lead to career stress known as "burnout" (Box 6-1).

The issue of balancing life to find time for self-care is likely to remain at the forefront of health and fitness counseling for years to come. With technology advances, people can be available to everyone, everywhere, 24 hours a day, unless they set clear boundaries. Clients report feeling that the pace of life quickens each year. Many are single parents, work multiple jobs, commute long distances, or face other significant challenges that result in a truly overwhelming time bind (Behavior Change in Action 6-1).

Box 6-1. Coping With Burnout: Advice for Health and Fitness Professionals

Burnout is career code for stressed out. Burnout generally results when people feel overwhelmed and that they do not have the resources to cope with all the demands they face. People in helping professions, such as health and fitness professionals, often complain of burnout, since it takes a great deal of energy to work with people, and they often find themselves in stressful situations. Professionals in caregiving roles with very-needy people may lose patience. The excess stress that can trigger burnout leads to a plethora of symptoms, from negative health effects such as high blood pressure and digestive complaints, to emotional symptoms such as irritability, anger, anxiety, and depression.

At work, excess stress can lead to symptoms of burnout. When people feel that trying hard at work is not leading to desirable results, they sometimes give up and stop trying at all. They stop caring about the quality of their work. They may become bored, sloppy, and negative. Productivity declines and absenteeism rises.

People generally think of burnout as resulting from too much stress at work. However, stressful situations at home can trigger burnout as well because home stress reduces people's ability to cope with stress at work; their energy is already depleted when they arrive at work.

Professionals who feel that stress overload is leading to career burnout in their lives should examine their work and personal lives and try to create a better balance. Here are some suggestions for stopping burnout.

Make Time for Self-care
When people get too busy, often the first thing to go is their exercise program. However, when their stress load increases, people need physical activity more than ever to help reduce feelings of stress and the risk of stress-related illness. Make good health your first priority because, without it, your stress will be greater than ever. It is also important to model self-care behavior for your clients.

In addition to regular physical activity, be sure you are getting adequate sleep, eating nutritious meals, and spending quality time with loved ones. Squeeze pleasurable activities into your day, such as taking a few minutes to enjoy a cup of tea or share a funny story with a friend.

Find or Create Meaning in Your Work and in Your Life
The worst symptoms of burnout are helplessness and hopelessness. People need to find or create meaning in their personal and professional lives. Spend some time reconnecting with the values and ideals that led you to choose your line of work or your particular lifestyle. If you do not find satisfaction in your work, you need to develop interesting activities outside of work and find meaning in other ways.

Develop Your Career Skills
If work is stressful, putting more energy into professional development may reduce stress because it may lead to more options, a change in job description, or even a promotion. Professional development can also help you connect with your original passion for the work you do, nurture your creative spirit, and make your work more interesting and satisfying.

> ### Box 6-1. Coping With Burnout: Advice for Health and Fitness Professionals—cont'd
>
> **Address Job Issues That Are Creating Stress**
> Take a problem-solving approach to job stress, working with supervisors and coworkers to address the problems causing the stress. Can you reconfigure workloads? Are there better ways to do certain tasks? Could work hours be more flexible? Good suggestions and a positive approach are key.
>
> **Address Personal Issues That Contribute to Job Stress**
> Take the same approach to personal stress issues. What are your options? What resources do you have at your disposal? How can you get help from family members or friends? If stress is a significant problem, talk to a counselor or therapist who can help you find some answers.

 BEHAVIOR CHANGE IN ACTION 6-1

Working With Clients Who Have No Free Time

▉ CHALLENGE
Health and fitness professionals often find themselves working with clients who are juggling multiple priorities and simply do not have the time for self-care.

▉ PLAN
Suggestions for helping stressed-out clients who have no time include:

Encourage clients to see that some self-care is a priority. The biggest hurdle facing many clients is overcoming the notion that exercising, eating well, and getting enough sleep are extravagant luxuries, rather than essential behaviors. People's health must be a priority, so that they have the energy, creativity, and drive to be a good worker, parent, friend, partner, and citizen.

A client once asked a personal trainer, "How much should I exercise?" The personal trainer's wise reply: "About 30 minutes a day is good, except when you are really busy. Then you should try to exercise for at least an hour." When clients are busy, they need self-care more than ever, yet that is when they are least likely to get it.

Start with small, simple changes. After seeing how little free time a client has, ask questions to elicit ideas for small, easy changes. Explore multitasking opportunities. For example, perhaps the client would be able to walk on the weekend while young children ride their bikes or are in the stroller, combining self-care with family time. Maybe busy workers have a fitness center at work or near work they could use before or after work or during their lunch hour? A client could use an exercise bike at home while watching television. And clients working to improve eating behaviors can save time by creating a weekly meal plan and shopping just once a week.

Educate clients about the stress-reduction benefits of physical activity and a healthful lifestyle. Clients who feel stressed by life overload may especially appreciate the stress-reduction benefits of physical activity, adequate sleep, and good eating habits. Share information about these benefits and encourage clients to notice how they feel after their workouts, healthy meals, or a good night's sleep.

Do not cut into sleep. Busy, productive clients often decide the only time they have for self-care is before work or late at night, cutting into sleep time. Clients getting up at 5 a.m. to commute to work may decide getting up an hour earlier to use the treadmill at home is their only option. Discourage this line of thought and educate clients about the importance of adequate restorative sleep.

Be understanding and sympathetic but refer clients if stress is a problem. Sometimes life just snowballs, and there really is barely time to breathe much less enjoy recreational pursuits. All these clients can do is address today's demands and do their best to work toward a better balance tomorrow. If they can squeeze in a few simple changes, fine. If not, let them know you understand and will welcome them back in the future.

Health and fitness professionals should express understanding and sympathy but withhold judgment. It is inappropriate to push clients to make big changes in work and relationships that could have enormous and undesirable repercussions. For example, encouraging someone to quit their job or leave a partner is unethical and outside of the scope of practice of most health and fitness professionals. They should be ready to refer clients to helping professionals for assistance in dealing with stress that is interfering with daily life or causing significant distress.

Often people feel stressed when combining work with attending school and/or parenting young children. Most job descriptions evolved at a time when the breadwinner had a supporter at home, usually a wife, who handled the shopping, cooking, cleaning, childcare, and the many details that keep a family functioning. Homemaking was a full-time, albeit low-status, job. Much of the conflict that working parents experience arises from expectations regarding career success and family function carried over from a time when someone was home taking care of the details. Unrealistic expectations about various life roles can create stress. Finding a balance involves addressing expectations to bring them more in line with present reality.

Redefining role expectations is essential when roles become impossible to fulfill. People and organizations may need to redefine a "good worker" or a "good parent." For example, a person might believe good workers can take time off to bring a sick child to the doctor or attend a school meeting. Or maybe good parents can prepare family dinners most but not all evenings. Working parents must consider their personal goals and try to balance these with family and work responsibilities.

Guilt and frustration arise when people fail to meet their goals, even if these goals are impossible. They blame themselves for not working hard enough or for failing to be there for their children or partner. As a result, they feel inadequate, helpless, and depressed—and more stressed than ever.

Societal supports have not kept pace with changing family structures, and people often do not have the tools needed to care for aging parents, help children who are struggling in school, or deal with other problems that arise. Sometimes people find themselves in difficult situations that take a lot of creativity and energy to solve (Behavior Change in Action 6-1). Talking to others in similar situations is helpful and is conducive to helping people realize that they are not alone. People can certainly work together to construct community and worksite supports for those facing challenges.

STRESS AND HEALTH

Although a strong stress response is helpful for stressors best faced with fight or flight, constant activation of the stress response, referred to as a chronic stress response, can have negative health effects over time. Understanding the physiology of the acute stress response helps predict the effects of chronic stress on health. For example, since blood pressure elevation is a significant component of the acute stress response, it makes sense that chronic stress can result in hypertension. The chronic stress response and its health effects vary widely. For example, not everyone experiencing chronic stress develops hypertension. This is because the psychophysiology of the chronic stress response varies depending on a person's genetic predisposition and health behaviors. A person with a genetic predisposition to hypertension might develop hypertension with chronic stress if he is overweight and consuming a lot of caffeine, but not if he is exercising regularly and maintaining a healthful body weight. It is important to remember these complex interactions of lifestyle, genetics, and stress. The following sections discuss the effect of chronic stress on the various body systems.

Effects on the Immune System

Chronic activation of the stress response has a number of immune system effects. It suppresses some aspects of the immune response and stimulates others. The result can be an imbalanced immune system, with inadequate defense against pathogens such as cold and flu viruses, but higher levels of inflammatory cytokines and systemic inflammation.

Some studies have examined the effect of stress on antibody production in response to a vaccine. Ideally, after vaccination, the body recognizes the pathogen, produces a good supply of antibodies, and is thus armed for resistance should the pathogen appear in the future. Several research groups have found that subjects reporting more stress tend to mount a less vigorous immune response to a vaccine, suggesting an immune-suppression effect of chronic stress (Pedersen, Zachariae, & Bovbjerg, 2009).

Other studies have examined pro- and anti-inflammatory cytokine concentrations in subjects reporting chronic stress. Higher levels of stress are associated with dysregulation of both pro- and anti-inflammatory cytokines (Miller, Cohen, & Ritchey, 2009). Higher stress levels are often associated with worsening symptoms of autoimmune disorders such as rheumatoid arthritis, asthma, and psoriasis. Autoimmune disorders often involve an inappropriate inflammatory response as the body mistakenly attacks its own cells and tissues. Because some of the stress hormones, such as the glucocorticoids, are associated with immune-system suppression, scientists were at first puzzled as to why inflammation is often higher, rather than lower, as might be expected in response to stress. (And, indeed, occasionally severe acute stress does temporarily suppress autoimmune symptoms.) Research suggests that with chronic stress, the body's response to the glucocorticoid hormones may become dampened, so that a sort of glucocorticoid resistance occurs, making immune regulation abnormal (Miller et al., 2002; Pace, Hu, & Miller, 2007).

Cardiovascular Effects and the Metabolic Syndrome

Most severe of the cardiovascular effects are those leading to a heart attack, or myocardial infarction. Many researchers and medical practitioners have wondered whether chronic stress increases heart attack risk. A large international study collected data on about 25,000 people from 52 countries to examine this relationship (Rosengren et al., 2004). The researchers defined stress as "feeling irritable, filled with anxiety, or having sleeping difficulties as a result of conditions at work or at home." When data were adjusted for other variables known to affect heart attack risk, such as age, gender, and smoking, the study found that subjects reporting "permanent stress" were over two times as likely to suffer a myocardial infarction. Other studies have found similar results for both acute and chronic stress (Dimsdale, 2008).

Chronic stress harms the cardiovascular system in several ways (Fig. 6-9). The cardiovascular system is a target of the acute stress response, as its activation is essential for physical activities such as fleeing and fighting. Sustained activation for a long time may cause the following problems.

Hypertension

Chronic stress increases risk of hypertension through two pathways (Fig. 6-10). Central to the acute stress response is an increase in heart rate and the contractile force of the heartbeat. As the heart beats faster and harder, blood pressure rises. Second, to compound the problem, the stress response also stimulates contraction of the small muscles that regulate dilation of the arteries. When these arteries narrow, the result is peripheral resistance. Peripheral resistance means that there is more resistance to the blood flow because the area through which it flows is smaller. This increases the pressure of the blood in the arterial system. Peripheral resistance may be at least partly a result of endothelial dysfunction. (The endothelium is the artery lining.) Studies measuring the response of arteries to a stimulus designed to trigger vasodilation, or a widening of the

artery diameter, have found an association between psychosocial stress and impaired vasodilation (Cooper et al., 2010). Hypertension increases risk for both heart disease and stroke.

Increased Blood Sugar and Risk of Type 2 Diabetes

The acute stress response is designed to make plenty of energy available to the muscles and brain, raising levels of blood sugar and blood lipids to supply this energy. The observation that blood sugar increases in response to stress has raised many questions about a possible link between stress and blood sugar regulation. Several researchers believe that the effect of stress on the nervous and endocrine systems contributes to type 2 diabetes. A group led by epidemiologist Michael Marmot examined the relationship between employment level (code for social class) and a variety of health outcomes. Marmot's first cohort, recruited in 1967, consisted of over 18,000 male civil servants (government employees) in London. The study was called the Whitehall Study. Marmot and his team collected information about employment category, demographic variables, health behaviors, and health problems every few years over a 10-year period. The prospective nature of this epidemiological research allowed researchers to observe the development of health problems over time and to analyze the relationship of these problems to several variables. This first Whitehall study demonstrated an association between employment level and a number of health problems, including coronary heart disease. In fact, men in the lowest employment category suffered over two times the risk of coronary artery disease as men in the highest employment category (Marmot, Rose, Shipley, & Hamilton, 1978). The higher risk held even when other variables such as smoking,

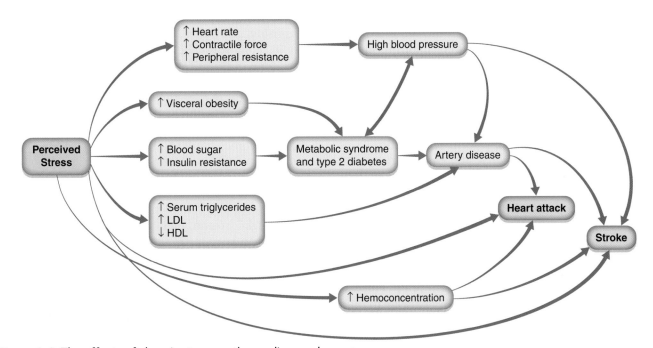

Figure 6-9. The effects of chronic stress on the cardiovascular system.

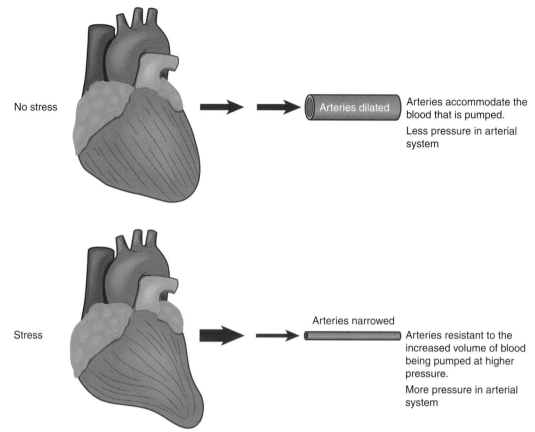

Figure 6-10. The effects of chronic stress on blood pressure.

physical activity, and amount of leisure time were controlled for statistically.

Marmot and colleagues believed that psychosocial stress might account for some of the increased health risks associated with low employment level. To investigate this further, they initiated the Whitehall II Study, or the Stress and Health Study, in 1985. The researchers recruited another group of civil servants, including 6,895 men and 3,413 women at all employment levels. Data were collected every few years, including information on perceived job stress and perceptions regarding the opportunity to socially interact at work. Several publications reported results from this group.

The Whitehall II Study found a relationship between work stress and risk of developing type 2 diabetes (Heraclides, Chandola, Witte, & Brunner, 2009). The study team examined stress in the form of job strain. Prior research suggested that jobs are especially stressful when they involve high demands but low levels of control. Workers with high levels of job stress combined with low opportunities for social interaction experienced the highest levels of stress. Female workers who fit this profile had double the risk of developing type 2 diabetes over the study period as workers with lower stress levels. This relationship was strong despite the fact that the researchers controlled for body composition, smoking, physical activity, and other variables known to increase diabetes risk. The data in men were less conclusive. The authors speculated that since a much lower percentage of the men in their subject

group held low-level jobs, where the most stress is found, the numbers were too small to find a difference. (Specifically, 35% of the women were employed in the lowest grade, whereas only 5% of the men were in that grade.) However, men at the lowest employment level did show a significant relationship between perceived stress and risk for developing type 2 diabetes (Heraclides et al., 2009).

A relationship between stress and diabetes is not surprising, given that the stress hormones stimulate a rise in blood sugar. Research also suggests that under conditions of chronic stress, sustained elevations in cortisol can interfere with the normal regulation of blood glucose by decreasing the body's sensitivity to insulin (Qi & Rodrigues, 2007).

People with type 1 diabetes often find that their condition becomes harder to manage when they experience chronic stress. Management of type 1 diabetes depends on a strict routine of diet, physical activity, and the administration of insulin (given at the right time to maintain the correct blood sugar). Since stress raises blood sugar, insulin, diet, and exercise may need adjustment to keep blood sugar in balance during times of increased stress.

Obesity and the Metabolic Syndrome
The Whitehall II research team examined rates of obesity and metabolic syndrome in their subjects, correlating the development of these problems with stress level. The researchers found that chronic job stress doubled risk for

development of the metabolic syndrome (Chandola, Brunner, & Marmot, 2006). Chronic stress also increased the likelihood of subjects gaining fat on the torso, as measured by a high waist circumference (Brunner, Chandola, & Marmot, 2007). An interesting study from the United States found a similar result (Hunte, 2011). Rather than measuring job stress, these researchers asked subjects about their perceptions of daily interpersonal discrimination. Interpersonal discrimination refers to feeling that one is receiving disadvantageous treatment from other people because of one's personal characteristics, such as religion, ethnic background, gender, and so forth. A positive association was found between perceived discrimination and a high waist circumference over the 9 years of the study for both men and women. Some researchers believe that the stress hormones, especially the glucocorticoids, contribute to visceral obesity and the metabolic syndrome (Anagnostis, Athyros, Tziomalos, Karagiannis, & Mikhailidis, 2009), whereas others suggest that an imbalance between sympathetic and parasympathetic output may be to blame (Licht et al., 2010). Either way, stress appears to be a contributing factor to visceral obesity and the metabolic syndrome.

Blood Lipid Levels

Several studies have shown a relationship between stress and a blood lipid profile associated with increased risk of artery disease. These proatherogenic lipid levels manifest as higher measures of blood triglycerides and LDL cholesterol and lower levels of helpful HDL cholesterol. Research suggests that greater levels of SNS activation are associated with both sustained hypertension and higher LDL cholesterol levels (Palatini et al., 2006). Higher levels of serum epinephrine are associated with lower levels of HDL cholesterol (Flaa, Mundal, Eide, Kjeldsen, & Rostrup, 2006). One study of 199 middle-aged men and women found that subjects who showed a greater change in lipid levels with acute stress were more prone to exhibit chronic elevations in harmful blood lipids 3 years after the initial testing (Steptoe & Brydon, 2005).

Risk of Artery Disease

Hypertension, poor blood lipid profile, insulin resistance, visceral obesity, and increased inflammatory response all contribute to the progression of artery disease. Chronic, unrelenting stress can promote the continuing development of these risk factors over time. Artery disease develops over a lifetime, compounded not only by stress, as discussed here, but by many other risk factors, as discussed in Chapter 1.

Increased Blood Clotting Rate

The process of blood clotting helps the body heal blood vessel breaks resulting from wounds. The clot forms a temporary patch to prevent blood loss, keep out pathogens, and stimulate the cells to initiate repair. Unfortunately, clotting can also happen when there is no wound to heal. Instead, a blood clot can form inside the circulatory system and subsequently block blood flow. Stress appears to increase the risk of this response for two reasons.

First, in response to stress, the blood becomes more concentrated as fluid is removed from the circulatory system—a process known as hemoconcentration. Hemoconcentration results in a higher concentration of blood cells to plasma volume. Plasma is the liquid portion of the blood. This results in "thicker" blood and an increased likelihood of blood clots forming within the circulatory system. A blood clot that forms within a blood vessel or in one of the chambers of the heart is called a thrombus. A thrombus can interfere with blood flow. An embolus is a blood clot that moves through the bloodstream until it lodges and blocks circulation.

In addition to increasing hemoconcentration, stress also appears to increase clotting speed independent of its effects on hemoconcentration (von Känel et al., 2009). This makes sense in terms of survival: when coping with stressors results in injury, a faster clotting rate would reduce blood loss. Unfortunately, the net effect of increased hemoconcentration and clotting rate today is an increased risk for heart attack, stroke, and other health problems.

Sam observes a strong link between his coffee consumption and stress and is gradually reducing his intake. But he has been having difficulty getting to the club more than once or twice a week, and Morgan is disappointed that Sam often seems stressed and distracted during his workouts. Morgan has been learning about the effects of stress on hypertension in his Stress and Health class. The evidence for the harmful effects of stress is so strong that Morgan wonders why more people are not talking about the importance of stress reduction.

Morgan asks Sam how the exercise is going. Sam admits that sometimes fitting exercise into his day just creates more stress for him. Morgan listens carefully as Sam describes the many factors that prevent him from exercising more often. Morgan learns that Sam feels he should be spending more time with his family, so Morgan asks Sam to think about ways to be active with his family and ways exercise could be more enjoyable for him. Morgan also discusses with Sam the negative effects that stress can have on blood pressure and suggests that he might benefit from talking to a therapist. Morgan describes how even a few sessions could help Sam clarify better ways of coping with stress in his life. ∎

Musculoskeletal Effects

The acute stress response signals muscles to brace for action. The postural muscles, including muscles of the head, neck, shoulders, and back, tense up to prepare the body for action. Chronic stress often creates tension and pain in these same muscle groups. Some of the pain syndromes found in the head and postural muscles appear to be related to chronic stress, although as with other health problems discussed in this section, stress may not always be the original cause. Stress may contribute to pain by increasing muscle tension but also by increasing inflammation and possibly by lowering the pain threshold, so pain is perceived with tension levels that would not usually cause pain (Fig. 6-11).

Headache

Excess muscle tension in the forehead, face, jaw, and neck can cause tension headaches. Excess muscle tension often results from stress, and most headache sufferers report a relationship between feelings of stress and the occurrence of tension headache; stress seems to increase the likelihood of headaches (Cathcart, Petkov, Winefield, Lushington, & Rolan, 2010; Chen, 2009). Excess sympathetic output maintains higher levels of tension in the muscles, causing pain. Researchers believe that people who experience recurrent tension headaches may originally have normal pain thresholds but become more sensitive to pain over time (Buchgreitz, Lyngberg, Bendtsen, & Jensen, 2008). This means they experience more pain, even with relatively low levels of muscle tension.

Migraine headaches result from vascular changes that lead to increased blood volume in the blood vessels of the head, causing pressure and pain. Symptoms of migraine include intense throbbing in one area of the head, nausea, vomiting, and sensitivity to sound and light. Scientists do not completely understand the causes of migraine. Many migraine sufferers are able to discern links between certain foods and substances such as caffeine that seem to trigger headache onset. Stress is a common trigger for migraine onset in people predisposed to migraines (Sauro & Becker, 2009). Stress may exacerbate migraine pain through a number of pathways, including stress hormones that provoke vascular changes associated with migraine, as well as muscle tension that may worsen pain.

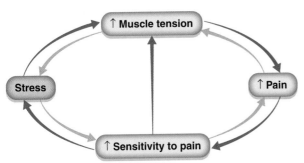

Figure 6-11. The effects of chronic stress on musculoskeletal pain.

Temporomandibular Joint Dysfunction

The temporomandibular joint is where the jawbone meets the skull, and movement in this joint is required for talking, chewing, and yawning. The symptoms of temporomandibular joint dysfunction (TMD) are tenderness, tension, and pain. Although sometimes TMDs relate to observable problems with this joint, most of the time there is no apparent reason for pain. As with headache, researchers believe that the pain of TMDs is at least partly related to increased pain sensitivity (Cairns, 2010). As with other pain syndromes, feelings of stress tend to worsen pain. Some studies suggest that stress may also play a role in the development of TMDs (Cairns, 2010).

Back, Neck, and Shoulder Pain

A variety of problems—from structural disorders to neurological issues—can cause back, neck, and shoulder pain. Chronic stress can lead to muscle tension that in turn can lead to pain, especially in areas already compromised by previous injury or other causes of pain. Research on psychosocial stress and pain, such as back pain, typically finds that perceived stress is related to both onset and intensity of pain (Saastamoinen, Laaksonen, Leino-Arjas, & Lahelma, 2009).

Effects on the Digestive System

When people are feeling stressed, they report "butterflies," or a sinking feeling in the pit of the stomach—a typical effect of stress on the digestive system. Many people experience abdominal sensations resulting from a variety of emotions—from anger and hate to love and joy. These sensations reflect the acute stress response, which can have significant effects on digestive function and health. For most people, these "gut reactions" are a harmless response; but for some, chronic stress easily upsets the digestive system and can lead to several health problems. During the acute stress response, the body neglects digestive function while it tends to the needs of the cardiovascular and musculoskeletal systems. Sometimes maladaptive coping behavior provides additional digestive system stress. Drinking countless cups of coffee irritates the stomach and intestines. Alcohol is also an irritant. Smokers have higher ulcer rates than nonsmokers, and their ulcers heal more slowly. When intake of junk food low in fiber and high in fat is greater than usual, digestive function will reflect this change. Skipping meals means an empty stomach, which can exacerbate an already-irritated stomach lining. Eating well can be a challenge during stressful periods, especially for people who experience nausea, loss of appetite, or indigestion. Some of the health problems of the digestive system that can worsen with chronic stress include the following.

Gum Disease

Gum disease, also known as gingivitis, results when the gum tissue around the teeth becomes inflamed and bleeds easily. Inflammation is caused by the same bacteria that are responsible for dental caries, or tooth decay. As the bacteria act on sugars, they give off acids that penetrate the tooth's enamel. Other bacteria produce a sticky substance that combines with bacterial and other debris to form dental plaque, which adheres to the tooth surface, especially along the gum line. If one does not remove plaque by brushing and flossing, it can build up and harden. Normally, saliva reduces acidity and protects the teeth, but plaque prevents saliva from reaching the surface of the teeth and providing these benefits. Plaque also provides a place for bacteria to thrive and inflame gum tissue.

Researchers offer these hypotheses to explain why stress might exacerbate gingivitis: a reduction in saliva (resulting from stress or other factors) favors the growth of harmful bacteria and subsequent plaque production; proinflammatory cytokines, which increase in response to stress, may exacerbate gum inflammation; or people may neglect oral hygiene and healthful eating during periods of stress (Rosania, Low, McCormick, & Rosania, 2010). Tobacco products also contribute to gum disease, so people who smoke more when stressed may experience an increased incidence of gum disease during stressful times.

Esophageal Spasms

Spasm of the smooth muscle of the esophagus produces pain in the chest, which many people mistake for heart attack. These spasms are the result of abnormal peristalsis, the slow wave contractions produced by the smooth muscles of the digestive system that move food along the gastrointestinal tract. Stress can interfere with the normal motility, or movement, of these muscles. Esophageal spasms are also sometimes produced by gastroesophageal reflux, a condition in which stomach contents escape through the esophageal sphincter, which normally stays closed except to allow food to pass into the stomach. The acidic contents of the stomach irritate the esophagus, which can interfere with normal peristalsis. Gastroesophageal reflux may also cause heartburn. Like other gastrointestinal symptoms, esophageal spasms may worsen during stressful times, even though their causes may be factors other than stress (Talley, DeVault, & Fleischer, 2010).

Ulcers

Ulcers are breaks in the lining of the stomach or other parts of the gastrointestinal tract that create sores. Early studies in animals, including those performed by Hans Selye, found stomach ulcers to be a common stress response, especially when the animals had no control over stressors (Selye, 1956).

The stomach produces hydrochloric acid, which speeds up digestion. Hydrochloric acid is such a strong acid that it would damage the tissue of the stomach itself if the stomach did not produce a protective mucus coating. It is possible that during stress, norepinephrine causes blood vessels in the stomach lining to constrict,

decreasing mucus production and leaving the stomach wall vulnerable to the destructive action of hydrochloric acid. Ulcers may occur anywhere along the gastrointestinal tract but are most common in the stomach and the upper portion of the small intestine.

A bacterial strain, *Helicobacter pylori* (*H. pylori*), appears to be associated with the development of ulcers in many people. *H. pylori* is believed to inflame the stomach lining or stimulate excess acid production, or both. *H. pylori* bacteria infect approximately half of the human population, in most cases causing no symptoms. It is possible that other microorganisms in the stomach help keep the population of *H. pylori* at a reasonable level. Research in vitro has demonstrated that norepinephrine encourages the growth of *H. pylori* and may thus precipitate ulcers in vulnerable people (Doherty, Tobias, Watson, & Atheron, 2009). Antibiotics may effectively treat some ulcers. An accurate diagnosis and appropriate medical treatment are essential for people with ulcers.

Nervous Stomach and Nausea

Many people experience nausea, a loss of appetite, and stomachaches when feeling stressed. Extreme stress can even lead to vomiting. Stomach pain associated with stress is not necessarily indicative of ulcer development but may result from the same factors that cause stomach ulcers. Indigestion or strong spasms of the stomach muscles may also cause symptoms. People who find that stomach problems signal excess stress are likely to benefit from relaxation techniques that help reduce sympathetic arousal and increase the parasympathetic "rest-and-digest" response. These people also tend to develop fewer digestive problems when they consume their meals slowly in a relaxing environment, rather than eating when they feel stressed.

Irritable Bowel Syndrome

In some people, chronic stress may alter peristalsis. When peristalsis speeds up too much, diarrhea results; when it slows down too much, constipation occurs. Symptoms of irritable bowel syndrome (IBS) include abdominal pain and irregular bowel habits, including constipation and/or diarrhea. Indigestion and excess gas cause some of the pain, as do spastic contractions of the large colon. Some people with IBS find that certain foods are associated with symptoms.

Stress seems to exacerbate IBS in at least two ways. Recent research has found that people with IBS have excess sympathetic nervous system activity compared with those without IBS (Manabe, Tanaka, Hata, Kusunoki, & Haruma, 2009). Other research in rats found that stress alters motor function in the colon because of elevated plasma levels of norepinephrine (Choudhury, Shi, & Sarna, 2009). The changes in motor function result in increased motility and thus faster colonic transit and an increased defecation rate. Studies in rats have also shown a variety of tissue and cellular responses to stress hormones, including an increase in inflammation of the intestinal lining and increased mucus production (Vicario et al., 2011). IBS often responds well to lifestyle treatment, including dietary changes, regular physical activity, and stress management (Tavassoli, 2009).

Inflammatory Bowel Diseases

Although inflammatory bowel diseases (IBDs) such as ulcerative colitis and Crohn's disease do not appear to be caused by stress, most people who have IBDs find that their symptoms worsen when they are feeling stressed, perhaps because of an increase in inflammatory cytokines associated with stress. One review of the literature concluded that evidence is weak for stress as a cause of IBDs but that psychosocial stress appears to play a significant role in disease severity (Maunder & Levenstein, 2008).

Effects on the Reproductive System

Stress appears to interfere with normal functioning of the reproductive system in several ways. Chronic stress can reduce libido (sex drive) in vulnerable individuals. In women, chronic stress can suppress the menstrual cycle, causing amenorrhea or oligomenorrhea. Stress can also inhibit fertility in some women or lead to problems during pregnancy, including premature birth. In men, chronic stress is associated with decreased sperm count, erectile dysfunction, and premature ejaculation. The stress hormones, such as the glucocorticoids, appear to inhibit the body's production of gonadotropin-releasing hormone (GnRH), which drives the reproductive system in both sexes. In addition, stress may induce the brain to produce another hormone, gonadotropin-inhibitory hormone (GnIH), which inhibits reproductive function (Kirby, Geraghty, Ubuka, Bentley, & Kaufer, 2009).

Effects on the Central Nervous System

Research shows chronic stress exerts negative effects on both cognitive function (especially memory) and mood disorders, including anxiety and depression. Receptors for the stress hormones, including the glucocorticoids, are found throughout the brain, and the stress hormones affect gene expression in the cells to which they bind (Lupien, McEwen, Gunnar, & Heim, 2009). Neuroscientists believe that stress thus impacts brain structures, along with cognitive function and mental health (Lupien et al., 2009).

Cognitive Function, Memory, and Dementia

It makes intuitive sense that cognitive function might decline with stress overload. As a person's cognitive capacity becomes crowded with stressors crying for a solution, less room is available for attention to other areas of life. Athletes and sports psychologists know the critical importance of staying focused on one's performance during a contest. The same principle is at work for

students writing a paper or giving a presentation. Chronic stress is often responsible for accidents and injury, as people feel distracted and do not pay attention to what they are doing.

The Whitehall II study compared employees working 40 hours a week with those working more than 55 hours a week (Virtanen et al., 2009). Subjects completed a battery of tests on cognitive function. The middle-aged employees working longer hours saw a greater decline on reasoning test scores over a 4-year period. Studies in both laboratory rodents and humans have found that psychosocial stress interferes with the activity of the prefrontal cortex and impairs attentional control and functional connectivity (Liston, McEwen, & Casey, 2009). Attentional control refers to the process of deciding which thing, among the wide array of stimuli coming into the brain through the sensory organs and other parts of the brain, needs one's focus. Attentional control involves both the decision to focus on something and the ability to maintain that focus. For example, attentional control for a student might mean deciding to work on a certain assignment and making oneself stay focused on that task even though other thoughts and diversions surface. Functional connectivity refers to the coordination of various cognitive processes in order to accomplish complex cognitive tasks, such as solving challenging problems. People take a more-creative approach to solving problems when feeling less stressed. Creativity requires a high level of functional connectivity.

Research in both laboratory animals and humans has demonstrated an association between psychosocial stress and dementia. Researchers suggest that this risk probably relates to both neurological and vascular changes associated with chronic stress (Nation et al., 2011; Fig. 6-12). Impaired blood flow to the brain accelerates dementia. In addition, stress is associated with reduced levels of brain-derived neurotrophic factor (BDNF) and reduced cell volume in certain areas of the brain, including the hippocampus, an area important for memory. People with Alzheimer's disease have elevated levels of stress hormones such as cortisol, and higher levels of these hormones have been associated with disease progression (Nation et al., 2011). Of course, experiencing Alzheimer's disease creates stress

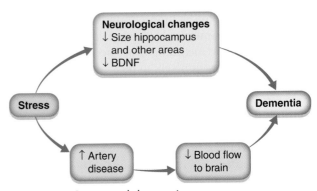

Figure 6-12. Stress and dementia.

for patients trying to deal with a brain that is not working correctly, so some of the increase in stress hormones might be caused by the disease itself. However, animal studies have found that the experience of stress and elevated stress hormones affects neurological structure and function in several brain areas, especially the hippocampus (Conrad, 2008).

Emotional Health

The relationship between stress and emotional health is complex and involves the physical, psychological, and emotional components of the stress response, as well as coping behaviors. One uses all three components to build stress resistance. These components can also develop in ways that worsen emotional health disorders. The two most common emotional health disorders associated with stress are anxiety and depression.

Anxiety is a feeling of worry and apprehension. Some of the more-common anxiety disorders are presented in Chapter 3. People bothered by anxiety do not need much stimulus to become worried. In fact, for many people, anxiety and stress are synonymous. People with any form of anxiety disorder or even mild anxiety symptoms generally feel more anxious and experience more symptoms when highly stressed. Depressed people feel hopeless, helpless, and lacking in drive, energy, and interest in life. Stressors usually require energy and involvement, which can make a depressed person feel even more inadequate, depressed, and incapable of meeting the new demands. The downward spiral of depression, with depression leading to withdrawal leading to more depression, seems to speed up when additional stressors arise.

FACTORS THAT INFLUENCE THE STRESS–HEALTH RELATIONSHIP

Why do some people seem to fall apart under what appear to be very mild levels of stress, whereas others persevere through unbelievable difficulties? Why do some people develop stress-related illnesses, whereas others are able to put stress in perspective and do what they need to do? Although researchers still have much to learn about stress resistance and the variations in people's stress tolerance and coping, interesting research is beginning to illuminate the psychophysiological factors that mediate the stress–health relationship.

Anger, Hostility, and Cynical Outlook

Research on Type A Behavior Pattern (TABP) in the 1960s brought the importance of personality factors, such as hostility and a cynical outlook, to the attention of the medical community (Game Changers 6-2). The relationship between TABP and heart disease interested practitioners and researchers alike. Many researchers were Type As themselves and wondered whether all Type A traits were to blame for elevated heart disease

risk or whether the negative health effects were more strongly related to a subset of variables within the TABP. Several researchers have shown that the components of TABP that appear to be the strongest predictors of poor health outcomes are feelings of anger and hostility and a negative, cynical outlook (Williams, 2008). Redford B. Williams, one of the leading researchers in this area, showed that feelings of anger are associated with both negative health behaviors (more smoking, alcohol abuse, etc.) and with chronic stress. Chronic anger and feelings of hostility trigger the neuroendocrine and autonomic nervous system responses associated with stress-related illness, especially cardiovascular disease (Williams, 2008). (See also "What's the Evidence?" in Chapter 1.)

Depression

Depression is strongly related to poor health. Depression has been associated with higher levels of physical distress, pain, and anxiety, as well as decreased quality of life, decreased social support, and increased disability (Strine et al., 2009). Depression's physical symptoms can be complicated by lack of motivation to engage in positive health behaviors. People suffering from depression show greater risk of stress-related illness.

Loneliness

James J. Lynch began writing about the importance of social support and close relationships in the 1960s. His first book, published in 1977, was called *The Broken Heart: The Medical Consequences of Loneliness* (Lynch, 1977). In this book, he spelled out the many ways that feelings of loneliness and lack of connection to others cause health problems, both physical and psychological. A great deal of research supports his conclusions (Lynch, 2000). Cardiologist Dean Ornish believes that teaching his patients to "open their hearts" to others and nurture loving relationships is the most important component of his cardiac-rehabilitation programs (Ornish, 1998). Social support, connection to others, and loving relationships are important foundations of wellness and promote quality of life.

Type D Personality

The description of Type D personality comes from the work of Johan Denollet and colleagues in the Netherlands. Like Friedman and Rosenman, Denollet observed a cluster of behavior traits in his patients, which he called Type D for "distressed." According to Denollet, Type D patients are anxious, irritable, and insecure. They want people to like them but are tense and inhibited around others, which creates further anxiety (Denollet et al., 1996). In the first study of Type D, published in 1996 (Denollet et al., 1996), Denollet and his colleagues tested 286 men and women enrolled in a cardiac-rehabilitation program and categorized them

Game Changers 6-2. Meyer Friedman, Ray Rosenman, and the Type A Behavior Pattern

The concept of Type A Behavior Pattern (TABP) was first defined by two San Francisco cardiologists, Meyer Friedman and Ray Rosenman. They had observed that their patients with coronary artery disease tended to share a number of traits that they called the Type A Behavior Pattern (TABP). These traits included a hard-driving competitiveness, hostility, a sense of time urgency, and a concern with achievement and acquisition of objects. According to the cardiologists, Type B people came less frequently to the ward and had a more-easygoing attitude.

Friedman and Rosenman decided to test their theory. They came up with the "structured interview," which categorized subjects into Type A or Type B groups according to their response style. They were Type A if they spoke quickly and loudly, finished the investigator's sentences, and exhibited impatient mannerisms. The researchers categorized 3,524 male volunteers into Type A and B groups, and about half the men fell into each group. If these behavior patterns had no relationship to artery disease, one would expect that over time both groups would show similar rates of artery disease development. This was not the case. The research team followed the men for over 8 years, during which time twice as many men in the Type A group experienced coronary artery disease (Rosenman, et al., 1975). Convinced of the strength of the relationship between TABP and coronary artery disease, Friedman and Rosenman wrote a book called *Type A Behavior and Your Heart*, which was published in 1974. They also created behavior-change programs designed to help people change Type A traits (Friedman et al., 1984). In these programs, people practiced becoming more patient and relaxed.

Friedman and Rosenman were some of the first biomedical researchers to draw attention to the importance of personality traits for understanding health outcomes, especially heart disease. Subsequent research has focused on further refining the specific Type A traits most predictive of artery disease, the measurement of these traits, the physiological mechanisms through which these traits lead to artery disease, and possible treatment modalities for individuals with these traits. Thus, early research on TABP has led to the interesting investigations linking hostility, depression, loneliness, and other emotional experiences with a variety of health outcomes.

Sources: Friedman, M., & Rosenman, R. H. (1974). *Type A Behavior and Your Heart*. Greenwich, CT: Fawcett; Friedman, M., Thorensen, C. E., Gill, J. J., Powell, L. H., Ulmer, D., Thompson, L., ... Dixon, T. (1984). Alteration of Type A behavior and reduction in cardiac recurrences in postmyocardial infarction patients. *American Heart Journal, 108*(2): 237-248; Rosenman, R. H., Brand, R. J., Jenkins, C. D., Friedman, M., Straus, R., & Wurm, M. (1975). Coronary heart disease in the Western Collaborative Group Study: final follow-up of 8 1/2 years. *Journal of the American Medical Association, 233*: 872-877.

into Type D and non–Type D groups. Eight years later, the researchers found that 27% of the people in the Type D group had died, mostly from heart disease and strokes, whereas only 7% of the non–Type D patients had died.

In 2010, Denollet's group published a follow-up study that examined the results of nine prospective studies on Type D personality and heart disease (Denollet, Schiffer, & Spek, 2010). They studied 6,121 patients with cardiovascular conditions and found that people who fit the Type D description had a three-fold risk of cardiac events, such as a heart attack. Type D provides a double hit to the heart. Anxiety and feelings of social isolation are both risk factors for heart disease, and their combination may be what makes Type D personality so risky. Type D is different from depression, although the two can overlap. Depression is even riskier than Type D personality for the development of heart disease (Denollet et al., 2009).

Resilience

Resilience is a state of successful adaptation to stressful events and circumstances (Juster, McEwen, & Lupien,

2010). Resilient people are able to "bounce back" from stress (Smitha, Tooleya, Christophera, & Kay, 2010). Researchers believe that genetics, behavior, and the environment affect resilience. Certain life circumstances, such as low socioeconomic status, poverty, and discrimination, seem to reduce the likelihood that people will develop resilience, whereas other situations increase the chance for its development (McEwen & Gianaros, 2010). Too much stress can create feelings of helplessness and hopelessness—the opposite of resilience. Exposure to traumatic stress early in a person's development can produce enduring changes in the stress response, making the hypothalamus more likely to set the stress response in motion (Gillespie, Phifer, Bradley, & Ressler, 2009). Researchers believe that early traumatic experiences may affect development of the neural pathways regulating emotion (Gillespie et al., 2009). Trauma seems to affect these neural pathways in a manner that increases risk for emotional health disorders, such as anxiety and depression.

On the other hand, research with primates has shown that early experiences with moderate levels of stress may actually build resilience and better coping

(Katz et al., 2009). In monkeys, practice coping with stress leads to better development of neural pathways in the prefrontal cortex and other cortical regions that control arousal regulation and resilience (Katz et al., 2009). Some researchers, working with laboratory rodents, have begun to identify mechanisms at the molecular level in the CNS that appear to be associated with resilient behavior (Vialou et al., 2010).

Several factors have a great deal of research support as important components of resilience. These include a sense of control, self-esteem, and social support.

Control

A sense of control over the circumstances of one's life, or at least a sense of options, is an important component of resilience (Thoits, 2010). Of course, no one has total control over events, but resilient people at least feel that they have some control and can take action to cope with stressors as they arise. A sense of control goes along with feeling as if one is able to muster some resources to cope with the demand of a given stressor. A sense of control is an important component of Self-determination Theory, because feeling that one is making choices in line with one's priorities is important for behavior change and life in general. Attribution Theory posits that an internal locus of control is crucial for successful behavior change. Self-efficacy also embodies a sense of having control, as control is necessary for feeling efficacious.

Self-esteem

Self-esteem refers to the degree to which a person values himself. Self-esteem encompasses self-confidence and self-efficacy and means valuing one's personal assets and abilities. A healthy self-esteem means that a person feels relatively competent at meeting life's challenges. Self-esteem relates to control, as a healthy self-esteem includes feeling one has resources in terms of skills and abilities, which in turn engenders a greater sense of having options or control. A healthy self-esteem enhances coping ability by giving people the confidence they need to confront and solve, rather than avoid, difficult problems. A healthy level of self-esteem is essential for changing problematic behavior patterns.

Social Support

Social support is an essential stress reducer and health promoter. As discussed in Chapter 5, social support refers to a person's perception of having a connection with others. It increases resilience in several ways. First, people often feel less stressed when they disclose their worries and concerns to others, such as family members and close friends. Second, social support expands a person's perception of resources that are available to meet a stressful demand. Social support might mean a friend who can provide a ride to a medical appointment, a neighbor who can feed the cat while one is in the hospital, or a relative who can give advice on a difficult situation. Third, social support simply helps

people feel connected to others, even those they do not know very well. Social support, which helps someone feel part of a community, can include a teacher who praises a student's good work, the server who already knows how a person likes her coffee, or the other dog walkers one passes in the park every afternoon. Clients and patients often experience feelings of social support from health and fitness professionals (Fig. 6-13).

Hardiness

Another model of resilience or stress resistance is a cluster of attributes called hardiness. Suzanne Kobasa originally proposed the concept of hardiness in 1979 (Kobasa, 1979). Kobasa had studied the research linking stressful life events and illness. She conducted her first study to determine why some people were more resistant to the negative health effects of stress than others (Kobasa, 1979). Soon after this initial study, Kobasa and colleagues studied men experiencing occupational stress and compared subjects who developed stress-related illness with those who did not (Kobasa et al., 1982). Subsequent research by others, including Salvatore Maddi and colleagues (Maddi, Khoshaba, Harvey, Fazel, & Resurreccion, 2011), has built on this original research to apply the hardiness concept to a broader demographic and devise tools for measuring hardiness.

Kobasa found that hardy people displayed attributes she called control, commitment, and challenge. She also found that engagement in regular exercise and good social support are characteristic of people

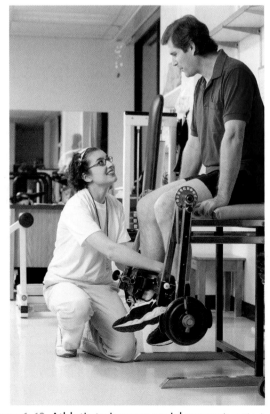

Figure 6-13. **Athletic trainers as social support.** © Thinkstock

scoring high on hardiness (Kobasa, 1979). Maddi later described hardiness as a cluster of attributes "that together provide the existential courage and motivation to turn stressful circumstances from potential disasters into growth opportunities" (Maddi, 2011). Maddi defines existential courage as the courage that grows out of creating meaning in an otherwise meaningless world. According to Maddi, existential psychologists study a person's "ongoing search for meaning in life" (Maddi, 2004). Existential psychology, which has its roots in existential philosophy, studies how people come to terms with the facts of human existence. These include coping with the anxiety of one's eventual mortality, constructing meaning out of daily existence, and making choices based on constructed meaning, often in the face of challenging circumstances and situations.

The concept of control in the hardiness model contrasts with feelings of powerlessness or hopelessness and helplessness as previously discussed in this chapter. The concept of commitment contrasts with feelings of alienation and an inability to relate to a purpose, organization, or group of people. Alienation can feel similar to loneliness and a lack of social connection—a powerful variable in many models. The concept of challenge contrasts with that of security. According to the hardiness model, people who are able to feel challenged by future demands are less likely to suffer from stress, whereas those afraid to leave the security of the known will inevitably be stressed (since the future always brings the unexpected).

Optimism and Positive Emotions

Research has shown that optimism, as opposed to cynicism, is associated with better long-term health (Seligman, 2008; Boehm & Kubzansky, 2012). Studies have also shown that people can learn optimism and that stress-resistant people can consciously develop the habit of perceiving potential stressors in ways that give life meaning and give them a sense of control (Seligman, 2006).

Research in the field of positive psychology has shown that experiencing positive emotions helps people recover more quickly from stress and reduces risk of stress-related illness (Fredrickson, Cohn, Coffey, Pek, & Finkel, 2008). Barbara Fredrickson, a leading researcher in this area, has demonstrated that experiencing positive emotions broadens people's thinking, allowing them to solve problems more creatively and effectively (What's the Evidence? 6-1). Positive emotions also generate the energy required for self-control, thus fueling further attempts at behavior change or coping with stressors. Other researchers in positive psychology have shown that happy people are healthier. They practice better health behaviors, have stronger immune systems, and experience less pain (Kesebir & Diener, 2008).

Interestingly, Fredrickson has shown that increasing experiences of positive emotion may not decrease the frequency or intensity of negative emotions, such as anger, sadness, or anxiety. She argues that these negative emotions are an important source of information

WHAT'S THE EVIDENCE? 6-1

Positive Emotions, Personal Resources, and Life Satisfaction

Fredrickson, B. L., Cohn, M. A., Coffey, K. A., Pek, J., & Finkel, S. M. (2008). Open hearts build lives: positive emotions, induced through loving-kindness meditation, build consequential personal resources. *Journal of Personality and Social Psychology, 95*(5): 1045-1062.

■ PURPOSE

Previous correlational research had found associations between the experience and expression of positive emotion and personal resources, such as social support, mental health, and resilience. Researchers did not know whether personal resources caused positive emotions or the other way around. Fredrickson and colleagues wanted to find out whether experiencing positive emotions might enhance the development of personal resources.

■ STUDY

Fredrickson and colleagues solicited volunteers for a 9-week loving-kindness meditation (LKM) workshop as part of an employee-wellness program at a software and information technology services company. A total of 202 men and women volunteered and were randomly assigned to the workshop or a wait-list control group, which participated in the workshop after the first group's study was finished. The subjects who actually completed the study numbered 139.

The LKM group attended six weekly meetings to learn LKM. In addition, subjects practiced the LKM daily for about 15 to 20 minutes. All subjects in both groups completed a battery of standard psychological questionnaires at the beginning and end of the study, daily measures of positive and negative emotions, and a record of LKM practice. Emotions that were evaluated included amusement, anger, awe, compassion, contempt, contentment, disgust, embarrassment, gratitude, hope, joy, interest, love, pride, guilt, sadness, shame, fear, and surprise.

Subjects in the LKM group initially experienced fewer positive emotions than the control group. The researchers hypothesized that this is typical of people's experiences in behavior-change programs, since changing behavior is

WHAT'S THE EVIDENCE? 6-1–cont'd

initially difficult. However, after a few weeks, the LKM group reported experiencing more positive emotions each day on average than the control group. A comparison of questionnaire results found that the LKM group increase in the experience of positive emotions was associated with an increase in 9 of the 18 personal resources measured, including mindfulness, savoring the future, environmental mastery, self-acceptance, purpose in life, social support received, positive relations with others, and illness symptoms. An increase in positive emotion also increased a measure called "pathways thinking," which refers to a person's perceived ability to find routes to desired goals. Improvement in personal resources, in turn, predicted improvement in measures of life satisfaction. (Improvement in positive emotions alone did not predict life satisfaction, so the researchers concluded that building personal resources is required for increasing life satisfaction.)

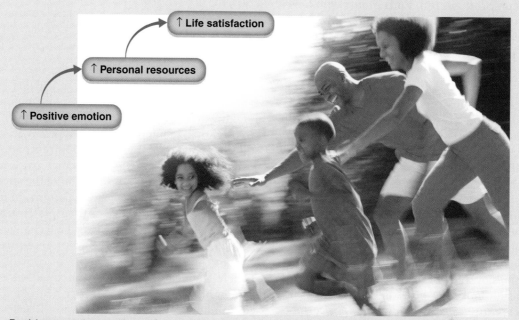

Positive emotions, personal resources, and life satisfaction. Photograph © Thinkstock

■ IMPLICATIONS

The research of Fredrickson and colleagues remains central to the field of positive psychology, which focuses on the importance of cultivating positive emotions and experiences to create optimal health and well-being. This study found that increasing one's daily experience of positive emotions leads to an increase in personal resources. This buildup of personal resources is associated with life satisfaction.

The results of this study have important application for health and fitness professionals as they help people build positive emotion through beneficial lifestyle change. Such work can help clients improve their lives in many important ways.

for people and an important part of life. The goal of stress management, discussed below, is not to eliminate stress (since this is impossible and probably undesirable) but to improve people's ability to let go of stress once they have addressed a stressor and not spend excess time in prolonged periods of chronic stress. Cultivating more experiences of positive emotions can help address problems made worse by negative emotions, such as depression, chronic anger, and anxiety. Fredrickson notes that it is impossible to "will" positive emotions to occur. Instead, people must elicit them with a memory, thought, image, or other experience

such as film, writing, or physical activity. Humor used in positive ways can generate positive emotions and reduce stress.

MOTIVATING CHANGE: Using Humor to Promote Positive Emotions

Introducing humor into work situations is not as easy as it sounds. Humor only promotes positive emotions when it is the right kind of humor used appropriately in the right situation with the right people. In the work setting, humor should be used in the spirit of kindness and connection. When working with clients, funny stories and jokes can nurture clients' self-esteem or connect with their personal interests. Avoid sarcasm and destructive forms of humor. This type of "humor" alienates people and blocks constructive problem solving. Also destructive is using humor to insult individuals or groups. Recognize that sense of humor varies considerably from person to person. What some people find funny others find insulting or irritating. If you are using humor with clients, you must work with them to discover what makes them smile. Wait until you know clients better before telling too many jokes. You should certainly be friendly but also respectful. With clients who have no sense of humor, focus instead on positive emotions. Instead of telling jokes, get them to talk about their children, pets, and other passions.

Hope

Hope is the cornerstone of optimism. It is the belief that a positive outcome is possible despite evidence to the contrary. Hope is an important component of resilience, especially in difficult or traumatic situations because it allows people to persevere at problem solving. The quality of hope is what helps people see future demands as challenges (as in the hardiness model). According to the work of Martin Seligman and colleagues, hope is a distinguishing characteristic of happy people (Seligman, 2006).

A sense of hope is associated with more positive health outcomes. A study of veterans of the wars in Iraq and Afghanistan looked at how these veterans coped with their exposure to armed conflict (MacDermott, 2010). Not surprisingly, this population is vulnerable to post-traumatic stress disorder, depression, and suicide. This study suggested that veterans' ability to construct meaning from their experience contributed to their

sense of hope or hopelessness and, consequently, to risk of future suicide. Veterans able to construct meaning and had a sense of hope had lower risk of suicide.

Gratitude

Gratitude means feeling thankful for the benefits one has received or may receive in the future. Seligman's work on happiness has shown that people who frequently experience feelings of gratitude tend to report higher levels of well-being and lower levels of stress (Seligman, 2006). Gratitude is not just an intellectual experience; it involves feeling true thankfulness that increases positive outlook and counteracts feelings of stress.

STRESS MANAGEMENT

Stress management refers to the use of a variety of techniques that can enhance one's ability to cope with stress (Fig. 6-14). The word "management" suggests taking action or gaining some control over a situation. Stress-management programs typically teach people to become aware of their personal stress patterns and design ways to intervene and change patterns to reduce unnecessary stress and activation of the stress response. Individuals can manage stress patterns in many different ways, and they vary in their preference for stress-management strategies. Even small changes in the way people organize their days or interpret events around them can improve their sense of control and reduce their feelings of being overwhelmed. Stress-management practices can have positive neurobiological effects on the brain, its neural pathways, BDNF, and the signaling molecules, including the endorphins, serotonin, and other neurotransmitters. Researchers have called stress management "an endogenous potential" (Esch & Stefano, 2010), meaning that stress-reduction effects,

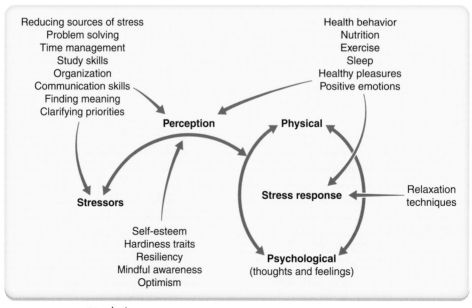

Figure 6-14. Stress-management techniques.

what others have called "the relaxation response" (Benson, 1975), create a state the mind and body can learn to produce. Although stress-management practices can help reduce stress, it is important to note that stress management is not the same thing as counseling or therapy, although it can complement work done in a therapeutic setting (Box 6-2). Some of the more widely used approaches for managing stress include the following.

Finding Meaning and Clarifying Priorities

People who feel overwhelmed with their many roles and obligations often feel better when they can connect those roles and obligations to the big picture of their lives. Time-management exercises always begin by asking people to take some time to make a list of their lifetime priorities, along with short- and long-range plans. Students, for example, sometimes feel overwhelmed with classes and assignments. Those who can connect all of their schoolwork with meaningful long-term goals at least feel that what they do matters.

Clarifying priorities also helps people decide whether there are stressors in their lives that they could eliminate. It is easy to get involved in too many activities. Although each is worthwhile, interesting, or fun, participating ceases to be when the activity becomes "one more thing" to do. It is important to keep good friends in one's life and build meaningful social connections, but it is best to do this in a way that balances one's work and other obligations. Clarifying priorities and thinking about time management can also help people identify time wasters, such as watching television when nothing

good is on or spending too much time online. After clarifying priorities, people often clear their schedules out a bit and make more time for rewarding experiences with the people they care about and the activities that are most important to them.

Reducing Sources of Stress

People who participate in stress-management workshops or classes often keep track of the sources of stress in their lives. Sometimes taking a step back and looking at sources of stress from a new perspective or even discussing them with others triggers new thoughts about changing or eliminating some of them. Stress-management programs are not the place to decide to leave a marriage, quit a job, or make big life changes. However, simple changes often reduce feelings of stress. Getting more organized can save time and aggravation. Deciding to discuss a chronic job-related problem with a coworker or boss can help solve it. Asking for help with a project, finding the resources needed to complete an assignment, or creating a budget can all reduce sources of stress. Figuring out where to go for help with difficult, stress-producing issues and making an appointment for counseling, legal advice, or financial planning can help tackle these problems. Improving skills in problem solving, communication, and time management can help people more effectively deal with sources of stress in their lives.

Improving Coping Skills

Unfortunately, many times people cannot eliminate or dramatically change sources of stress. However, the way they cope with these problems can reduce the impact of stressors in their lives. Coping skills refer to behaviors used by people to deal with difficult situations. Difficulties are a part of life, and resilience grows when people develop coping skills that allow them to thrive and grow even in challenging circumstances. When people examine their own stress patterns, they can often discern maladaptive and adaptive coping strategies and choose to further develop adaptive strategies, thus improving their coping skills. For example, a student might decide that her procrastination habit has gotten out of control and is creating too much stress and mediocre academic performance as she scrambles to complete assignments at the last minute. She might reduce feelings of stress by taking control of her work—improving her study skills, organization, scheduling, and time management. Eventually, instead of coping with school stress by avoiding her work and procrastinating, she would cope by getting organized and doing her work on a regular schedule.

Increasing Mindful Awareness

Mindfulness practices can be helpful techniques for managing stress. Mindfulness means present moment,

> ## Box 6-2. The Limitations of Stress Management
>
> Stress management is not a substitute for medical treatment. People with physical symptoms such as back pain or hypertension should check with their health-care providers and receive appropriate medical care. Many symptoms may be indicative of something other than stress. However, many health-care providers do recommend stress-management techniques to complement standard medical care or professional counseling for stress-related disorders. Psychologists, social workers, and other therapists can assist people struggling with too much stress or other emotional health issues.
>
> Stress management can be very effective, but it is not magic. Some people try yoga, meditation, or some other stress-reduction practice hoping for quick results. Stress management is not instant self-transformation. Reducing one's stress patterns takes practice and mindful awareness.

nonjudgmental awareness of one's physical and psychological experience. Mindful awareness, practiced over time, can lead to insight regarding one's motivations, emotions, and habitual physical and psychological response patterns. Present-moment mindful awareness can be practiced during simple activities such as walking, eating, and performing chores. Mindfulness meditation grows out of Buddhist meditation practice. Practitioners try to keep their focus on their breathing and occurrences in the present moment. Various programs of mindfulness training are available. Best known is the Mindfulness-Based Stress Reduction (MBSR) program designed by Jon Kabat-Zinn at the University of Massachusetts Medical Center for patients coping with chronic pain and illness (Kabat-Zinn, 1990). Many research studies have documented positive emotional and physical changes with regular practice of mindfulness in a variety of populations (Bohlmeijer, Prenger, Taal, & Cuijpers, 2010; Carmody, Baer, Lykins, & Olendzki, 2009; Dobkin & Zhao, 2010). Mindfulness can also affect a person's perception of stressors, often decreasing the perceived severity of minor stressors.

Promoting Positive Emotions

Interesting research on compassion meditation suggests that it reduces stress arousal and inhibits the negative health effects of stress (Pace et al., 2009). In addition to calming the mind or developing mindfulness, compassion meditation strives to generate feelings of compassion for other people. People practicing this type of meditation visualize a person toward whom they feel loving kindness, such as their child or partner, and attempt to elicit this emotion. The practitioner then expands the focus to include him or herself and eventually strangers and even people the practitioner dislikes. Feeling the positive emotions of loving kindness and compassion reduces the negative physiological effects of stress, such as high levels of stress hormones and negative changes in the immune system (Pace et al., 2009).

MOTIVATING CHANGE: Building Positive Stories to Bolster Self-esteem, Positive Emotions, and Motivation

When you work with clients for a while, you have the opportunity to hear their stories about past attempts at behavior change. You may also hear about their successes in life and get a sense of what makes them feel good. Which stories seem associated with positive emotions, such as pride and self-confidence? Repeat these stories back to clients when they are feeling stressed or are telling you why they may fail. For example, a client may have shown that she feels very strong in her parenting role. Perhaps she has told stories that indicate she is organized, loving, and proud of her family. When she tells you that she has trouble fitting exercise in because she is a disorganized person, show her in a supportive and encouraging way that she has great organization skills in the parenting area. How does she manage this? Explore her answers in ways that help her feel good about her skills.

Find opportunities to remind clients of previous successes, large and small. These can be successes in their behavior-change programs as they work with you or other successes you become aware of over time. Link these accomplishments to their personal strengths and point out what you see as their assets. If clients have been successful before, they may feel more able and motivated to be successful again. Increased self-confidence for their behavior-change programs can fuel motivation and enhance the likelihood of future success.

Engaging in Healthy Pleasures

One of the simplest ways to help clients manage stress and have more positive emotional experiences is to help them discover how to increase simple, healthy pleasure in their daily lives. Generating moments of enjoyment and peace throughout the day can reduce chronic stress arousal and recharge energy levels. Health and fitness professionals can ask clients to generate a list of 20 things they enjoy doing (Health Psychology in Your Life 6-1). They should guide clients to think of things they can do daily or almost every day. For example, although mountain climbing or wind surfing can be on the list, at least 10 of the 20 items should be easily accessed on a daily basis. Clients should be encouraged to enjoy simple pleasures, such as a delicious cup of coffee or tea, watching birds at the feeder, sending a funny e-mail to a friend, or enjoying a favorite physical activity. Many clients will list listening to music, reading, and watching a good movie. Health and fitness professionals who work regularly with clients can assign them "homework"—to experience a certain number of pleasurable moments each day. They should emphasize the stress-reduction and health-promoting benefits of *healthy* pleasures.

HEALTH PSYCHOLOGY IN YOUR LIFE 6-1.
Healthy Pleasures

One way of reducing stress is to increase pleasure. Make a list of 20 little and big things that you enjoy doing—at least 10 of which you can do several times a week.

Next to each item, write how often you use that activity for relaxation and enjoyment.

Circle those things you might like to use more often for relaxation and enjoyment.

If other ideas for enjoyable activities come to you later, add them to your list.

◼ *The following week, Sam seems much more focused and relaxed. He tells Morgan that he took a mental health day off from work, took a long walk, and then spent after-school time with his kids. His blood pressure readings at home have finally started to show some improvement, and he has resolved to continue to improve his lifestyle. Sam reports that he has switched from coffee to tea and feels much better.*

Morgan increases Sam's exercise intensity and encourages him to add a third day of activity a week, such as a walk on the weekends. Sam decides to walk around the soccer field in the park while his kids have practice, since he has to drive them there anyway. Morgan gives Sam the Healthy Pleasures exercise to complete for their next session together. ◼

Reducing Unnecessary Stress Arousal

Stress management is also about learning to reduce unnecessary reactions to stress or at least reduce the intensity of one's stress response. Relaxation and stress-reduction techniques such as physical activity, breathing exercises, and meditation can help people learn to let go of an acute stress response and reduce chronic stress. They can also learn to encourage feelings of relaxation and well-being to counteract the stress response. Those who are prone to stress-related symptoms such as tension headaches, digestive problems, and high blood pressure benefit greatly from learning to relax. This usually requires daily practice of one or more techniques to get good results.

Many effective relaxation practices are available online, in workshops, or from books and magazines. These range from simple breathing exercises to body-awareness practices to various types of meditation and visualization. Some people find that participation in activities such as yoga or tai chi helps reduce unnecessary stress arousal (Box 6-3; Health Psychology at Work 6-1).

The Role of the Health and Fitness Professional in Stress Management

Many health and fitness professionals have practiced various relaxation techniques as part of exercise classes or sport experiences. They are qualified and experienced enough to lead group exercise classes or to teach the techniques to clients for at-home practice. Common techniques that are widely supported and available are safe and helpful.

Most clients will probably have difficulty enough just finding time to exercise, and exercise generally produces better outcomes than relaxation techniques. So, if time is in short supply, recommend exercise first. Emphasize the emotional-health and stress-reduction benefits of physical activity, as described in Chapter 3. If stress is a problem, encourage present-moment

---

Box 6-3. Mind–Body Activities for Stress Reduction

Many clients are interested in exploring physical activities that promise to reduce stress, calm the mind, and promote inner peace. Activities such as yoga, tai chi, and many forms of martial arts have become popular around the world. Often called mind–body activities because they combine mental and physical capacities, these activities usually include the cultivation of an internal meditative state. Mind–body activities such as tai chi and yoga employ mindful awareness, a nonjudgmental observation of what is occurring in the present moment. The person focuses awareness on breathing, body sensations, thoughts, and feelings.

Many mind–body activities also include a spiritual component. This is especially true for activities such as yoga, tai chi, and many forms of martial arts, which have their roots in Eastern philosophy. Although most of these activities do not require that participants espouse a specific religion, they promote certain moral values such as integrity and respect for others. They emphasize people's connectedness to each other and their environment. Many clients appreciate the spiritual component of mind–body activities as a balance to a primarily sectarian culture.

Studies show that activities such as yoga and Pilates produce therapeutic results for some people. These health benefits seem to stem from improved posture, core strength, body mechanics, and the stress-reduction benefits of the activities. Many mind–body activities use a mindful focus combined with stretching and strengthening exercises to help people develop better posture and alignment both during exercise and in daily life. Pilates, the Feldenkrais method, and the Alexander technique are well known for their therapeutic success due to improved core strengthening and/or body mechanics (Adelman, 2006).

All of the mind–body activities (and in fact, most exercise) can improve mood and reduce feelings of stress. Reducing stress in turn lowers risk of stress-related illnesses and reduces symptoms of stress such as high blood pressure and low back pain (Sherman, Cherkin, Erro, Miglioretti, & Deyo, 2005). It is important, however, for health and fitness professionals not to overstate these therapeutic claims and to urge clients to use therapeutic exercise in conjunction with standard medical treatment for health problems.

HEALTH PSYCHOLOGY AT WORK 6-1. Yoga, Stress, and Compassion

Abigail Clarke is a yoga instructor, teaching a form of yoga known as Embodyoga. Abi began practicing yoga in 2000 and began teaching it in 2008. As a certified Embodyoga® RYT 500 level teacher, she places a strong emphasis on mind–body awareness, self-acceptance, and individualization of the student's experience. After teaching for several years, Abi returned to college and received her B.A. in Health Behavior from Smith College in 2012.

"Stress is one of the main reasons people decide to try yoga—stress and back pain. (And the two often go together.) Yoga helps reduce feelings of stress in many ways. First, the combination of movement, breath, and meditation leads to changes in the autonomic nervous system that reduce stress arousal. So each practice session or class can reduce feelings of stress.

"Second, yoga is a life-affirming practice. Stress often results from turning away from the sources of stress in your life, kind of like procrastinating on studying for an exam. Procrastination and worrying about the exam just make the experience worse, causing so much stress! But, if we had just turned towards our books weeks ago, the exam would feel more like a challenge, perhaps even an exciting one, and less like an insurmountable task. In yoga, we encourage our students to turn toward the experience, whatever is coming up for them in the moment, whether that is physical, emotional, or mental. Often the only way through the stress is to go through the experience: the stretch or the muscle fatigue of the posture, or facing an issue that is bothering you. Yoga practice cultivates mindfulness—a present-moment awareness. Being in the present moment is usually a lot nicer than being in your anxiety about the future.

"My own experience taught me the power of yoga practice. I first began practicing yoga as a way to achieve perfection—of both body and mind. I spent my adolescence struggling with an eating disorder, and yoga seemed like a life raft with the practices of breathing and meditation, but it also held the promise of a perfect body as a result—and how could I breathe and meditate without a flat belly and the perfect set of thighs? I felt that contentment would be a result of achieving this perfection. Because of this, for the first years of my practice, I did yoga because it seemed like something I should do; and although I did enjoy some benefits—I was calmer, more relaxed, stronger, and more flexible—I didn't really begin to practice for the pure joy of it until I met my teacher, Patty Townsend, founder of Embodyoga®, and I realized that my yoga practice offered a new way of seeing myself. I gradually transitioned from trying to achieve someone else's (impossible) idea of perfection and instead worked toward optimizing my own experience.

"There are many different approaches to teaching yoga. Some approaches resemble physical gymnastics. I find a yoga of integration and embodiment much more interesting. This mind–body awareness and integration is available to everyone, not just the super-fit and flexible. The more we come into a place of compassion within ourselves, the more compassion we can find for others."

Information on Embodyoga® is available at www.embodyoga.com.

---

awareness during exercise and advise clients to use exercise as a break from problems. Exercising with a friend can be very therapeutic for some. Healthy pleasures can allow busy clients to "multitask" their stress reduction, building social support and reducing stress by doing something enjoyable with friends. People experiencing symptoms of depression are usually better off leaving the house and doing physical activity rather than staying home and relaxing. However, some clients, especially those with stress-related pain or health concerns, may be willing to carve out 10 to 15 minutes a day to practice a stress-reduction technique.

When clients complain of "stress-related" symptoms, such as digestive complaints or headaches, health and fitness professionals must not diagnose (unless qualified as medical professionals) but instead refer clients to their providers. Relaxation is usually helpful, and clients can often combine it with standard medical care. Clients should tell their providers they are practicing a new activity, such as yoga, or even meditation or

relaxation techniques, just to be safe. It is possible that stress reduction will enhance treatment, and medication dosages may need adjustment in some cases, as for hypertension.

Health and fitness professionals make great cheerleaders, promoting lifestyle improvements and wellness practices such as effective exercise programs, healthful eating habits, and stress reduction. They can recommend relaxation techniques without being perceived by clients as giving advice on personal issues better handled by professionals licensed to provide psychological counseling and therapy (Box 6-4).

Guidelines for Relaxation Practice

Most relaxation techniques work best when people follow a few simple guidelines, including the following:

- Schedule a convenient time and place and practice regularly—not just when stress hits full force. Be as comfortable as possible. Loosen tight

Box 6-4. Best Practices for Helping Clients Address Stress in Behavior-Change Programs

Health and fitness professionals can help clients address stress in several helpful ways, including:

- Educate about the stress-reduction and emotional-health benefits of exercise. Encourage clients to be aware of feeling less stressed after exercise or on days when they exercise.
- If clients are coping with stress-related illness, be sure they are receiving good medical care and that you are not working outside of your scope of practice.
- If clients complain of stress, ask about other health behaviors that might be promoting stress. Encourage them to get adequate sleep, consume less caffeine, and exercise regularly. Discuss how a healthy lifestyle reduces stress-related illness. Acknowledge that stress is a fact of life.
- Remind clients that their health and well-being are priorities.
- If stress interferes frequently with behavior-change plans, help clients come up with ways to deal with stress and to connect behavior change with stress reduction.
- Keep your focus on helping clients build positive emotions and personal resources. Rather than addressing particularly difficult stressors such as a critical boss or depressed spouse (refer if clients have such problems), help clients use exercise and healthy pleasures to reduce feelings of chronic stress and generate positive emotions.
- Help clients feel they are in control of their behavior-change programs.
- Help clients feel they are making progress in their lifestyle-change programs and achieving feelings of self-efficacy in this area.
- Encourage social connection. Maintain a respectful positive regard for clients and encourage enjoyment at your worksite, without compromising quality of work. Encourage clients to exercise with a friend or family member.
- Model resilience in your own life. Model optimism and a positive outlook. Use appropriate humor and commit to your own optimal health journey. Express hope, gratitude, and enthusiasm as much as possible.

clothing, remove eyeglasses, use a supportive chair, and have warmer clothes on hand.

- Try not to try. The harder people try to relax, the tenser and more distracted they become. Many techniques ask the mind to imagine a special place or focus on the breath. The mind, however, tends to wander. When this happens, gently bring attention back to the technique without judgment, simply letting go of extraneous thoughts and regaining focus.
- Avoid falling asleep. Relaxation techniques require concentration and active awareness. If sleepy, practice with the eyes open, in a well-lighted place, and practice seated rather than lying down.

Easy Relaxation Techniques

Relaxation techniques usually begin with deep breathing. Some people find that breathing slowly and deeply for 5 to 15 minutes reduces feelings of stress (Box 6-5). One can also alternately tense and relax each muscle group, a technique called progressive relaxation pioneered by Edmund Jacobson (Jacobson, 1929). Jacobson recommended tensing for about 5 to 7 seconds, then relaxing for 20 to 30 seconds. Another easy-to-teach technique is Benson's relaxation response (Benson, 1975; Box 6-6).

Box 6-5. Deep Breathing Exercise

One can practice deep breathing in either a sitting or reclining position. If you start to feel dizzy or short of breath, you may be hyperventilating or breathing too quickly. Resume normal breathing if this occurs. Let your breathing be slow and smooth.

1. Place one hand on your abdomen and one hand on your chest. As you inhale, allow your abdomen to rise and expand.
2. After filling the lower portion of your lungs with air, keep inhaling, filling the middle portion of your lungs in your lower chest. You will feel the hand on your chest rise and your ribs expand.
3. Continue to inhale and feel the air filling your upper lungs. You will feel your collarbone rise as your lungs fill completely. After practicing this exercise a few times, you can perform these first three steps in a smooth, continuous motion in just a few seconds.
4. Exhale slowly, from the top of your lungs to the bottom. Near the end of your exhalation, allow your abdominal muscles to contract slightly, pushing out the last bit of air.
5. The exhalation phase of the breath is when relaxation occurs. To increase relaxation, gradually lengthen the exhalation. Once the deep breathing feels somewhat natural, try letting the exhalation phase take twice as long as your inhalation.

Box 6-6. The Relaxation Response

During the relaxation-response exercise, you focus on a particular word or phrase with each exhalation. When Herbert Benson first studied this practice, he recommended using the word "one" or any other relaxing word or phrase. However, after time, he found that his patients who used meaningful words, such as a line from a prayer or poem, had better improvements in health (Benson, 1984). Other meaningful words might include the words "relax" or "peace." Here are the instructions for this exercise:

1. Pick a focus word or phrase.
2. Sit quietly in a comfortable position.
3. Close your eyes or focus them gently on a point in front of you.
4. Relax your muscles.
5. Become aware of your breathing, letting the breath come slowly and naturally. Repeat your word or phrase as you exhale.
6. Maintain a passive attitude. If other thoughts come along, gently let them go and turn your attention back to your focus word.
7. Continue for 10 to 20 minutes.

Relaxation Anxiety

Some people experience feelings of anxiety when trying to relax. This may involve a discomfort with "letting go" and a fear they are losing control. Such clients may wish to use healthy pleasures or exercise to reduce stress instead.

People prone to panic attacks may even experience panic when relaxing. If this happens, the client should breathe deeply, stop the practice, and self-calm by doing something "normal," such as reading a book, talking to a friend, or doing some routine household chores.

■ *Morgan has been working with Sam for over 4 months. Sam's slow-but-steady progress with lifestyle change continues. He exercises at the health club twice a week but now often brings his children along, as Morgan urged him to do. The younger one enjoys the free childcare activities, and the older one is starting to work out with his dad. This slows Sam down somewhat, but he feels less stressed about taking time for exercise. Sam and his family have started taking short hikes on the weekend, visiting local parks and rail trails. Sam is enjoying getting outdoors more often and spending more time with his family.*

Sam has also met with the dietitian recommended by his doctor and Morgan, and he is trying to add more fruits and vegetables to his diet. His wife Lisa has gone to these appointments with him, and they are trying to replace salty snacks like potato chips with vegetable sticks and fruit. Sam and Lisa know this change will benefit everyone in the family, not just Sam.

Sam tells Morgan his doctor is pleased with his blood pressure readings. He continues to monitor his blood pressure at home and finds that this reinforces his resolve to leave work at work and enjoy life more. Ironically, deciding to stress less about work has actually improved Sam's work life, and his supervisor praised his more positive attitude during his last performance review.

Morgan reflects on the powerful effect stress has on health, and the benefits of lifestyle change. Morgan has to write a case study for his Stress and Health class and asks Sam's permission to use his story. Sam agrees but only if Morgan will tell him more about what he has learned in class. ■

KEY TERMS

acute stress response

adaptive coping responses

adrenal cortex

adrenal glands

adrenal medulla

adrenocorticotropic hormone (ACTH)

aldosterone

attentional control

burnout

catecholamines

chronic stress response

coping

coping skills

corticosterone

corticotropin-releasing hormone (CRH)

cortisol

cortisone

embolus

emotion-focused coping

epinephrine

eustress

functional connectivity

gingivitis

glucocorticoids

gonadotropin-inhibitory hormone (GnIH)

gonadotropin-releasing hormone (GnRH)

hardiness

hemoconcentration

homeostasis

hypothalamic-pituitary-adrenal (HPA) axis

inflammatory bowel disease (IBD)

irritable bowel syndrome (IBS)

maladaptive coping responses

migraine headache

mineralocorticoids

norepinephrine

oxytocin

peripheral resistance

peristalsis

pituitary gland

plasma

positive reappraisal

problem-focused coping

progressive relaxation

relaxation response

resilience

stress

stress management

stressor

sympathomimetic

tension headache

thrombus

thyrotropic hormone

thyrotropic hormone-
releasing factor (TRF)

thyroxin

Type A Behavior Pattern

Type D personality

ulcer

vasopressin

CRITICAL THINKING QUESTIONS

1. Create a table like Table 6-1. Imagine that you are a college senior worried about finding a job after graduation. List adaptive and maladaptive coping responses for this stressor. Include examples of both problem-focused and emotion-focused coping.

2. A Chinese proverb states, "Where the mind goes, the body follows." Explain how the acute and chronic stress responses might illustrate this proverb.

3. Cardiologist Dean Ornish has said that when he presents his lifestyle-change programs for the treatment of artery disease at medical conferences, his physician colleagues want to discuss the diet and exercise recommendations in detail but are less interested in talking about stress reduction and emotional health. Why do you think it is easier to talk about diet and exercise than stress?

4. Practice the deep breathing or the relaxation-response exercise every day for a week. Describe how the exercise made you feel. Were you able to reduce feelings of stress?

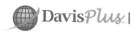 For additional resources log in to Davis*Plus* (**http://davisplus.fadavis.com**/ keyword "Brehm") and click on the Premium tab. (Don't have a *Plus*Code to access Premium Resources? Just click the Purchase Access button on the book's Davis*Plus* page.)

REFERENCES

Adelman, E. M. (2006). Mind-body intelligence: a new perspective integrating Eastern and Western healing traditions. *Holistic Nursing Practice, 20*(3): 147-152.

Anagnostis, P., Athyros, V. G., Tziomalos, K., Karagiannis, A., & Mikhailidis, D. P. (2009). The pathogenic role of cortisol in the metabolic syndrome: a hypothesis. *Journal of Clinical Endocrinology and Metabolism, 94*(8): 2692-2701.

Bennett, M. P., & Lengacher, C. A. (2009). Humor and laughter may influence health. IV. Humor and immune function. *Evidence-Based Complementary and Alternative Medicine, 6*(2): 159-164.

Benson, H. (1975). *The Relaxation Response*. New York: Morrow Press.

Benson, H., with Proctor, W. (1984). *Beyond the Relaxation Response*. New York: Berkeley Books.

Boehm, J., & Kubzansky, L. D. (2012). The heart's content: the association between positive psychological well-being and cardiovascular health. *Psychological Bulletin, 138*: 655-691.

Bohlmeijer, E., Prenger, R., Taal, E., & Cuijpers, P. (2010). The effects of mindfulness-based stress reduction therapy on mental health of adults with a chronic medical disease: a meta-analysis. *Journal of Psychosomatic Research, 68*: 539-544.

Brown, T. M., & Fee, E. (2002). Walter Bradford Cannon: pioneer physiologist of human emotions. *American Journal of Public Health, 92*(10): 1594-1595.

Brunner, E. J., Chandola, T., & Marmot, M. G. (2007). Prospective effect of job strain on general and central obesity in the Whitehall II Study. *American Journal of Epidemiology, 165*(7): 828-837.

Buchgreitz, L., Lyngberg, A. C., Bendtsen, L., & Jensen, R. (2008). Increased pain sensitivity is not a risk factor but a consequence of frequent headache: a population-based follow-up study. *Pain, 137*(3): 623-630.

Cannon, W. B. (1915). *Bodily Changes in Pain, Hunger, Fear, and Rage*. New York: D. Appleton & Co.

Cannon, W. B. (1936). The role of emotions in disease. *Annals of Internal Medicine, 9*: 1453-1465.

Cannon, W. B. (1945). *The Way of an Investigator: A Scientist's Experiences in Medical Research*. New York: W.W. Norton.

Carmody, J., Baer, R. A., Lykins, L. B., & Olendzki, N. (2009). An empirical study of the mechanisms of mindfulness in a mindfulness-based stress reduction program. *Journal of Clinical Psychology, 65*(6): 613-626.

Cathcart, S., Petkov, J., Winefield, A. H., Lushington, K. & Rolan, P. (2010). Central mechanisms of stress-induced headache. *Cephalalgia, 30*(3): 285-295.

Chandola, T., Brunner, E., & Marmot, M. (2006). Chronic stress at work and the metabolic syndrome: prospective study. *British Medical Journal, 332*(7540): 521-525.

Chen, Y. (2009). Advances in the pathophysiology of tension-type headache: from stress to central sensitization. *Current Pain and Headache Reports, 13*(6): 484-494.

Choudhury, B. K., Shi, X.-Z., & Sarna, S. K. (2009). Norepinephrine mediates the transcriptional effects of heterotypic chronic stress on colonic motor function. *American Journal of Physiology: Gastrointestinal and Liver Physiology, 296*(6): GI238-GI247.

Conrad, C. D. (2008). Chronic stress-induced hippocampal vulnerability: the glucocorticoid vulnerability hypothesis. *Reviews in the Neurosciences, 19*(6): 395-411.

Cooper, D. C., Milic, M. S., Mills, P. J., Bardwell, W. A., Ziegler, M. G., & Dimsdale, J. E. (2010). Endothelial function: the impact of objective and subjective socioeconomic status on flow-mediated dilation. *Annals of Behavioral Medicine, 39*(3): 222-231.

Denollet, J., de Jonge, P., Kuyper, A., Schene, A. H., van Melle, J. P., Ormel, J., & Honig, A. (2009). Depression and type D personality represent different forms of distress in the Myocardial INfarction and Depression—Intervention Trial (MIND-IT). *Psychological Medicine, 39*(5): 749-756.

Denollet, J., Rombouts, H., Gillebert, T. C., Rombouts, H., Gillebert, T. C., & Brutsaert, D. L. (1996). Personality as independent predictor of long-term mortality in patients with coronary heart disease. *The Lancet, 347*(8999): 417-421.

Denollet, J., Schiffer, A. A., & Spek, V. (2010). A general propensity to psychological distress affects cardiovascular outcomes. *Circulation: Cardiovascular Quality and Outcomes, 3*(5): 546-557.

Dimsdale, J. E. (2008). Psychological stress and cardiovascular disease. *Journal of the American College of Cardiology, 51*(13): 1237-1246.

Dobkin, P. L., & Zhao, Q. (2011). Increased mindfulness—the active component of the mindfulness-based stress reduction program? *Complementary Therapies in Clinical Practice, 17*(1): 22-27.

Doherty, N. C., Tobias, A., Watson, S., & Atheron, J. C. (2009). The effect of the human gut-signaling hormone, norepinephrine, on the growth of the gastric pathogen *Helicobacter pylori*. *Helicobacter, 14*(3): 223-230.

Esch, T., & Stefano, G. B. (2010). The neurobiology of stress management. *Neuroendocrinology Letters, 31*(1): 19-39.

Flaa, A., Mundal, H. H., Eide, I., Kjeldsen, S., & Rostrup, M. (2006). Sympathetic activity and cardiovascular risk factors in young men in the low, normal, and high blood pressure ranges. *Hypertension, 47*: 396-402.

Fredrickson, B. L., Cohn, M. A., Coffey, K. A., Pek, J., & Finkel, S. M. (2008). Open hearts build lives: positive emotions, induced through loving-kindness meditation, build consequential personal resources. *Journal of Personality and Social Psychology, 95*(5): 1045-1062.

Friedman, M., & Rosenman, R. H. (1974). *Type A Behavior and Your Heart.* Greenwich, CT: Fawcett.

Friedman, M., Thorensen, C. E., Gill, J. J., Powell, L. H., Ulmer, D., Thompson, L., ... Dixon, T. (1984). Alteration of Type A behavior and reduction in cardiac recurrences in postmyocardial infarction patients. *American Heart Journal, 108*(2): 237-248.

Gillespie, C. F., Phifer, J., Bradley, B., & Ressler, K. J. (2009). Risk and resilience: genetic and environmental influences on development of the stress response. *Depression and Anxiety, 26*(11): 984-992.

Greenglass, E. R., & Fiksenbaum, L. (2009). Proactive coping, positive affect, and well-being. *European Psychologist, 14*(1): 20-39.

Hatch, S. L., & Dohrenwend, B. P. (2007). Distribution of traumatic and other stressful events by race/ethnicity, gender, SES, and age: a review of the research. *American Journal of Community Psychology, 40*(3-4): 313-332.

Heraclides, A., Chandola, T., Witte, D., & Brunner, E. J. (2009). Psychosocial stress at work doubles the risk of type 2 diabetes in middle-aged women: evidence from the Whitehall II Study. *Diabetes Care, 32*(12): 2230-2235.

Hunte, H. E. R. (2011). Association between perceived interpersonal everyday discrimination and waist circumference over a 9-year period in the midlife development in the United States Cohort Study. *American Journal of Epidemiology, 173*(11): 1232-1239.

Jacobson, E. (1929). *Progressive Relaxation.* Chicago: University of Chicago Press.

Juster, R.-P., McEwen, B. S., & Lupien, S. J. (2010). Allostatic load biomarkers of chronic stress and impact on health and cognition. *Neuroscience and Biobehavioral Reviews, 35*: 2-16.

Kabat-Zinn, J. (1990). *Full Catastrophe Living: Using the Wisdom of Your Body and Mind to Face Stress, Pain, and Illness.* New York: Delacorte Press.

Katz, M., Liu, C., Schaer, M., Parker, K. J., Ottet, M. C., Epps, A., ... Lyons, D. M. (2009). Prefrontal plasticity and stress inoculation-induced resilience. *Developmental Neuroscience, 31*: 293-299.

Kelly, M. M., Tyrka, A. R., & Anderson, G. M. (2008). Sex differences in emotional and physiological responses to the Trier Social Stress Test. *Journal of Behavior Therapy and Experimental Psychiatry, 39*(1): 87-98.

Kesebir, P., & Diener, E. (2008). In pursuit of happiness: empirical answers to philosophical questions. *Perspectives on Psychological Science, 3*(2): 117-125.

Kirby, E. D., Geraghty, A. C., Ubuka, T., Bentley, G. E., & Kaufer, D. (2009). Stress increases putative gonadotropin inhibitory hormone and decreases luteinizing hormone in male rats. *Proceedings of the National Academy of Science, 106*(27): 11324-11329.

Kobasa, S. C. (1979). Stressful life events, personality, and health—inquiry into hardiness. *Journal of Personality and Social Psychology, 37*(91): 1-11.

Kobasa, S. C., Maddi, S. R., & Kahn, S. (1982). Hardiness and health: A prospective study. *Journal of Personality and Social Psychology, 42*:168-177.

Lazarus, R. S., & Folkman, S. (1984). *Stress, Appraisal, and Coping.* New York: Springer.

Licht, C. M. M., Vreeburg, S. A., van Reedt Dortland, A. K. B., Giltay, E. J., Hoogendijk, W. J. G, DeRijk, R. H., ... Penninx, B. W. J. H. (2010). Increased sympathetic and decreased parasympathetic activity rather than changes in hypothalamic-pituitary-adrenal axis activity is associated with metabolic abnormalities. *Journal of Clinical Endocrinology and Metabolism, 95*(5): 2458-2466.

Liston, C., McEwen, B. S., & Casey, B. J. (2009). Psychosocial stress reversibly disrupts prefrontal processing and attentional control. *Proceedings of the National Academy of Science, 106*(3): 912-917.

Lupien, S. J., McEwen, B. S., Gunnar, M. R., & Heim, C. (2009). Effects of stress throughout the lifespan on the brain, behaviour and cognition. *Nature Reviews Neuroscience, 10*: 434-445.

Lynch, J. J. (1977). *The Broken Heart: The Medical Consequences of Loneliness.* New York: Basic Books.

Lynch, J. J. (2000). *A Cry Unheard: New Insights into the Medical Consequences of Loneliness.* Baltimore: Bancroft Press.

MacDermott, D. (2010). Psychological hardiness and meaning making as protection against sequelae in veterans of the wars in Iraq and Afghanistan. *International Journal of Emergency Mental Health, 12*(3): 199-206.

Maddi, S. R. (2004). Hardiness: an operationalization of existential courage. *Journal of Humanistic Psychology, 44*(3): 279-298.

Maddi, S. R., Khoshaba, D. M., Harvey, R. H., Fazel, M., & Resurreccion, N. (2011). The personality construct of hardiness, V: relationships with the construction of existential meaning in life. *Journal of Humanistic Psychology, 51*(3): 369-388.

Manabe, N., Tanaka, T., Hata, J., Kusunoki, H., & Haruma, K. (2009). Pathophysiology underlying irritable bowel syndrome: from the viewpoint of dysfunction of autonomic nervous system activity. *Journal of Smooth Muscle Research, 45*(1): 15-23.

Marmot, M. G., Rose, G., Shipley, M., & Hamilton, P. J. (1978). Employment grade and coronary heart disease for British civil servants. *Journal of Epidemiology and Community Health, 32*(4): 244-249.

Marziali, E., McDonald, L., & Donahue, P. (2008). The role of coping humor in the physical and mental health of older adults. *Aging and Mental Health, 12*(6): 713-718.

Maunder, R. G., & Levenstein, S. (2008). The role of stress in the development and clinical course of inflammatory bowel disease: epidemiological evidence. *Current Molecular Medicine, 8*(4): 247-252.

McEwen, B. A., & Gianaros, P. J. (2010). Central role of the brain in stress and adaptation: links to socioeconomic status, health, and disease. *Annals of the New York Academy of Sciences, 1186*: 190-222.

McLean, C. P., & Anderson, E. R. (2009). Brave men and timid women? A review of the gender differences in fear and anxiety. *Clinical Psychological Review, 29*(6): 496-505.

Miller, G. E., Cohen, S., & Ritchey, A. K. (2002). Chronic psychological stress and the regulation of pro-inflammatory cytokines: a glucocorticoid resistance model. *Health Psychology, 21*(6): 531-541.

Miller, G. E., Rohleder, N., & Cole, S. W. (2009). Chronic interpersonal stress predicts activation of pro- and anti-inflammatory signaling pathways 6 months later. *Psychosomatic Medicine, 71*(1): 57-62.

Nation, D. A., Hong, S., Jak, A. J., Delano-Wood, L., Mills, P. J., Bondi, M. W., & Dimsdale, J. E. (2011). Stress, exercise, and Alzheimer's disease: a neurovascular pathway. *Medical Hypotheses, 76*(6): 847-854.

Ornish, D. (1998). *Love and Survival: 8 Pathways to Intimacy and Health*. New York: HarperCollins.

Pace, T. W. W., Hu, F., & Miller, A. H. (2007). Cytokine-effects on glucocorticoid receptor function: relevance to glucocorticoid resistance and the pathophysiology and treatment of major depression. *Brain, Behavior, and Immunity, 21*(1): 9-19.

Pace, T. W. W., Negi, L. T., Adame, D. D., Cole, S. P., Sivilli, T. I., Brown, T. D., ... Raison, C. L. (2009). Effect of compassion meditation on neuroendocrine, innate immune and behavioral responses to psychosocial stress. *Psychoneuroendocrinology, 34*: 87-98.

Palatini, P., Longo, D., Zaetta, V., Perkovic, D., Garbelotto, R., & Pessina, A. C. (2006). Evolution of blood pressure and cholesterol in stage 1 hypertension: role of autonomic nervous system activity. *Journal of Hypertension, 24*: 1375-1381.

Pedersen, A. F., Zachariae, R., & Bovbjerg, D. H. (2009). Psychological stress and antibody response to influenza vaccination: a meta-analysis. *Brain, Behavior, and Immunity, 23*(4): 427-433.

Qi, D., & Rodrigues, B. (2007). Glucocorticoids produce whole body insulin resistance with changes in cardiac metabolism. *American Journal of Physiology: Endocrinology and Metabolism, 292*(3): E654-E667.

Rosania, A. E., Low, K. G., McCormick, C. M., & Rosania, D. A. (2009). Stress, depression, cortisol, and periodontal disease. *Journal of Periodontology, 80*(2): 260-266.

Rosengren, A., Hawken, S., Ounpuu, S., Sliwa, K., Zubaid, M., Almahmeed, W. A., ... the INTERHEART Investigators. (2004). Association of psychosocial risk factors with risk of acute myocardial infarction in 11,119 cases and 13,646 controls from 52 countries (the INTERHEART study): case–control study. *The Lancet, 364*(9438): 953-962.

Rosenman, R. H., Brand, R. J., Jenkins, C. D., Friedman, M., Straus, R., & Wurm, M. (1975). Coronary heart disease in the Western Collaborative Group Study: final follow-up of 8 1/2 years. *Journal of the American Medical Association, 233*: 872-877.

Saastamoinen, P., Laaksonen, M., Leino-Arjas, P., & Lahelma, E. (2009). Psychosocial risk factors of pain among employees. *European Journal of Pain, 13*(1): 102-108.

Sauro, K. M., & Becker, W. J. (2009). The stress and migraine interaction. *Headache, 49*(9): 1378-1386.

Seligman, M. E. P. (2006). *Learned Optimism: How to Change Your Mind and Your Life*. New York: Vintage Books.

Seligman, M. E. P. (2008). Positive health. *Applied Psychology, 57*(S1): 3-18.

Selye, H. (1936). A syndrome produced by diverse nocuous agents. *Nature, 138*: 32.

Selye, H. (1956). *The Stress of Life*. New York: McGraw-Hill.

Selye, H. (1982). History and present status of the stress concept. In: Goldberg, L., & Breznitz, S., eds. *Handbook of Stress: Theoretical and Clinical Aspects*. New York: Free Press.

Sherman, K. J., Cherkin, D. C., Erro, J., Miglioretti, D. L., & Deyo, R. A. (2005). Comparing yoga, exercise, and a self-care book for chronic low back pain: a randomized, controlled trial. *Annals of Internal Medicine, 143*(12): 849-857.

Smeets, T., Dziobek, I., & Wolf, O. T. (2009). Social cognition under stress: differential effects of stress-induced cortisol elevations in healthy young men and women. *Hormones and Behavior, 55*(4): 507-513.

Smitha, B. W., Tooleya, E. M., Christophera, P. J., & Kay, V. S. (2010). Resilience as the ability to bounce back from stress: a neglected personal resource? *Journal of Positive Psychology, 5*(3): 166-176.

Steptoe, A., & Brydon, L. (2005). Associations between acute lipid stress responses and fasting lipid levels 3 years later. *Metabolism, 25*:601-607.

Strine, T. W., Kroenke, K., Dhingra, S., Balluz, L. S., Gonzalez, O. & Berry, J. T. (2009). The associations between depression, health-related quality of life, social support, life satisfaction, and disability in community-dwelling U.S. adults. *Journal of Nervous and Mental Disease, 19*(1): 61-64.

Talley, N. J., DeVault, K. R., & Fleischer, D. E. (2010). Esophageal motility disorders. In: Talley, N. J., DeVault, K. R., & Fleischer, D. E., eds. *Practical Gastroenterology and Hepatology: Esophagus and Stomach*. West Sussex, UK: Blackwell Publishing.

Tavassoli, S. (2009). Yoga in the management of irritable bowel syndrome. *International Journal of Yoga Therapy, 19*(1): 97-101.

Taylor, S. E., Klein, L. C., Lewis, B. P., Gruenewald, T. L., Gurung, R. A., & Updegraff, J. A. (2000). Biobehavioral responses to stress in females: tend-and-befriend, not fight-or-flight. *Psychological Review, 107*(3): 411-429.

Thoits, P. A. (2010). Stress and health: major findings and policy implications. *Journal of Health and Social Behavior, 51*(suppl 1): S41-S53.

Vialou, V., Robison, A. J., LaPlant, Q. C., Covington, H. E., 3rd, Dietz, D. M., Ohnishi, Y. N., ... Nestler, E. J. (2010). ΔFosB in brain reward circuits mediates resilience to stress and antidepressant responses. *Nature Neuroscience, 13*: 745-752.

Vicario, M., Alonso, C., Guilarte, M., Serra, J., Martínez, C., González-Castro, A. M., ... Santos, J. (2012). Chronic psychosocial stress induces reversible mitochondrial damage and corticotropin-releasing factor receptor type-1 upregulation in the rat intestine and IBS-like gut dysfunction. *Psychoneuroendocrinology, 37*(1): 65-77.

Virtanen, M., Singh-Manoux, A., Ferrie, J. E., Gimeno, D., Marmot, M. G., Elovainio, M., ... Kivimäki, M. (2009). Long working hours and cognitive function: the Whitehall II Study. *American Journal of Epidemiology, 169*(5): 596-605.

von Känel, R., Kudlelka, B. M., Haeberli, A., Stutz, M., Fischer, J. E., & Patterson, S. M. (2009). Prothrombic changes with acute psychological stress: combined effect of hemoconcentration and genuine coagulation activation. *Thrombosis Research, 123*(4): 622-630.

Williams, R. B. (2008). Psychosocial and biobehavioral factors and their interplay in coronary heart disease. *Annual Review of Clinical Psychology, 4*: 349-365.

CHAPTER OUTLINE

LEARNING OBJECTIVES

After reading this chapter, you will be able to:

1. Describe the concepts of cultural sensitivity and cultural competence.

2. Explain some of the variables that help clarify the relationship between socioeconomic status (SES) and health.

3. Summarize the reasons that poverty is associated with an increased risk for obesity.

4. Discuss how spirituality and religion may affect health.

5. Explain some of the important factors that affect health and behavior for children and adolescents.

6. Describe some of the ways in which pregnancy influences behavior-change recommendations.

7. Suggest motivational strategies that might be helpful for new parents and other adults struggling with work and parenting responsibilities.

8. List several factors that affect behavior-change recommendations for midlife and older adults.

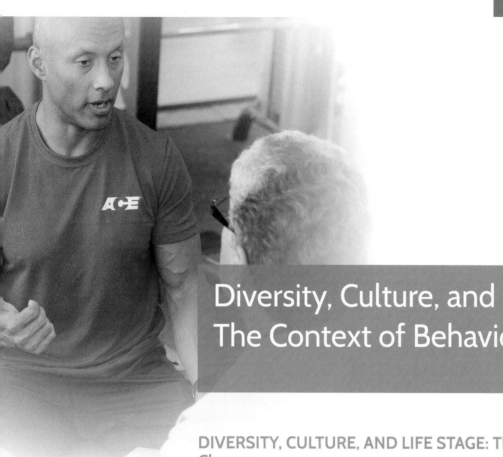

CHAPTER 7

Diversity, Culture, and Life Stage: The Context of Behavior Change

DIVERSITY, CULTURE, AND LIFE STAGE: The Context of Behavior Change

Katie has just graduated with a master's degree in athletic training. She worked as a graduate assistant in the athletic training facility at her university for the past year, and now the head athletic trainer has hired her for a summer job. The athletic training facility provides consultation and treatment services to a number of summer programs each year. These include youth sport camps as well as summer fitness programs for adults of all ages, including an alumni group with participants as old as 90. Katie is excited to begin her new job and hopes that working with a wider variety of people this summer will expand her skills. She is a little nervous, though, as up to this point she has only worked with college athletes.

The first program begins tomorrow. It is a soccer program for high-school-aged teens from immigrant families in the area, many of whom are refugees from various countries in Africa, Southeast Asia, and Eastern Europe. Most have only spoken English for a year or two. In addition to working with the athletes who become injured during the program, Katie is going to teach an injury-prevention program for the group. She decides to make the program mostly demonstration and participation, with only a little talking. ■

213

Behavior-change recommendations are most effective when they are individualized for specific clients. Just as no two people are alike, so no two sets of behavior-change recommendations will be identical. Health and fitness professionals must craft recommendations that take into consideration the many details of clients' lives. The greater the ability of health and fitness professionals to communicate and work effectively with a wide range of clients, the more successful they will be in promoting positive health-behavior change.

Many countries, including the United States and Canada, are home to diverse collections of people. In this context, diverse describes groups of people that are different from each other. Groups of people can be diverse in many ways. One of the most noticeable ways in which people differ from one another is in terms of their countries and cultures of origin. Sometimes these differences are manifest in appearance and speech. Diversity is also seen in how long people have lived in their present locations. For example, two people whose families were originally from the same country will be very different from each other if one has recently arrived in the new country, whereas the other has been there for several decades. People differ in ethnicity, color, national origin, religion, education level, SES, gender, sexual orientation, age, size, disability, and in many other ways. Health and fitness professionals observe diversity in motor skill ability, athletic background, and fitness levels in their clients. All of these factors influence health behavior and the motivations that influence behavior change.

Communication about health and behavior change can lead to misunderstanding, even when the people communicating have similar cultural backgrounds. It becomes even more complex when the people communicating are from very different cultures. Language is not the only problem. Cultural expectations regarding health and fitness professionals, gender roles, appropriate behaviors in certain settings, and even body language can cause people to misinterpret what others are saying and doing.

This chapter presents an overview of a few of the most important ways in which culture affects health and health behavior and how health and fitness professionals can learn to work appropriately with people from other cultures and backgrounds. The first part of this chapter also explores the complex relationship between SES and health and the many variables that may influence this relationship. A special section on poverty, obesity, and health will help health and fitness professionals gain some understanding of how SES influences obesity. This chapter also looks at the relationships among spirituality, religion, and health.

Everyone can attest that working with a 7-year-old is different from working with a 17-year-old. People who are 27 generally have different psychological and physical health issues than people who are 57. Developmental stage influences people's physical abilities, psychological traits, and life priorities. The second half of this chapter reviews some of the considerations that may arise at various stages throughout the life span and how these influence client motivation and the work of health and fitness professionals.

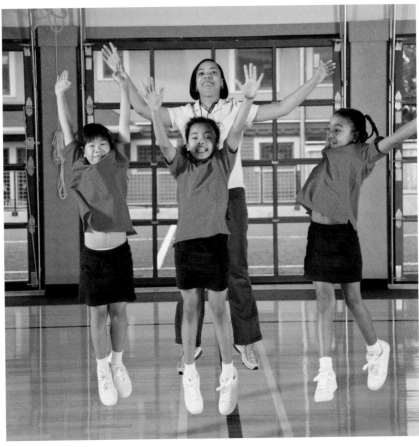

© Thinkstock

CULTURE, DIVERSITY, AND BEHAVIOR CHANGE

Cultural norms and values shape the salient variables found in most models of health behavior. These norms and values also influence people's perceptions of illness and health and their beliefs regarding their susceptibility to health problems. Cultural influences also contribute to people's feelings of self-efficacy regarding health-behavior change. Culture contributes to the formation of health behaviors themselves: what people eat, how they perceive physical activities, how they regulate emotions, and how they perceive and cope with stress (Health Psychology in Your Life 7-1). Cultural norms and values influence perceptions of body size and ideas regarding physical attractiveness and body image. Culture influences how people interpret symptoms and the meaning of illness.

Purnell and Paulanka (2008) define culture as "the totality of socially transmitted behavioral patterns, arts, beliefs, values, customs, lifeways, and all other products of human work and thought characteristics of a population of people that guide their worldview and decision making." Cultural beliefs and practices surround a baby at birth and develop in people throughout their lives. Culture is acquired at both conscious and subconscious levels. Culture influences all health behaviors, including physical activity, eating habits, stress patterns, and substance use (Fig. 7-1).

A critical point to remember is that although cultural forces create differences between cultural groups, the variation within a given group is often greater than differences between groups. This means that health and fitness professionals can never make assumptions about a given client based on cultural background. Health and fitness professionals must meet each client as an individual, without letting stereotypes and prejudice interfere with the relationship (Health Psychology at Work 7-1).

Cultural Sensitivity and Cultural Competence

Individuals often take their own cultural beliefs for granted and assume that their way of seeing things is the right way. They may even assume that others have the same beliefs or feel superior to people who don't share those beliefs. When health and fitness professionals have incorrect assumptions about clients or feelings of superiority to clients, barriers to effective communication emerge. Health and fitness professionals and clients may not understand one another, and clients feel insulted, judged, and then unmotivated to consider the professional's recommendations.

People exhibit cultural awareness when they notice the external signs indicating that another person may be from a different cultural background. That person may look different, dress or speak differently, or have different mannerisms. People also exhibit cultural awareness by not assuming that another person shares their background, even though no visible signs suggest a difference. People show cultural sensitivity when they are not only aware of others' cultural differences but they also try to behave in ways that do not offend others. A culturally sensitive person appreciates the importance of diversity and the implications of diversity for interactions with others. People with cultural sensitivity realize that another person's values and beliefs may differ from their own, and they are careful not to make assumptions about that person. Health and fitness professionals should continually work to increase both their cultural awareness and sensitivity, especially regarding the groups with whom they often work.

Health and fitness professionals who frequently work with clients from particular cultural groups may have the opportunity to develop cultural competence. Cultural competence means having the knowledge and skills to interact with people from another culture in culturally appropriate ways. Health and fitness professionals who are culturally competent are able to incorporate clients' cultural beliefs and practices into behavior-change recommendations. Culturally competent professionals know how to "fit in" and communicate effectively with people from the target group (Rose, 2010).

All health and fitness professionals should strive to develop cultural sensitivity, so that they do not offend clients with whom they work. Cultural sensitivity is important not only for dealing with people from other cultural and religious backgrounds but also for being aware of how people with any kind of difference might perceive another. Health and fitness professionals

HEALTH PSYCHOLOGY IN YOUR LIFE 7-1.
How Culture Shapes Beliefs About Physical Activity

Explain how your own beliefs about physical activity have been influenced by your culture, including beliefs you have adopted from your family, school, and community. If you have received different messages from different people that you consider to be part of your culture, describe. In particular, what does your culture teach about the importance of physical activity? What are the goals of physical activity? How do people in your culture view the relationship between physical activity and health?

If you know someone from a cultural background different from yours, ask him or her to explore these questions. How did this person's answers differ from yours? You might also get different answers from a classmate of the opposite sex or someone much older than you.

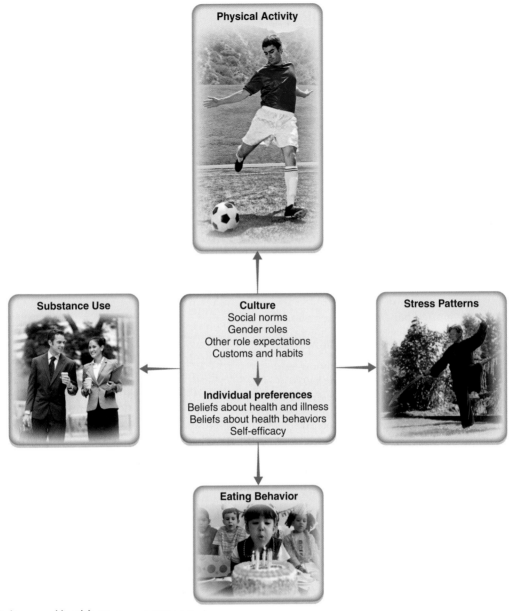

Figure 7-1. Culture and health. Photograph © Thinkstock

HEALTH PSYCHOLOGY AT WORK 7-1. Cultivating Youth Resilience in Resource-Poor Environments

Ashley Niles, M.A.T., has worked with disadvantaged adolescents and youth in a variety of behavior-change contexts. She has led wilderness-backpacking trips for adolescents with behavior disorders, helping them to redefine themselves and build self-efficacy as they face and grow from challenging experiences. Niles also worked for a year with AmeriCorps, serving as Youth Services and Activities Coordinator for a transitional living program that helped 18- to 21-year-olds who were homeless or at risk of becoming homeless. She planned and taught life skills courses to help these young adults acquire the knowledge and skills needed to transition from this residential program to independent living. During Niles's graduate work, she served at an exciting youth-development after-school program called Project Coach. Project Coach works with community leaders to address the needs of children and teens. Rather than viewing youth as a "problem to be managed," Project Coach seeks to develop youth as a community resource. Project Coach teaches high school students in economically disadvantaged areas of Springfield, Massachusetts, to be sport coaches and to organize youth-sports programs for third-, fourth-, and fifth-grade children in their neighborhoods. In addition to learning how to coach sports, the high school students provide literacy tutoring for their young

HEALTH PSYCHOLOGY AT WORK 7-1. Cultivating Youth Resilience in Resource-Poor Environments—cont'd

athletes to help them succeed in school. Although Niles is from a rural community many miles away from the Project Coach schools, she is able to work effectively in this diverse community.

"The challenge of working with people different from myself is not knowing what to expect. You can read all the literature you want about your target population and still be totally surprised. You can't assume anything. I never go into this work assuming I know a person's story. Instead, I work to create relationships that let people teach me about themselves and about their lives. This takes time, and being open, day after day.

"What helps kids change? Providing them with experiences that develop life skills and show them what more they can be. Creating connections—these kids don't know what resources are available to help them get through school, get job training, and even get into college. Positive role models, so the kids can see different ways of living. And having a safe place in a community where they feel like they belong.

"It can be discouraging to work intensely with kids and then watch life circumstances overwhelm your efforts. But you have to keep trying. The students in Project Coach come from environments where it is normal to not attend school, to get bad grades, and drop out of school. Family problems, health issues, crime, and chaotic lives create real barriers to healthy development. Project Coach runs an after-school Coaching Academy for these high school students and closely monitors their academic performance, encouraging the kids to stay in school so they graduate. The Coaching Academy teaches skills the teens need as student coaches and as people: communication skills, self-awareness, conflict resolution, group management, time management, and study skills. We hope that the project will help some of these kids be more successful in school and in life and that they in turn can help the younger kids in their communities.

"This work is very rewarding and meaningful to me. Adolescence is rarely an easy time. It can be especially difficult for disadvantaged kids. I love being able to guide someone through those years, especially someone from an underserved community or someone with a lack of family support. This kind of work can really make a difference in a young person's life. Much of what I strive for in working with adolescents is to create a safe space while providing them with challenging experiences that will foster growth and change.

"My advice for people considering work in youth development: Be sure you are going into this work for the right reasons. Don't go in thinking you have all the answers, and you are going to change their world. You must work to build strong relationships with people. You do that by being open-minded and willing to learn from people about their lives and what they need. Young people don't need more people telling them what is wrong with their life; they need mentors who can lead them to a state of well-being."

References on Project Coach:

Smith College. Project Coach. http://projectcoach.smith.edu/. Accessed 7/5/12.

Intrator, S. M., & Siegel, D. (2010). Project Coach: a case study of a college-community partnership as a venture in social entrepreneurship. *Perspectives on Urban Education, 7*(1), 66-72.

Intrator, S. M., & Siegel, D. (2008). Project Coach: youth development and academic achievement through sport. *Journal of Physical Education, Recreation, and Dance, 79*(7), 17-23.

show cultural sensitivity when they dress more modestly at work than they might among their peers or when they take clients' dietary restrictions into account when ordering food for an event. Box 7-1 highlights some of the most important ways in which health and fitness professionals can demonstrate cultural sensitivity and avoid offending the clients with whom they work.

Immigrant Cultures

Cultural sensitivity can be especially challenging when health and fitness professionals are working with clients who have recently moved from other countries. Both the United States and Canada have a long history of serving as a destination for people

leaving other countries. In the United States, as of 2010 about 12.9% of residents are foreign born. And about 20.1% speak a language other than English at home (U.S. Census Bureau, 2011). Over half of the immigrants arriving in the United States come from the Americas, especially Mexico, but also El Salvador, Cuba, and other countries. About one-fourth emigrate from Asian countries, including India, the Philippines, China, Vietnam, and South Korea. About one-eighth move from European countries, and only about 4% come from Africa (Fig. 7-2).

In Canada, 19.8% of residents were foreign born in 2006 (Statistics Canada, 2006). Over 40% of immigrants are originally from countries in Asia, including China, India, the Philippines, the Hong Kong region of China, and Vietnam. About 37% are from Europe,

Box 7-1. Cultural Sensitivity in Action

Health and fitness professionals who try to display professional behavior at all times will be less likely to offend clients and coworkers, whether from another country or the house next door. Making a good first impression is especially important, when clients are initially forming an opinion of the professional. Some of the more common issues requiring cultural sensitivity include the following.

Attire: Young people often dress casually. Students on college campuses may spend much of their day in sweatpants, shorts, and athletic apparel. Such attire may be perceived by some people (including potential employers) as sloppy and too casual. In addition, fitness center attire is often quite revealing, as skintight clothes may be recommended so that instructors can correct problems with body position and alignment. People from more conservative backgrounds may be offended by what they perceive as a lack of modesty. Health and fitness professionals should develop an appropriate wardrobe for their work lives, seeking direction from supervisors regarding work expectations. Those who work with people from cultures who value modesty would do well to choose less-revealing clothing. Professionals, especially women, who often work with people from another culture may wish to learn about specific areas that should be covered, such as the shoulders, upper arms, and thighs.

Formality of professional–client interactions: When meeting a new client, it is better to err on the side of being a little too formal than too informal. North Americans often begin new relationships, even with people much older than themselves, on a first-name basis. Professionals should learn about their clients' preferences here. Treating clients more politely and formally may be seen as more professional. People from many cultures expect a relationship more formal in tone when working with a professional. For example, professionals should use a title and last name to address clients: Mr. Diaz or Mrs. Wu. The health and fitness professional can be friendly and formal at the same time, conveying sincere interest and respect.

Physical contact: Many clients are uncomfortable with physical contact for numerous reasons. An introductory handshake is usually fine, although even shaking hands may be awkward for some people, especially people of the opposite sex, if they are from cultures where contact between men and women is strictly proscribed. If this may be the case, health and fitness professionals should check with their coworkers about these situations. Professionals who need to touch clients as part of assessment or training should explain these procedures ahead of time and ask permission before proceeding. Even people culturally similar to professionals may not want to be touched, for a variety of personal reasons.

Voice and speech: If English (or whatever language is chosen for communication) is a foreign language for clients, health and fitness professionals should speak a little more slowly and clearly. Many young people have to make a real effort to slow their speech. A translator should be available if clients and professionals do not speak a common language. Health and fitness professionals should modulate speech volume. Others frequently stereotype Americans as talking too loudly and aggressively. People from other cultures are often more soft spoken. Professionals should also avoid peppering their speech with empty words such as "like" and "you know."

Pace of conversation: When working with clients from very different backgrounds, health and fitness professionals may want to slow the pace of the conversation to be sure of clarity. They should paraphrase more often to ensure that they are understanding their clients. The OARS communication skills described in Chapter 5 work well when professionals and clients differ in background. Health and fitness professionals should not force clients to answer questions quickly. If clients don't understand the question, or are reluctant to answer, they may just pretend to agree or say what they think is the right answer, rather than sharing important information. Professionals should give clients enough time to think and to speak. Slowing the pace of conversation gives clients more time to ask questions.

including the U.K., Italy, Germany, and Poland. More than 15% are from the Americas. And approximately 6% come from Africa, especially Egypt, Morocco, South Africa, and Algeria.

Cultural ideas and values influence how clients perceive their own health behaviors and the fitness professionals with whom they work. Health and fitness professionals working with clients from other cultures should try to find out as much as they can about that culture. What is the best way to learn about another culture? First, health and fitness professionals should

talk to supervisors and coworkers who are already working in the setting, asking about the challenges involved and seeking advice on working and communicating effectively. Second, professionals may find helpful literature on cultural competency for their target clients. For example, the U.S. Centers for Disease Control and Prevention website (CDC, 2012b) has helpful materials for working with a number of different immigrant groups. These ethnographic guides were originally developed for health workers diagnosing and treating tuberculosis but they are applicable in any

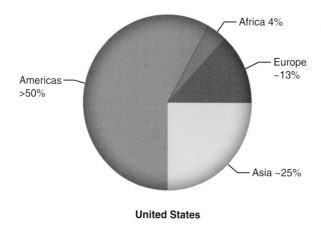

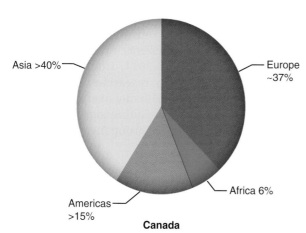

Figure 7-2. Area of origin for foreign-born residents of the United States and Canada.

health-education context. The Australian government has also produced brief, readable guides to the immigrant groups common in Australia, many of whom have also made homes in North America (Queensland Government, 2011). Books on a variety of cultural groups are also available (Purnell & Paulanka, 2008). Although many of these were written for health-care professionals, they provide pertinent information on cultural beliefs and practices related to health and health behaviors.

When working with clients from other cultures, health and fitness professionals should observe and listen with an open mind and note how clients behave. They should also remember that the variation in beliefs and behaviors among members of a given group is far larger than variations among groups. Having some idea of a client's cultural background may help professionals avoid the most egregious errors and be ready to incorporate cultural preferences into behavior-change recommendations, as appropriate. But professionals should still be guided in their recommendations by the health, fitness, hopes, and dreams of each individual client.

■ *On the second day of the program, one of the coaches brings in a boy, Nikola, who is hopping on one foot, leaning heavily on the coach. The 14-year-old has suffered an ankle sprain. Nikola has already been taken to the hospital, and x-rays showed no broken bones. The ankle is swollen and painful. As she gives Nikola a bag of ice, Katie tries to explain that caring for the ankle is very important and that failure to treat the ankle may jeopardize Nikola's sport participation this fall. She asks Nikola if he understands; he smiles and nods but does not say much. After the ice treatment, Katie shows Nikola how to wrap his ankle with the elastic bandage, not too tight and not too loose. As Katie watches him, she sees he is wrapping his ankle too tightly. She makes him take it off and start over. He is impatient to join his friends but he finally succeeds on his third attempt. He hurries out of the athletic training facility on a pair of crutches; Katie hopes he has understood her directions to stay off the foot for a few days and to continue icing.*

Nikola is out of practice and games for the rest of the program, although he enjoys the social events. Katie works with him twice a day in the athletic training facility, teaching him exercises to strengthen the ankle. Hopefully, it will be strong enough for him to play soccer this fall. After his initial enthusiasm for the BAPS (balance) board, Nikola quickly tires of the exercises. Katie is worried that he will neglect the rehabilitation instructions she has so carefully worked up for him. She would like to go over them with Nikola's mother, but she never comes to the program, as Nikola takes the bus with a friend. Katie asks her supervisor, Dan, the head athletic trainer, for advice on how to be sure Nikola receives adequate follow-up care after the program is over. He compliments Katie on the thoroughness of the instructions she has written up and gives her the name and address of Nikola's regular youth soccer coach. Hopefully, the coach will help Nikola return to play at the right time. ■

Socioeconomic Status and Health

Much has been written about the relationship between SES and health. SES itself is a complex variable and includes influence from a person's income level, employment variables, and education level (Adler & Stewart, 2010). SES also strongly influences where people may live and thus the services available in the community, the types of restaurants and food markets to which people have access, and the schools that their children attend. SES appears to influence health and health behaviors through a complex interaction of many factors.

Culture, Socioeconomic Status, Ethnicity, and Health Disparities

Chapter 6 discussed some of the results from the Whitehall Studies, which found that workers in lower employment categories in the U.K. experienced a greater incidence of stress-related illness, including obesity, type 2 diabetes, hypertension, and cardiovascular disease. U.S. health statistics often examine health data by race/ethnic group. In these data, rates of morbidity and premature mortality often differ with race/ethnic group category (U.S. Department of Health and Human Services, 2010). For example, within the United States, rates of cardiovascular (CV) disease and rates of CV disease risk factors differ significantly by racial and ethnic group (Kurian & Cardarelli, 2007). The independent effect of race/ethnic group can be confounded by the influence of SES and its associated variables, such as income, education level, neighborhood, school environments, and access to/quality of medical care. In other words, whereas race/ethnic group may exert independent effects on health, many of the observed discrepancies may be caused by these other variables alone, or in combination with race/ethnicity. It is important to note that many health sociologists have proposed that the use of race/ethnic categories in the analysis of health data has both risks and benefits (Box 7-2). For this reason, Canada does not currently collect data on patients' ethnicity in most health-care contexts. Some of the variables that may contribute to health disparities among groups are shown in Fig. 7-3.

Perceived Stress

Level of perceived stress is one of the most salient factors that may at least partially explain links among SES, race/ethnicity, and health (Thoits, 2010). Chronic, uncontrollable stress exerts strong biological effects on human physiology, as explained in Chapter 6, mediated by the nervous, endocrine, and immune systems (Miller, Chen, & Cole, 2009). Exposure to chronic stress often varies with life circumstances, and these circumstances may be influenced by SES and race/ethnicity. Life circumstances are also influenced by other variables such as gender and marital status. Different stress loads can contribute to health disparities. Minority groups experience the additional stress of discrimination (Hunte, 2011; Hunter & Schmidt, 2010). Stress and health researcher Peggy Thoits explains that "stressors proliferate over the life course and across generations, widening gaps between advantaged and disadvantaged group members" (Thoits, 2010).

Box 7-2. Examining Health With Racial and Ethnic Categories: Helpful or Harmful?

Race and ethnicity are both socially constructed categories, rather than biologically defined descriptors. Race refers to groups defined by physically visible differences that are biologically inherited, such as skin color and type of hair. Race is not biologically defined, as separate genetic races do not exist. So, whereas the physical characteristics on which concepts of race are based have biological roots, race itself does not (Bradby, 2012). The concept of race, however, and assigning people to groups based on certain distinguishing characteristics have a long history, usually resulting in discrimination on many levels. Ideas of race and racial categories affect people's assessment and treatment of each other. Thus, racial categories often exert an influence on health.

Ethnicity refers to a cultural group, defined by factors such as language, country of origin, religion, family ethnic identification, or other cultural categories. Because racial and cultural categories can overlap, the United States and other countries often combine race and ethnicity together in the term "racial/ethnic group."

Various countries, including the United States, use racial and/or ethnic categories to examine public-health data. Countries following this practice hope that by studying differences among groups, experts will be able to discern important patterns in health and thus target prevention and treatment methods more effectively. They also hope that by bringing health disparities among groups into the public eye, measures can be taken to correct these disparities and improve the health of disadvantaged groups.

Critics of this practice argue that since race and ethnicity are social constructions that perpetuate the idea that groups differ significantly from one another, using these categories further stereotypes groups and the individuals in them (Proctor, Kurmeich, & Meershoek, 2011). For example, when medical research finds that Caucasians have higher rates of depression than other groups, will all Caucasians be seen as fragile and vulnerable neurotics? If public-health professionals find that rates of HIV infection are higher in certain groups, will everyone in those groups be stigmatized? Does the use of racial and ethnic categories perpetuate the very discrimination that public-health experts hope to fight?

As more is learned about the relationship of race and ethnicity to specific health variables, it is likely that researchers will uncover the underlying variables, such as SES, access to employment, educational background, and so forth that are more closely related to health. And, while it is true that certain genetic markers are associated with disease risk and that these markers may be more common in certain groups, genetic testing should eventually supersede racial/ethnic categorization for helping people understand their personal disease-risk profile.

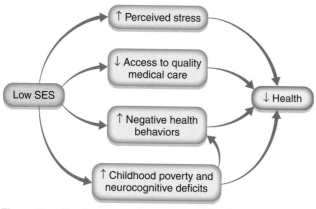

Figure 7-3. Socioeconomic status and health.

Medical Care: Access and Quality

Public-health experts have wondered whether some of the health discrepancies observed among racial/ethnic groups in the United States might be caused by variations in access to medical care. Access to medical care does vary greatly in most countries and especially in the United States. Researcher Ichiro Kawachi believes that access to medical care might be part of the explanation for health disparities among groups but cautions that more important to keep in mind is that disparities in access to health care reflect disparities in access to jobs, income, credit, and education (Kawachi, 2005). Even in countries with universal health care, one finds disparities in the quality of medical care and the geographic distribution of medical facilities and caregivers. Kawachi argues that the social determinants of health include access to safe neighborhoods and employment, lack of discrimination, and "full participation in the life of communities" (Kawachi, 2005).

Research suggests that patients with minority status are more likely to be pleased with the health care they receive when their provider is of the same race or ethnic background (Saha, Komaromy, Koepsell, & Bindman, 1999). In one study, African American patients reported better care if their physician was also African American. Similarly, Hispanic patients reported better care if their physician was Hispanic. This study reinforces the importance of increasing diversity within the ranks of health-care providers.

Researchers have also explored whether some health discrepancies could result from differences in advice and treatment received from health-care providers. The Institute of Medicine of the National Academies has issued a number of reports on disparities in health care. Variations in health are apparent from life expectancy statistics. For example, life expectancy at birth is about 6 years longer for white men than for African American men (Institute of Medicine, 2011). Although some of this difference may be related to stressful life circumstances, as discussed above, the report found that in many instances, minorities may receive less aggressive treatment for certain illnesses and thus have higher

mortality rates. In addition, minorities sometimes harbor distrust toward the medical establishment and seek care later in the course of illness, when fewer effective treatment options are available.

Variations in advice received within racial/ethnic groups appear to be as great as differences in health advice received between groups. For example, one study found that for a group of adults recently diagnosed with type 2 diabetes, recommendations on behavior change (diet and exercise) were similar across racial/ethnic groups (Gavin, Fox, & Grandy, 2011). However, in all groups, only about half of the patients reported that providers told them exercise would be helpful. In this study, reported intentions varied somewhat among groups, with slightly more minorities reporting an intention to follow exercise recommendations than Caucasians. Actual exercise behaviors were not examined. This study underscores the observation that advice from health-care providers varies widely in all population groups and that health and fitness professionals cannot make assumptions about clients based on their ethnic backgrounds.

Health Behavior

Some researchers have explored whether differences in health behavior might partly explain the effect of SES on health. A longitudinal study of the Whitehall subjects suggests that some of the health disparities observed among people of different socioeconomic groups may indeed be due to differences in health behaviors (Stringhini et al., 2010). The investigators monitored four health behaviors over 24 years and looked at the associations between these behaviors and causes of death. The four health behaviors were smoking, alcohol consumption, diet, and physical activity. Subjects with the lowest SES experienced all-cause mortality rates 60% higher than those of subjects in the highest SES group. Health behaviors explained about 72% of this discrepancy, according to the researchers. Smoking explained about 35% of mortality differences, physical inactivity 21%, diet 17%, and alcohol consumption 12% (Stringhini et al., 2010).

Experts in health and culture have cautioned that these results do not negate the effect of stressful life circumstances on health (Dunn, 2010). Stress may be the cause of negative health behaviors in lower SES groups, since individuals may use some behaviors such as alcohol consumption to cope with feelings of stress, or behaviors may be harder to change when individuals feel stressed (Rod Gronbaek, Schnohr, Prescott, & Kristensen, 2009). Research following 7,066 women and men in the Copenhagen City Heart Study found that people reporting higher levels of stress were less likely to quit smoking, more likely to become physically inactive, and less likely to limit alcohol consumption. In addition, women reporting higher levels of stress were more likely to become overweight during the course of the study (Rod et al., 2009).

Kawachi (2005) does not support the idea that poorer health in low-SES individuals is caused by "poor people behaving badly." He suggests that higher rates of negative health behaviors reflect the response of people to their environments. He points out that the tobacco industry targets advertising to low-income and ethnic minorities. Fast-food establishments are more common than grocery stores in poorer communities. And neighborhoods where lower-SES groups reside generally offer fewer opportunities to be physically active.

Childhood Poverty and Neurocognitive Deficits

Another view of the SES, stress, and health-behavior associations proposes that childhood poverty may set the stage for neurocognitive deficits that make people more prone to stress and negative health-behavior patterns. Self-regulation and executive function develop in childhood and become the foundation for future stress-management skills and other health behaviors (Dunn, 2010). Children from lower-SES families are more likely to show deficits in self-regulation and executive function (Farah et al., 2006). Researchers have suggested targeting these critical skills in programs designed to improve health behaviors, especially in children and young people. Some evidence suggests that including development of these skills in behavior-change curricula improves program success (Riggs, 2007).

Poverty, Obesity, and Health

One of the most pressing health issues around the world is the rapid rise of obesity and obesity-related illnesses. In resource-rich countries, rates of obesity tend to be highest among the most disadvantaged groups. Although one might expect that people with the fewest resources would have less to eat, the conditions created by poverty in the richer countries encourage obesity, a phenomenon called the poverty–obesity paradox. The poverty–obesity paradox is probably attributable to a number of interacting factors, including the following (Fig. 7-4).

- **Low-income families consume more energy-dense foods and fewer fruits and vegetables.**

   Several researchers have found evidence to support this hypothesis (Aggarwal, Monsivais, Cook, & Drewnowski, 2011; Drewnowski, 2009). Some researchers have found there is an inverse relationship between a food's energy density (calories per unit weight) and cost; that is, cheaper foods tend to have more calories per unit of volume. For example, cookies and potato chips supply about 1,200 calories per dollar, whereas fresh carrots provide only 250 calories per dollar (Drewnowski & Specter, 2004). If dollars are in short supply and a person has a family to feed, it makes sense that economic pressures will affect shopping choices. The cost of food has risen sharply over the past several years, with increased demand for food from developing countries and

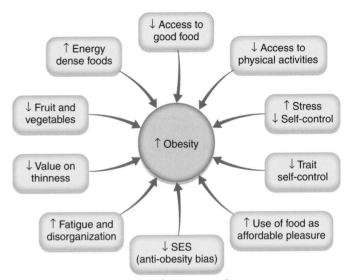

Figure 7-4. The poverty–obesity paradox.

the diversion of crops for the manufacture of biofuels (*The Economist*, 2008). If food prices push consumers to choose filling but less nutritious foods, the rising costs of food may mean that more people than ever will find it difficult to avoid obesity.

Brooks and colleagues have suggested that overconsumption of calories may be partially driven by the need to consume adequate protein (Brooks, Simpson, & Raubenheimer, 2010). Protein is the most expensive fuel, compared with fats and carbohydrates. People with inadequate resources may tend to choose cheaper foods with low protein levels and must thus consume more food to get enough protein.

- **Resource-poor neighborhoods offer less access to good food and fewer opportunities for physical activity.**

   Poor neighborhoods tend to have fewer supermarkets and more convenience stores, liquor stores, and fast-food establishments (Stafford et al., 2007). Food costs more when purchased at convenience stores rather than large supermarkets, and the selection is poor. Whereas people in poor areas may walk more for transportation, other options for physical activity are generally more limited, with less access to parks, recreation centers, and swimming pools (Diez Roux & Mair, 2010). People who fear neighborhood crime restrict outdoor time for themselves and family members. Some experts have argued, however, that in some cases, people do exercise preferences in choosing their neighborhoods, with those who like to walk moving to more walkable neighborhoods (Frank, 2007).

- **Poverty is stressful and feelings of deprivation decrease self-control.**

   Readers will recall from Chapter 5 that self-control is a limited resource and that coping with stress depletes the energy available for self-control (Hagger, Chantelle, Stiff, & Chatzisarantis, 2010). Feelings of deprivation are associated with overconsumption of calories when food is available (Crescioni et al., 2011).

- **Lower levels of self-control are associated with the downward spiral of poverty.**

Some research has looked at a concept called trait self-control. Trait self-control reflects an individual's general level of self-control. Research suggests that individuals with low levels of trait self-control are less likely to do well in school or in the workplace and are more likely to overeat (Casey et al., 2011; Moffit et al., 2011). Low levels of success in school and work may partly explain lower SES and, hence, the link between poverty and obesity.

Self-control can be improved through training and practice. Children in better schools practice self-control in their educational systems. Children also gain self-control ability through family child-rearing practices, recreational sports programs, after-school activities, and in a variety of other ways. A scarcity of opportunity for the acquisition of self-control may contribute to both obesity and poverty in adulthood.

- **Anti-fat bias may push obese people into lower-status positions.**

People who are obese may have access to fewer educational, employment, and social opportunities than others. If people experience health problems along with obesity, they have even fewer opportunities for employment. Such discrimination could exert pressure over time that causes obese people to be less successful and to move into the lower social classes (Puhl & Brownell, 2001). Since body size has strong genetic links, children of obese parents are more likely to be obese and, like their parents, face limited opportunities to improve SES.

- **People of higher SES value thinness and behaviors promoting healthy body weight.**

People of higher SES are exposed to more pressure to maintain a healthy body weight. They monitor their weight more frequently and hear more messages promoting the associations between weight and health (McLaren, 2007). They experience more workplace and societal norms that exert pressure to control body weight and are likely to perceive healthy eating and regular physical activity as normal and positive behaviors.

- **People often respond to chronic stress and poor health with fatigue and disorganization.**

Disorganized households have less energy to put toward long-term planning and shopping. For many people, eating reduces feelings of stress. Such people may eat more comfort foods to cope with stress (Olson, Bove, & Miller, 2007).

Some researchers have suggested that stress may alter metabolic pathways and lead to more visceral obesity, which increases obesity-related health problems (van Reedt Dortland et al., 2012). Poor health often accompanies excess body fat, as discussed in Chapter 1. Once disorders such as diabetes and heart disease are added to the poverty mix, household organization and finances are further stressed.

- **Preparing nutritious meals at home requires planning ahead and organization.**

Cooking at home requires grocery shopping, planning meals ahead of time so that the necessary ingredients are on hand, time to prepare the meal, and then time and energy for cleaning up after the meal has been eaten (Fig 7-5). When people do not have enough time and energy, they may choose to buy prepared foods or to eat out. Eating out can be an affordable luxury, especially at fast-food restaurants.

- **Food is an affordable pleasure, and people like the taste of fat and sugar.**

People enjoy food, and parents providing meals want to please their families. When access to food is limited, people preparing meals want to be sure that no one feels hungry at the end of a meal (Drewnowski & Specter, 2004). Filling bellies and satisfying those at the table comes ahead of nutrition recommendations. Food is used as a reward in many families (Olson, Bove, & Miller, 2007).

Most people, especially children, enjoy the taste of foods high in fat and sugar. Food product manufacturers have invested time and money to devise products that please the palate and can be sold at an affordable price. About half the calories in the U.S. diet come from added sugars and fat (Drewnowski & Specter, 2004). Although people's tastes for fatty and sweet foods may have provided an evolutionary advantage, driving humans to eat enough to avoid starvation, in an environment with abundant food choices, people consume too many calories. People

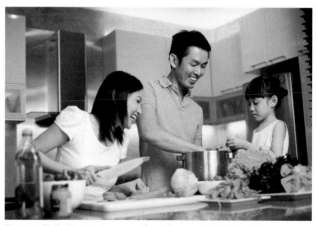

Figure 7-5. **Preparing meals at home.** © Thinkstock

purchasing food generally value taste more highly than health and nutrition (Drewnowski, 2009). When financial pressures reduce spending power, they may not buy vegetables.

The exact contribution made by each of the above factors is unclear and often confusing. Results of longitudinal studies do not always support the conclusions reached in cross-sectional observations (Hruschka, 2012). Addressing the poverty–obesity paradox will require interventions at all levels of ecological models, from public policy and legislative action, to neighborhood interventions increasing access to good food and physical activity, and finally, to support for individual behavior change.

■ *The next group that Katie works with is attending a week-long alumni wellness program. Katie is available to meet with participants concerned about accommodating old injuries and adapting general exercise recommendations to their health limitations. The alumni participants of all ages seem to enjoy being back on campus and are a motivated and cheerful group. They attend lectures and workshops on a wide range of wellness topics and participate in a variety of exercise classes in the athletic center. The alumni athletes have especially enjoyed visiting the athletic training facility and admiring how much it has changed since they were student athletes.*

Katie's last participant of the day, Diane, comes to ask Katie for advice on heel pain. Diane's doctor back home has diagnosed plantar fasciitis. Diane is a large woman; Katie estimates that she is probably about 50 pounds heavier than the BMI charts want her to be. Diane walks about an hour a day before work in a park near her home. Diane's physical therapist at home has advised Diane to cut back on the walking until her heel pain goes away. Diane shows Katie her current physical therapy exercises. Katie confirms for Diane that the exercises will help but that healing may take several months. Katie wonders if anyone has talked to Diane about how excess weight might be contributing to the problem. But Diane brings up the subject herself. "I know what you're thinking. Please don't tell me to lose weight. I am so tired of the fact that, every time I go to the doctor, my problem ends up being about my weight. This is my size; that's it. I have a healthy diet, I exercise, and my blood pressure and blood sugar are fine. Everyone in my family is big but healthy. The more I diet and try to lose weight, the bigger I get. So I'm done with that." Instead, Katie asks Diane how she might cut back on her daily walking and find activities that will allow her foot to heal. After some

discussion, Diane decides to replace walking with bicycling several mornings a week. ■

Accommodating Size

One of the most challenging diversity issues faced by health and fitness professionals is relating effectively to people who are significantly overweight. Most fitness centers are temples to the sleek physique. Even the most overweight clients and employees are still relatively lean in comparison with the general population. Fitness assessments often include measurement of body weight (sometimes in public) and body composition. Pictures of athletic models adorn the walls. The XL T-shirts are still too small. Many clients are exercising to lose weight, and the subject of weight loss is on everyone's mind.

Health and fitness professionals are usually willing to help overweight and obese clients but may simply not know how. Most professionals live in a "thin" world, often with dance or sports backgrounds and physical education environments. Many have had limited relationships with obese people, except perhaps to advise them on weight reduction. They may have difficulty relating to obese clients without patronizing or embarrassing them.

Health and fitness professionals have studied obesity as a disease state and are familiar with the treatment options, especially diet and exercise. But, beyond this, their understanding stops, and the problem relating to obese clients begins; for them, fatness has a great deal of meaning beyond its association with health risks. For many health and fitness professionals, obesity represents a lifestyle of gluttony and sloth, and they look down on clients who are overweight. Fatness is harshly judged, and people who are overweight are thought to be weak-willed, undisciplined, or lazy.

Many health and fitness professionals wonder why obese people do not just lose some weight. Instead, they should familiarize themselves with the dismal obesity statistics. A majority of people who lose weight on a weight-control program are unable to keep the weight off for even a year. Losing weight is not easy. Some people are genetically prone to obesity, modern cultures are prone to overeating, and a history of dieting (a common experience for many overweight people) can make people gain more body fat than ever.

The worst thing about weight-loss programs is that they may reinforce a negative self-image: People are repeatedly told that they are too heavy and they must do something about it. Dieters who fail at their attempts lose self-esteem rather than weight, and food becomes the enemy, with eating an act of self-destruction or balm for an aching heart.

This is not to say that weight-loss programs always fail; some people do succeed in maintaining long-term weight loss through changes in diet and exercise (see Chapter 10). But some obese people have decided to get off the weight-loss merry-go-round and focus on fitness rather than weight loss, to make the most of their potential. Some obese people have commented they were waiting to start exercising until they lose some weight. Eventually, many discover that if they want to exercise, they'd better go ahead and start now. The problem is often how to get started.

Although physical educators advocate exercise for everyone, they have been a little slow in helping special populations. Most fitness centers can increase the level of hospitality offered to obese people. One of the most important elements in the fitness center experience is the attitude of the health and fitness professionals working there. Many fitness instructors have found that a little consciousness-raising about the special needs of any given population goes a long way in helping them become more effective teachers. Think for a minute about the experience of being an overweight person in a culture that values thinness. One of the qualities of body size is high visibility. Being obese is not easy to hide. It's there, and it's judged.

Accepting the existence of obesity does not mean one must go out and gain 50 pounds. It simply means acknowledging that some people are obese, and their size does not necessarily mean they are any less disciplined than anyone else or looking for sympathy. It means conducting fitness programs in a way that respects the dignity of obese people (and everyone else, for that matter). Some suggestions for working effectively with overweight and obese clients include the following:

- Avoid assumptions about health. Although, in general, extra body fat is associated with certain health risks, not every fat person is unhealthy. Some overweight people are quite healthy and active. Like all clients, obese people may or may not have health risks or even be appropriate for fitness programs. Health and fitness professionals should follow normal medical-clearance procedures.
- Avoid assumptions about health and fitness goals. Many overweight people come to the fitness center to improve their fitness. Health and fitness professionals should not make the mistake of assuming they have come to lose weight; these clients may be tired of hearing about weight loss.
- Individualize recommendations and advice. Like other clients, obese people may have special needs, such as knee problems, back problems, or high blood pressure. The key to effective communication is challenging one's own biases concerning obesity and treating each client as an individual, not as an obese person. It may be tempting to say, "Your knees will feel better if you'd just lose some weight." Overweight clients have probably heard this a million times already, and at this point they simply need help designing a program that will not stress problematic joints.

Obese people want to be treated like a person with a knee problem, not an obese person with a knee problem.

- Consider size in activity recommendations. Large people do take up more space and generally move more slowly than smaller people. Whether an exercise activity or class suits a particular client will depend on his or her size and fitness level. A fast-paced, high-impact aerobics class may or may not work. Fitness centers that have enough low-fitness clients (of any size) might consider a special class geared to this level. Some obese people want to join the mainstream, and others appreciate a special environment with others of their fitness level. Health and fitness professionals must consider a person's larger size when making activity recommendations, as a very large or obese person may simply not fit the exercise machines or enjoy the exercise classes at the fitness center. Swimming can be one of the most comfortable exercise modes for obese people but the pool can be an intimidating place. Finding water exercise apparel that fits and is attractive is hard enough; going into the pool area dressed in it can be even harder. Slower swimmers of any size appreciate designated slow lanes.
- Design fitness centers to accommodate disability and diversity in size. Some fitness centers are difficult to navigate unless one is lean. An environment that is wheelchair friendly will generally accommodate large people as well. Locker rooms can be crowded and lockers hard to reach. Most people prefer private changing areas and showers to open areas.
- Consider changing embarrassing fitness testing or making it optional. If fitness testing is mandatory in certain programs, health and fitness professionals should consider adapting procedures to avoid embarrassing obese clients. If clients are not trying to slim down, consider eliminating weigh-ins and body-composition assessments.
- Promote fitness at every size. Fitness centers interested in recruiting a wider variety of clients can increase marketing strategies targeting these populations. For example, promotional material can feature people of all sizes and fitness levels having fun.

Spirituality, Religion, and Health

Many people include spiritual practices, such as prayer and meditation, in their daily lives and look for answers to their spiritual questions. Many people say that their spiritual beliefs and practices improve their health. After decades of avoiding spirituality and religion as a difficult-to-measure and potentially divisive phenomenon, medical research has begun to study the role of spiritual belief in health and healing.

Spirituality refers to the quality of being spiritual or concerned with the nature of spirit or soul, the intangible and immaterial essence of a person. Religion refers to a set of beliefs, values, and practices related to belief in a higher power and usually based on the teachings of a spiritual leader. Spirituality and religion are closely related, as both include practices designed to help followers experience the transcendence of daily life, communicate with a higher power, develop ethical practices, and discover the meaning of one's life. Religions are by definition spiritual in orientation but people can be spiritual without subscribing to a particular religion. People experience transcendent states in a variety of nonreligious ways, such as when being outdoors in nature or while helping others.

Throughout human history, people in every culture have searched for explanations for existence. Many religions arose to help explain the meaning of life, often in terms of people's relationship with a divine force and with each other. The effect of religion on health has not always been positive. For example, "witches" have been burned at the stake, and numerous wars have been fought in the name of religion. Some religious beliefs may interfere with the pursuit of positive health behaviors, as practitioners believe illness is one's destiny and that people do not have the ability to change what God has willed. Some people even see illness and other negative outcomes as divine punishments one must endure. Religious groups sometimes turn to prayer, rather than diet and exercise, for help with health problems such as obesity and diabetes that are better treated with lifestyle measures.

Spirituality and Religion: Positive Effects

But spirituality and religion can also serve as positive forces for health and for promoting positive health behaviors. Several studies examining the link between spiritual practices and health have found intriguing results (Guilfoyle & St. Pierre-Hansen, 2012). A number of practices connected with spiritual health, including prayer, meditation, attendance at religious services, and participation in service groups based in religious communities, have been associated with improved health outcomes. In one study of 232 heart patients, death rates during the 6 months following surgery were substantially lower for subjects who said they participated in group activities and for those who said they had a strong religious faith. In fact, the subjects who said they did not participate in group activities had a four times higher risk of death, on average, than subjects reporting participation in group activities. Those who participated in regular (at least once a week) religious group activities and who said they had a strong religious faith had the lowest death rate of all (Oxman, Freeman, & Manheimer, 1995). Subjects reporting no group activities and no religious involvement had a death rate seven times higher than subjects reporting both group and religious involvement.

Researchers studying the faith–health connection have come up with several ideas that may help explain these interesting findings. Spirituality and religious practices may positively affect health for many reasons, including the following (Fig. 7-6).

Clean Living

Some religions discourage unhealthy habits such as smoking, drinking alcohol, and taking drugs. Some even endorse healthy eating and other positive self-care behaviors. In addition to healthy habits, the routine of attendance at worship/religious services may be part of a weekly rhythm and schedule that helps make life feel more stable and manageable.

Relaxation Response

Many religious practices elicit the relaxation response that counteracts the fight-or-flight response. As discussed in Chapter 6, the relaxation response reduces the negative health effects of chronic overactivation of the sympathetic nervous system. The relaxation response reduces pain and blood pressure and improves mood and immune response. Prayer, meditation, singing, performing altruistic activities, and feeling connected to others can elicit the relaxation response.

Social Support

Spiritual and religious practices often promote feelings of connectedness to others and a sense of social support. Social support is a powerful buffer against stress-related illness. In many spiritual and religious groups, members provide strong emotional support for one another, and, in times of stress and illness, people feel comforted by the knowledge that others in the group care. When serious health or other problems arise, members provide supportive services for

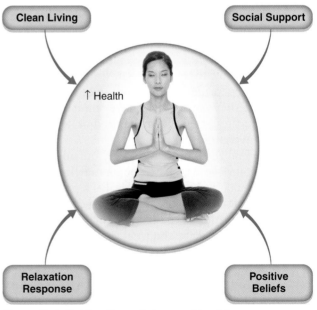

Spirituality, Religion, and Health

Clean Living

Social Support

↑ Health

Relaxation Response

Positive Beliefs

Figure 7-6. Spirituality, religion, and health. Photograph © Thinkstock

each other, such as meals, housekeeping assistance, childcare, and transportation.

Positive Beliefs

A Chinese proverb states, "Where the mind goes, the body follows." This proverb illustrates many scientific observations from the placebo effect to self-efficacy. Many religions and other spiritual traditions encourage the mind to go in helpful directions that nurture positive emotional states and counteract the negative thoughts and feelings that exacerbate the stress response. Remember from Chapter 6 that research has found that a hostile, cynical outlook on life, associated with frequent feelings of anger, increases risk for heart disease. Forgiveness, compassion, and love can "open the heart" and are associated with a lower risk of heart disease (Ornish, 1998). Similarly, feelings of isolation, hopelessness, and helplessness are associated with many negative health effects. Their opposites—a sense of connection to others, feelings of hope, and a sense of control over events—reduce stress and chronically elevated levels of stress hormones. If spiritual beliefs nurture these helpful feelings, this could at least partly explain some of the health benefits associated with spirituality and religion.

Researchers have observed that having a sense of meaning and purpose in life reduces stress. This sense of meaning and purpose counteracts harmful feelings of alienation. Many psychologists believe that humans are "hard-wired" for religion, that searching for answers to the immense questions of "Who am I?" and "Why am I here?" is part of what makes people human. Wellness writers, who have always included spiritual health as an important part of each person's health, emphasize that spiritual questing enriches and strengthens an individual's life (Travis & Ryan, 2004).

Faith-Placed Health Promotion

Faith-placed health-promotion programs utilize the existence of religious groups to promote positive behavior change. Sternberg and colleagues (2007) define faith-placed programs as including spiritual reinforcement for behavior change, taking place in a religious setting, and being organized and run with significant involvement of a faith group. Faith-placed health-promotion programs can be effective for reaching groups that have a strong religious affiliation. For example, various churches have conducted programs for African Americans, especially African American women. Faith-placed programs can provide strong social support for participants (Sternberg, Munschauer, Carrow, & Sternberg, 2007). In addition, church pastors and other leaders can serve as influential forces to motivate positive behavior change.

MOTIVATING CHANGE: Motivating Behavior Change in a Diverse World

Health and fitness professionals who easily develop rapport with clients similar to themselves may find that it takes a little longer to build trust with people who differ in age, gender, ethnicity, size, SES, educational background, ability, or fitness level. As fitness centers reach out to a more diverse range of clients to broaden their market, some fitness professionals must work a little harder to learn more about clients from different walks of life. It is easy to develop a rapport with clients similar to yourself and your family. As you expand your client base and reach out to a wider variety of people, it could take longer before you and your clients communicate on the same wavelength.

Learn About Your Clients' Backgrounds

Who are your clients? What are they like? If they differ from you in age, ethnicity, gender, size, SES, or educational background, do a little research. If you find significant cultural differences between you and your clients, try to learn about their beliefs, attitudes, and lifestyles. Talk to others who work with this population. Spend time with your clients and listen to what they have to say.

Some clients may not talk very much or ask very many questions. Older people and some cultural groups may believe that asking questions is rude and indicates that you have not been clear. To find out if clients understand instructions, watch them perform the exercises or ask them questions. Are they more comfortable writing? Perhaps they can fill out a form. Older people often need glasses to read, however, so don't expect them to fill in forms with you unless they have their reading glasses handy.

Encourage clients to participate in behavior-change program design. You need information from them so that your recommendations fit their lifestyles. Some clients may expect you to be the expert and not offer much input. They may not realize that behavior change is most successful when professionals and clients work together to craft an effective plan. Simple handouts and written feedback forms may be helpful in this situation.

Suspend Judgment

People's lives are complicated. Although you might find many logical reasons to criticize the decisions your clients make, forgive them for being human. Clients may be struggling with low self-esteem, addiction, stress, depression, anxiety, health problems, or issues with food that you don't understand. You don't have to endorse counterproductive behavior but you can be supportive and patient as you encourage clients to stick to their behavior-change plans.

Help Clients Feel Safe Exercising

It's easy to market exercise programs to people who love to work out and enjoy the fitness center environment. It's also easy to forget that this describes a small minority of the population. For many, fitness centers feel foreign and intimidating.

People who have health problems or other physical limitations face extra barriers when beginning an exercise program. Help them feel safe emotionally ("I belong here") and physically ("I won't get hurt"). Share your training, credentials, and experience working with clients similar to them. And always refer clients to a more experienced personal trainer or health-care provider if you learn they have health problems beyond your scope of practice.

BEHAVIOR CHANGE THROUGHOUT THE LIFE SPAN

People's chronological age influences their health and their motivations for behavior change in many ways. As people age, their health changes, particularly as they reach midlife and old age. People's motivations and activity preferences also change as the years go by. The following sections present brief snapshots of the major life stages and the most important variables that may influence behavior-change recommendations.

Childhood

Childhood generally refers to the developmental period between birth and puberty. During this time, children go through enormous changes, so programs should be designed for a specific target age range. For example, younger children, such as those aged 4 to 5, have very different developmental needs and behaviors from older children aged 9 to 10. Children are usually separated into programs based on age or school grade level. Programs should accommodate developmental readiness and psychosocial as well as physical needs. Health and fitness professionals working with children should learn as much as possible about the developmental needs of the age group they serve. Several important variables that influence professionals' work with children include the following.

Family Influences

One of the biggest differences between working with children and working with adults is that children are almost totally dependent on their families. Families exert strong influences, both positive and negative, on how children spend their time, their access to physical activities, and what they eat. Families also influence children's attitudes toward negative health behaviors such as cigarette smoking and alcohol use. Families provide the environment and role modeling that guide development of children's health habits, both good and bad. Establishing good habits in childhood influences children's psychological and physical health.

Many studies have examined the relationship between family characteristics and children's health behaviors. In general, children exhibit better health behaviors in families with adequate parent/guardian involvement. For example, one study followed children aged 10 and 11 for 18 months (Ray & Roos, 2012). The researchers were interested to see how behaviors such as sleep duration, eating habits, and screen time changed during this time. In general, children's health behaviors tend to worsen as they approach adolescence. They become less physically active, sleep fewer hours, eat fewer fruits and vegetables, drink more soft drinks, and increase screen time. This study found that in families who shared a meal at the end of the day, children showed a smaller increase in screen time over the 18-month follow-up. Children who spent less time alone at home after school showed smaller reductions in sleep duration and less of an increase in soft drink consumption (Ray & Roos, 2012). Another study examining parenting practices and their association with changes in childhood weight found that several practices were associated with lower risk of developing obesity (Avula et al., 2011). These practices included providing children with cognitively stimulating activities, setting limits on screen time, monitoring bedtimes, and showing greater expressions of emotional warmth.

Parents and guardians can help their children form positive eating behaviors in many ways, including making healthy food available; developing good food practices, so that children feel they have some choice in what they consume; monitoring children's behaviors; and modeling healthy eating (Savage, Fisher, & Birch, 2007). Similarly, parents and guardians can model healthy levels of physical activity, provide the transportation children need to after-school sports and activities, and establish positive expectations and attitudes about physical activity (Cottrell et al., 2012).

Health and fitness professionals working to change the health behavior of children must communicate with both the children and their parents or guardians. This is especially important if target behaviors are to be performed at home or outside of an organized program.

School Performance

Children's school performance is generally one of the highest priorities for their families and society at large. The goal of the educational system is to mold highly functioning people who are prepared to take on productive roles in society. Families want their children to do well in school so that they will develop satisfying lives and rewarding careers. A great deal of research has focused on parenting and educational methods that will nurture the qualities related to good academic performance.

Home environment is extremely important for good school performance. Children need a stable environment where they know what to expect and where stressful circumstances do not deplete their energy. Children show better school performance when they have a routine that reinforces good sleep habits, accommodates homework demands, and rewards good behavior.

The behaviors related to good health in adulthood, including adequate sleep, plenty of physical activity, good eating behaviors, coping effectively with stress, and avoiding negative behaviors such as smoking, are also related to good academic performance in children. The abilities to sit still, concentrate, remember, synthesize knowledge, and think creatively are dependent on good health and brain function.

Several studies have linked regular physical activity with better school performance. A recent meta-analysis found strong support for this relationship and concluded that the relationship was independent of other factors associated with school performance, including family SES (Roberts, Freed, & McCarthy, 2010; Singh, Uijtdewilligen, Twisk, van Mechelen, & Chinapaw, 2012). Singh and colleagues summarized the existing research, concluding that exercise may improve school performance for several reasons, including the following:

- Emotional health benefits of physical activity: The emotional health benefits of exercise discussed in Chapter 3 are apparent in children as well as adults. Children appear to experience increased blood flow and oxygen to the brain and changes in neurotransmitter activity associated with stress reduction and better mood (Singh et al., 2012).
- Better classroom behavior: Children who get more exercise seem to have a better ability to sit still and focus on class material. Children have a great need for physical activity, and it is likely that when deprived of sufficient exercise they have difficulty not moving.
- Higher levels of executive control and memory: Active children have more developed prefrontal cortexes and hippocampuses than inactive children. These brain areas are not only larger but show greater activity in neural imaging studies (Chaddock, Pontifex, Hillman, & Kramer, 2011). School behavior requires high levels of inhibition (inhibiting impulses to get up and walk around or behave in a disruptive fashion) as well as concentration. Concentration itself requires inhibiting impulses to think about more pleasant and entertaining subjects. A good working memory supports learning and thinking, since recalling information is necessary for reasoning and constructing knowledge.

Research suggests that good dietary habits are also related to better school performance (Benton, 2010; Florence, Asbridge, & Veugelers, 2008). The brain appears to be sensitive to the availability of a variety of nutrients, which may explain why consuming breakfast and regular meals enhances brain function. Children need the same variety of foods as adults with a calorie intake that meets the needs of daily energy expenditure along with growth and development. Children are particularly vulnerable to the effects of iron-deficiency anemia, so food sources of iron should be included in their daily diet.

Screen Use

Screen use refers to the time spent viewing or using electronic devices such as televisions, computers, video games, and so forth. Early concerns regarding too much screen use tended to focus on the sedentary nature of these pursuits. Although this is still an issue, screen time has also been associated with a variety of psychological difficulties regardless of children's physical activity level (Page, Cooper, Griew, & Jago, 2010). In other words, even children who participate in plenty of vigorous physical activity show more psychological problems with increased screen time. Strasburger and colleagues (2010) have reviewed the evidence supporting the American Academy of Pediatrics' recommendations that parents limit screen time in children of all ages (AAP, 2011a, 2011b). Important research findings include the following:

- Exposure to screen time in infancy is associated with a possible delay in language development. Researchers found no benefits for media exposure in children less than 2 years old.
- Heavy media viewing (more than 2–3 hours per day) in childhood has been associated with increased incidence of attention deficit disorders in the early school years.
- Greater screen time is associated with higher risks for sleep disorders, mood disorders, depression, and other forms of psychological distress.
- Media exposure, especially exposure of young children to PG-13 and R-rated material, increases the likelihood of aggressive behavior disorders, early sexual behaviors, substance abuse, and disordered eating behaviors.
- Greater screen time is associated with a higher risk for obesity, perhaps mediated through the advertisement of food products that prompts overeating.

The American Academy of Pediatrics (AAP) recommends avoiding media exposure for children under age 2 (AAP, 2011b). It also advises limiting screen time to less than 2 hours for older children and choosing appropriate material for young children (AAP, 2011a). The AAP recommends that parents view programs with young children and discuss content. Televisions and other screen media should be kept out of children's bedrooms, so that parents can more easily monitor use and so children get more sleep.

Psychophysical Development and Obesity Prevention

A healthy lifestyle allows children to maximize their potential for physical growth and psychophysical health and prevents the development of obesity. Young children, from infancy through elementary school, need plenty of unstructured playtime to develop their bodies and minds (AAP, 2011a). A well-balanced diet that provides for adequate nutrition is important for growth and development, as discussed above, as is good parenting and a stable home life.

Some experts on childhood health and body composition believe that over an hour per day of vigorous physical activity is required for normal growth and development in childhood (Gutin, 2008). Larger amounts of mechanical stimulation supplied by vigorous activity appear to cause stem cells to differentiate into bone and muscle rather than fat (Rosen & Bouxsein, 2006). Thus, vigorous activity over the two decades of childhood and adolescence may lead to more favorable body composition (Fig. 7-7) (What's the Evidence? 7-1).

Health professionals have expressed alarm at the rising obesity rates in all segments of the population, including children and adolescents. In less than 30 years, the obesity rates for children and teens have doubled, and rates have tripled for children aged 6 to 11 (Centers for Disease Control and Prevention, 2012a). Obesity in children is determined by checking a child's weight against the weight of other children his or her age and sex. Some parents see their children as fat even though they are of normal weight, whereas others overlook obesity problems. Both are problematic, and parents should seek the opinion of a health-care provider if questions arise as to whether they should be concerned about obesity in their children.

Much has been written about the probable short- and long-term health consequences of this obesity epidemic. In addition to obesity-related metabolic disorders, obesity increases children's risk of developing emotional health problems, such as low self-esteem,

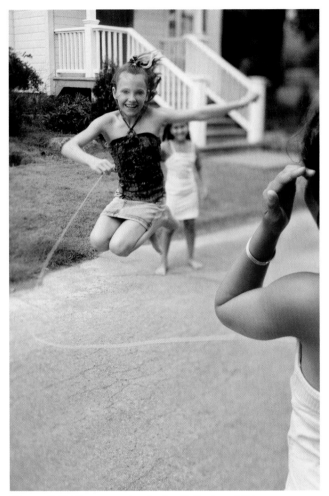

Figure 7-7. Vigorous physical activity for children.
© Thinkstock

WHAT'S THE EVIDENCE? 7-1

A High-Energy Lifestyle Is Associated With Less Body Fat in Adolescents

Stallmann-Jorgensen, I. S., Gutin, B., Hatfield-Laube, J. L., Humphries, M. C., Johnson, M. H., & Barbeau, P. (2007). General and visceral adiposity in black and white adolescents and their relation with reported physical activity and diet. *International Journal of Obesity, 31*, 622–629.

■ PURPOSE
The purpose of this study was to examine diet and exercise factors potentially related to body composition in young people. The researchers wanted to find out which factors were most strongly related to body fat levels.

■ STUDY
A total of 661 adolescents (aged 14–18) volunteered to participate in this study. The researchers collected data on food intake and physical activity level. They also measured body composition using a technique with good accuracy—dual-energy x-ray absorptiometry. Visceral adipose tissue (VAT) was assessed in 434 subjects using magnetic resonance imaging.

The study showed that greater amounts of vigorous physical activity were associated with lower levels of body fat. Vigorous physical activity was defined as having an average intensity of greater than 6 METS*. Examples of vigorous activities include jogging at 6 mph or faster; shoveling; bicycling at 14 to 16 mph or faster; and basketball, soccer, and tennis (singles) games. Amount of moderately vigorous physical activity was not significantly related to the percentage of body fat.

An interesting thing about this study was that the authors did not find that subjects with higher body fat levels ate more. In fact, the only diet variable that was related to percentage of body fat was energy intake, and that was *negatively* related, which means that the more calories consumed, the leaner the child. Interestingly, energy intake

WHAT'S THE EVIDENCE? 7-1–cont'd

was positively associated with participation in vigorous physical activity. In other words, the most active adolescents also consumed more calories. The researchers suggest that higher energy intake may be a marker for high-energy lifestyles, with higher levels of vigorous physical activity.

■ IMPLICATIONS

The results of this study suggest that the traditional focus on restricting food intake to prevent obesity may be misguided, especially for children and adolescents. Encouraging a healthy diet in children is still a good idea in terms of nurturing good health and positive eating behaviors. But equally if not more important is encouraging children and adolescents to engage in high volumes of vigorous physical activity. Sports, games, and dance activities appear to provide a better stimulus to optimal body-composition development than less vigorous exercise modes such as walking.

*A MET is a measure of exercise intensity that allows for comparison of people of different sizes. Caloric expenditure is harder to compare, since big people expend more calories performing most activities than small people. One MET is the energy expenditure for a person at rest, which is about 60 to 70 calories per minute for an average adult. Thus, 6 METS means the exercise intensity is six times higher than energy expenditure at rest.

negative body image, and depression. Obesity is also associated with poorer school performance and lower standardized test scores in children (Roberts, Freed, & McCarthy, 2010). Many overweight children can attest to the observation that they are likely to be the object of bullying and discrimination. As obese children develop anxiety about physical education classes, sports participation, and exercising in public, they may become increasingly sedentary and overweight.

Not every overweight child becomes an overweight adult. Many children "grow out of" obesity at some point. And many children who are thin or normal weight will become obese during their adult years. Helping children develop healthy lifestyles that include good food choices, lots of social support, and plenty of physical activity helps prevent obesity, gives overweight kids a chance to "grow out of" their obesity, and provides kids with the skills they need to nurture good health throughout their lives.

Many parents and caregivers seek the advice of health and fitness professionals to help their obese children. Advice for helping overweight children differs somewhat from advice for overweight adults. General guidelines include the following:

- Examine the child's lifestyle and try to determine the cause of obesity. What habits need correcting?
- Increase physical activity gradually to at least an hour per day. Young children prefer active games with stop-and-start bursts of activity, whereas older children and teens may enjoy continuous activities such as cycling and running. Many older children and teens enjoy strength training and working out at the fitness center. Strength-training guidelines for children differ from those for adults, so health and fitness professionals should be familiar with these if working with children (Faigenbaum et al., 2009). Children

with low fitness levels will need to start slowly and build fitness gradually to avoid injury.
- Provide healthy food choices at home and at school. Empty-calorie foods, especially sugary beverages such as soft drinks, should be avoided. Restrictive diets have not been shown to be particularly effective in children. Children generally need to eat more servings of fruits and vegetables. Good advice on helping children eat well can be found at the U.S. Department of Agriculture ChooseMyPlate website (www.choosemyplate.gov/healthy-eating-tips/ten-tips.html).
- Reduce screen time.
- Offer children opportunities to participate in enjoyable groups and activities that build self-esteem, such as boys' and girls' clubs; community service opportunities; music, theater, and art classes; and youth sport and activity programs.

Emotional Vulnerability

Children are often more influenced than adult clients by interactions with health and fitness professionals. This means that professionals should treat children with respect and kindness. Children's self-concepts are still developing, and their self-esteem is often very fragile. A thoughtless or rude comment by a professional may feel overwhelming to a child and even set negative behaviors, such as eating disorders, in motion. Children want to belong and feel accepted. They look to caring adults for guidance and feedback on how they are doing.

Behavior-Change Models and Children

Many studies have examined the efficacy of behavior-change models to predict behavior change in children. The variables that have been most predictive for changes in dietary behavior and physical activity have been self-efficacy and outcome expectations (Paw, Singh, Brug,

& van Mechelen, 2008). Researchers also find social norms to be significant, including family, peer, and school norms (McClain, Chappuis, Nguyen-Rodriguez, Yaroch, & Spruijt-Metz, 2009). These variables appear in Social Cognitive Theory, the Theory of Planned Behavior, and the Health Belief Model. Although many behavior-change programs for children tend to focus on parental behavior, some investigators argue that professionals should also focus on children's intentions to change. One research group used the Theory of Planned Behavior to examine intentions to change weight-control behaviors in children aged 10 to 14 (Cottrell et al., 2012). The researchers found children's perceptions and beliefs about obesity and weight-control behaviors helped to predict future eating and exercise behaviors. Children's perceived behavioral control (or self-efficacy) about implementing the desired behaviors was also predictive.

The Stages of Change Model from the Transtheoretical Model seems to apply fairly well to children and their engagement in moderate and vigorous physical activity (Haas & Nigg, 2009). Children old enough to read can use the Stages of Change questionnaire for behaviors such as physical activity and consumption of fruits and vegetables.

Because children are so dependent on their families, other caregivers, communities, and the educational system (once they are in school), most programs targeting behavior change in children rely on a holistic behavior-change perspective. This encompasses an ecological approach that includes biological, psychological, and sociological factors relevant to the behavior change in question (Wilson & Lawman, 2009).

What motivates children? Young children tend to be naturally curious and engaged, spending more time "in the moment" than older people. They may chase one another, mimic others, and join in on whatever activities are occurring around them. Older children enjoy being part of a group and are able to play more complicated games. Children seek to have fun and experience positive emotions that reinforce the behaviors with which they are associated.

The drives important in Self-determination Theory motivate children as well as adults. Children seek connection and enjoy being competent and mastering skills. Anyone who has witnessed a 2-year-old throwing a tantrum because she did not get things her way knows that the drive for autonomy develops at a very early age. Children, like everyone else, prefer to do things because they want to, rather than because they have to. However, compulsory education, parental guidance, and even sports coaches often rely more on extrinsic or controlled motivation than intrinsic or other forms of autonomous motivation for getting children to do what they should. Some extrinsic motivation is inevitable, as children don't always know what is best for themselves. But research suggests that giving children some choice with regard to lifestyle behaviors such as what they eat or what physical activities they

participate in may enhance motivation (Deforche, Haerens, & de Bourdeaudhuij, 2011). Very young children need less choice. The older the child, the more latitude with choice may be given. Lack of choice or participating in activities such as sport training with little autonomous motivation predicts a greater likelihood of burnout and dropping out of activities (Harris & Watson, 2011). A preference for autonomous rather than controlled motivation appears to occur in children (and adults) of all cultures (Ryan. Ortmeyer, & Sorkin, 2011). Certainly, culture influences what people perceive as desirable activities to pursue. But people still want to feel like they have choices or options. One study of young Chinese students found that autonomous versus controlled motivation predicted interest in school courses (Zhou, Ma, & Deci, 2009).

Katie is enjoying her meetings with the alumni. What a high-energy group! Each person she sees is like a puzzle that needs to be solved. And Katie has found that these adults are much more open to her advice than college athletes. Her next client, Cindy, is seeking Katie's advice for exercising with knee pain. Cindy was a sprinter as an undergraduate but stopped running once she had kids. Recently diagnosed with prediabetes, Cindy was told to increase her physical activity and to lose 20 pounds to prevent her prediabetes from getting worse. Cindy decided to start running again, picking up where she left off 12 years ago. Katie cautions Cindy that she has probably increased her exercise volume too quickly, likely doing too much, too soon. They come up with a more reasonable program of physical activity that includes more exercise variety and fewer miles of running. "Switch to swimming for the next few days while you are here. If your knee is still hurting when you get home next week, be sure to check in with your doctor. Don't ignore this!"

Cindy also asks Katie for suggestions on improving her family's eating habits. "I'm not sure how it's happened," Cindy laments. "I used to be so careful about what the children ate when they were very young. I guess over the years I have slacked off, and little by little our eating habits have declined without my really noticing. The kids pester me into buying high-sugar breakfast cereals and snack bars; they say all their friends are drinking soda for lunch. 'Just this once,' has turned into a daily routine. Those kids know how to wear me down!

"But after speaking with a nutritionist about my own diet, I am trying to eat more fruits, vegetables, and whole grains and less junk. My blood sugar was a little high at my last physical, and I am concerned about diabetes and *heart disease. The kids also seem to be a little pudgier than their friends. They hardly ever eat fruits or vegetables. They'll be teenagers in a few years, and I know that then it will be even harder to influence their diet. Do you have any suggestions for improving my family's eating habits without having a nervous breakdown in the process?"*

Since Cindy has already met with a dietitian and has good guidelines on what to eat, Katie is comfortable helping Cindy brainstorm ways to implement the dietitian's suggestions. Cindy decides to talk with her children and explain why they need to make changes in the kinds of food they eat at home. Cindy also decides to go grocery shopping without the kids, cut back on the amount of sugary foods she buys, and introduce more vegetable servings with dinner. Katie has explained that sports beverages are designed for athletes at risk for dehydration and are not a good snack beverage for kids. Cindy decides to switch her kids back to milk or water with meals and save the sports beverages for hot summer practices. ■

Adolescence

Adolescence refers to the stage of development between the onset of puberty and the completion of physical growth, roughly ages 11 to 19. Adolescents, like people in all age groups, are an extremely diverse group. Needs, abilities, and motivations vary enormously with age and life circumstances. Working with middle-school teens requires a different skill set from working with 18- and 19-year-olds who are practically adults.

Most of the variables discussed above in the context of childhood are still important to some degree in adolescence. Families still provide important resources, structure, and role models for their adolescent members. Families continue to purchase and provide food and supply transportation and access to activities for many teens. Parents and caregivers still set limits and try to reinforce them. During adolescence, the influence of peer groups strengthens. As discussed in several behavior-change models, social norms are predictive of behavior-change success; this is especially true for adolescents.

School performance strongly influences adolescent development. Adolescents who drop out of school generally have fewer employment options, although many bounce back later in life, obtaining job skills and higher education in a variety of ways. Some students enjoy their middle and high school years, participating in activities that they find rewarding and making lifelong friendships. Many young people experience a great deal of academic stress, as they struggle to achieve the highest grades and test scores possible in order to gain admission to top colleges and universities. Why do some teens drop out, and others strive for top performance? Peer norms, family expectations, SES, aptitude, motivation, and other variables all play into this complicated issue.

Lifestyles continue to have a major effect on teens' psychophysical development and obesity prevention. Families have less control over eating and exercise behaviors at this stage. Some teens become very careful about their lifestyles, even to the extent of overmonitoring diet and exercise. Others give little thought to food and physical activity. Most adolescents want to be physically attractive and may strive to meet societal ideals of beauty, although these efforts can backfire into unhealthy patterns. Other teens develop good eating, exercise, and stress-management behaviors, enjoying the activities that they find rewarding and meaningful.

Health Behavior and the Challenges of Adolescence

During adolescence, the body develops into that of an adult, and the brain undergoes enormous change. Researchers have made much of the observation that in general, the emotional brain develops more quickly than the prefrontal cortex, which does not mature until around the age of 25. Teens can still be intelligent, perceptive thinkers but emotions may be more important to them. This means that although teens understand the risks of behaviors, such as smoking or driving fast, they sometimes weigh emotional benefits of a given behavior more heavily (Steinberg, 2007).

Adolescents probably tire from the conversations initiated by well-meaning parents and educators about their lack of executive function. Psychologists have also commented that casting adolescents as "all gas and no brakes" may underestimate the capabilities of young people and even create self-fulfilling prophecies (Payne, 2012). Psychological development is complex, and the brain cannot be neatly divided into purely psychosocial or purely cognitive areas (Banich, 2009; Fischer, Stein, & Heikkinen, 2009).

A variety of risky behaviors may emerge during adolescence, many of which are responsible for the leading causes of death in this age group. Some negative behaviors continue into adulthood, setting the stage for chronic disease and reducing quality of life. Families' and societies' concerns for developing healthy lifestyles in some adolescents may shift at this time from a concern for developing healthy eating and exercise behaviors to simply trying to help adolescents survive their teenage years.

Information on the prevalence of risky behaviors among adolescents is collected in the United States by the Centers for Disease Control and Prevention's Youth Risk Behavior Surveillance System (YRBSS) (Centers for Disease Control and Prevention, 2012c). The YRBSS compiles data on the most important high-risk behaviors in this age group and presents results by grade level, sex, and ethnic background. The behaviors are divided into six categories, including the following:

- Behaviors that can lead to injury and violence, including failure to use seat belts; driving after drinking or riding with a driver who had been drinking alcohol; carrying a gun; getting into a physical fight; experiencing dating violence; being bullied at school; not attending school because of safety concerns; considering or attempting suicide; and feeling so sad or hopeless that one stops doing some of one's usual activities
- Tobacco use, including use of all types of tobacco products
- Alcohol and other drug use
- Sexual behaviors that contribute to sexually transmitted diseases (STDs) and unintended pregnancy; use of condoms and other forms of contraception
- Dietary behaviors, including fruit and vegetable intake and consumption of soft drinks
- Physical activity measures, including whether students exercised for at least an hour a day, at least 5 days a week; participation on sports teams; and measures of screen time

The questionnaire also asks about body weight and weight-control behaviors, including disordered eating behaviors.

The data collected by this survey reinforce the importance of appropriate interventions directed to help adolescents develop safer and healthier behaviors. For example, in 2011, during the 30 days before taking the survey, over 32% of high school students said they had texted or e-mailed while driving. Almost a third of high school students reported that they had been in a physical fight, almost 17% said they had carried a weapon on at least one day, and approximately 7.8% said they had attempted suicide. About 18% had smoked cigarettes in the previous 30 days. All of the behaviors examined are changeable, and many are interrelated. These data illustrate the need for effective programs and efforts to help teens find a place in the world where they can live positively and productively.

Promoting Positive Health Behaviors in Adolescents

Health and fitness professionals may work with adolescent clients in a number of ways. Some, like Ashley Niles (Health Psychology at Work 7-1), may work in programs and classes for teens. Others may have adolescent clients in their work as personal trainers, fitness instructors, health educators, athletic trainers, dietitians, or other professionals. Behavior-change theories can guide work with adolescents. Suggestions for working effectively with adolescents in behavior-change programs include the following:

- First, do no harm. Adolescents can be open to the advice of adult mentors. Professionals working with this age group must be especially careful to keep the focus positive and the big picture

in mind. Although the professional may be working with teen athletes to prevent injury and improve performance, the big picture is still optimal health and well-being, essential for all performance. For example, if the adolescent client is trying to lose weight, health and fitness professionals should encourage a healthy diet and cutting back on empty calories such as soft drinks, fried foods, and desserts. It is desirable to help teens develop a healthy concern regarding their lifestyle behaviors, but adolescents sometimes take health behaviors to extremes. Keeping a positive focus on health, performance, and the activities that the adolescent client enjoys can help prevent eating disorders, steroid abuse, and body-image problems. Young athletes should seek to improve sport performance through well-designed training programs and sport-nutrition practices rather than supplements or drugs.

- Prevent injury. The National Athletic Trainers' Association estimates that over half of the sports injuries occurring in children and adolescents are preventable (McLeod et al., 2011). According to one study, high school athletes are treated for over 2 million sports injures yearly, and another 3.5 million sports injuries are treated in children under 14 (Powell & Foss, 1999). Injury related to sport training and exercise has been increasing in children and teens over the past few decades (CDC, 2012d). Children often begin specializing in a single sport at a young age, rather than playing a variety of sports in different seasons. Training volume for some children and teens is quite high, increasing risk of overuse injury (Luke et al., 2011). Teens may not see the long-term problems that can result from ignoring signs of injury. Coaches and parents may not realize the extent of an athlete's injury, as athletes may not mention their symptoms or may make them seem less serious than they are. Athletes and coaches may focus on the next contest, and athletes may not want to let team members down by not competing. The National Athletic Trainers' Association and other sports medicine organizations have urged health-care professionals to do more to prevent overuse injuries in children and adolescents (McLeod, Decoster, Loud, et al., 2011; Veigel & Pleacher, 2008). Health and fitness professionals who become aware of injury symptoms in a young client should refer the athlete to an athletic trainer or other medical professional for advice.

- Help adolescents build autonomous motivation. Health and fitness professionals should begin their work with young clients by talking with them and discovering what is important in their lives. Sometimes parents set their child and teen athletes up with personal trainers to get an edge on the competition. But the young athlete's agenda may not always match the parent's. Health and fitness professionals may be able to improve the athlete's competitiveness but also link the training to what is important to the young athlete. Building autonomous motivation for lifestyle change increases the likelihood that young clients will stick to their behavior-change programs.

- Build on young clients' passions, interests, and character strengths. Health and fitness professionals can often use a young person's interest in sport, dance, or other activities to encourage a healthy lifestyle: getting enough sleep, eating well, and staying active. Involvement in compelling activities may help teens quit smoking and overcome other addictions and negative health behaviors. Professionals should help adolescents discover and build on their personal character strengths and cultivate positive emotions. Strengthening self-esteem, hope, and other positive emotions increases life satisfaction in teens, which serves as a protective factor to increase resilience and promote healthy development (Suldo & Huebner, 2004). Positive sport experiences can be very motivational for adolescents (Box 7-3) (Fig. 7-8).

- Keep expectations realistic about changes in size and appearance. Teens can be very self-focused and worry a great deal about their appearance. Media sources influence young clients' ideals of

---

Box 7-3. Youth-Sport Programs: Opportunities and Challenges

The interest in youth sports among school-aged boys and girls has never been stronger. Many health and fitness organizations are responding to this interest by offering a wide variety of youth-sport programs, from clinics and camps to sport teams that compete in local, state, and national contests. But this growth in youth sport comes with a full set of growing pains, and youth-sport coaches and administrators face a variety of challenges. Some of the most important issues that are prompting heated discussions among youth-sport coaches and administrators follow.

Coaching Qualifications

Many people become youth-sport coaches because they have some playing experience in the sport they are coaching, along with a child or two on the team. Sometimes they have little background in physical education or coaching and often coach on a volunteer basis. Many of these volunteer coaches do a great job despite their lack of education or certification. A majority of youth-sport programs would fold without them, especially programs for younger children.

As the competitive level of the team and the age of the players increase, the demands of athletes, parents, and employers grow as well. Some countries, including Canada, have developed nationwide coaching certification programs. Several organizations in the United States offer certification programs for youth-sport coaches, including the National Youth Sports Coaches Association, American Sports Education Program, National Coaching Certification Program, and the American Coaching Effectiveness Program. All coaches should have some basic first-aid training and be able to demonstrate good organization, sportsmanship, and leadership. A good coach is a good teacher and should be adept at demonstrating and teaching sport skills.

Program Philosophy

Coaches and administrators of youth-sport programs must have a clear coaching philosophy that guides their decision-making and coaching behavior. Some of this philosophy must be based on program goals and procedures. For example, a common problem is finding a balance between equal playing time for all players and winning contests. Is the program designed to give all players a similar experience? Or does the team need to have a competitive edge to attract talented players and thus use some players more than others? Will the program reward effort, talent, or both? How will the organization teach sportsmanship?

How important is "fun"? Having fun is the number-one reason children and adolescents join a sports team. What do players in the program call "fun"? Players often cite improving their skills, being part of a team effort, and winning as fun. Players also like being with their friends and being recognized for their effort and performance.

Concepts of fun vary tremendously with age and ability. Younger children are less likely to enjoy the stress of competition and may drop out when sports are no longer a game. Even older children may prefer a light level of involvement. Communities need to offer both competitive and recreational levels of play for popular sports, so that sport experiences are available to all levels of interest and ability.

Players say that the coach has a key role in determining whether they have fun during practice and competition. Coaches should run informative, well-organized practices and contests, reward effort and ability, and encourage players to improve their skills. They should communicate in a supportive, positive manner as much as possible. Coaches should model a good attitude and good sportsmanship.

Continued

Box 7-3. Youth-Sport Programs: Opportunities and Challenges—cont'd

Positive Parent Involvement

Youth-sports programs have begun to pay more attention to educating parents about sportsmanship expectations for both players and their families. Coaches should give parents guidelines for their behavior at practices and contests and tell them where to sit and what to do (and what not to do) during competitions. Programs may wish to establish consequences for poor behavior from parents as well as players, if negative behavior is a problem.

Supportive parents can be a strong asset to any program. Usually, they fund their children's participation and provide the transportation and organization that gets young players to sport programs. Parents may also volunteer to help with many organizational details.

Good communication can get parents off on the right track. Parents need to know what is required of players and what kind of experience their sons and daughters can expect to have in a sports program. Coaches should inform parents about the program philosophy, how practices are run, how contests are structured, and how playing time is decided. Most coaches transmit this information via handouts, although some coaches hold a meeting with parents at the beginning of the season. Parents often have very strong opinions about their children's sport experiences, and coaches should be experienced in dealing firmly but positively with parent concerns.

More information on coaching in ways that promote positive youth-sport experiences can be found on the website for the Positive Coaching Alliance, www.positivecoach.org.

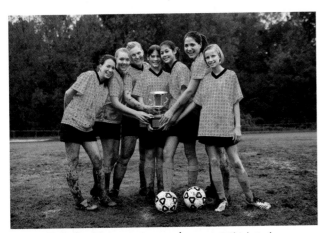

Figure 7-8. **Positive sport experiences.** © Thinkstock

a perfect body and suggest that the right kinds of eating behaviors and exercise can "sculpt" a desirable physique. Adolescents are disappointed when their bodies are not as changeable as those they see in the media. Health and fitness professionals should encourage young clients to tune into improvements in emotional well-being, sleep quality, and stress reduction that come with a healthy lifestyle. Professionals can help teens see improvement in sport performance, strength, and/or endurance. Those working with adolescents should model a healthy criticism of media efforts to instill feelings of inferiority in consumers to entice them to purchase more beauty products. Adolescents often enjoy practicing their critical skills in this area.

• Communicate effectively with parents and guardians. Health and fitness professionals working with adolescents must strike a balance

between maintaining the right level of confidentiality with their young clients, while also communicating effectively with parents and guardians. Although parents and guardians are usually supportive of the professional's work, this is not always the case. Professionals who believe that parents are putting too much pressure on their children may need to meet with the parents and express concern. At the other extreme, professionals may feel parents should be doing more to support their adolescents' efforts to develop positive behaviors. For example, parents may need advice on shopping, meal planning, and other activities to help their children develop better eating habits. Parents may need to be encouraged to help (and pay for) their teens to enroll in activity programs. Teen clients usually prefer to work with health and fitness professionals independently, rather than with their parents on hand. Professionals may let adolescents know they will maintain the client's confidentiality, unless they become worried that a young client is in danger or may pose a danger to others.

Behavior-Change Models and Adolescents

An ecological perspective provides the best starting point for behavior-change work with adolescents (Wilson & Lawman, 2009). Like children, adolescents still rely a great deal on families and communities for support and on peer groups for deciding what is normal. Self-identity and self-esteem can be somewhat fluid and fragile throughout adolescence, and building self-efficacy for target behaviors is essential (Parker, Martin, Martinez, Marsh, & Jackson, 2010).

Health and fitness professionals can discuss the variables from the Health Belief Model and the Theory of Planned Behavior if relevant for an adolescent's behavior-change program. For example, a teen newly diagnosed with type 2 diabetes has the capacity to gain a better understanding of the disease and its progression, along with the behaviors that can control it. Professionals can help adolescents form an intention to become more active, quit smoking, eat better, and manage illnesses in effective ways.

Research suggests that the Stages of Change Model predicts a variety of health behaviors in adolescents (Lee, Nigg, DiClemente, & Courneya, 2001; Parker et al., 2010). Assessing stage of change in adolescent clients can help health and fitness professionals match interventions to client readiness to change.

Self-determination Theory should guide work with adolescents. As noted above, self-efficacy, or competence, is extremely important in this age group. Connection with others, especially friends, is critical to adolescent motivation. Group activities can be motivational at this age. Autonomous motivation is the most effective driver of behaviors in adolescence. Health and fitness professionals should work creatively to help connect productive behaviors to the goals important to adolescent clients.

The field of positive psychology offers a great deal to health and fitness professionals striving to promote positive behaviors in adolescents. Because emotions are especially salient in teens' lives, building positive emotion is a prerequisite for creating and sustaining behavior-change motivation. Constructs especially associated with good emotional health and academic achievement include hope, life satisfaction, and self-esteem (Marques, Pais-Ribeiro, & Lopez, 2001). One interesting study from Portugal compared 218 adolescents who received a treatment called "Strengths Gym" with 101 controls who did not receive the training (Proctor et al., 2011). The program consisted of character strength–based exercises, designed to build self-esteem and nurture positive emotions. The study found that students receiving the Strengths Gym treatment reported greater increases in life satisfaction and feelings of well-being than the control students.

Early to Mid-adulthood: Special Issues

Like all age groups, people in early to mid-adulthood are an extremely diverse group. One of the time-consuming and potentially most interesting issues in this group is professional development and the pursuit of employment. For some adults, employment is about getting a job in order to have access to necessary resources, whereas for others work is a meaningful path to self-fulfillment and community participation. Most adults provide unpaid labor in various ways as volunteers and caretakers.

Building social connections, including close relationships such as romantic partners, is important for most

people in this group. Family responsibilities emerge for many. Although there are many exceptions, level of physical activity generally declines during the transition from adolescence to adulthood, and BMI increases (Zick, Smith, Brown, Fan, & Kowaleski-Jones, 2007).

The models of behavior change discussed in Chapter 4 and the motivational strategies explored in Chapter 5 were designed primarily from research on people in this age group. Health and fitness professionals should individualize their approach to each client as they apply these models and theories. Some of the special issues likely to affect behavior change in this age group include issues related to childbearing and parenting, as these exert significant physical and psychological demands. Balancing work, family, self-care, and other responsibilities is another common theme for clients in this stage of life.

Pregnancy

Women contemplating becoming pregnant and women who have already conceived often consider changes in their health behaviors. Some women begin planning for pregnancy in advance, seeking recommendations from their health-care providers on what they can do to increase the likelihood of a healthy pregnancy and delivery and to contribute to the health of their future children. They may improve their diets, exercise regularly, quit smoking, and manage stress. They may make changes in their home and work environments, seek the assistance of relatives and friends for support during and following pregnancy, and consult books and other media for advice on pregnancy and childbirth. Women may increase their readiness to change health behaviors and seek help from health and fitness professionals in their behavior-change endeavors.

Behavior change during pregnancy has been the focus of many public health efforts, as research is revealing the long-term effects of maternal health on birth outcomes and the health of offspring (Prochaska, Mauriello, Dyment, & Gokbayrak, 2011). The United States has one of the highest rates of low infant birth weight (which increases risk of health problems in infants) and maternal mortality of resource-rich countries. Some of these risks are related to changeable health behaviors, such as tobacco use. One study in West Virginia, for example, followed women who smoked or quit smoking (Chertok, Luo, & Anderson, 2011). On average, women who quit smoking gave birth to infants with higher and thus healthier birth weights. Comparisons in this study were interesting, as some mothers gave birth while still smoking regularly and then again after quitting. Women who did not quit smoking were more likely to deliver babies of low birth weight.

A great deal of publicity has been given to the effect of alcohol consumption during pregnancy on the developing fetus, and pregnant women are urged to avoid or at least severely limit alcohol consumption while pregnant, since safe levels of consumption have not been established (Carter et al., 2012; Kesmodel et al., 2012). Similarly, the effects of prescription medicines, over-the-counter medications, and illegal drugs can be negative and irreversible.

Some behaviors and risks are less easily controlled through behavior change. For example, exposure to stress and elevated feelings of stress during pregnancy are associated with long-term negative health consequences in offspring. Researchers have found that prenatal stress increases the risk of mental health disorders in these mothers' children years later, between the ages of 2 and 14 (Robinson et al., 2011). The effects of prenatal stress appear to be independent of postnatal stress exposure. In other words, children are more likely to develop mental health issues even though the stressors may have been resolved by the time of their birth. Especially sobering have been the associations demonstrated for the negative effects of perceived racial discrimination during pregnancy on birth outcomes and subsequent child health (Pachter, 2009).

Obesity increases risk of several medical problems that can develop during pregnancy, including gestational diabetes and hypertension. Because obesity rates have been rising in the general population, increasing numbers of women begin their pregnancy considerably overweight. Behavior-change interventions can help women reduce body fat before becoming pregnant and avoid excessive weight gain during pregnancy (Weisman et al., 2011). Women seeking guidance on changing dietary behaviors during pregnancy should be referred to a dietitian for diet planning, as nutrition needs during pregnancy must be met in order to avoid compromising the developing infant's health. Once pregnant women have a sound plan, health and fitness professionals can support them in trying to improve their eating habits, such as reducing soda intake, drinking more water, taking prescribed prenatal supplements, and consuming adequate servings of fruits and vegetables.

What about physical activity? Women in good health with uncomplicated pregnancies and no contraindications are generally urged to exercise for at least 30 minutes a day (Zavorsky & Longo, 2011). Guidelines for exercise during pregnancy are spelled out by the American College of Obstetricians and Gynecologists (ACOG, 2011). Exercise offers many benefits for healthy women with uncomplicated pregnancies. Exercise generally improves sleep quality, appetite, energy level, self-image, and sense of well-being in pregnant women. It may also help protect against back pain and gestational diabetes, two problems that commonly develop during pregnancy. Women who exercise during pregnancy can maintain or improve fitness indices such as muscle strength and aerobic endurance (Price, Amini, & Kappeler, 2012). A recent study compared 62 healthy, sedentary pregnant women randomly assigned to participate in an exercise program or to serve as controls. The researchers found that women in the exercise group (45–60 minutes, 4 days a week) not

only improved fitness but had a significantly lower rate of cesarean (surgical) deliveries: 6% in the exercise group compared with 32% in the control group (Price, Amini, & Kappeler, 2012).

Although theoretical concerns remain regarding the potential dangers of heavy exercise, clinical studies have not found increased risk of health problems for mothers or babies of moms who exercise during pregnancy (ACOG, 2011). These studies have been reassuring to athletic women who wish to maintain high levels of fitness during pregnancy. Nevertheless, pregnancy complications do occur in both exercising and sedentary pregnant women and at similar rates. Pregnant clients should have their physician's clearance to exercise and understand which symptoms mean that they should stop exercising and seek medical attention (Box 7-4). During prenatal exams, doctors and midwives screen for possible complications that could have negative health consequences for the mother and/or baby. Identifying such conditions as early as possible in pregnancy can improve pregnancy outcome and even save the life of the mother or the baby. When complications such as pregnancy-induced hypertension are present, exercise taxes a system that is already overly stressed. Thus, exercise is contraindicated for several conditions (Box 7-5).

Teaching prenatal exercise classes requires special training, so health and fitness professionals who work with pregnant clients either in a group exercise or personal training format should learn as much as they can about exercise physiology during pregnancy (Fig. 7-9). Certain exercises and exercise positions should be avoided, and changes in balance must be accommodated as bellies expand.

Box 7-4. Pregnancy and Exercise: Warning Signs to Stop Exercise

Pregnant women who experience any of the following symptoms should stop exercising and be referred to their health-care providers for medical evaluation.

- Vaginal bleeding
- Fluid leaking from the vagina
- Dizziness
- Uterine contractions
- Unusual shortness of breath
- Chest pain
- Headache
- Calf swelling or pain
- Decreased fetal movement

Source: American College of Obstetricians and Gynecologists. (2011). Exercise during pregnancy. www.acog.org/~/media/For%20Patients/faq119.pdf?dmc=1&ts=20120424T1109367337. Accessed 7/5/12.

Box 7-5. Contraindications for Exercise During Pregnancy

Most healthy women with uncomplicated pregnancies can exercise safely. Certain conditions, however, make exercise dangerous to the mother. These include the following:

- Pregnancy-induced hypertension
- Preterm rupture of membranes. This is the "bag of water" or amniotic fluid that surrounds the baby, which must stay intact until delivery.
- Preterm labor in current pregnancy or in a previous pregnancy
- Incompetent cervix or cerclage. In this condition, the cervix is in danger of opening prematurely, leading to a preterm delivery. A cerclage is a minor surgical procedure that helps keep the cervix closed.
- Intrauterine growth retardation. Doctors are concerned when the baby is not growing as quickly as it should and may direct the mother-to-be to take precautions to reduce any possible sources of stress, such as exercise.
- Placenta previa. This refers to a placenta located near or on top of the cervix, which can lead to bleeding and preterm labor.
- Persistent bleeding.

Source: American College of Obstetricians and Gynecologists. (2011). Exercise during pregnancy. www.acog.org/~/media/For%20Patients/faq119.pdf?dmc=1&ts=20120424T1109367337. Accessed 7/5/12.

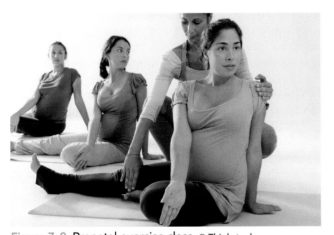

Figure 7-9. **Prenatal exercise class.** © Thinkstock

The next alumna to come to the athletic training facility, Lara, is 7 months pregnant, and she wants Katie's advice on her low-back pain and recommendations for staying active throughout her pregnancy. She has been *very fit and active all her life. Her last medical appointment was a month ago, and everything looked fine. But, as they begin reviewing Lara's exercise program, Lara mentions casually that she stopped at the drugstore on the way to see Katie and took her blood pressure. It was 160/110. She asks Katie if that is too high. Alarmed, Katie gets out her blood pressure cuff and stethoscope and takes Lara's blood pressure again. Katie takes it a second time to be sure she is correct. Sure enough, it is quite high: 150/110. Katie tells Lara she needs to see a doctor right away and that her high blood pressure needs to be evaluated. Since Lara is far from home, she will need to go to the emergency department at the local hospital. Lara shrugs and tells Katie that since the hospital is only a mile away, she will walk over. "The walk will be good for me," Lara says. Katie disagrees. She urges Lara to accept a ride to the hospital. Katie calls Dan as she walks Lara to the car and cancels her next appointment in order to drive Lara to the hospital right away.*

The emergency department staff finds that Lara is in preterm labor. They are able to stop the labor, but Lara is hospitalized. Lara's husband will be flying out tomorrow to be with Lara and to drive her home, once she is able to travel. Katie is relieved that she got Lara to the hospital in time. ■

Postpartum and New Parent Challenges

New parents face many joys but also many challenges once a new baby or adopted child joins the family. It can take some time for a new routine to become established, and the new responsibilities of parenting can feel overwhelming for many. Women undergoing postchildbirth psychophysiological changes experience additional demands as their bodies and brains adapt to a new nonpregnant state. Health and fitness professionals working with new parents should be compassionate and understanding with them since they may be experiencing a number of new stressors (Behavior Change in Action 7-1).

Behavior-change programs are easier to implement when they require minimal self-control and can quickly be transformed into habits that do not require a great deal of self-regulation. Unfortunately for new parents, disrupted routines are the hallmark of parenting, especially when children are very young. Sleeping schedules change, babies get fussy or sick, and some days it seems like a miracle that the dishes even get washed. New parents may abandon an exercise program or eating plan when interruptions arise. A sense of disorganization and too little sleep cause many of them to feel out of control, especially regarding self-care. New parents may need to plan ways to implement physical activity and other behavior-change options

BEHAVIOR CHANGE IN ACTION 7-1

Motivating New Parents

■ CHALLENGE

New parents' lives are often chaotic and stressful as they adapt to their new roles and priorities. In addition, many women find that they are still carrying extra weight for a year or more after delivering their babies and may be at risk for future obesity.

■ PLAN

Health and fitness professionals should show empathy and understanding for clients adjusting to this new life stage. When building on the motivation that new parents often feel to serve as good role models for their children, behavior-change programs should also be somewhat flexible to accommodate the disruptions common in the lives of these clients. Specific suggestions include the following.

Be gentle with new moms. The early postpartum period is not the time to rush into a demanding exercise program or a restrictive diet, as the mother's body needs time to heal during the first few months after the baby's birth. During these early weeks, new mothers should get plenty of rest, napping as much as possible. Women recovering from surgeries will need more time for healing. During the early postpartum period, women should add exercise slowly, following their doctor's recommendations for resuming activity. Women should be encouraged to eat as healthfully as possible. Breastfeeding mothers should be sure to drink plenty of water.

Help new parents see that self-care is family care. Becoming a parent can provide a healthy motivation to lose weight and develop a healthful lifestyle. Parents often want to be healthy so that they have the energy to enjoy their kids. A lifestyle that incorporates regular physical activity can help reduce stress and increase energy levels.

Most parents say that they want to be good role models for their children. Health and fitness professionals may be able to help parenting clients see that self-care is not selfish, as many adults seem to think but rather that it is family care. Parents need to show their children by their example that healthy people make time to take care of themselves. They choose good food, eat for the right reasons, and make time to enjoy physical activity.

Work with new parents to establish a feasible exercise routine. Regular physical activity should be the cornerstone of behavior-change programs. Exercise will help strengthen muscles, reduce fatigue, improve mood, and promote health in many other ways. It will also burn some calories and enhance weight-loss efforts.

What kind of activity can fit into clients' new lives? Which activities are most enjoyable? Ask open-ended questions and listen carefully as clients discuss their options. Let clients take the lead in figuring out what will work for them, keeping in mind that even a small amount of exercise is better than none and may at least help clients establish an exercise habit. Walking is often the most accessible form of exercise, with or without baby in tow.

Help clients anticipate disruption and recover from lapses quickly. It may take a while for new parents to establish a daily routine that makes time for self-care. Even then, parenting requires an enormous amount of flexibility and adaptability. If you are working with new parents, help them brainstorm ways to accommodate the disruptions that a new baby brings to the household. Help them design a realistic behavior-change routine that will make exercise and good food choices habitual as quickly as possible. If you are working with parents of young children, help your clients create contingency plans for those days when sleepless nights, sick children, and the extra demands of parenting will interrupt their normal routine. It is especially important for new parents to cut themselves some slack and not view disruptions as personal failures.

Create social support. Since new parents often feel the need for more support, many fitness centers have stepped in to provide helpful options. Some offer pregnancy and postpartum exercise classes where mothers-to-be and new moms can work out together under the guidance of qualified instructors. Many fitness centers provide childcare or incorporate babies into the class format.

Encourage new parents to think of ways to reduce fatigue and stress. Fatigue and stress are the most common reasons people fail to stick to their behavior-change plans. They are also two of the things that all new parents seem to have in common. Encourage new parents to do everything they can to get enough rest and to reduce stress. They may need to lower their expectations of what they can accomplish in a day. Be sure that they experience exercise as refreshing and invigorating rather than exhausting.

Advise clients seeking weight loss to eat sensibly and avoid restrictive diets. The best way to lose weight is to eat less and exercise more. The best way to eat less is to reduce the amount of empty-calorie "junk" food in one's diet. Advise clients to try for a well-balanced diet that includes protein foods at each meal and to eat plenty of fruits and vegetables. Chapters 9 and 10 will explain in more detail the kinds of advice health and fitness professionals should give regarding healthy eating and weight loss.

Help clients address emotional eating behaviors. Parents of babies and young children may struggle with stress overload, feeling that they can never meet all of the expectations placed on them. Balancing work, childcare, and

BEHAVIOR CHANGE IN ACTION 7-1–cont'd

household responsibilities can create feelings of stress for even the most organized parents. In addition, early-postpartum hormonal and social changes can trigger the "baby blues" and other symptoms of depression in some women.

Many people overeat in response to emotional states such as stress, fatigue, anger, depression, anxiety, and even boredom. Eating helps people feel soothed and relaxed. Ask overweight parents about emotional eating and, if this is a problem, help them explore this issue. Help them discover better ways to feel nurtured and deal with stress. The self-monitoring records they create as they work with you can help you guide the problem-solving techniques. Of course, you will want to refer your clients to professional help when they say that emotional eating and the feelings that trigger it are a significant problem for them.

Encourage realistic expectations regarding behavior-change efforts and a focus on good health. Encourage new parents to focus on lifelong good health, rather than short-term goals such as quick weight loss. Losing weight may be challenging for some clients, especially those who tend to gain weight easily, who gained more than an average amount of weight during pregnancy, and who are still carrying extra weight 6 months or more after the baby's birth.

when problems arise and to accept the fact that some days may not be perfect.

Parents, especially new ones, cite a lack of support as a barrier to participation in physical activity (Bellow-Riecken & Rhodes, 2008). Lack of social support is also one of the primary sources of stress for parents. It takes a village not only to raise a child but to support new parents as well. A network of extended family, friends, and neighbors makes parenting less stressful by giving parents a break. For example, Grandma watches the baby while Mom takes a walk. Social support can also provide perspective as parents feel part of a larger social network.

A healthy weight gain supports a healthy pregnancy and fetal development. But, once the baby is born, most women are eager to regain their prepregnancy figures. Following the birth of a baby, most women lose weight fairly quickly for the first 3 months. Weight loss then slows to about 1 or 2 pounds per month, until normal weight is achieved by about 6 months after the baby's birth. Weight loss patterns vary greatly, however, with some women losing pregnancy weight very easily and quickly, whereas others seem to struggle to lose the extra pounds. Women who have a history of obesity and those who gain a great deal of extra weight during their pregnancies have a greater risk of postpartum weight retention and later weight gain. Indeed, medical researchers believe that pregnancy and the postpartum period are times of increased risk for the development of long-term obesity for many women (Gore, Brown, & West, 2003; Rooney. Schauberger, & Mathiason, 2005). One study found that excess gestational weight gain, failure to lose weight after delivery, lack of exercise, and breastfeeding for fewer than 3 months all predicted obesity 10 years later (Rooney & Schauberger, 2002).

Women struggling to lose weight after they give birth cite a number of barriers to weight-control behaviors, such as diet and exercise. In addition to wishing they had more support from friends, family members, and society at large, many women feel that they have too little time to take on a behavior-change program (Montgomery, Bushee, & Phillips, 2011). Some women also experience low motivation and low self-efficacy for overcoming barriers to self-care behaviors (Montgomery, Bushee, & Phillips, 2011).

Women who are breastfeeding their babies sometimes worry that diet, exercise, and weight loss may compromise their milk supply and the health of their babies. But research shows that as long as weight is lost slowly and women are consuming a well-balanced diet, milk supply does not suffer (McCrory, Nommsen-Rivers, Mole, Lönnerdal, & Dewey, 1999). Exercise should be moderate and balanced with adequate rest. Lactating mothers should wear a supportive bra and nurse their babies before exercising, so breasts will be more comfortable during exercise.

Another concern for lactating women is the possibility that calorie restriction might compromise bone density. Bone mineral content declines during lactation for all women, as calcium is drawn from the bones to make milk and as estrogen levels decline. Most, although not all, studies suggest that this bone loss is reversed after weaning, as estrogen rises with the resumption of the menstrual cycle (More, Bettembuk, Bhattoa, & Balogh, 2001). Because exercise has been shown to help improve bone mineral density, one research group examined whether engagement in exercise during the postpartum period in breastfeeding women might reduce the loss of bone mineral (Lovelady, Bopp, Colleran, Mackie, & Wideman, 2009). Researchers compared bone density change in breastfeeding subjects who exercised (45 minutes of walking and 30 minutes of resistance training, 3 days a week) with control subjects. Neither group was dieting, although subjects in both groups lost on average about 3.5 kg. Women in the exercise group lost less bone mineral (group average 4.7%) than the nonexercising group (7.0%).

A similar study examined the effect of adding calorie restriction to exercise to help postpartum mothers lose excess weight. Women who reduced calorie intake (500–600 kcal less per day) and engaged in resistance training did not lose any more bone than controls who did not diet or exercise (Colleran, Wideman, & Lovelady, 2012). These studies suggest than breastfeeding moms should exercise and consume plenty of calcium and not be surprised if bone density declines temporarily. New moms can at least engage in appropriate weight-loss behaviors such as modest calorie restriction and regular physical activity, knowing that these behaviors will not make the situation worse.

Work-Life Balance

A majority of working adults express concern about achieving a balanced, healthy lifestyle in the face of a perceived lack of time. This concern is widespread among both men and women and affects all age groups, even teens and seniors. Men and especially women with young children seem to experience the most acute time crunch, coupled with feelings of guilt and frustration at not being able to "do it all." Issues of finding time for self-care while balancing work and family commitments are likely to remain at the forefront of health-behavior counseling for years to come. Many employers have increased the availability of flexible work schedules; these are helpful but not a complete solution. The work still has to get done, and people's expectations of what they should be able to accomplish in a day are often unrealistic. Clients report feeling that the pace of life accelerates each year. Many people are single parents, work multiple jobs, commute long distances, or face other significant challenges that result in a truly overwhelming time bind. Role overload predicts a decrease in physical activity as people move through their adult years (Bellows-Riecken & Rhodes, 2008).

Helping clients find time for self-care while balancing the demands of work and family requires an understanding of the many issues that arise when people attempt to juggle multiple priorities. Health and fitness professionals who keep these in mind will be in a better position to understand clients' challenges as they try to stick to their behavior-change programs. The most commonly cited barriers to physical activity for adults include lack of time, lack of social support, fatigue, childcare issues, obligations to other roles, and lack of money (Bellow-Riecken & Rhodes, 2008).

Parenting demands continue throughout the child-raising years and do not cease once children begin school. Caring for children can be time consuming and stressful. Some research suggests that mothers are more likely to have a higher BMI and lower levels of physical activity than women of the same age who are not parents (Berge, Larson, Bauer, & Neumark-Sztainer, 2011). Some fitness centers offer parallel programs for children

and parents in the late afternoon. Moms and dads are able to work out while children enjoy after-school games, sports, or swimming. Offering family-friendly programs allows some fitness centers to attract adults trying to juggle family, work, and self-care.

Midlife and Older Adults

Adults over 50 can be delightful clients who truly appreciate the efforts of the health and fitness professionals with whom they work. Many in this group begin to feel the need to make time for self-care and even have a little more free time as children grow up and become more independent. Adults often retire at some point in their 60s and look for meaningful activities to fill their days. Older adults may especially value the sense of connection they find in physical activities, group exercise classes, and fitness centers. Some of the most important issues that affect behavior-change motivation in midlife and older adults include health problems, declining physical fitness and ability, changes in body composition, and for midlife women, the psychophysiological changes associated with menopause.

Health Issues

As men and women approach their 50s and 60s, they usually become increasingly concerned about their health and the development of real or potential health problems, including the leading causes of death and disability discussed in Chapter 1. Older adults are even more conscious of the limitations imposed by the aging process and have developed or watched their peers cope with a variety of illnesses, many related to lifestyle and health behaviors. Midlife and older adults may have watched their parents' health decline and thus are motivated to avoid or delay the onset of any heritable illnesses, if possible.

The Health Belief Model and Theory of Planned Behavior offer valuable direction for behavior-change conversations with midlife and older adults. Clients who have sought a health and fitness professional's help in addressing concerns such as diabetes, hypertension, osteoporosis, and other chronic health problems may be very receptive to discussions about lifestyle changes to prevent or slow the progression of these conditions. Such clients are usually in the contemplation or preparation stage of change. Health and fitness professionals should ask open-ended questions and listen carefully to understand how much clients know about the relationship between lifestyle and chronic health problems and do everything they can to help clients see the importance of health behaviors for their individual situations.

Decline in Physical Fitness and Ability

Many measures of physical fitness begin to decline once people reach young adulthood, especially if they become less active. Speed, power, and force of movement begin to decrease, and reflexes may slow. These changes occur gradually over the years and often go unnoticed in young adults. Some midlife adults may notice losses in muscle size, strength, and power at this time, whereas these symptoms may not become apparent to others until later.

The term sarcopenia refers to a loss of muscle mass. Although sarcopenia is a type of muscle atrophy, it differs from the atrophy experienced with inactivity that is observed in younger adults (Altun et al., 2010). Originally, experts attributed the age-related decline in muscle strength and power to sarcopenia; but researchers now believe that sarcopenia is only part of the explanation, as loss of strength and power are often proportionally greater than loss of muscle mass. This means that with aging and inactivity, people experience not only a loss of muscle mass but also relative weakness in the remaining muscle tissue. Researchers Manini and Clark (2012) coined the term dynapenia to refer to this loss of muscle strength and power that often occurs with aging. Dynapenia, more than sarcopenia per se, contributes to a decline in physical function and increased rates of disability. Dynapenia appears to be caused by a number of age- and inactivity-related metabolic changes, including the impairment of several metabolic pathways responsible for the production of adenosine triphosphate (ATP) (Russ & Lanza, 2011). Dynapenia can eventually lead to a significant loss of physical ability for even the activities of daily living (ADLs), such as standing from a sitting position, grocery shopping and cooking, and performing basic household chores. Regular strength training is the most effective way to prevent or reverse this decline in physical ability (Game Changers 7-1).

Changes in Body Composition

Along with the loss of muscle tissue come losses in other structural tissues as well. Bone density declines, and joints become weaker. Osteoarthritis is diagnosed as cartilage is lost from the surfaces of bones in synovial joints. The nature of flesh changes with age: skin and subcutaneous adipose tissue sag, and muscles feel less firm as they lose muscle tissue and accumulate intramuscular fat deposits. Such changes in body composition are compounded to some extent by sedentary behaviors. An active lifestyle that includes strength training can significantly delay the loss of bone, muscle, and joint tissues and prevent the accretion of excess fat.

Too much excess fat, especially visceral fat, increases risk for developing obesity-related health problems in midlife adults. Many clients in this age group may want to lose weight both to look and feel better and to reduce health risks or control conditions such as diabetes and hypertension.

Studies show that caloric restriction and weight loss result not only in fat loss but also in loss of muscle tissue and bone mineral (Ensrud et al., 2003; Villareal, Fontana, & Weiss, 2006). This is true for both young and old, but young people at least have higher levels of anabolic hormones such as testosterone and estrogen,

---

Game Changers 7-1. Miriam Nelson: Promoting Physical Fitness for Older Adults

No one has done more than Miriam E. Nelson to change the way people think about physical fitness for older adults. Her scientific research has helped to demonstrate the beneficial effect of exercise, especially strength training, in elderly people. Her books for the lay public, including *Strong Women, Strong Bones* (2000) and *Strong Women and Men Beat Arthritis* (2002), have inspired the adoption of strength-training exercise programs in people who had never before, even in their wildest dreams, considered the idea of lifting weights.

At one time, scientists believed that older people were unable to respond physically to exercise training programs, especially if they had been previously sedentary. In addition, scientists thought even moderate physical activity unnecessarily increased an older person's risk of injury, heart attack, and stroke. Doctors believed exercise hastened the progression of arthritis. Health-care providers advised seniors to take it easy, advice now thought to accelerate physical decline and make older adults even more prone to injury and cardiovascular disease and less inclined to exercise. Providers attributed the physical decline associated with a sedentary lifestyle not to a lack of exercise but to the aging process.

Miriam Nelson helped to change these mistaken beliefs and practices. Research by Nelson and colleagues helped to establish the fact that older adults respond well to appropriate levels of strength training. Building on prior research examining strength training in older adults (Evans, 2002), Nelson helped to promote these findings in the scientific community (Seguin & Nelson, 2003). Her research examined the effects of strength training on a variety of fitness and health variables. Nelson and colleagues (2004) demonstrated that a home-based exercise program could improve functional performance in elderly subjects. Her randomized controlled trial of resistance training for older Latino adults with type 2 diabetes demonstrated that strength training improved glycemic control (Castaneda et al., 2002).

Miriam Nelson is also well known outside of the laboratory. Her *Strong Women* books have been translated into 14 languages and have inspired older adults all over the world. Her Strong Women Program has

Continued

Game Changers 7-1. Miriam Nelson: Promoting Physical Fitness for Older Adults—cont'd

groups in a number of states, where group exercise leaders, trained by Nelson and her team, offer two different curricula (www.strongwomen.com). A program in strength training helps women maintain muscle mass, strength, and function as they age. A heart-disease-prevention program focuses on heart-healthy nutrition and aerobic exercise to reduce cardiovascular disease risk. Data collected on volunteers participating in these programs support the idea that such programs lead to improvements in several measures of physical fitness (Seguin, Heidkamp-Young, Kuder, & Nelson, 2012). A firm believer in the ecological model of behavior change, Nelson has focused much of her public-health work on helping people, especially older women, form networks for health-behavior change. These projects help people build strong social support along with personal self-efficacy for behavior change.

Sources: Castaneda, C., Layne, J. E., Munoz-Orians, L., Gordon, P. L., Walsmith, J., Foldvari, M., . . . Nelson, M. E. (2002). A randomized controlled trial of resistance exercise training to improve glycemic control in older adults with type 2 diabetes. *Diabetes Care, 25*(12), 2335-2341; Evans, W. J. (2002). Exercise as the standard of care for elderly people. *Journal of Gerontology: Medical Sciences, 57A*(5), M260-M261; Nelson, M. E., with Wernick, S. (2000). *Strong Women, Strong Bones: Everything You Need to Know to Prevent, Treat, and Beat Osteoporosis.* New York: The Berkley Publishing Group; Nelson, M. E., Baker, K., & Roubenoff, R., with Lindner, L. (2002). *Strong Women and Men Beat Arthritis.* New York: G. P. Putnam's Sons; Nelson, M. E., Layne, J. E., Bernstein, M. J., Nuernberger, A., Castaneda, C., Kaliton, D., . . . Fiatarone Singh, M. A. (2004). The effects of multidimensional home-based exercise on functional performance in elderly people. *Journal of Gerontology Series A: Biological Sciences and Medical Sciences, 59*(2), 154-160; Seguin, R. A., Heidkamp-Young, E., Kuder, J., & Nelson, M. E. (2012). Improved physical fitness among older female participants in a nationally disseminated, community-based exercise program. *Health Education and Behavior, 39*(2), 183-190; Seguin, R., & Nelson, M. E. (2003). The benefits of strength training for older adults. *American Journal of Preventive Medicine, 25*(3 suppl 2), 141-149; StrongWomen Program (2012). Information on Nelson's public-health programs. www.strongwomen.com/strongwomen-programs/program-description. Accessed 7/5/12; StrongWomen (2012). Strong Women: Lifting Women to Better Health. List of all books. www.strongwomen.com/books/. Accessed 7/5/12.

which can help them recover somewhat from these losses, given good exercise and nutrition most of the time. However, in midlife and older adults, losses may never be regained and may speed the course toward osteoporosis and sarcopenia.

Rather than just trying to lose weight, overweight clients should focus on improving body composition by building strength and general fitness and decreasing calories somewhat by eliminating less nutritious foods while increasing vegetable intake. Some research suggests that resistance training can help dieting older adults preserve muscle and bone mass. One study of sedentary, overweight adults with type 2 diabetes randomly assigned half of the volunteers to a moderate weight-loss program only, whereas the other half received the same program plus resistance training (Daly et al., 2005). After 6 months, both groups showed similar losses in weight and fat mass. The resistance training groups showed small but significant increases in lean mass as well. Over the following 6 months, resistance trainers switched to a home-based program, and all subjects resumed normal eating. At the end of this period, control subjects showed a slight decrease in lean mass, whereas the resistance trainers maintained lean mass. This study underscores the benefits of including resistance training in weight-control programs for older adults. In addition, even if clients do not lose weight, a healthy lifestyle may help address chronic

health problems associated with obesity, such as hypertension and diabetes.

Cognitive Decline

Adults over 50 often notice some decline in their abilities to recall information. They may have more trouble finding the word they want when speaking or writing, remembering names, and learning new information. Many adults worry that such changes herald the development of Alzheimer's disease or other forms of dementia. Knowing that exercise increases cognitive function, or at least delays its loss, is very meaningful to them. Exciting studies have provided good evidence that aerobic exercise can increase cognitive ability and even brain volume in aging humans (Colcombe et al., 2006). Strength training has also been shown to improve some indicators of cognitive function (Hurley, Hanson, & Sheaff, 2011; Nagamatsu et al., 2012). Studies suggest that higher levels of fitness are associated with lower risk of dementia, including death from dementia (Liu et al., 2012).

Menopause

Menopause refers to the cessation of the menstrual cycle in women and occurs because the ovaries decrease their production of the sex hormones estrogen and progesterone. Menopause is defined as the time when a woman has had no menstrual periods for

1 year, and the cessation of the menstrual cycle is not due to other factors, such as illness or eating disorders. Natural menopause refers to menopause that occurs because the ovaries naturally decrease their sex hormone production as women age. Induced menopause occurs when the ovaries are removed surgically or are inhibited from producing hormones by drugs. Menopause usually occurs between the ages of 45 and 55. A woman is said to have early menopause when it occurs before age 40. Perimenopause refers to the years leading up to menopause, during which symptoms such as irregular menstrual cycles, hot flashes, and mood swings may emerge. Perimenopause is also called the menopause transition. The term premenopausal describes women who have not yet reached menopause, whereas postmenopausal describes women who have already gone through the menopause transition.

The menopause transition is a good example of the mind-body connection, as most women experience both psychological and physical changes during these years. In addition to the symptoms mentioned above, many women experience night sweats (waking up feeling hot and sweaty), difficulty sleeping, fatigue, fluctuations in sexual desire, and forgetfulness. Risk for several health problems begins to increase after menopause, partly from hormonal changes and partly just from aging. The rate of bone mineral loss increases for several years at menopause. Blood lipid levels also tend to shift to a more atherogenic profile, with decreases in HDL and increases in LDL cholesterol. Risk for type 2 diabetes and hypertension increases, especially with changes in body composition (Polotsky & Polotsky, 2010). But the menopause transition may bring positive changes as well. Many women breathe a sigh of relief to be done with menstrual periods and concern about unwanted pregnancy. Some women become more dedicated to their work in the world at this time as family responsibilities decline.

Some of the most unwanted changes for many women seeking the advice of health and fitness professionals are shifts in body composition, with increasing abdominal fat and weight gain, along with muscle loss. Researchers believe that the body composition changes that accompany menopause in most women are the result of a combination of hormonal changes along with normal age-related changes. Alterations in lifestyle, such as a reduction in physical activity or a shift in eating behaviors, can compound the effects of menopause and aging. But even nonobese women who exercise and have a healthy diet generally experience a significant increase in visceral and abdominal fat during the first few years after menopause (Abdulnour et al., 2012).

Women vary widely in the way they perceive and experience the menopausal years. Whereas some women experience few difficulties, others find menopausal symptoms severe and disruptive. Particularly difficult are sleep problems that can develop during this period.

Fatigue increases feelings of stress and interferes with good intentions to exercise regularly and eat a well-balanced diet. Women who find that menopausal symptoms interfere significantly with their quality of life may consider various medications. Although hormone therapy is no longer recommended as a preventive measure, many women still opt for some form of hormonal treatment to quell sleep problems and other serious symptoms. Decisions about medical treatment for menopausal symptoms are often difficult, since none are without risk, so clients should discuss these with a health-care provider.

Regular exercise can help prevent obesity and other chronic health problems for midlife clients and improve quality of life for women experiencing difficult menopause symptoms. Research has found that higher levels of physical activity are associated with fewer physical and psychological symptoms during the menopause transition (Sternfeld & Dugan, 2011). A healthy lifestyle can improve body composition and reduce health risks at any age. Postmenopausal women experience the same benefits of exercise and a healthy diet as their male peers and premenstrual women. For example, research demonstrates that exercise and a modest calorie restriction leads to a decrease in visceral, subcutaneous, and intramuscular fat and an increase in insulin sensitivity in obese postmenopausal women (aged 49–76) with impaired glucose tolerance (Ryan, Ortmeyer, & Sorkin, 2012).

Older Adults

Adults 65 and older are a growing segment of the population in many countries. In the United States, 20% of the population is expected to be in this age bracket by 2030, up from 12% in 2000 (He, Sengupta, Velkoff, & DeBarros, 2005). The number of people 85 and older, often called the oldest old, is expected to double by then.

As clients reach their 70s, 80s, and beyond, their behavior-change motivation often centers on improving or preserving physical and psychological functioning and quality of life. Health problems and limitations in many areas may also strongly influence behavior-change motivation and program design. About 80% of people over 65 contend with at least one chronic health condition; half of the people in this age group have two or more chronic health conditions (He, Sengupta, Velkoff, & DeBarros, 2005). The most common health problems appearing in this group include arthritis, hypertension, heart disease, stroke, cancer, and type 2 diabetes (Houston, Nicklas, & Zizza, 2009).

Obesity rates peak in the United States at around age 60. After this age, BMIs tend to be lower, although for some people BMI may decline because of loss of lean body mass. In fact, in older adults, BMI may not be a good indicator of obesity. Many older adults experience sarcopenic obesity, excess body fat accompanied by a loss of lean body mass. People with sarcopenic obesity may or may not be classified as obese according to their BMIs.

Experts are unclear as to the benefits of weight loss in the elderly. Studies have failed to show a clear benefit of weight loss in terms of health (Decaria, Sharp, & Petrella, 2012). Several factors may complicate the obesity–health relationship in older adults, including the following:

- Survival of the healthy obese. Older obese people may be less prone to develop obesity-related health problems. Their survival into old age may indicate that for them, extra body fat is less risky than for most other people.
- Weight loss in the elderly is often due to underlying illness. When this is the case, weight loss is statistically associated with health problems. Although the weight loss may not have caused the health problem, in epidemiological studies, weight loss will be associated with health risk or at least confound the effect of intentional weight loss that might improve health markers.
- Some excess body fat may be protective in old age. Some studies have found that obesity is associated with reduced mortality, although this effect may be influenced by the above factors and not necessarily causative (Artham, Lavie, Patel, & Ventura, 2009). In other words, the excess fat may itself be protective, or it may be simply an indicator that the person is not sick.

How should health and fitness professionals advise older adults who are obese or who express a desire to lose weight? Most experts recommend focusing on improving fitness, increasing physical activity, and eating well rather than on weight loss per se (Decaria, Sharp, & Petrella, 2012). Health and fitness professionals should individualize behavior-change recommendations based on each client's unique health concerns. For example, an overweight client with diabetes may benefit from a small weight loss achieved through exercise and diet modifications (Houston, Nicklas, & Zizza, 2009).

People in many countries are living longer, but in their later years, the oldest old often become weak and dependent on others for care. People with sarcopenic obesity may look strong enough but have difficulty with ADLs, as their relatively weak muscles are unable to move their excess mass. Many older adults seek help from health and fitness professionals to make beneficial lifestyle changes.

In general, people become less active as they grow older (Davis, Fox, Hillsdon, et al., 2011). This is unfortunate, as sedentary habits compound the natural decline in function associated with the aging process. Sarcopenia, dynapenia, and other physical limitations can make it impossible for vulnerable seniors to live independently. As scientists continue to explore the psychophysiology of aging, it is becoming clear that appropriate exercise can slow and even reverse many components of the aging process. Exercise can improve cardiovascular health and fitness; increase muscular strength, power, and endurance; and improve joint mobility and flexibility, balance, and coordination. Metabolic markers including insulin sensitivity and blood lipid levels improve. Regular physical activity can improve mood; combat anxiety and depression; and enhance one's daily energy level, self-esteem, and general enthusiasm for life. Older adults are likely to be motivated by the hope that regular physical activity may slow or even reverse the cognitive decline associated with the aging process, as discussed above.

Eating well can be difficult at any age, and older people are likely to have even more barriers that interfere with plans to consume a healthy diet. Health problems may limit shopping and cooking, and living alone may reduce motivation to cook meals. Sense of taste and smell, along with appetite, may decline with age. Some older adults have dental problems such as missing or painful teeth that decrease their ability to chew. One of the biggest nutrition problems for older adults is that they generally need fewer calories per day, but their need for several nutrients increases. In addition, the GI tract's nutrient-absorption ability declines with age. This means that older adults must make calories count by choosing nutritious foods as often as possible and avoiding empty-calorie foods that offer energy but little nutrition.

MOTIVATING CHANGE: Individualizing Your Exercise Recommendations for Midlife and Older Adults

Mainstream culture in most parts of North America is biased against midlife and older adults, tending to more highly value a youthful appearance and productivity. Midlife and older people tend to be patronized, misunderstood, dismissed, and ignored. Just as the fitness center can be unfriendly to larger people, it can often cause older adults to feel out of place as well.

Health and fitness professionals should treat midlife and older adults as individuals. Gather data on health concerns and fitness goals as you would for any other client. Use good communication skills and listen carefully to understand what recommendations might work best for each client. Cultivate a feeling of connection with clients, build their competence, and inspire intrinsic motivation for behavior change. As adults get older, they may be concerned both with preserving health and building quality of life.

Most midlife and older exercisers benefit greatly from strength-training programs that help build or at least preserve lean body mass and strengthen bones and joints. Remember that older joints may adapt more slowly to strength training than younger joints. As you work with older exercisers, keep in mind that many will come to you with prior injuries that you must accommodate in your exercise recommendations. Start people new to strength training slowly and build gradually to prevent injury.

Some midlife and older adults should be concerned about functional fitness that improves their ability to perform ADLs (Fig. 7-10). Older adults low in strength may be motivated to exercise regularly to reduce risk of falling. If this is the case, work on strength and balance. Some older adults should learn how to recover from a fall and get back on their feet. Frail elders may be motivated to increase strength so that they can get up from a sitting position, walk a given distance, lift groceries, and perform other daily tasks.

One of the most valuable effects of regular physical activity is mood improvement. Increased exercise self-efficacy and strength can enhance confidence for other activities, such as joining an exercise class or walking group or going out to events. Exercise classes and groups can provide social contact, which is especially therapeutic for people with limited opportunities for companionship.

The organizer of the alumni group has asked Katie to give a lecture on the benefits of strength training for older adults. The group attending her lecture ranges in age from around 50 to 90. Perfect, thinks Katie. This is just what they need. After the instructional session, Katie takes the group over to the weight room to let them try the machines. She is amazed at how weak most of the participants are—very different from her student athletes! She realizes that she does not know how to judge their capabilities. So she has everyone start with just one plate to learn how the machines work. The weight room monitor comes over to give her a hand, and they split the group in half. The alumni take turns on the machines and cheer one another on. They thank Katie warmly when the session is over and promise to check out their local fitness centers when they return home.

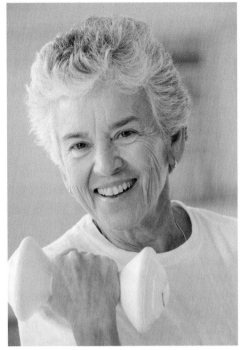

Figure 7-10. Exercise to improve functional fitness.
© Thinkstock

KEY TERMS

cerclage	perimenopause
cultural awareness	placenta previa
cultural competence	postmenopausal
cultural sensitivity	poverty–obesity paradox
diverse	premenopausal
dynapenia	race
energy density	religion
ethnicity	sarcopenia
faith-placed programs	sarcopenic obesity
induced menopause	screen use
menopause	spirituality
menopause transition	trait self-control
MET	
natural menopause	

CRITICAL THINKING QUESTIONS

1. Imagine that you are an exercise physiologist and part of a cardiac-rehabilitation team. One of your jobs is to meet with patients and help them design an exercise program they can continue once the official cardiac-rehabilitation program ends. You have a 70-year-old female client who recently moved to your town from Saudi Arabia. She has improved her fitness in your program. Her husband comes with her to every session and walks with her. He comes to all of her meetings with you as well, although he sits off to the side and lets her do the talking. What are five open-ended questions that you might ask your client as you gather information to help her design a program for continued exercise? Your goal is to understand what types of exercise might be culturally appropriate as well as motivating, for your client.

Continued

CRITICAL THINKING QUESTIONS–cont'd

2. How active were you as an elementary school child? What kinds of activities did you and your friends enjoy in fourth and fifth grade? Do you think your activity level met the recommendation of 1 hour per day of vigorous exercise? Remember that activity need not be continuous but may occur in a variety of ways over the course of the day. What percentage of your classmates do you think met the hour-per-day guideline? If you were a physical education teacher now, how would you encourage fourth and fifth graders to increase their performance of vigorous physical activity?

3. Imagine that you are working with two personal training clients. One is pregnant for the first time and wants to exercise to have a healthy pregnancy and childbirth. The other has two young children and a full-time job outside of the home. Her goal is to exercise to reduce stress. Describe how the exercise programs for these two women might differ.

4. How would you respond to the following client: a 65-year-old man with a normal BMI but sarcopenic obesity and low levels of strength. He is concerned about his excess abdominal fat and walks about 3 miles a day to try to reduce this excess fat. He enjoys the walking but does not see any changes in his weight or body shape. He wants to know what you would recommend in terms of diet and exercise to improve his body composition.

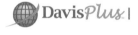 **DavisPlus** | For additional resources log in to DavisPlus (**http://davisplus.fadavis.com**/ keyword "Brehm") and click on the Premium tab. (Don't have a *Plus*Code to access Premium Resources? Just click the Purchase Access button on the book's *DavisPlus* page.)

REFERENCES

Abdulnour, J., Doucet, E., Brochu, M., Lavoie, J. M., Strychar, I. Rabasa-Lhoret, R., & Prud'homme, D. (2012). The effect of the menopausal transition on body composition and cardiometabolic risk factors: a Montreal-Ottawa New Emerging Team group study. *Menopause, 19*(7), 760-767.

Adler, N. E., & Stewart, J. (2010). Preface to the biology of disadvantage: socioeconomic status and health. *Annals of the New York Academy of Sciences, 1186,* 1-4.

Aggarwal, A., Monsivais, P., Cook, A. J., & Drewnowski, A. (2011). Does diet cost mediate the relation between socioeconomic position and diet quality? *European Journal of Clinical Nutrition, 65*(9), 1059-1066.

Altun, M., Besche, H. C., Overkleeft, H. S., Piccirillo, R., Edelmann, M. J., Kessler, B. M., . . . Ulfhake, B. (2010). Muscle wasting in aged, sarcopenic rats is associated with enhanced activity of the ubiquitin proteasome pathway. *Journal of Biological Chemistry, 285*(51), 39597-39608.

American Academy of Pediatrics, Council on Communication and Media. (2011a). Children, adolescents, obesity, and the media. *Pediatrics, 128*(1), 201-208.

American Academy of Pediatrics, Council on Communication and Media. (2011b). Media use by children younger than 2 years. *Pediatrics, 128*(5), 1040-1045.

American College of Obstetricians and Gynecologists. (2011). Exercise during pregnancy. www.acog.org/~/media/For%20Patients/faq119.pdf?dmc=1&ts=20120424 T1109367337. Accessed 7/5/12.

Artham, S. M., Lavie, C. J., Patel, D. A., & Ventura, H. O. (2009). Obesity paradox in the elderly: is fatter really fitter? *Aging Health, 5*(2), 177-184.

Avula, R., Gonzalez, W., Shapiro, C. J., Fram, M. S., Beets, M. W., Jones, S. J., . . . Frongillo, E. A. (2011). Positive parenting practices associated with subsequent childhood weight change. *Journal of Primary Prevention, 32*(5-6), 271-281.

Banich, M. T. (2009). Executive function: the search for an integrated account. *Current Directions in Psychological Science, 18*(2), 89-94.

Bellows-Riecken, K. H., & Rhodes, R. E. (2008). A birth of inactivity? A review of physical activity and parenthood. *Preventive Medicine, 46*(2), 99-110.

Benton, D. (2010). The influence of dietary status on the cognitive performance of children. *Molecular Nutrition & Food Research, 54*(4), 457-470.

Berge, J. M., Larson, N., Bauer, K. W., & Neumark-Sztainer, D. (2011). Are parents of young children practicing healthy nutrition and physical activity behaviors? *Pediatrics, 127*(5), 881-887.

Bradby, H. (2012). Race, ethnicity and health: the costs and benefits of conceptualising racism and ethnicity. *Social Science & Medicine, 75*(6), 955-958.

Brooks, R. C., Simpson, S. J., & Raubenheimer, D. (2010). The price of protein: combining evolutionary and economic analysis to understand excessive energy consumption. *Obesity Reviews, 11* (12), 887-894.

Carter, R. C., Jacobson, J. L., Molteno, C. D., Jiang, H., Meintjes, E. M., Jacobson, S. W., & Duggan, C. (2012). Effects of heavy prenatal alcohol exposure and iron deficiency anemia on child growth and body composition through age 9 years. *Alcoholism: Clinical & Experimental Research, 36*(11), 1973-1982.

Casey, B. J., Somerville, L. H., Gotlib, I. H., Ayduk, O., Franklin, N. T., Askren, M. K., . . . Shoda, Y. (2011). Behavioral and neural correlates of delay of gratification 40 years later. *Proceedings of the National Academy of Sciences USA, 108*(36), 14998-15003.

Castaneda, C., Layne, J. E., Munoz-Orians, L., Gordon, P. L., Walsmith, J., Foldvari, M., . . . Nelson, M. E. (2002). A randomized controlled trial of resistance exercise training to improve glycemic control in older adults with type 2 diabetes. *Diabetes Care, 25*(12), 2335-2341.

Centers for Disease Control and Prevention. (2012a). Adolescent and School Health: Childhood Obesity Facts. www.cdc.gov/healthyyouth/obesity/facts.htm. Accessed 7/5/12.

Centers for Disease Control and Prevention. (2012b). Ethnographic Guides. www.cdc.gov/tb/publications/guidestoolkits/EthnographicGuides. Accessed 7/5/12.

Centers for Disease Control and Prevention. (2012c). Youth Risk Behavior Surveillance—United States, 2011. *Morbidity and Mortality Weekly Report, 61*(No. SS-4), 1-168. www.cdc.gov/mmwr/pdf/ss/ss6104.pdf. Accessed 12/6/12.

Centers for Disease Control and Prevention. (2012d). Protect the Ones You Love: Child Injuries Are Preventable. www.cdc.gov/safechild/Sports_Injuries/index.html. Accessed 12/12/12.

Chaddock, L., Pontifex, M. B., Hillman, C. H., & Kramer, A. F. (2011). A review of the relation of aerobic fitness and physical activity to brain structure and function in children. *Journal of the International Neuropsychological Society, 17*(6), 975-985.

Chertok, I. R. A., Luo, J., & Anderson, R. H. (2011). Association between changes in smoking habits in subsequent pregnancy and infant birth weight in West Virginia. *Maternal & Child Health Journal, 15*(2), 249-254.

Colcombe, S. J., Erickson, K. I., Scalf, P. E., Kim, J. S., Prakash, R., & McAuley, E., (2006). Aerobic exercise training increases brain volume in aging humans. *Journal of Gerontology: Medical Sciences, 61A*(11), 1166-1170.

Colleran, H. L., Wideman, L., & Lovelady, C. A. (2012). Effects of energy restriction and exercise on bone mineral density during lactation. *Medicine and Science in Sports and Exercise, 44*(8), 1570-1579.

Cottrell, L., Harris, C. V., Bradlyn, A., Gunel, E., Neal, W. A., Abildso, L., & Coffman, J. W. (2012). Identifying the people and factors that influence children's intentions to make lifestyle changes. *Health Promotion Practice, 13*(2), 183-189.

Crescioni, A. W., Ehrlinger, J., Alquist, J. L., Conlon, K. E., Baumeister, R. F., Schatschneider, C., & Dutton, G. R. (2011). High trait self-control predicts positive health behaviors and success in weight loss. *Journal of Health Psychology, 16*, 750-759.

Daly, R. M., Dunstan, D. W., Owen, N., Jolley, D., Shaw, J. E., & Zimmet, P. Z. (2005). Does high-intensity resistance training maintain bone mass during moderate weight loss in older overweight adults with type 2 diabetes? *Osteoporosis International, 16*(12), 1703-1712.

Davis, M. G., Fox, K. R., Hillsdon, M., Sharp, D. J., Coulson, J. C., & Thompson, J. L. (2011). Objectively measured physical activity in a diverse sample of older urban UK adults. *Medicine and Science in Sports and Exercise, 43*(4), 647-654.

Decaria, J. E., Sharp, C., & Petrella, R. J. (2012). Scoping review report: obesity in older adults. *International Journal of Obesity (London), 36*(9), 1141-1150.

Deforche, B., Haerens, L., & de Bourdeaudhuij, I. (2011). How to make overweight children exercise and follow the recommendations. *International Journal of Pediatric Obesity, 6*(suppl 1), 35-41.

Diez Roux, A. V., & Mair, C. (2010). Neighborhoods and health. *Annals of the New York Academy of Sciences, 1186*, 125-145.

Drewnowski, A. (2009). Obesity, diets, and social inequalities. *Nutrition Reviews, 67*(suppl 1), S36-S39.

Drewnowski, A., & Specter, S. E. (2004). Poverty and obesity: the role of energy density and energy costs. *American Journal of Clinical Nutrition, 79*(1), 6-16.

Dunn, J. R. (2010). Health behavior vs the stress of low socioeconomic status and health outcomes. *Journal of the American Medical Association, 303*(12), 1199-1200.

Economist, The. (2008). The food industry: tightening belts. *The Economist,* April 10, 71-72. www.economist.com/node/11021146. Accessed 7/5/12.

Ensrud, K. E., Ewing, S. K., Stone, K. L., Cauley, J. A., Bowman, P. J., Cummings, S. R., & Study of Osteoporotic Fractures Research Group. (2003). Intentional and unintentional weight loss increase bone loss and hip fracture risk in older women. *Journal of the American Geriatrics Society, 51*(12), 1740-1747.

Evans, W. J. (2002). Exercise as the standard of care for elderly people. *Journal of Gerontology: Medical Sciences, 57A*(5), M260-M261.

Faigenbaum, A. D., Kraemer, W. J., Blimkie, C. J. R., Jeffreys, I., Micheli, L. J., Nitka, M., & Rowland, T. W. (2009). Youth resistance training: updated position statement from the National Strength and Conditioning Association. *Journal of Strength and Conditioning Research, 23*(suppl 5), S60-S79.

Farah, M. J., Shera, D. M., Savage, J. H., Betancourt, L., Giannetta, J. M., Brodsky, N. L., . . . Hurt H. (2006). Childhood poverty: specific associations with neurocognitive development. *Brain Research, 1110*(1), 166-174.

Fischer, K. W., Stein, Z., & Heikkinen, K. (2009). Narrow assessments misrepresent development and misguide policy: comment on Steinberg, Cauffman, Woolard, Graham, and Banich (2009). *American Psychologist, 64*(7), 595-600.

Florence, M. D., Asbridge, M., & Veugelers, P. J. (2008). Diet quality and academic performance. *Journal of School Health, 78*(4), 209-215.

Frank, L. D., Saelens, B. E., Powell, K. E., & Chapman, J. E. (2007). Stepping towards causation: do built environments or neighborhood and travel preferences explain physical activity, driving, and obesity? *Social Sciences and Medicine, 65*(9), 1898-1914.

Gavin, J. R., 3rd, Fox, K. M., & Grandy, S. (2011). Race/ethnicity and gender differences in health intentions and behaviors regarding exercise and diet for adults with type 2 diabetes: a cross-sectional analysis. *Biomedcentral Public Health, 11*, 533-541.

Gore, S. A., Brown, D. M., & West, D. S. (2003). The role of postpartum weight retention in obesity among women: a review of the evidence. *Annals of Behavioral Medicine, 26*(2), 149-159.

Guilfoyle, J., & St. Pierre-Hansen, N. (2012). Religion in primary care: let's talk about it. *Canadian Family Physician, 58*(3), 249-251.

Gutin, B. (2008). Child obesity can be reduced with vigorous activity rather than restriction of energy intake. *Obesity, 16*(10), 2193-2196.

Haas, S., & Nigg, C. R. (2009). Construct validation of the stages of change with strenuous, moderate, and mild physical activity and sedentary behaviour among children. *Journal of Science and Medicine in Sport, 12*(5), 586-591.

Hagger, M. S., Chantelle, W., Stiff, C., & Chatzisarantis, N. L. D. (2010). Ego depletion and the strength model of self-control: a meta-analysis. *Psychological Bulletin, 136*(4), 495-525.

Harris, B. S., & Watson, J. C., II. (2011). Assessing youth sport burnout: a self-determination and identity development perspective. *Journal of Clinical Sport Psychology, 5*(2), 117-133.

He, W., Sengupta, M., Velkoff, V., & DeBarros, K. (2005). *65+ in the United States: 2005*. Washington, D.C.: U.S. Department of Health and Human Services.

Houston, D. K., Nicklas, B. J., & Zizza, C. A. (2009). Weighty concerns: the growing prevalence of obesity among older adults. *Journal of the American Dietetic Association, 109*(11), 1886-1895.

Hruschka, D. J. (2012). Do economic constraints on food choice make people fat? A critical review of two hypotheses for the poverty–obesity paradox. *American Journal of Human Biology, 24*(3), 277-285.

Hunte, H. E. (2011). Association between perceived interpersonal everyday discrimination and waist circumference over a 9-year period in the Midlife Development in the United States cohort study. *American Journal of Epidemiology, 173*(11), 1232-1239.

Hunter L. R., & Schmidt, N. (2010). Anxiety psychopathology in African American adults: literature review and development of an empirically informed sociocultural model. *Psychological Bulletin, 136*(2), 211-235.

Hurley, B. F., Hanson, E. D., & Sheaff, A. K. (2011). Strength training as a countermeasure to aging muscle and chronic disease. *Sports Medicine, 41*(4), 289-306.

Institute of Medicine. (2011). *State and Local Policy Initiatives to Reduce Health Disparities—Workshop Summary*. Washington, D.C.: National Academy of Sciences.

Intrator, S. M., & Siegel, D. (2010). Project Coach: a case study of a college-community partnership as a venture in social entrepreneurship. *Perspectives on Urban Education, 7*(1), 66-72.

Intrator, S. M. & Siegel, D. (2008). Project Coach: youth development and academic achievement through sport. *Journal of Physical Education, Recreation, and Dance. 79*(7), 17-23.

Kawachi, I. (2005). Why the United States is not number one in health. In: Brown, L. D., Jacobs, L., & Morone, J. (eds.). *Healthy, Wealthy and Fair: Health Care for a Good Society*. New York: Oxford University Press.

Kesmodel, U. S., Bertrand, J., Stovring, H., Skarpness, B., Denny, C. H., Mortensen, E. L., & Lifestyle During Pregnancy Study Group. (2012). The effect of different alcohol drinking patterns in early to mid pregnancy on the child's intelligence, attention, and executive function. *British Journal of Obstetrics and Gynaecology, 119*(10), 1180-1190.

Kurian, A. K., & Cardarelli, K. M. (2007). Racial and ethnic differences in cardiovascular disease risk factors: a systematic review. *Ethnicity & Disease, 17*(1), 143-152.

Lattanzi, J. B., & Purnell, L. D. (2006). *Developing cultural competence in physical therapy practice,* Philadelphia: F.A. Davis Company.

Lee, R. E., Nigg, C. R., DiClemente, C. C., & Courneya, K. S. (2001). Validating motivational readiness for exercise behavior with adolescents. *Research Quarterly for Exercise and Sport, 72*(4), 401-410.

Liu, R., Xuemei, S., Laditka, J. N., Church, T. S., Colabianchi, N., Hussey, J., & Blair, S. N. (2012). Cardiorespiratory fitness as a predictor of dementia mortality in men and women. *Medicine and Science in Sports and Exercise, 44*(2), 253-259.

Lovelady, C., Bopp, M. J., Colleran, H. L., Mackie, H. K., & Wideman, L. (2009). Effect of exercise training on loss of bone mineral density during lactation. *Medicine and Science in Sports and Exercise, 41*(10), 1902-1907.

Luke, A., Lazaro, R. M., Bergeron, M. F., Keyser, L., Benjamin, H., Brenner, J., . . . Smith, A. (2011). Sports-related injuries in youth athletes: is overscheduling a risk factor? *Clinical Journal of Sports Medicine, 21*(4), 307-315.

Manini, T. M., & Clark, B. C. (2012). Dynapenia and aging: an update. *Journal of Gerontology: Medical Sciences, 67A*(1), 28-40.

Marques, S. C., Pais-Ribeiro, J. L., & Lopez, S. J. (2011). The role of positive psychology constructs in predicting mental health and academic achievement in children and adolescents: a two-year longitudinal study. *Journal of Happiness Studies, 12*(6), 1049-1062.

McClain, A. D., Chappuis, C., Nguyen-Rodriguez, S. T., Yaroch, A. L., & Spruijt-Metz, D. (2009). Psychosocial correlates of eating behavior in children and adolescents: a review. *International Journal of Behavioral Nutrition and Physical Activity, 6*:54.

McCrory, M., Nommsen-Rivers, L., Mole, P., Lönnerdal, B., & Dewey, K. G. (1999). Randomized trial of the short-term effects of dieting compared with dieting plus aerobic exercise on lactation performance. *American Journal of Clinical Nutrition, 6* (5), 959-967.

McLaren, L. (2007). Socioeconomic status and obesity. *Epidemiologic Reviews, 29*:29-48.

McLeod, T. C. V., Decoster, L. S., Loud, K. J., Micheli, L. J., Parker, J. T., Sandrey, M. A., & White, C. (2011). National Athletic Trainers' Association Position Statement: Prevention of Pediatric Overuse Injuries. *Journal of Athletic Training, 46*(2), 206-220.

Miller, G., Chen, E., & Cole, S. W. (2009). Health psychology: developing biologically plausible models linking the social world and physical health. *Annual Review of Psychology, 60*, 501-524.

Moffitt, T. E., Arseneault, L., Belsky, D., Dickson, N., Hancox, R. J., Harrington, H., . . . Caspi, A. (2011). A gradient of childhood self-control predicts health, wealth and public safety. *Proceedings of the National Academy of Sciences, 108*(7), 2693-2698.

Montgomery, K. A., Bushee, T. D., & Phillips, J. D. (2011). Women's challenges with postpartum weight loss. *Maternal and Child Health Journal, 15*(8), 1176-1184.

More, C., Bettembuk, P., Bhattoa, H. P., & Balogh, A. (2001). The effects of pregnancy and lactation on bone mineral density. *Osteoporosis International, 12*(9), 732-737.

Nagamatsu, L. S., Handy, T. C., Hsu, C. L., Voss, M., & Liu-Ambrose, T. (2012). Resistance training promotes cognitive and functional brain plasticity in seniors with probable mild cognitive impairment; a 6-month randomized controlled trial. *Archives of Internal Medicine, 172* (8), 666-668.

National Center for Health Statistics. (2011). *Health, United States, 2010: With Special Feature on Death and Dying*. Hyattsville, MD: Centers for Disease Control and Prevention.

Nelson, M. E., with Wernick, S. (2000). *Strong Women, Strong Bones: Everything You Need to Know to Prevent, Treat, and Beat Osteoporosis*. New York: The Berkley Publishing Group.

Nelson, M. E., Baker, K., & Roubenoff, R., with Lindner, L. (2002). *Strong Women and Men Beat Arthritis*. New York: G.P. Putnam's Sons.

Nelson, M. E., Layne, J. E., Bernstein, M. J., Nuernberger, A., Castaneda, C., Kaliton, D., . . . Fiatarone Singh, M. A. (2004). The effects of multidimensional home-based exercise on functional performance in elderly people. *Journal of Gerontology Series A: Biological Sciences and Medical Sciences, 59*(2), 154-160.

Olson, C. M., Bove, C. F., & Miller, E. O. (2007). Growing up poor: long-term implications for eating patterns and body weight. *Appetite, 49*(1), 198-207.

Ornish, D. (1998). *Love & Survival: 8 Pathways to Intimacy and Health.* New York: HarperCollins Publishers.

Oxman, T. E., Freeman, D. H., & Manheimer, E. D. (1995). Lack of social participation or religious strength and comfort as risk factors for death after cardiac surgery in the elderly. *Psychosomatic Medicine, 57*(1), 5-15.

Pachter, L. M. (2009). Racism and child health: a review of the literature and future directions. *Journal of Developmental and Behavioral Pediatrics, 30*(3), 255-263.

Page, A. S., Cooper, A.,R., Griew, P., & Jago, R. (2010). Children's screen viewing is related to psychological difficulties irrespective of physical activity. *Pediatrics, 126*(5), e1011-e1017.

Parker, P. D., Martin, A. J., Martinez, C., Marsh, H. W., & Jackson, S. A. (2010). Stages of change in physical activity: a validation study in late adolescence. *Health Education and Behavior, 37*(3), 318-329.

Paw, M. J. M. C. A., Singh, A. S., Brug, J., & van Mechelen, W. (2008). Why did soft drink consumption decrease but screen time not? Mediating mechanisms in a school-based obesity prevention program. *International Journal of Behavioral Nutrition and Physical Activity, 5*, 41.

Payne, M. A. (2012). "All gas and no brakes": helpful metaphor or harmful stereotype? *Journal of Adolescent Research, 27*(1), 3-17.

Polotsky, H. N., & Polotsky, A. J. (2010). Metabolic implications of menopause. *Seminars in Reproductive Medicine, 28*(5), 426-434.

Powell, J. S., & Barber Foss, K. D. (1999). Injury patterns in selected high school sports: a review of 1995–1997 seasons. *Journal of Athletic Training, 34*, 277-284.

Price, B. B., Amini, S. B., & Kappeler, K. (2012). Exercise in pregnancy: effect on fitness and obstetric outcomes—a randomized trial. *Medicine and Science in Sports and Exercise, 44*(2), 2263-2269.

Prochaska, J. M., Mauriello, L., Dyment, S., & Gokbayrak, S. (2011). Designing a health behavior change program for dissemination to underserved pregnant women. *Public Health Nursing, 28*(6), 548-555.

Proctor, A., Kurmeich, A., & Meershoek, A. (2011). Making a difference: the construction of ethnicity in HIV and STI epidemiological research by the Dutch National Institute for Public Health and the Environment. *Social Science and Medicine, 72*(11), 1838-1845.

Proctor, C., Tsukayama, E., Wood, A. M., Maltby, J., Fox Eades, J., & Linley, P. A. (2011). Strengths Gym: the impact of a character strengths–based intervention on the life satisfaction and well-being of adolescents. *Journal of Positive Psychology, 6*(5), 377-385.

Puhl, R., & Brownell, K. D. (2001). Bias, discrimination, and obesity. *Obesity Research, 9*, 788-805.

Purnell, L. D., & Paulanka, B. J. (2008). *Transcultural Health Care: A Culturally Competent Approach.* Philadelphia: F.A. Davis Company.

Queensland Government. (2011). Cultural Profiles: Community Profiles for Health Care Providers. www.health.qld.gov.au/multicultural/health_workers/cultdiver_guide.asp. Accessed 7/5/12.

Ray, C., & Roos, E. (2012). Family characteristics predicting favourable changes in 10 and 11-year-old children's lifestyle-related health behaviours during an 18-month follow-up. *Appetite, 58*(1), 326-332.

Riggs, N. R., Sakuma, K. L., & Pentz, M. A. (2007). Preventing risk for obesity by promoting self-regulation and decision-making skills: pilot results from the PATHWAYS to health program (PATHWAYS). *Evaluation Review, 31*(3), 287-310.

Roberts, C. K., Freed, B., & McCarthy, W. J. (2010). Low aerobic fitness and obesity are associated with lower standardized test scores in children. *Journal of Pediatrics, 156*(5), 711-718.

Robinson, M., Mattes, E., Oddy, W. H., Pennell, C. E., van Eekelen, A., McLean, N. J., . . . Newnham, J. P. (2011). Prenatal stress and risk of behavioral morbidity from age 2 to 14 years: the influence of the number, type, and timing of stressful life events. *Development and Psychopathology, 23*(2), 507-520.

Rod, N. H., Gronbaek, M., Schnohr, P., Prescott, E., & Kristensen, T. S. (2009). Perceived stress as a risk factor for changes in health behaviour and cardiac risk profile: a longitudinal study. *Journal of Internal Medicine, 266*(5), 467-475.

Romanello, M. L., & Holtgrefe, K. (2009). Teaching for cultural competence in non-diverse environments. *The Internet Journal of Allied Health Sciences and Practice, 7*(4), 1-8.

Rooney, B. L., Schauberger, C. W., & Mathiason, M. A. (2005). Impact of perinatal weight change on long-term obesity and obesity-related illnesses. *Obstetrics and Gynecology, 106*(6), 1349-1356.

Rooney, B. L., & Schauberger, C. W. (2002). Excess pregnancy weight gain and long-term obesity: one decade later. *Obstetrics and Gynecology, 100*(2), 245-252.

Rose, P. R. (2012). *Cultural Competence for the Health Professional.* Burlington, MA: Jones & Bartlett Learning.

Russ, D. W., & Lanza, I. R. (2011). The impact of old age on skeletal muscle energetics: supply and demand. *Current Aging Science, 4*(3), 234-247.

Ryan, A. S., Ortmeyer, H. K., & Sorkin, J. D. (2012). Exercise with calorie restriction improves insulin sensitivity and glycogen synthase activity in obese postmenopausal women with impaired glucose tolerance. *American Journal of Physiology: Endocrinology and Metabolism, 302*(1), E145-E152.

Ryan, R. M., Lynch, M. R., Vansteenkiste, M., & Deci, E. L. (2011). Motivation and autonomy in counseling, psychotherapy, and behavior change: a look at theory and practice. *The Counseling Psychologist, 39*(2), 193-260.

Saha, S., Komaromy, M., Koepsell, T. D., & Bindman, A. B. (1999). Patient-physician racial concordance and the perceived quality and use of health care. *Archives of Internal Medicine, 159*(9), 997-1004.

Savage, J. S., Fisher, J. O., & Birch, L. L. (2007). Parental influence on eating behavior: conception to adolescence. *Journal of Law and Medical Ethics, 35*(1), 22-34.

Seguin, R. A., Heidkamp-Young, E., Kuder, J., & Nelson, M. E. (2012). Improved physical fitness among older female participants in a nationally disseminated, community-based exercise program. *Health Education and Behavior, 39*(2), 183-190.

Seguin, R., & Nelson, M. E. (2003). The benefits of strength training for older adults. *American Journal of Preventive Medicine, 25*(3 suppl 2), 141-149.

Singh, A., Uijtdewilligen, L., Twisk, J. W. R., van Mechelen, W., & Chinapaw, M. J. (2012). Physical activity and performance at school: a systematic review of the literature including a methodological quality assessment. *Archives of Pediatrics and Adolescent Medicine, 166*(1), 49-55.

Stafford, M., Cummins, S., Ellaway, A., Sacker, A., Wiggins, R. D., & Macintyre, S. (2007). Pathways to obesity: identifying local, modifiable determinants of physical activity and diet. *Social Science and Medicine, 65*(9), 1882-1897.

Stallmann-Jorgensen, I. S., Gutin, B., Hatfield-Laube, J. L., Humphries, M. C., Johnson, M. H., & Barbeau, P. (2007). General and visceral adiposity in black and white adolescents and their relation with reported physical activity and diet. *International Journal of Obesity, 31*, 622-629.

Statistics Canada. (2006). Immigrant population by place of birth and period of immigration, 2006 Census of Population, last updated 10/14/09. www.statcan.gc.ca/tables-tableaux/sum-som/l01/cst01/demo24a-eng.htm. Accessed 7/5/12.

Sternfeld, B., & Dugan, S. (2011). Physical activity and health during the menopausal transition. *Obstetrics and Gynecology Clinics of North America, 38*(3), 537-566.

Strasburger, V. C., Jordan, A. B., & Donnerstein, E. (2010). Health effects of media on children and adolescents. *Pediatrics, 125*(4), 756-767.

Steinberg, L. (2007). Risk taking in adolescence: new perspectives from brain and behavioral science. *Current Directions in Psychological Science, 16*(2), 55-59.

Sternberg, Z., Munschauer, F. E., III, Carrow, S. S., & Sternberg, E. (2007). Faith-placed cardiovascular health promotion: a framework for contextual and organizational factors underlying program success. *Health Education Research, 22*(5), 619-629.

Stringhini, S., Sabia, S., Shipley, M., Brunner, E., Nabi, H., Kivimaki, M., & Singh-Manoux, A. (2010). Association of socioeconomic position with health behaviors and mortality. *Journal of the American Medical Association, 303*(12), 1159-1166.

Suldo, S. M., & Huebner, E. S. (2004). The role of life satisfaction in the relationship between authoritative parenting dimension and adolescent problem behavior. *Social Indicators Research, 66*, 165-195.

Thoits, P. A. (2010). Stress and health: major findings and policy implications. *Journal of Health and Social Behavior, 51*(1 suppl), S41-S53.

Travis, J. W., & Ryan, R. S. (2004). *The Wellness Workbook: How to Achieve Enduring Health and Vitality.* Berkeley, CA: Ten Speed Press.

U.S. Census Bureau. (2011). 2010 American Community Survey. Washington, D.C.: U.S. Census Bureau.

U.S. Department of Commerce, U.S. Census Bureau. (2012). State and county QuickFacts. http://quickfacts.census.gov/qfd/states/00000.html. Updated 12/10/12. Accessed 12/12/12.

U.S. Department of Health and Human Services. (2010). *Healthy People 2020.* Washington, D.C.: U.S. Department of Health and Human Services. www.healthypeople.gov/2020/TopicsObjectives2020/pdfs/HP2020_brochure_with_LHI_508.pdf. Accessed 7/5/12.

van Reedt Dortland, A. K. B., Vreeburt, S. A., Giltay, E. J., Licht, C. M., Vogelzangs, N., & van Veen, T., (2012). The impact of stress systems and lifestyle on dyslipidemia and obesity in anxiety and depression. *Psychoneuroendocrinology.* http://dx.doi.org/10.1016/j.psyneuen.2012.05.017.

Veigel, J. D., & Pleacher, M. D. (2008). Injury prevention in youth sport. *Current Sports Medicine Reports (American College of Sports Medicine), 7*(6), 348-353.

Villareal, D. T., Fontana, L., & Weiss, E. P. (2006). Bone mineral density response to caloric-restriction-induced weight loss or exercise-induced weight loss. *Archives of Internal Medicine, 166*(22), 2502-2510.

Weisman, C. S., Hillemeier, M. M., Downs, D. S., Feinberg, M. E., Chuang, C. H., Botti, J. J., & Dyer, A. M. (2011). Improving women's preconceptual health: long-term effects of the Strong Healthy Women behavior change intervention in the Central Pennsylvania Women's Health Study. *Women's Health Issues, 21*(4), 265-271.

Wilson, D. K., & Lawman, H. G. (2009). Health promotion in children and adolescents: an integration of the biopsychosocial model and ecological approaches to behavior change. In: Roberts, M. C., & Steele, R. G. (eds.). *Handbook of Pediatric Psychology,* ed. 4, 603-607. New York: Guilford Press.

Zavorsky, G. S., & Longo, L. D. (2011). Exercise guidelines in pregnancy: new perspectives. *Sports Medicine, 41*(5), 345-360.

Zick, C. D., Smith, K. R., Brown, B. B., Fan, J. X., & Kowaleski-Jones, L. (2007). Physical activity during the transition from adolescence to adulthood. *Journal of Physical Activity and Health, 4*(2), 125-137.

Zhou, M., Ma, W. J., & Deci, E. L. (2009). The importance of autonomy for rural Chinese children's motivation for learning. *Learning and Individual Differences, 19*(4), 492-498.

CHAPTER OUTLINE

LEARNING OBJECTIVES

After reading this chapter, you will be able to:

1. Apply an ecological perspective to better understand physical-activity behavior.

2. Apply the Stages of Change Model to physical-activity behavior.

3. Identify the factors that motivate people to consider becoming more active, applying the Health Belief Model and Chaos Theory.

4. Discuss factors that motivate people to form an intention or decision to increase physical activity, applying the Theory of Planned Behavior.

5. Describe the influence of self-efficacy on exercise adherence, the factors influencing exercise self-efficacy, and self-efficacy for overcoming barriers.

6. Set effective exercise program goals.

7. Apply self-regulation concepts and behavior-change methods for modifying behavior and increasing exercise adherence.

8. Explain factors associated with long-term exercise adherence.

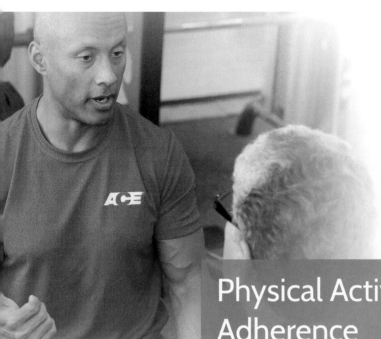

CHAPTER 8

Physical Activity and Exercise Adherence

PHYSICAL ACTIVITY AND EXERCISE ADHERENCE

◼ *Jessica graduated from college last year and has just started a new job as a personal trainer and exercise instructor at a busy fitness center in a large city. One of the most-important benefits associated with her new job is access to the state-of-the-art fitness center where she works, so Jessica can continue her exercise training. Jessica did well in several bodybuilding competitions last year, and she wants to continue training and competing this year. This means several hours in the gym most days. Working at the fitness center seems to be a great way to support her exercise habit. She has to work with a few clients this morning, but then she can get on with her real work: bodybuilding.*

Her client Sheila is small, 55 years old, and with a family history of osteoporosis. In fact, her mom is quite bent over, so Sheila is terrified of the condition. She has been monitoring her bone density since she was in her late 40s. After her third bone density test, Sheila received a diagnosis of mild, gradually worsening osteopenia. Her doctor explained that osteopenia is like preosteoporosis and that her bones have lost some mineral, but her risk of fracture is still low. A battery of tests found normal calcium metabolism and no other explanation for her bone mineral loss other than normal aging. Her doctor did not recommend any drug treatment at this point but did recommend that Sheila increase her intake of calcium and vitamin D and also increase her level of physical activity.

Sheila has always enjoyed walking and already walks several times a week for 60 minutes per session. She knows that walking is at least a "weight-bearing" exercise and is helpful for preventing bone loss. Sheila has also read in several magazine articles that weight training is supposed to be very good for keeping bones strong. She has joined the fitness center in order to start a weight-training program. Sheila's membership fee includes one personal training session to help her get started. When Jessica asks Sheila what she is looking for, she says she wants help setting up a weight-training routine to improve her bone density. ◼

Healthy adults need at least 30 minutes of moderately intense physical activity almost every day to stay healthy. A varied exercise program that includes strength training is helpful for most health and fitness goals. Many people have difficulty achieving even the minimal amount of physical activity, and unfortunately, the people who need physical activity the most seem to have the greatest difficulties working exercise into their lives. Designing exercise recommendations is the easy part; getting people to stick to their exercise programs is the hard part. Why is it so difficult for people to be physically active? This chapter examines issues related to exercise adherence, discusses how people change their physical-activity behaviors, and reviews the factors that promote successful maintenance of a physically active lifestyle.

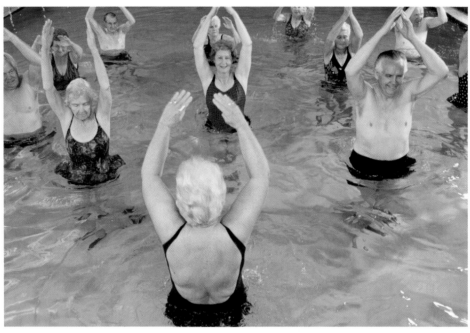

© Thinkstock

FACTORS AFFECTING PHYSICAL ACTIVITY

An ecological perspective provides a big picture of the many factors that influence a person's physical-activity level. It looks at individual characteristics along with the relationship between the individual and his or her environment, including the influence exerted by interpersonal relationships as well as by the organizations and communities in which the individual participates. An ecological perspective also examines the influence that larger social and cultural forces may exert on people's behavior (Fig. 8-1). The exact domains examined in ecological perspectives often vary, as they are dependent upon the nature of the model's use (Golden & Earp, 2012). Ecological perspectives include both factors that promote physical activity and those that reduce physical activity. An ecological perspective helps health and fitness professionals understand a given client's particular situation. Ecological perspectives have been used in many research settings to understand physical-activity patterns in various individuals and groups, including children and adolescents (Dunton, Intille, Wolch, & Pentz, 2012; Perry, Garside, Morones, & Hayman, 2012; Zhang, Solmon, Gao, & Kosma, 2012) and adults (Bennie, Timperio, Crawford, Dunstan, & Salmon, 2011; Li, et al., 2012; Lopez, Bryant, & McDermott, 2008).

In general, people have cleverly found ways to make life less physically taxing. Instead of shoveling coal or chopping wood to heat homes and businesses, people turn up the thermostat. Instead of walking, most people board buses and trains and drive cars. Homemakers are grateful that they no longer have to carry water up to the house, walk miles to gather food and fuel, or wash clothes down at the river. Laborers are more likely to operate machinery to construct buildings or to dig ditches than to carry heavy loads or shovel by hand. Sedentary recreational pursuits lure people into their chairs; they may spend more time watching television and movies than dancing and playing sports.

Of course, there are many exceptions to this generalization. Some workers perform a great deal of physical activity as part of their jobs. Mail carriers still walk many miles a day. Nursing professionals in hospitals walk from room to room and expend energy assisting patients. Wait staff in restaurants are on their feet for hours a day. Some household and yard care tasks still take energy: chasing children, mowing the lawn, and washing the windows. Many

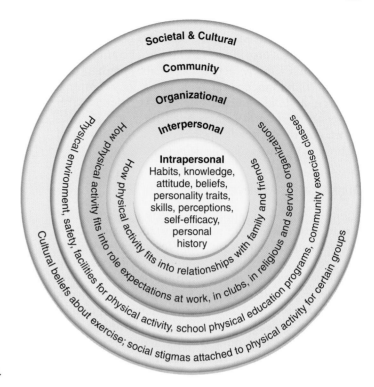

Figure 8-1. Ecological model of exercise behavior.

people enjoy active leisure pursuits. But, for most people, creating opportunities for physical activity and developing exercise habits are like swimming upstream in a heavy cultural current. Ecological perspectives can be very helpful for identifying barriers to physical activity and for developing programs and strategies to promote increased levels of physical activity (Cerin, Leslie, Sugiyama, & Owen, 2010; O'Connor, Alfrey, & Payne, 2012).

Intrapersonal Level

Changing exercise behavior means significant changes in every part of a person's life, beginning with the intrapersonal level. People may lack the necessary knowledge and skills needed to begin exercising. Particularly important are personal values and beliefs. For example, in many economically developed countries, people value making money and being productive more than self-care. Although people understand on a rational level that their health is important, many have deep-seated beliefs that it is selfish to take time to exercise when so many other things need to be done. On the other hand, some people are raised to value sport and physical activity and find exercise inherently enjoyable. They may grow up in active families and absorb the idea that engagement in activity is a good use of time.

In addition to swimming upstream in a world that urges a sedentary lifestyle, many people have difficulty sticking to an exercise program because exercising requires a significant amount of time and energy, and both time and energy may be in short supply. People who have difficulty sticking to exercise programs often cite lack of time and energy as their reasons for quitting (Cerin, Leslie, Sugiyama, & Owen, 2010). The greater the time and energy required for a behavior-change goal, the more personal resources, such as self-control, organization, and stress management that people must summon.

Change goes against human nature. People need some degree of stability, predictability, and comfort in their lives. For many, becoming more active "feels bad." Adding exercise to life disrupts the routine and may even cause physical discomfort.

Interpersonal Level

Interpersonal relationships exert a strong influence on lifestyle behaviors (Smith & Holm, 2011). Many people face barriers to exercise from important interpersonal relationships. When family members and friends discourage physical activity, people have more difficulty sticking to an exercise program. Sometimes marital partners resent a change in the family schedule or feel that the newly active partner disdains the old family ways. Inactive partners may feel judged when their mate becomes more active. Children may complain about babysitters, or friends may complain that the newly active person has less time for them. Interpersonal relationships thrive on habitual behaviors performed together. If these are sedentary in nature, such as watching television or movies or eating out, where will exercise fit in? Does exercising mean the disruption of relationships? Such worries can create barriers to change.

Family and friends can also provide helpful support in maintaining active lifestyles. For some people, recreational activities provide rewarding social connections. Some families enjoy active vacations together that include activities such as camping, hiking, or swimming. Children and adolescents often make friends with others on their sports teams or in their activity programs, and these friendships help keep them involved in the activity and make the activity more fun.

Organizational Level

Attempts to become more active may conflict with a person's role expectations in important organizations and institutions, such as workplaces, clubs, or volunteer groups. For example, sometimes supervisors at work frown on employees "wasting time" exercising, and they suggest that having priorities other than work may interfere with performance reviews and promotions or even lead to termination of employment. Social groups based on sedentary activities, such as book clubs, religious or service organizations, or any groups focused on sit-down meetings, may not promote physical activity.

Organizations can also encourage physical activity (Lucove, Huston, & Evenson, 2007; Tamers et al., 2011). Many workplaces offer discounts to fitness centers or even provide on-site exercise programs. Some insurance companies promote active lifestyles by offering discounts to participants who exercise regularly or maintain a healthy weight. People may join organizations such as community centers, YMCAs, and fitness centers that offer a variety of opportunities to be active. Children and teens often benefit from groups, school activities, and camps that focus on outdoor challenge and recreational activities.

Community Level

People often have to work around barriers to physical activity coming from the community, such as a lack of safe or convenient places to exercise. An absence of sidewalks, parks, and sports facilities limit exercise venues. High crime rates and an absence of public-safety personnel keep people indoors. Urban designs based on automobile transportation often eliminate opportunities to walk.

Communities can do a great deal to become friendlier to exercisers. Some towns have developed walking trails, bike paths, parks, and community gardens. When it is time to build a new school, communities can look for locations that allow more students to walk or bike to school. Developers can be sure to make sidewalks and parks part of the plan.

Societal and Cultural Level

Sometimes people must contend with barriers that come from society, such as cultural beliefs that exercise is not appropriate for certain people (Caperchione, Kolt, & Mummery, 2009). For example, people who are significantly overweight are often shamed when they exercise in public, such as when walking in a town or park. Old people may feel uncomfortable joining exercise classes or sport activities filled with young people. Mothers may be told they should not take time away from their young children. Some groups believe participation in sport or exercise is frivolous and a waste of time.

Societal and cultural beliefs can also promote active lifestyles. Some groups value self-care and encourage healthful behaviors. Some religious groups practice good dietary and exercise behaviors. In many cultures people feel that physical activities and sports are important for the development of young people. At some schools, it is cool to be an athlete, and students who are lucky enough to become athletes receive reinforcement from their peers.

MOTIVATING CHANGE: Understanding the Big Picture

When working with people to change physical activity, it is important to look at the big picture of their lives. Health and fitness professionals who have always enjoyed exercise and easy access to sports and physical activity may have to stretch their imaginations to relate to people who have never had the desire or opportunity to be active. Learning about clients' families, work, neighborhoods, and culture can enhance your understanding of the challenges that clients face in trying to become more active and can help you create more-realistic and successful recommendations.

STAGES OF CHANGE MODEL: Understanding Exercise Behavior Change

Despite numerous challenges and barriers, many people do succeed in becoming more active. Even very busy people with demanding jobs and family situations find ways to work exercise into their lives. Such change rarely happens overnight. Because exercise requires so much time and energy, people hardly ever become more active without a great deal of willpower and effort. Exercise psychologists have found that the Stages of Change Model, from Prochaska's Transtheoretical Model, provides a helpful description of how people generally proceed with changing their exercise behavior (Garber, Allsworth, Marcus, Hesser, Lapane, 2008; Haas & Nigg, 2009; Prochaska & Marcus, 1994). Chapter 4 introduced the Stages of Change Model (Fig. 8-2). Each stage is described below and used throughout the chapter to explore how health and fitness professionals can best work with clients who wish to improve their physical-activity programs. It is important to remember that Prochaska's Stages of Change Model theorizes that people move at different speeds and in different directions, from one stage to another. Fluctuation among the

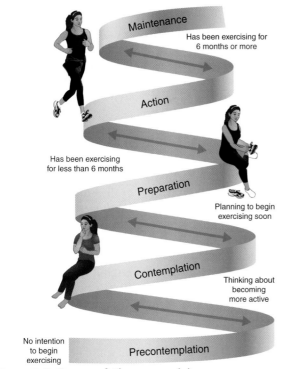

Figure 8-2. **Stages of Change model.**

Maintenance
Has been exercising for 6 months or more

Action
Has been exercising for less than 6 months

Preparation
Planning to begin exercising soon

Contemplation
Thinking about becoming more active

Precontemplation
No intention to begin exercising

(Box 8-1)

stages is especially prevalent when looking at people's physical-activity levels. Health and fitness professionals may find that knowing exactly what stage a person is in is less important than recognizing that activity levels, motivation, and commitment may change frequently for any given person (Box 8-1).

Precontemplation

The Stages of Change Model begins with people who are not even thinking about becoming more active, a stage called precontemplation. Precontemplators do not exercise and have no intention of starting. Precontemplators are sometimes divided into two groups, based on their beliefs about the value of physical activity (Gonzalez & Jirovec, 2001; Kotecki, 2011; Reed, 1999).

Precontemplation Nonbelievers

Precontemplation nonbelievers may not realize that a sedentary lifestyle is problematic. This has become less common as public-health campaigns promoting the health benefits of physical activity have increased their visibility and outreach in the past decade. However, some people still think exercise health benefits are not personally relevant. For example, some thin people believe the only reason to exercise is to lose weight, and because they don't need to lose weight, they don't need to exercise. In fact, some people still believe that exercise might make them become too thin. Other misconceptions may prevent nonbelievers from becoming more active. For instance, many people experience fatigue during the day and worry that exercise will worsen their daily fatigue levels. They don't realize that

BOX 8-1. Does Use of Stage Models Improve Exercise Adherence?

Although research supports the utility of applying stage models to behavior-change work, not everyone has found stage models helpful for increasing exercise adherence (e.g., Jones, Harris, Waller, & Coggins, 2005). Sometimes interventions based on stage of change have been no more successful at improving exercise adherence than standard exercise recommendation procedures. This may be because stage of change may vary for some people from day to day, depending on what else is going on in their lives. So, for example, people filling out a questionnaire about how ready they are to begin an exercise program might complete it in a way that indicates a readiness to change on a day when everything is going well and they feel in control. They might complete the questionnaire very differently on a bad day, when they can't possibly imagine squeezing exercise into their schedules. In other words, stage of change may change from time to time, especially for clients who have not yet reached the action or maintenance stages.

One of the most accepted concepts from the Stages of Change Theory is readiness to change. People are more successful in sticking to an exercise program if they are ready to change. Whether people are in preparation or action or on the cusp is not as important as understanding whether they are ready, and thus motivated to change.

Using the Stages of Change Model is helpful in a one-on-one situation or with a small group, where the health and fitness professional has plenty of contact with clients. Over time, the health and fitness professional can get a better sense of clients' lives, barriers to exercise, and motivations to increase physical activity. Even more important than figuring out which stage a client is in is having a deep understanding that changing habits is a process. Assigning a client to an actual stage becomes less important than understanding clients' thoughts and feelings about sticking to an exercise program and helping them address problems that seem to be interfering with motivation and commitment to regular physical activity.

an appropriate amount of exercise might actually reduce daily fatigue. They might think exercise is not appropriate for people their age, their size, or with their health risks.

Nonbelievers may have no idea that a sedentary lifestyle is a serious risk factor for chronic disease. They may be unaware that their sedentary ways increase risk for hypertension, type 2 diabetes, heart disease, osteoporosis, and colon cancer. Some precontemplation nonbelievers may feel that the dangers of a sedentary lifestyle have been exaggerated and may become defensive when others try to explain that a sedentary lifestyle is a problem.

Precontemplation Believers

Precontemplation believers accept, at least to some degree, that exercise is a valuable and reasonable thing to do, but the idea of taking steps to become more active is just not something they are thinking about. While they may have heard or read about the importance of physical activity, they have not considered incorporating exercise into their own lives. The ideas and forces that reinforce their sedentary lifestyles are stronger than factors motivating change. They may have many misconceptions about exercise. But they may at least recognize that physical activity has value.

Contemplation

People in the contemplation stage are still sedentary but thinking about becoming more active. Contemplators are aware of at least some of the benefits of regular exercise and are considering ways to work exercise into their lives. Many have had prior experience with exercise or sports, and their positive and negative experiences become part of the contemplation process. Contemplators are weighing the pros and cons of beginning an exercise program. They may be wondering how to begin but have not yet made the decision to change.

> **MOTIVATING CHANGE:** Match Motivational Approach to Stage of Change
>
> The idea that people go through a series of stages as they attempt to adopt an exercise program has great implication for health and fitness professionals. Clients usually seek the advice of an exercise instructor or personal trainer when they are already in the preparation stage and are getting ready to start exercising. Providing appropriate exercise program advice for these clients is helpful. But sometimes you may find yourself facing clients or groups of people who have not yet even made the decision to begin exercising. In this situation, your exercise recommendations will probably not result in much behavior change. Your time would be better spent helping people make the decision to change, so that they are ready to commit themselves to increasing their levels of physical activity.

Preparation

As the name of the stage suggests, people in the preparation stage are preparing to make a change in their physical-activity levels. They have decided to become more active and are preparing to begin. People in preparation might sign up for exercise classes, hire a personal trainer, make a doctor's appointment to get advice on exercising safely, buy new clothes or equipment, or even start exercising sporadically.

Action

People in the action stage of change are carrying out their plans to exercise. While they may miss a session now and then, they are generally doing what they decided to do. People in the action stage have started to exercise but have not yet maintained their exercise program for 6 months. Why 6 months? Researchers have found that the first 6 months of an exercise program are the most challenging (Marcus et al., 2006). During the first 6 months of a behavior-change program, people may struggle to stick to their plans. Health and fitness professionals often work with people in the action stage and are very familiar with the diversity of this group. While some become regular exercise members, others will drop out over the following months.

People in the action stage vary enormously in their confidence, skills, and ability to stick to an exercise program. While some people may be coming to every exercise class or working out as planned, their motivation and commitment to change may be very fragile. Psychologically, they still bear a strong resemblance to people in the preparation stage, questioning their ability to exercise, weighing the pros and cons of exercise, and worrying about whether their exercise plans will prove worthwhile. At the other end of the spectrum, some people in action are making great strides toward a long-term commitment to exercise and are motivated to make lifestyle changes. And, of course, people with various levels of motivation and commitment are scattered all along the action spectrum (Fig. 8-3).

Maintenance

People are in the maintenance stage when they continue to exercise according to their plans for 6 months or more. The longer people have been exercising, the more likely they are to continue to exercise. Although their exercise program and activities may change over time, they are likely to have found rewards in their programs that make participation worthwhile, even in the face of difficulties. For example, one interesting research study found that people in the maintenance stage of change actually *increased* their exercise adherence when feeling stressed, while people in the other stages exercised less frequently than usual when stressful conditions arose (Lutz, Stults-Kolehmainen, & Bartholomew, 2010).

Nevertheless, because regular exercise requires so much time and energy, and because exercise programs

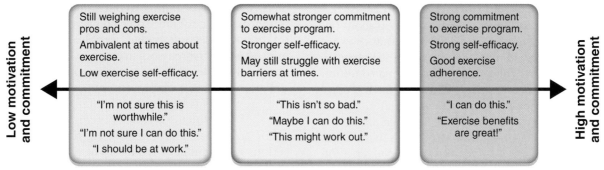

Figure 8-3. The action stage spectrum.

are so easily disrupted by changes in other areas of life, even people in the maintenance stage are at some risk of being unable to stick to their exercise programs at various times in their lives. Therefore, people rarely use Prochaska's "termination" stage with exercise adherence. Termination refers to a stage where people are very unlikely to return to the former behavior—in this case, a sedentary lifestyle. While the termination stage might make sense with addiction behaviors (people might reach a stage where they no longer ever have a desire for a cigarette, for example), relapse in exercise behavior is usually a risk.

Jessica talks with Sheila briefly about the weight room policies and gives her a couple of handouts on strength training. Sheila feels pretty uncomfortable in the weight room. She thinks that she is the only new person there; everyone else looks like they know what they are doing. Her eyes sweep the room for people her age or older. There aren't very many, and they look pretty strong and confident. Sheila realizes that Jessica is talking to her, but she is too distracted by her discomfort to listen carefully. Jessica and Sheila fly from station to station. They only have an hour together, and Jessica is anxious to give Sheila as much information as possible. But Sheila feels overwhelmed with the equipment, and she has trouble understanding much of what Jessica is saying. At the end of their hour together, Jessica hands Sheila a workout card with a long list of exercises written on it, but Sheila is not sure what everything means. ■

FROM PRECONTEMPLATION TO CONTEMPLATION: What Makes People Start Thinking About Becoming More Active?

People start thinking about becoming more active for many reasons. The motivation to become more active usually grows out of both intellectual understanding and emotional need. People may begin thinking about

becoming more active when they receive new information about themselves or about exercise that moves them to consider the pros and cons of becoming active. Three theoretical models explain some of the factors that stimulate people to consider the possibility of increasing physical activity.

Health Information as a Motivator

People may be motivated to change when they receive information about a health problem affecting them or people close to them or information about exercise benefits that are relevant to a personal health issue (Gammage & Klentrou, 2011). As discussed in Chapter 4, the Health Belief Model is one of the models most commonly used to understand health behavior. The Health Belief Model illustrates how health beliefs may nudge people to begin thinking about becoming more active (Fig. 8-4). Some research suggests that concepts from the Health Belief Model may be helpful for motivating people with illnesses such as diabetes to increase physical-activity level (Speer et al., 2008). According to this model, people will be more likely to consider adding exercise to their lives under certain conditions.

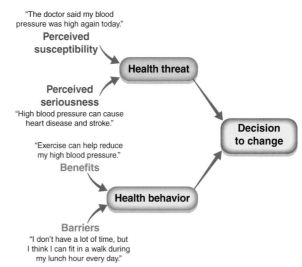

Figure 8-4. The Health Belief Model: Motivating the decision to exercise.

Perceived Susceptibility to a Health Problem

People may be more likely to begin thinking about becoming more active when they perceive that they are susceptible to a health problem. A person may receive a diagnosis from a health-care provider for a condition such as type 2 diabetes or hypertension. Such a diagnosis can be a shock that has the potential to initiate change thinking. While negative feelings about the diagnosis may cause the person to block thought about change, in many cases a diagnosis and a conversation with a health-care provider will at least get a person moving toward such thinking.

Clients sometimes perceive themselves to be susceptible to a health problem when a family member or friend receives a medical diagnosis, and the client feels similar to the person diagnosed. For example, when a sister is diagnosed with heart disease, the sibling may realize she is also at risk. Perception is critical here. People must perceive that they are similar enough to the other people receiving the diagnosis to begin thinking about the potential health problem.

Public-health campaigns sometimes nudge a person in precontemplation to feel vulnerable to a certain health problem. This might occur due to a program at work, an ad on television, or a story in a magazine or on the Internet. For example, overweight people may have lived with their condition most of their adult lives, considering it more an aesthetic concern than a health problem. But hearing about the health risks of obesity might make people begin to feel susceptible to future health problems and motivate them to become more active.

> **MOTIVATING CHANGE:** Combine Fear of a Health Risk With Hope for Exercise Benefits
>
> How much fear is best for motivating people to think about becoming more active and to carry through with their plans? Research shows that some level of stress and arousal motivates people to pay attention and to deal with a source of stress (Rothman, Bartels, Wlaschin, & Salovey, 2006). But too much fear, especially about an ongoing situation that has no easy solution, actually causes people to ignore the problem. When patients receive a scary diagnosis, they must also receive hope. If the hope is built on realistic lifestyle change, patients may be motivated to become active. But, if the scary diagnosis is accompanied by feelings of helplessness and hopelessness, patients may shove lifestyle-change recommendations aside as being unachievable. In applying this to clients, a little worry is fine but it should be linked to a positive solution and the buildup of a client's self-efficacy.

Perceived Seriousness of a Health Problem

People are more likely to begin thinking about change if a health problem is perceived to be serious. For example, people experiencing chest pain associated with heart disease can hardly avoid thinking about their symptoms. In addition to receiving whatever medical treatment is recommended, people with chest pain may be ready to reassess their health behaviors and perhaps consider changes in activity level.

Patients often underestimate the severity of chronic illness (Livneh, 2009). Many of the chronic illnesses for which exercise is recommended as part of the treatment plan have a long-term course until serious consequences are likely to result and no immediate symptoms. For example, while hypertension increases risk for stroke, many patients feel that the risk is small and far away. The same goes for the health risks associated with type 2 diabetes and obesity. And for all three of these, patients may feel few or no symptoms. The lack of immediate symptoms can make it easy for people to downplay the seriousness of their conditions and forget about the importance of lifestyle change.

People's perceptions of the seriousness of many chronic illnesses often change over time. People may feel the disease is very serious when they receive their initial diagnosis but then become accustomed to the idea as the weeks go by. They may never get around to exercising, and as the weeks and months roll by they feel no worse. Their perceptions of the condition's seriousness fades, and they may feel less motivated to think about becoming more active.

Perceived Exercise Benefits and Barriers

As people who feel susceptible to a serious health problem are motivated to look for ways to deal with the problem, they examine the benefits and barriers of behaviors recommended to prevent or treat the health problem. They are more likely to consider exercising if they perceive exercise to have significant beneficial effects. As discussed in Chapter 1, many of today's most-common chronic health disorders, such as type 2 diabetes or hypertension, have no simple or permanent cure. Exercise may be prescribed as part of the treatment plan and be recommended as one of the steps that can be taken for preventing long-term complications.

This is where education is essential. Many precontemplators are not aware of the effectiveness of regular exercise for controlling blood sugar, blood pressure, or improving blood lipid profile. If precontemplators are looking for options, the benefits of physical activity need to be clearly presented. The perceived benefits must be strong and relevant to attract the precontemplator's attention.

Many precontemplators, however, say no to exercise before they have even had a chance to think it over (Health Psychology in Your Life 8-1). The barriers to exercise are numerous and complex. For many precontemplators, even those who believe in the benefits of exercise, the perceived barriers hold them back from entering the contemplation stage and seriously considering the pros and cons of becoming more active. Contemplators are open to the idea of exercise, and they

HEALTH PSYCHOLOGY IN YOUR LIFE 8-1. Relating to People Who Hate Exercise

Do you have a sedentary friend or relative, especially someone who professes to hate exercise? Have you ever wondered how someone could *hate* exercise? Many health and fitness professionals have difficulty relating to self-avowed exercise haters.

But every life has a story. Make an opportunity to interview an exercise hater to discover his prior experiences with and his thoughts and feelings about physical activity. Suspend judgment, expressing only interest and curiosity. Listen empathetically. Try to really understand the person. Do not make recommendations, express your opinions, argue, or even think. Just listen. Did you learn anything?

Practicing this type of exploration will increase your communication skills, and you may even gain a deeper understanding of your friend or relative.

Box 8-2. Exercise Is Medicine

Several exercise organizations have teamed up with physicians' organizations to promote the importance of physical activity throughout the life span. One such effort is the "Exercise Is Medicine" campaign. The goal of this campaign is to encourage health-care providers to ask patients frequently about their participation in physical activity. The initiative seeks to educate providers on the importance of using their authority to urge patients to make exercise a part of daily life. It is hoped that by raising awareness of the link between physical activity and disease prevention, providers can help more people become active, leading to less chronic lifestyle-related disease and lower health-care costs. At the local level, many health and fitness professionals are joining with health-care providers to raise patient awareness about the importance of regular physical activity. Providers counsel patients to prevent disease and improve health by becoming more active. Providers also provide information to patients on community resources such as fitness centers and recreational programs. For more information, go to http://exerciseismedicine.org.

begin weighing exercise costs and benefits. All types of situational variables can influence precontemplators to consider thinking about becoming more active.

Cues to Action

The perceived susceptibility to a health problem and the perception of the seriousness of a health problem are reinforced by cues to action. Cues to action include things like medical advice, conversations with friends or family members, and information found in the media. These cues may only start people thinking about change. Sometimes cues seem to have no effect on precontemplators; they may block out advice to become more active even with a diagnosis of a serious health problem. But sometimes those initial cues may sensitize people to subsequent cues: more family members and friends developing the health problem, media campaigns, or reminders from a health-care provider that they need to be exercising. Cues to action from health-care providers and allied health professionals often carry heavy weight for precontemplators (Greenlund, Giles, Keenan, Croft, & Mensah, 2002; Box 8-2). The concerns of nagging family members may be shoved aside, but when doctors tell precontemplators to become more active, they may be more likely to listen, although actual behavior change may require more support (Woolf, Dekker, Byrne, & Miller, 2011).

Processes of Change

The Transtheoretical Model includes not only descriptions of the stages a person passes through while moving from not thinking about change to actually changing, but it also includes descriptions of several processes of change (see Chapter 4). In general, the cognitive processes of change are most helpful in the early stages of change, as people weigh the pros and cons of changing (Plotnikoff, Lippke, Johnson, & Courneya, 2010). Two of these processes, consciousness raising and emotional relief, are particularly relevant to the precontemplation stage and may motivate people in this stage to think about changing exercise behavior.

Consciousness Raising

Health information often contributes to an overall increase in awareness, or consciousness raising, regarding one's vulnerability to health problems and one's realization that exercise might be a helpful preventive or treatment option. At other times, consciousness raising occurs in response to factors other than health, where exercise is perceived to be helpful. Consciousness raising about exercise benefits may occur in response to something as simple as a conversation with a good friend who now feels so much better since he began working out or watching a movie that somehow motivates the viewer to revisit a sport she once loved. A consultation with a health and fitness professional might raise a client's consciousness (Behavior Change in Action 8-1). People may be suddenly struck with a decline in their stamina or difficulty fitting into their

BEHAVIOR CHANGE IN ACTION 8-1

Working With Clients in the Precontemplation and Contemplation Stages

■ CHALLENGE

How do I motivate change in a client who is not yet thinking about changing?

■ PLAN

The best approach is to use OARS communication skills, discussed in Chapter 5.

Explore preconceptions about health and exercise. With regard to physical activity, your goal is to listen to what clients say about exercise and the things that are important to them. Sample questions include:

- What are your beliefs about exercise and health?
- What are your health concerns?

Explore both personal health issues and their family history.

Sample questions include:

- Do you know that exercise can help with health issues?
- Would you like more information?

When clients are fairly resistant, do more listening than talking and rein in your tendency to give advice. Demonstrate that you are trying to understand where they are coming from. Remember: they are the ones who must consider changing, not you.

Connect regular physical activity to getting them in shape for what they love to do. Sample questions include:

- What activities do you enjoy the most?
- Can regular physical activity help you become stronger so that you can pursue these goals?

Maybe they hate "exercise" but love to hunt. Would they like to hear some information on getting in shape for hunting? If so, how about regular walking, so that they can enjoy a day in the woods hunting with their friends? Some people love to dance. Would they like to learn about Zumba® or other exercise done to music? Salsa lessons or swing dancing? What about a new mother who has no time for self-care? What is most important for her? Does she want to set an example for her children? Would it be good for the kids to get some fresh air in the park? Can she suggest a way to make this work in her life?

Ask about other physical activity. Sometimes people who say they have never exercised have actually been active in other ways. Ask questions about these ways. People may realize they are not completely sedentary after all and build on their newly perceived strengths. Sample questions include:

- Do you regularly walk to work or walk your dog?
- Do you play outside with your young children?
- How often do you garden? Do lawn work?

Empower the client. Lectures about the benefits of exercise and complicated exercise program designs are likely to fall upon deaf ears for people who are not thinking about a connection between physical activity and their hopes and dreams. Help them feel you are on their side and that *they* are the ones in charge of changing their lives.

pants. A new grandchild may motivate adults to regain enough fitness to carry the baby and play games with the grandkids in coming years. An invitation to travel with friends may kindle a desire to improve walking endurance to be able to take advantage of hiking opportunities or to lose weight to better enjoy time on the beach in a bathing suit.

While the phrase "consciousness raising" suggests an intellectual realization, in reality consciousness often includes an emotional component. The consciousness-raising process, however it occurs, may precipitate movement from precontemplation to contemplation. Consciousness raising is frequently initiated by new

information about health and fitness factors and the likely benefits of exercise.

Emotional Relief

People in the early stages of behavior change, including precontemplation, commonly experience ambivalence toward exercise. While they have heard about possible exercise benefits, the barriers are perceived as being too difficult to overcome. As evidence continues to mount that people are out of shape or vulnerable to particular health problems for which exercise is recommended, this ambivalence becomes more uncomfortable. People in precontemplation may continue for a long time ignoring the suggestions of others that they need to exercise. While they may not be thinking about actually beginning an exercise program, the notion that they should be exercising may still be bothering them. As discomfort builds, they may finally feel pushed to consider the possibility that it is time to add physical activity to their lives. Needing to purchase clothing a size bigger, upcoming class reunions, or getting together with old friends may remind people that they have changed and not always for the better. Psychologists call this moment a "crystallization of discontent" (Hayes, Laurenceau, & Feldman, 2007). Such discomfort sometimes motivates people to consider behavior change.

Where is the emotional relief? The emotional relief occurs when people decide to become more active, and this decision eases the discomfort caused by the realization that their sedentary lifestyle jeopardizes their health. Once people experience discomfort about their lifestyles, the decision to exercise feels good and relieves stress (Prochaska & Marcus, 1994). Prochaska refers to emotional relief as "dramatic relief." For example, with New Year's resolutions, people feel great just resolving to exercise. The resolution itself dissolves the immediate discomfort.

Chaos Theory: Epiphanies and Motivation for Physical Activity

Resnicow and Page (2008) have suggested that psychologists may never be able to completely explain how people make a decision to change physical activity or eating behaviors or how likely that decision will be to lead to actual behavior change. Many health behavior–change models focus primarily on rational, cognitive processes, such as weighing costs and benefits, to describe how people form intentions to change. In real life, people often make decisions fairly impulsively. Chaos Theory, as applied to behavior change, suggests that the process of change is not linear, but rather progresses in fits and starts with people sometimes showing no movement at all and other times changing suddenly. The many factors described in this chapter influence the process of making a decision, but they do not tell the whole story. Behavior change is chaotic, in that while initial conditions influence decision-making, this process is highly variable, and the outcome is difficult to predict (Resnicow & Page, 2008).

Successful behavior change requires a great deal of motivation, and strong motivation is especially likely to come with very powerful realizations, which Resnicow and Page (2008) refer to as epiphanies. An epiphany refers to a sudden insight, revelation, or understanding. Epiphanies often create strong autonomous motivation to change. They may move a person very quickly from precontemplation to action and then help a person successfully maintain the decision to change. (Of course, epiphanies can also cause a person to quit exercising, such as when an emergency situation calls for a person's total attention.) Many health-behavior experts have observed that successful behavior change often follows an epiphany or a life-changing event of some sort (Ogden & Hills, 2008). People may have previously started and quit exercise programs many times, but then they suddenly make the decision that they must become more active and turn into lifelong exercisers.

Epiphanies may follow diagnosis of a health problem, death of a family member, birth of a new baby, or other life events. What's the difference between an epiphany and consciousness raising? An epiphany is experienced intensely. Consciousness raising does not always lead to an epiphany, but an epiphany always includes an intense emotional experience. That total cognitive and emotional experience can reorder a person's thinking, planning, and doing. It can provide strong motivation that helps people stick to their resolutions to increase physical activity.

FROM CONTEMPLATION TO PREPARATION: How Do People Make a Decision to Become More Active?

The process of becoming more physically active almost always includes some sort of decision to change, often a full-blown resolution to exercise more. Of course, a decision alone is not enough to create behavior change, but change rarely occurs without it. Both thoughts and feelings can motivate people to form a decision to increase physical activity.

Forming an intention to change is an important step in the behavior-change process. Many of the behavior-change models presented in Chapter 4 focus on this important point. The decision to become more active can move people from inactivity into a willingness to exercise and may motivate people to actually begin exercising. As people begin to weigh the costs and benefits of becoming more active, health and fitness professionals often hope to affect their decisional balance and to tip their decision away from inactivity and toward commitment to regular exercise.

Reasoning and Planning

The Theory of Planned Behavior suggests that humans sometimes try to rationally respond to information and make a plan to deal with the situation. An important part of this model is the idea that people form an intention to change as a first step to implementing a plan to do so. A strong decision to change behavior is more likely to actually result in change than a weak decision (Webb & Sheeran, 2006). Many variables influence the intention to change. These variables contribute to people's formulations of exercise costs and benefits

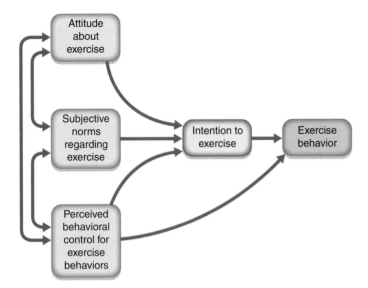

Figure 8-5. Theory of Planned Behavior: Motivating the decision to exercise.

(Fig. 8-5). With regard to changing physical-activity behaviors, the most salient of these variables are discussed in the following subsections.

Attitudes Toward Exercise, Health, and Fitness

Peoples' attitudes toward exercise are based on their expectations regarding the effects of exercise. Attitudes toward exercise are formed from people's total life experience, including their experiences with physical activity and things they have read, heard from friends, or seen on television or other media. These attitudes influence decisions about whether to become more active. Positive expectations must outweigh negative attitudes for a person to decide to exercise. Similarly, clients must place great value on health and fitness, or they will not perceive the health and fitness benefits of physical activity as worthwhile.

Other behavior-change models, including Social Cognitive Theory, also emphasize the importance of people's attitudes. Social Cognitive Theory has interesting applications for decisional balance. Social Cognitive Theory explains that attitudes are influenced by both expectations and expectancies about something, in this case, exercise. Expectations are what people think is going to happen if they exercise, and expectancies are the values people place on those things. So, if people expect that exercise will make them feel more energetic and they value feeling energized, their attitude toward exercise will tend to be positive. On the other hand, if people expect exercise to be painful or boring and if they value being comfortable and dread pain or boredom, their attitude toward exercise will probably be negative. Some research suggests that positive exercise expectancies may be more predictive of physical activity in older adults than younger adults (Williams, Anderson, & Winett, 2005).

Attitudes toward health and fitness vary as well. While almost everyone will say they want to be healthy, most healthy people take their health for granted. Many people value achievement over health, forgetting that a certain level of well-being supports achievement in one's various life roles. Younger, healthier clients tend to value appearance, and if they perceive that exercise will contribute to a positive appearance, their attitude toward exercise will generally be more positive.

Subjective Norms Regarding Physical Activity

Subjective norms are a person's perceptions of how strongly other people, such as family members and friends, want him or her to exercise. These subjective norms translate into people's perceptions of social pressure. Subjective norms have been found to be somewhat predictive of behavior change (McLachlan & Hagger, 2011; White, Smith, Terru, Greenslade, & McKimmie, 2009). Health and fitness professionals may find that social norms influence clients' attitudes about physical activity and self-care. Professionals may find it productive to explore which norms are important to clients. Gender roles? Roles as parent, worker, caregiver of aging parents, spouse? Do these norms reinforce the importance of physical activity? Or do these norms reinforce the idea that exercise is a waste of time? That self-care is not a priority?

MOTIVATING CHANGE: Tipping the Decisional Balance

How do you help clients who are on the fence make the decision to change? Professionals are sometimes tempted to offer quick solutions to concerns voiced by clients. But, unless clients are really looking for advice, ask questions to help clients explore these issues and come to their own conclusions. You are trying to figure out whether the exercise barriers, or cons, are excuses or real problems. What's behind the ambivalence? Low self-efficacy? Lack of information?

If the conversation starts to feel very repetitive like you are just hashing out the same excuses over and over, change tactics and ask clients about their passions. What do they really enjoy in life? What's important to them? Try to help clients find positive reasons to exercise. Point out their strengths and remind them of occasions when they have successfully changed their lives. Clients may tell you, for example, that they have no energy. You remind them that they told you just the other day about the family gatherings they host on the holidays and point out how these events must take energy and organization.

If you feel like clients are focusing primarily on exercise barriers, remind them of things they have previously said that support their intention to become more active. If the conversation falters, ask "How can I help you?" Get the conversation back to the client's goals.

What can the health and fitness professional do to tip the decisional balance in favor of exercise? Use your very best communication techniques, listening more than talking to get a good picture of how clients are thinking. Ask open-ended questions to uncover their thoughts about exercise, health, and fitness. People harbor many misconceptions about exercise and health. Correct these when possible. For example, many contemplators worry that exercise will make them tired. Suggest that a moderate amount of exercise (and you can help them figure out what that is) should help them feel energized, rather than exhausted. If they are interested, give them information on how exercise can help with their health problems or fitness goals. Don't overload them with educational materials, but if they have questions, get them answers geared toward their educational level and interest. Remember not to lecture, however. Let clients guide the conversation. Listen empathetically, with an open mind. The more you can understand clients who are trying to make a decision, the better you will be able to provide the most-helpful information. And, when clients sense that you are listening and trying to understand, they may pay more attention to you.

Sense of Control

People will not make a decision to change their behavior unless they see that behavior as something over which they have control. While exercise may seem to be a behavior under volitional control, many people see the barriers to exercise as out of their control. As they are trying to decide whether to become more active, feelings of control over the exercise situation and options increase the likelihood that contemplators will decide to give exercise a try. In terms of changing exercise behavior, a sense of control (perceived behavioral control) is one of the most strongly predictive

variables in the Theory of Planned Behavior Model (Husebo, Dyrstad, Soreide, & Bru, 2013).

The opposite of having a sense of control is feeling helpless and hopeless. People who feel helpless will have difficulty summoning the energy necessary to arrange their lives in a way that enables them to develop an exercise habit. But people are always full of surprises, so sometimes people who seem helpless manage to pull through and start exercising, if they have adequate resources and support.

Self-Efficacy for Exercise and Overcoming Exercise Barriers

Self-efficacy seems to find its way into almost every behavior-change model. Originally part of Social Cognitive Theory (Bandura, 1977), self-efficacy is so consistently related to a person's chance of successful behavior change that it is hard to talk about behavior change without this important variable (Game Changers 8-1). As discussed in Chapter 4, self-efficacy is the belief in one's ability to successfully accomplish a given task. Self-efficacy is situation specific. For example, people with strong exercise self-efficacy are more likely to decide to exercise, to stick to an exercise program, and to persist in the face of obstacles (Luszczynska, Schwarzer, Lippke, & Mazurkiewicz, 2011).

Several factors contribute to a person's self-assessment regarding exercise self-efficacy. Prior experiences with exercise, general self-confidence in the physical-activity realm, and other life situations shape people's beliefs about their exercise-adherence abilities. And as expected, success builds feelings of success. Self-efficacy increases likelihood of success, which in turn further increases self-efficacy. Similarly, being unsuccessful in sticking to an exercise program is associated with a decrease in exercise self-efficacy (Parschau et al., 2012).

Sometimes people have good exercise self-efficacy in general but find themselves in difficult life situations that preclude regular physical activity, at least temporarily. They may simply not have the time or energy because they are attending to an emergency situation or are overwhelmed at work or at home. Current barriers to regular exercise may lower exercise self-efficacy even in a very confident person. Barrier self-efficacy is a term used by health and fitness psychologists to indicate a person's feelings about how well they will be able to overcome barriers to exercise. People with higher barrier self-efficacy are more likely to develop better exercise adherence (Cramp & Bray, 2011).

Several factors have been shown to influence a person's self-efficacy, including the following (Bandura, 1997; Fig. 8-6).

Mastery Experiences

When people experience successful accomplishment of a skill, they build self-efficacy. Accomplishing a task or

Game Changers 8-1. Albert Bandura and Self-Efficacy

Albert Bandura created the concept of self-efficacy as part of his larger Social Learning Theory.
Bandura was a game changer in the field of psychology in that he helped to move the discipline away from the behaviorism of B. F. Skinner and others into the realm of human thoughts and feelings, a realm that came to be known as cognitive psychology. While behaviorism was based on the idea that people primarily react to outside forces, cognitive psychology devised experimental methods to not only study observable behavior (the hallmark of behaviorism) but also to evaluate people's thoughts and personality traits as well.

Bandura's Social Learning Theory explored the questions of how both children and adults learn behavior. Bandura proposed that people model their behavior on the behavior they observe in others. While this may sound obvious to readers today, at the time his landmark studies included new ways of measuring and supporting such psychological constructs. Bandura is well known for his "Bobo doll" experiments, which demonstrated that children exposed to an adult displaying aggressive behavior toward the Bobo doll were more likely themselves to act aggressively.

Bandura's early work on self-efficacy theory involved people's ideas regarding their ability to deal with phobias, anxiety-provoking fears, and irrational fears. In the abstract to his 1977 review of self-efficacy theory published in *Psychological Reviews* (Bandura, 1977), Bandura wrote:

> It is hypothesized that expectations of personal efficacy determine whether coping behavior will be initiated, how much effort will be expended, and how long it will be sustained in the face of obstacles and aversive experiences.... [E]xpectations of personal efficacy are derived from four principal sources of information: performance accomplishments, vicarious experience, verbal persuasion, and physiological states (p. 191).

Bandura's concept of self-efficacy is an important component of every behavior-change model. Whether people are trying to adopt new exercise behaviors or quit smoking, self-efficacy plays an important role.

Sources: Bandura, A. (1977). Self-efficacy: toward a unifying theory of behavioral change. *Psychological Review, 84*(2), 191-215; Bandura, A. (1997). *Self-efficacy: The Exercise of Control*. New York: Freeman.

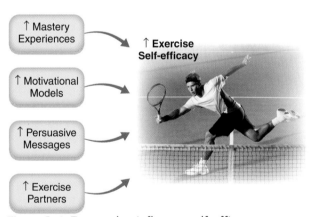

Figure 8-6. Factors that influence self-efficacy.
Photograph © Thinkstock

acquiring a new skill creates a mastery experience. As people master the skills they need to stick to an exercise program, their exercise self-efficacy grows. On the other hand, if they experience failure (note that both success and failure are subjective), their self-efficacy for that task declines.

Teachers and health and fitness professionals use this observation to structure learning experiences to provide early performance mastery experiences. Baby steps build confidence for clients to take giant steps.

Mastery experiences in the exercise realm can be very simple at first: learning to follow and fill out the workout card, coming to the fitness center twice a week, or learning to use a new piece of equipment.

Self-efficacy is all about perception. People may be performing physical activities correctly, but, if they don't *feel* successful, they will have poor self-efficacy. Positive feedback from others, especially from people considered to have expertise, can help people feel more successful. But in general, people with low self-efficacy may need to progress slowly and gradually so they are not overwhelmed by too many new demands.

Motivational Models

When clients see people similar to themselves being successful at exercise tasks that they themselves are trying to master, they feel more efficacious. Modeling increases client self-efficacy most when clients perceive models to be similar on those features about which clients feel most insecure. For example, if clients are low in exercise self-efficacy because they are "too old," they need to view older models. If clients feel low in exercise self-efficacy because they are overweight, they need overweight models. New mothers wondering how they will ever find the time to add activity to their crazy lives need to see new mothers model ways to be active.

Clients may especially have low exercise self-efficacy in fitness center settings. They may perceive themselves to be of a different social class, ethnic background, ability, age, or body type. To make matters worse, clients may mentally exaggerate the differences between themselves and the other people they see, especially if they already have low exercise self-efficacy. People can find motivational role models who increase their self-efficacy in many places. Real people near at hand are best; however, DVDs, magazine articles, movies, and other media may portray motivational models that increase exercise self-efficacy.

MOTIVATING CHANGE: Using Role Models to Strengthen Client Exercise Self-Efficacy

You can help expose clients to motivating role models in many ways. First, you must determine the defining variables that, in clients' eyes, limit their ability to be successful. Your clients may provide clues: "I don't want to be the oldest one here," or "I'm afraid I'll be the only beginner in the class."

Where do you find role models? Bring in former clients, other fitness professionals, friends, colleagues, or acquaintances who might serve as motivational role models. They might be willing to talk with your clients or to work out nearby. Maybe you can help clients locate a class that is designed for people like them, such as a class for older adults or people new to exercise. If you think there is a market, start your own group. Groups are especially powerful because they combine self-efficacy modeling and social support. If the group leader is similar to the members, so much the better. Group leaders who have successfully stuck to their exercise program model self-efficacy. If you can't find real people, give your clients magazine stories, DVDs, Internet video links, or other exposures. Talk about similar clients' success stories.

Persuasive Messages

Receiving persuasive messages from others also appears to enhance exercise self-efficacy. In one study, pregnant women exposed to persuasive messages designed to increase exercise self-efficacy showed greater increases in exercise self-efficacy following treatment than did the control group (Gaston, Cramp, & Propavessis, 2012).

Stress Arousal

Bandura has suggested that stress arousal is associated with decreased self-efficacy. People interpret stress symptoms as signs of inability. In terms of exercise, this might mean that people who experience anxiety walking into the weight room might interpret the anxiety as an indication of their low ability to perform strength-training exercise. Stress arousal can be reduced in an exercise setting in several ways. One of the best is with exercise partners. A good exercise partner can reduce feelings of stress

and boost exercise self-efficacy. Exercise partners work best when both people have compatible fitness or skill levels and enjoy similar physical activities. Exercise partners may work out together at a fitness center, join the same exercise class, or enjoy a walk or hike together. Good exercise partners tell each other how well they are doing and remind each other to come to their next workout. People see themselves reflected by their exercise partners, and this strengthens people's self-image as exercisers as well as their exercise self-efficacy.

Many people feel low exercise self-efficacy because they are worried about their appearance, especially if they are exercising in a public place (Box 8-3). While

Box 8-3. Worried About Appearance: Helping Clients With Social Physique Anxiety

Social physique anxiety refers to the feeling of anxiety that people experience when they worry that others are appraising their bodies (Hart, Leary, & Rejeski, 1989). Such anxiety may lead people to refuse to exercise in fitness centers or exercise classes or even to go for a walk in public. Social physique anxiety sometimes goes along with a distorted body image, so that even physically attractive people may still feel too fat and worry about how they look. Social physique anxiety may interact with motivation for exercise and be especially likely to cause exercise avoidance in people with low levels of autonomous motivation for participation in physical activity (Cox, Ullrich-French, Madonia, & Witty, 2011).

Anxiety about appearance is common in cultures that judge people on first impressions and on how they look. After all, people do check each other out in fitness settings or any other place for that matter. We form judgments about others based on their appearance. We think to ourselves in the grocery store, "That woman shouldn't be buying that ice cream." In the park, we might observe, "That man is too out of shape to be running."

Try to reassure clients that people come in all shapes and sizes and abilities. Most people's bodies are far from perfect. Give advice on finding comfortable, flattering exercise apparel. If you work in a facility that sells exercise clothing, stock flattering styles for all ages and sizes. If clients are reluctant to work out in the fitness center, they might attend during slow times with fewer patrons. If clients refuse to exercise in public, they may wish to use fitness equipment or videotapes at home. If body image is significantly interfering with a client's life, recommend professional help.

good clothes cannot make a person thinner or younger, they can improve appearance. Health and fitness professionals can recommend ideas for appropriate, attractive attire and footwear. While thin, young people may look nice in skin-tight clothing, most clients look and feel better in something looser with a nice fit. Clothes that are too small and too tight are especially demoralizing for people with low exercise self-efficacy.

Jessica's exercise training is going well, but at her next team meeting with the other personal trainers, she realizes that she is getting very few repeat clients compared to the others. Attracting clients to continue working with her is an important part of Jessica's job description. In fact, her supervisor asks her to meet with him briefly after the meeting. "The feedback we are getting from members suggests that you may need to work a little harder at connecting with them. Many say that you seem like you are in a hurry to finish with them and that your explanations are lengthy and hard to follow." Jessica explains that she is trying to give clients their money's worth in their single, 1-hour orientation. Her supervisor sets up a meeting for Jessica with their most-popular personal trainer, Susannah, who seems to have success at connecting with new clients.

"You're not going to be able to cover everything in 1 hour, so don't even try," Susannah explains. "The most important thing is to connect with clients, be sure they can work safely, and make them feel comfortable and welcome. If they only learn three machines, that's fine. If they benefit from their session with you, maybe they will book more sessions with you to learn more."

As she leaves her meeting with Susannah, Jessica notices that Sheila hesitates as she comes through the fitness center entrance. She looks lost and timid. Sheila notices that her stomach is in a knot. She realizes she is not sure how to begin and probably doesn't really belong at this fitness center. She has purchased a 3-month membership, however. "I'll do some more reading on weight training and try again next week," Sheila thinks. With a feeling of relief, she quickly turns around and leaves the fitness center. ■

Self-Determination Theory

When health and fitness professionals work with people who are thinking about exercising but have not really formed an intention to change, they often break into hard-sell mode. It's as though health and fitness professionals think that they can argue someone into exercising. Fitness professionals may be especially motivated to use this approach when their income is based on selling memberships.

Chapter 4 discussed the importance of intrinsic motivation, or at least integrated regulation, where exercise is linked with important personal goals for long-term behavior-change success (Deci & Ryan, 2008). Health and fitness professionals should keep Self-Determination Theory in mind when working with clients who are still weighing the costs and benefits of exercise and are not yet ready to commit to regular physical activity. Self-Determination Theory emphasizes three important concepts that guide human development and successful behavior change: autonomy, competence, and connection (Health Psychology at Work 8-1).

Autonomy

People probably won't follow an exercise program that is handed to them unless they have actively sought and asked for advice. Contemplators must make their own decisions to exercise regularly. No one else can do this for them, not the doctor, not the nurse, and not the personal trainer. In the contemplation phase, people need to come to the realization that exercise will help them achieve important goals.

Competence

People need to feel able to perform the recommended exercises and to carry out their exercise plans. Competence, in this context, may be experienced as exercise self-efficacy. When clients feel competent, they feel capable of carrying out the exercise plan. People who have not yet formed the intention to exercise may still be worried about many barriers to exercise participation.

Connection

People tend to seek relationships with other people. How does the motivation to connect with others apply in an exercise setting? Connection can reinforce competence in the exercise setting. Connection means that people feel they belong in a particular group or place. Connection means that clients appreciate the fitness instructor knowing their name, asking about their sick cat or whatever the last conversation was about, and seeing familiar faces. Clients appreciate health and fitness professionals who pay attention when clients are answering their questions. Clients like to feel understood and valued.

Positive or Negative Reasons for Exercise: Effect on Adherence

Research suggests that people who exercise for positive reasons tend to have better long-term exercise adherence than people who exercise for negative reasons (DiBartolo, Lin, Montoya, Neal, & Shaffer, 2007). Positive reasons for exercise include improving one's health, mood, energy level, and sleep quality. People who exercise to be able to carry their groceries, participate on a sports team, or go mountain climbing on their vacations are usually thought to be exercising for positive reasons. Positive reasons for exercise move a person closer to important goals. The person sees both

HEALTH PSYCHOLOGY AT WORK 8-1: Encouraging Patient Autonomy, Competence, and Connection

John J. O'Sullivan, PT, OCS, ATC, has been a physical therapist since 1986. He has worked in many settings, including industrial rehabilitation, hospitals, and outpatient clinics. John specializes in orthopedics and neurology as well as wellness and injury prevention. As an aspiring high school football star, John quickly realized that, at 140 pounds, he was unlikely to hurt anyone but himself on the football field, and he discovered a career in athletic training instead of professional sports. In addition to working with patients, John enjoys coaching youth soccer and teaching, and he serves as an adjunct professor at Springfield College in the Department of Physical Therapy in Springfield, Massachusetts.

"Physical therapists often give patients exercises to do at home. We also give them advice and strategies for coping with their pain and injuries and for preventing recurrences or future complications. Patients have to take an active role in their rehabilitation. I can help them figure out what to do, but I can't do it for them. Physical therapists sometimes see patients who are reluctant to change behavior. They may frequently not see a connection between their behavior and their problem.

"In the early years of my career as a physical therapist, whatever approach I was using was the approach everybody got. Over the years, I have learned to individualize my approach to each patient. I work hard to establish a helpful therapeutic relationship that puts the patient in charge of his or her recovery. I try to help the patient see the connection, that what they do and don't do makes a difference in their level of pain. I want patients to know that I am not the one in charge.

"I like to talk, which can be a problem. I have learned over the years it's more important to listen. Even after 20 years of practice, I am still working on how I listen. It is important for me to understand how patients see their problem and what in their life might motivate them to take more control of their situation.

"Sometimes, I realize I am talking with a patient as though I am trying to win an argument. My patients are telling me why they can't do this or that. But, if I am more invested in change than my patients, I'm on the wrong side of the equation. With some patients, if you argue for change, they argue against it. If I find myself arguing, then I shut up. I ask them, 'So what's the big deal if you don't change?' I have to let them tell me why they need to change. If the conversation really stalls, I just ask, 'What information can I give you? How can I help you?' That makes the patient take the lead again."

exercise and health as means to an end. People who participate in physical activity because it is fun and feels good are already intrinsically motivated.

Negative reasons for exercise include losing weight or improving appearance because people feel they are not "good enough" the way they are. Especially negative is trying to lose weight and improve appearance only to please someone else. In this context, people might see exercise as the result of a negative judgment, a reminder of their inadequacies, and even as a punishment. The difference between exercising to lose weight and exercising to improve health is the focus and emotion behind the goal. For example, weight loss can serve as either a positive or negative reason to exercise. On the positive side, weight loss can improve health. People exercising to lose weight and lower blood pressure might feel positively motivated to get healthier and feel good. In a negative context, people who want to lose weight because they feel pushed to exercise by a spouse or health-care provider may not yet really want to become active.

Processes of Change

The processes of change highlighted in the Transtheoretical Model are important at every stage. The processes

described in the section on precontemplation, consciousness raising, and emotional relief can motivate change in the contemplation stage as well. In addition, other processes are especially likely to support change in the contemplation stage (Pfeffer & Alfermann, 2008). These processes include the following.

Social Support

Social support is always helpful and appears in most behavior-change models. In the Transtheoretical Model, it is referred to as helping relationships. Social support may be enough to tip the decisional balance toward becoming more active for people who are on the cusp of changing. The encouragement of family, friends, and coworkers can provide the extra energy needed to make that decision to become active. In addition to emotional support, offers of logistical help may make exercise seem more feasible. An office coworker might work with a client to take turns covering the phones so each can take a walk over the lunch hour. A family member might offer help with childcare in the late afternoon so the client can attend an exercise class. A neighbor might become a walking partner. Clients still forming an intention to exercise might find such offers of help just enough to make exercise possible.

Self-Reevaluation

Self-reevaluation means a change in one's self-concept, from seeing oneself as a sedentary person to seeing oneself as an exerciser. A change in self-concept can occur in many ways. For example, it may come about as an epiphany, or it may slowly emerge out of discussions with a health and fitness professional. Self-reevaluation often includes a change in values, a change that supports a decision to begin exercising. People may change from not valuing health, fitness, or physical activity to believing "My health is a priority; I must make time for physical activity." The process of self-reevaluation may change people's self-concept from "I can't exercise because I am too busy doing important things," to "I must create time to exercise and take care of myself so that I can continue to do the things I need to do."

Social Liberation

Forming a commitment to regular exercise may require changing one's daily schedule, and thus social habits. In the context of exercise adherence, social liberation refers to changing social behavior to gather support for a new exercise program. These changes manifest as behaviors that seek support for the new exercise habit. Social liberation may take the form of joining an exercise class or fitness center, where a person would feel that exercise is a sanctioned behavior. Social liberation might also necessitate reducing sedentary behaviors, such as watching fewer hours of television each evening in order to walk after dinner.

The fitness center manager has observed that a majority of customers buying memberships do not renew after their first membership runs out. In addition, attendance by new members is poor. The manager decides to increase initial membership fees slightly but to offer three free personal training sessions. All personal trainers, including Jessica, send postcards to members who have joined in the past 3 months but never returned, offering two more free personal training sessions. Meanwhile, Jessica has pulled out the textbook she used for her exercise psychology course. As she reviews the sections on behavior-change theory, she thinks about the clients she will be seeing the next day. Sheila has signed up for a second session. "According to the Health Belief Model, she is probably pretty motivated to exercise regularly. I wonder what stage of change she is in?" Jessica wonders.

FROM PREPARATION TO ACTION: Planning for Success

Once people have formed an intention to exercise, the next step is for them to make some sort of plan to work physical activity into their lives. For some people, this is as simple as resuming a walking program that they abandoned several years ago. Those with extensive prior exercise experience may have strong exercise self-efficacy and the knowledge to make an effective plan. People with less confidence or those who wish to take a new approach to exercise training may enlist the help of a health-care provider or fitness professional.

Some psychologists have suggested that the factors important for making a decision and forming an intention to change behavior differ from those affecting and predicting the actual onset of the behavior-change program, in this case starting an exercise program (Rothman, Baldwin, & Hertel, 2004; Marcus et al., 2006). While many of the factors that led to a decision to exercise continue to be influential as they motivate people to pursue their physical-activity goals, the nuts and bolts of fitting exercise into life become very important as clients actually begin to exercise. The early steps in forming an exercise program provide experiences for clients that can serve either as energizing motivators or as excuses to quit.

Health and fitness professionals commonly work with clients in the preparation and action stages of change. These are often the clients who are buying fitness equipment, enrolling in exercise classes, or hiring a personal trainer. Clients moving into the preparation and action stages may seek professional advice on the best way to use their limited exercise time to meet their health and fitness goals. A good exercise plan addresses an individual's health concerns and fitness goals and accommodates personal preferences and constraints. Some of the common issues that tend to affect exercise planning and motivation in the preparation and early action stages include the following.

Medical Clearance

Many experts have commented that "people should get medical clearance to *not* exercise," since a sedentary lifestyle increases risk for many chronic illnesses. Nevertheless, because exercise can create health problems in a minority of cases, and because health and fitness professionals certainly do not want to cause any kind of injury or health problems for their clients, medical-clearance procedures are followed to minimize the risk of harm from physical activity. In addition, for clients with health risks, getting medical guidance on safe and effective exercise may be motivational because, hopefully, their health-care providers will encourage them to exercise. Providers' guidelines can also be helpful to fitness professionals for the design of exercise programs. Medical-clearance procedures give clients confidence that their exercise programs are safe and effective; and fitness professionals appreciate having medical expertise back up their recommendations.

Part of the medical-clearance procedure can be to obtain baseline values on health markers that may improve with regular exercise. Blood lipid profile, blood glucose levels, and other variables may provide helpful information for exercise program design and may improve over time if clients stick to their exercise programs.

Health and fitness professionals should follow the medical-clearance guidelines suggested by their employers or certifying organizations. An example of a popular medical clearance form in Canada is the Par-Q (Canadian Society for Exercise Physiology, 2002). The Par-Q is quick and easy to complete and flags possible concerns for follow-up. The Par-Q is widely accepted as an adequate first step in flagging clients who may be harmed by vigorous exercise or who would benefit from medical guidance regarding exercise program design. Since it is fairly brief, many health and fitness professionals gather additional information as well. The Par-Q medical-clearance form can be found at www.csep.ca/cmfiles/publications/parq/par-q.pdf.

Clients may perceive medical-clearance procedures as no problem, as a barrier to exercise, or as a motivational experience, depending on circumstances. Most certification and medical organizations do not recommend sending young, apparently healthy individuals to their physicians before beginning a vigorous exercise program because this is usually unnecessary, as risk of adverse events is very low in this population (Bryant, Franklin, & Newton-Merrill, 2007). In addition, finding the time and money for an appointment with a physician may cause some to abandon their idea of starting an exercise program.

Health Concerns

Health and fitness professionals should inquire about clients' health concerns before designing exercise recommendations. Health concerns may include information that comes up on the medical-clearance form as well as other issues about which clients are concerned. Even though a client may have completed medical-clearance and health-information forms, the health and fitness professional should discuss these with the client in person if possible. Many clients forget to write important information on their forms, especially if forms are filled out in a hurry. The health and fitness professional should inquire not only about current health concerns but family history of chronic illness as well. Clients may want their exercise programs to help prevent chronic health problems that run in their family.

Most people associate exercise with improvements in physical health but are less informed about the emotional health benefits of exercise. Health and fitness professionals should ask clients about feelings of stress, mood, sleep quality, and daily energy level. Because these variables may improve fairly quickly with exercise, it's important to get clients thinking about them and to get a baseline indication regarding how much they interfere with quality of life.

If health problems surface that are beyond the health and fitness professional's scope of practice, clients should be referred back to their providers or other specialists, and medical clearance for these concerns should be obtained. Depending on their training, certifications, and scope of practice, many health and

fitness professionals can then continue to work with such clients, accommodating the health concerns in their exercise recommendations.

MOTIVATING CHANGE: Link Exercise to Health
The first meeting with a new client should create a professional, positive emotional tone and engender feelings of confidence. Discussing health concerns can feel quite threatening to some clients. Health and fitness professionals should be respectful of the client's privacy, while gathering the information necessary to establish a safe and effective working relationship. This means being very careful about the questions you ask, and knowing which issues to explore and which to ignore. Ask only for information relevant to exercise program design and keep a professional emotional distance. If sad information comes up, such as when a client tells you about the recent death of a family member or a serious medical diagnosis, it is fine to express sympathy; a simple "I'm sorry" is usually enough.

When discussing physical and emotional health concerns with clients, take advantage of the motivation that may emerge as clients decide to address these issues. Give clients information on preventing or dealing with health problems that worry them. When clients understand how lifestyle measures may reduce their symptoms and improve quality of life, they may feel more in control of their health and more motivated to stick to their exercise and lifestyle-change programs.

Fitness Assessments

Many people find fitness assessments intimidating. The people who need exercise the most often receive poor scores on assessments, which can be demoralizing. Such clients may already have fairly low exercise self-efficacy, and receiving negative results on fitness tests may decrease motivation for physical activity. If a fitness assessment is required for beginning an exercise program, many people see this as one more reason to postpone getting started. Why increase the barriers to participation in regular physical activity? Starting an exercise program should be as easy and painless as possible, especially for clients with low self-confidence. In addition, fitness assessments, rather than the client, can end up dictating exercise program goals and design. Fitness assessments put the health and fitness professional in charge, not only of the client's body but also of the definition of fitness. If fitness assessments are used, the client's needs should remain central and fitness tests results used in ways that support the client's direction.

On the other hand, people with a strong history of physical activity may enjoy taking a battery of tests. For these people, the tests provide interesting information and serve as a benchmark for improvement. Fitness assessments may influence program design by uncovering weak areas that can be helped by exercise.

Health and fitness professionals should consider omitting comparison information on client test results for clients with low fitness levels. Learning that it takes a new client 25 minutes to walk a mile provides a helpful baseline for improvement, if the client does some walking as part of his fitness program. Telling the client his mile walk time is below average may not accomplish much, especially if the testing occurs early in the professional–client relationship.

Rather than administering a standard set of fitness tests, health and fitness professionals should tailor fitness testing (if any) to each client. What are the client's fitness goals? What improvements might be seen with the anticipated exercise program? What fitness tests are likely to show improvement or be motivational? What test results are helpful for writing exercise recommendations? For example, strength testing may be necessary to calculate starting weights for clients pursuing strength-training programs. However, maximal strength tests may leave older and out-of-shape clients in pain the next day or may even cause injury.

Many variables improve with regular exercise (Bryant, Franklin, & Newton-Merrill, 2007). Health and fitness professionals may wish to measure and record a selection of these variables when working with a new client. Progress on some of these measures might motivate clients to keep exercising. Common indicators of fitness improvement include the following:

- **Muscle strength and endurance.** Gains in muscle strength and endurance occur fairly quickly for most people during the first few months of a strength-training program. Most clients are happy to see their repetitions and weights go up on their workout cards. Initial repetitions and weights can serve as the baseline against which improvement is measured.
- **Walking speed.** Results on a timed walking test may reveal positive fitness improvement if clients have been walking for several weeks as part of their exercise programs.
- **Heart rate during a given submaximal workload.** Clients performing cardiovascular exercise are likely to see a decrease in exercise heart rate for exercise performed at a standard workload on a piece of equipment that reproduces the type of exercise training the client is performing (Fig. 8-7). For example, people who walk regularly on a treadmill may see a decrease in exercise heart rate when walking at a given workload but may not see a drop in exercise heart rate when pedaling a cycle ergometer. When submaximal exercise heart rate is used as a yardstick for improvement, the submaximal workload must be exactly reproduced each time the client is measured. A calibrated piece of equipment or a step bench with a controlled stepping rate is best. "Level 6" may vary from one machine to the next, and a given machine may perform differently over time.

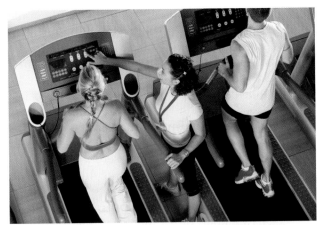

Figure 8-7. Many exercise machines have heart rate sensors. © Thinkstock

- **Resting heart rate.** Clients new to exercise often experience a decrease in resting heart rate after a few months of exercise. Resting heart rate must be taken in the same way and under the same conditions for each measurement. The most-reliable times are generally right before falling asleep or first thing in the morning (for people who wake up without an alarm). Clients should be aware of the variables that influence resting heart rate, including stress, noise, illness, menstrual cycle, and intake of alcohol, caffeine, and food.
- **Energy level.** A simple scale (for example, 1 to 10) can be used to capture perceptions of energy level. Many people feel energized after a workout or may even find they have more energy in general. Asking about this variable may help clients become aware of this important exercise benefit.
- **Emotional health indicators.** A simple scale can be used to measure emotional health indicators that are most likely to improve with regular physical activity. These include feelings of stress, anxiety, irritability, and depression, which may decrease. Clients may see improvements in mood and sleep quality.
- **Balance.** Balance measurements show the most improvement for people participating in balance training programs, but strength training and other exercise programs may also lead to improvements in balance for older adults.
- **Flexibility.** Flexibility measures are usually slow to improve, unless clients are stretching regularly for several weeks. Beginning exercisers may show flexibility improvements, however, simply because they learn not to "tense up" during flexibility testing.
- **Skill level.** Clients participating in sport-conditioning programs focused on activities such as tennis or golf are delighted when they find an improvement in sport skills. These clients may want help in establishing realistic ways to gauge skill improvement in a given activity.

- **Medical indicators, such as resting blood pressure, blood lipid profile, blood sugar levels, or bone density.** If any of these are important to clients or improvement is the goal of their exercise program, these should be measured regularly. Clients' health-care providers can help provide guidance on how frequently these should be checked. Many factors, including stress levels, diet, and changes in weight, can affect these variables and should be taken into consideration when evaluating exercise results.
- **Body weight.** Body weight is easily measured but not always a good indicator of body composition changes. Lean clients have been known to actually gain weight, mostly as muscle mass, as they increase exercise. In this case, female clients are sometimes dismayed. Body weight will also fluctuate with hydration levels. People who are overweight, however, may find weight a good indicator of progress in weight-control programs.
- **Waist circumference.** Waist and other circumferences may indicate change in body composition. A decrease in waist circumference can be reinforcing, especially if weight loss is not dramatic.
- **Body composition.** Body-composition measures are often very slow to change, so a focus on body composition can be pretty discouraging. If body-composition assessments are given, clients should be informed of the errors inherent in the measures. Repeated measures of body composition should be replicated as closely as possible by the same people on the same equipment.
- **Lab tests for maximal oxygen consumption, anaerobic threshold, and other metabolic variables.** These tests are useful for athletic clients training fairly intensely over a period of several months. Similarly, tests for speed, agility, and various measures of explosive power may improve if athletes perform training whose results might be captured by these tests.

Setting Motivational Goals

Health and fitness professionals should have a clear understanding of the goals motivating their clients. Open questions and effective listening can help expand and clarify clients' hopes and dreams. As discussed in Chapter 5, health and fitness professionals can help clients transform vague and unrealistic goals into more-measurable, reachable goals that can better guide exercise program design. Professionals can use S.M.A.R.T. goal guidelines to write motivational and effective exercise program goals (Bryant & Green, 2010).

Specific
Goals such as "exercise regularly" and "get in shape" need clarification to be sure that clients and health and fitness professionals are talking about the same thing. Professionals should encourage clients to take the lead in these discussions, guiding clients to become more specific. How specific is specific? Specific enough that progress toward the goal can be evaluated. Instead of "get in shape," specific goals might be to have enough endurance to be able to walk for several hours with the local hiking club or to be able to walk a mile in 20 minutes. Both of these goals help guide exercise recommendations and are specific enough that both the client and health and fitness professional know what they are talking about. Other examples of specific goals include completing a triathlon in the future, climbing the stairs without getting winded, or being able to fit into last year's jeans.

Measurable
Measurable goals allow clients to see that they are making progress toward their goals. The fitness variables discussed in the previous section are measurable. Scaling can be used to measure variables such as how difficult it feels to climb the stairs or perform other tasks of daily living, if those are important goals to clients.

Attainable
Health and fitness professionals should urge clients to look for gradual change in relevant fitness variables (variables likely to change with the given exercise program) over the next 6 months. Beginners and previously sedentary, out-of-shape clients will usually see progress more quickly than others as they begin to exercise. Large goals should be broken down into smaller goals, with all goals adjusted as clients are evaluated from time to time. While exercise physiology training studies have described the type of progress that health and fitness professionals are likely to see on different variables, each client is different, and no one can predict an individual's progress. Some individuals never show progress in certain areas. In these cases, health and fitness professionals can help set goals in other areas likely to show progress (Box 8-4).

Relevant
Health and fitness professionals usually have strong ideas about fitness and exercise program design. They may be tempted to look at clients and decide what clients need, the perfect exercise program already forming in their minds before clients have even introduced themselves. Clients may have different goals; however, and health and fitness professionals must suspend judgment and their own ideas early in their work with clients to understand what clients want.

Health and fitness professionals often assume, for example, that someone who appears to be overweight needs help with weight loss. But some clients who have struggled with diets and weight may have come to the conclusion that weight loss is out of reach for them. They may simply want advice on how to become more active to feel better and improve metabolic variables. These relevant goals will be more motivational (and probably more attainable).

Some clients may see fitness goals as pretty boring. For them, fitness must be connected to something more relevant, such as health: increasing strength means

Box 8-4. Exercise Training Nonresponders

Scientists reporting on the outcome of training studies give information on average improvements to a given training stimulus. Often left out of the discussion are the subjects who fail to improve. Averages and standard deviations rarely tell the whole story. Exercise training and adherence studies help build exercise-physiology theory and behavior-change models, but health and fitness professionals must always be aware that in any subject group there are outliers whose responses do not fit the models.

In almost every exercise training study, a minority of people fail to show improvement on certain fitness variables, even though they diligently perform their exercise programs (Karavirta et al., 2010; Timmons, 2010). For some reason, probably a mix of genetics and other variables, these people may see no improvements in aerobic capacity, muscle strength and endurance, or flexibility. Blood lipid levels do not budge, and blood pressure may not fall. What is the health and fitness professional to do with clients such as these?

Reassure such clients that they are not alone. Exercise is probably still beneficial for them. While some fitness variables may not improve, other variables may. Other measures, especially process goals, energy levels, and emotional health variables might demonstrate improvement. Researchers who have studied the issue of nonresponders still recommend regular exercise, since the health benefits are so wide-ranging (Timmons, 2010).

improving bone density, or increasing walking time means improving blood sugar regulation. Some people are able to link regular physical activity to fun goals like enjoying an upcoming hiking trip or learning to tango.

Time-Bound

People want to know when they can expect to see improvements in fitness variables. Time-bound means that the time it will take to reach specific goals should be spelled out. Health and fitness professionals should stress that the time it will take to see improvements are estimates that may need to be adjusted.

MOTIVATING CHANGE

While it is important to listen to clients and to be sure you are capturing their ideas about their goals, you can also suggest additional goals that are likely to have a high rate of success and thus be motivational for your clients. For example, be sure to ask clients about stress levels and daily energy level. Clients may not think of these when they are thinking about health and fitness; clients tend to think body when they think fitness. Help clients

understand that achieving emotional balance is as appropriate a goal as achieving a healthy weight or reducing risk of heart disease. (In fact, emotional balance will help with these other goals.)

Be sure to include process as well as product goals. In the context of physical activity, a product goal is a measurable change in a physical parameter, such as weight or strength. Clients do not always have much control over how quickly they progress toward product goals. A process goal is reached by simply completing the exercise recommendations; clients get credit for showing up. Examples of process goals include completing the strength-training workout twice a week, meeting with the personal trainer once a week, or attending a particular yoga class regularly.

Explain to clients how the exercise program recommendations will help them reach their goals. Break large goals down into smaller goals, so clients will see some progress in just a few weeks. Reevaluate and revise goals periodically to prevent discouragement because goals seem too far away. The workout record should include program goals and set dates for evaluating progress.

Jessica greets Sheila with a smile. "I'm sorry I was in such a hurry at our last session. An hour is not much time to tell you everything I want you to know. I'll try to go more slowly today and be sure you understand the equipment and exercises that will be most useful to you." Sheila explains that she has bought a book about weight training and has tried using the dumbbells her son left behind in the garage when he moved out. But the exercises are boring, and Sheila is not sure she is doing them correctly. "Preparation stage for weight training," Jessica thinks to herself. "Okay. Well, you seem ready to begin. You just need a little more experience with the equipment, so you will feel more comfortable," Jessica says.

Jessica has decided to start with five or six exercises that will be simple to learn. She teaches them to Sheila, who has a great deal of trouble following Jessica's confident demonstrations. But by the end of the hour, Sheila is relaxing and moving more smoothly. "Now you are getting the feel of this. Good for you! I think after we work together for your third free session, you'll be doing fine."

Effective Exercise Program Design

Effective exercise programs take into account people's health concerns, fitness goals, exercise preferences, and other personal variables. The structure of an exercise program influences people's abilities to stick to their exercise programs. While the perfect exercise program does not ensure adherence, psychologists have studied several factors that influence the likelihood that people will follow through with their exercise plans.

Clarity of the Action Plan

An effective exercise program provides a specific action plan that clearly spells out the details of the exercise program. Like good goals, an effective exercise program design is also S.M.A.R.T. The exercise program should be *specific*. It should also be *measurable*, in that it should delineate exercise mode (the type of exercise activity) as well as the frequency, intensity, and duration of performance. The exercise program should certainly be *attainable* and *relevant* for the client, in that it is designed to help the client reach his goals. The exercise program should be *time-bound*, in that exercise activities are scheduled into the client's week, so he knows when he is planning to do each activity.

Management of Expectations

Great expectations are a double-edged sword. Late-night abdominal crunching infomercials, bodybuilding supplements, and weight-loss programs promise quick and easy results that are, unfortunately, too good to be true. Such overselling of fitness programs and products can lead clients to have unrealistic expectations regarding exercise effects and exercise program design. Health and fitness professionals have observed that an exercise program that looks great on paper may turn out to require much more time and energy than clients actually have at their disposal. The planning fallacy and false hope theory, discussed in Chapter 5, can motivate clients to set lofty goals and begin an overly ambitious exercise program (Lovallo & Kahneman, 2003; Thaler & Sunstein, 2008; Trottier, Polivy, & Herman, 2009). But when people realize how much time their exercise program is actually taking, they may feel discouraged, especially if the spectacular results they were hoping for are not forthcoming. In many cases, they may give up and quit exercising. Health and fitness professionals should encourage positive, but realistic expectations about how much time and energy clients can really devote to an exercise program.

Self-Control

Adopting an exercise program takes a great deal of self-control. Self-control or self-regulation refers to the control people exert over their thoughts, feelings, and behavior (Baumeister, Gailliot, DeWall, & Oaten, 2006; Muraven, 2010), and was discussed in detail in Chapter 5. It takes self-control to change one's routine (Vohs et al., 2008). People use self-control when they roll out of bed in the morning and go for a walk, even though they would rather sleep another hour. Self-control is required to get to the fitness center after work when the television and dinner are calling. People use words such as willpower and determination when speaking of self-control, and most people feel like they never have quite enough of it, especially when trying to start an exercise program.

The less self-control energy an exercise program takes, the more likely people are to be successful in carrying out their plans. Coupled with the planning fallacy, this lack of energy for self-control is a leading cause of exercise nonadherence. Acknowledging that self-control is a limited resource can help people make more-effective exercise plans (Behavior Change in Action 8-2).

BEHAVIOR CHANGE IN ACTION 8-2

Understanding How Self-Control Influences Motivation

CHALLENGE
How can I apply the concept of limited self-control to increase exercise adherence?

PLAN
Fitness professionals are often guilty of designing behavior-change programs that look great on paper but don't match the amount of energy clients are able or willing to expend. This is partly because clients themselves don't really understand what they can realistically take on, and they underestimate the time and energy that an exercise or other behavior-change program will require. To improve the success of your clients, try to help them maximize their motivation and self-control, while reducing the self-control required by their exercise programs, using the following suggestions.

Help clients see that exercise gives them energy that helps them do the things that are important to them. Unless people see daily exercise as a priority, other commitments will consume their time and energy. Try to help clients link exercise and health to their personal priorities. People are willing to exert more energy when the activity in question helps them move toward important goals (Schmeichel & Vohs, 2009). Most clients will acknowledge that having more energy is important to them. Most clients will also agree that good health is a priority and that they need their health to do everything they want to do.

Acknowledge that daily exercise requires time and energy. People who mentally prepare for the challenge of taking on a program of daily exercise are better able to summon the self-control required to make their programs work. Rather than telling clients that exercise is easy and effortless, prepare them for the work as well as the rewards. Depending upon the exercise program, you might say, "An hour at the fitness center three times a week is a lot of time. Are you ready to make that commitment? How can you make this work?"

Continued

BEHAVIOR CHANGE IN ACTION 8-2–cont'd

Learn from past experience. If lack of willpower has been a problem in the past, keep exercise plans realistic. People vary in their levels of self-control. Professionals can try to help clients apply past experiences to their current programs. For example, if getting up an hour earlier to exercise has never worked in the past, maybe it will not work now, either.

Help clients make exercise a habit. Once exercise becomes a habitual routine, little self-control is required. Use the force of habit to increase exercise success. Encourage clients to quickly develop a weekly routine that is simple and repetitive, that doesn't take much thought. For example, clients might do strength workouts Tuesday and Thursday at the same time and the same place and walk Monday, Wednesday, and Sunday before dinner.

Recommend exercise early in the day, if this is feasible. People who exercise first thing in the morning tend to have the best adherence. Their goals have been accomplished before other demands eat up their time and wear away their self-control energy supply. Of course, the best time to exercise is whenever clients can work it into their schedules.

Increase exercise self-confidence with daily success. As clients become more confident in their abilities to stick to an exercise program, they will try harder to do so when obstacles arise. Start clients off with modest demands that they will really accomplish.

Help clients use exercise to reduce stress. Just as people can learn to overeat to reduce stress, so can they learn to exercise to reduce stress–a much more-adaptive response. Educate clients about the stress-reduction benefits of regular exercise. Encourage them to turn to exercise to reduce feelings of stress. Reducing stress with exercise does three great things: it reduces stress, creates incentives to exercise, and increases self-control energy.

Encourage social support. Clients need less self-control when that control is supplemented by encouragement from others. Recommend exercising with a friend. An exercise partner reduces the need for self-control. Instead of wasting time and energy thinking about whether to exercise or not, people must just show up because the exercise partner is expecting them.

Prior Exercise Experiences

Many people have tried to become more active at other times in their lives. Each attempt and each failure contains lessons for future efforts. Can variables associated with prior failure be avoided? Better dealt with? Can variables that supported success be incorporated into another attempt? Discussion of prior exercise experiences can help clients and health and fitness professionals design effective exercise programs together.

Pursuit of Happiness

Intrinsic motivation for physical activity occurs when people find pleasure, fun, and even meaning in their exercise program. People often think health clubs and fitness centers when planning a new exercise program, but many people find these environments boring. There are many types of physical activities, exercise settings, and options, and people should explore the kinds of exercise they find most enjoyable (or, for people who hate exercise, least onerous). Some considerations for matching exercise activities to personal activity preferences include the following (Brehm, 2004).

- **Outdoor options.** Many people find sunlight and fresh air therapeutic, especially if they spend most of their time indoors. Outdoor activities, also known as green exercise, have many emotional health benefits (Fig. 8-8; Pretty, Peacock, Sellens, & Griffin, 2005). Such activities include walking, bicycling, hiking, or skating. If there's

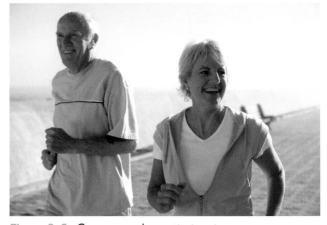

Figure 8-8. **Green exercise.** © Thinkstock

snow, Nordic or alpine skiing, snowshoeing, or sledding might be good choices.

- **Social support.** Some people enjoy exercising with a friend or family member. Many people enjoy the camaraderie of group exercise. Social support improves exercise adherence, and many people find that talking as they walk is great therapy.
- **Time alone.** Some people need a break from others and find that break in exercise. They may enjoy a solitary workout or being alone in a crowd.
- **Opportunities for problem-solving and creative thinking.** Repetitive exercise modes such

as walking, exercise machines, and swimming can give people time to ponder problems or think creatively.

- **Activities requiring concentration.** Some people enjoy activities that require total concentration, such as competitive sports like tennis, squash, and basketball. Rock climbing, whitewater kayaking, and other outdoor adventure-type activities require concentration as well. Such concentration forces one's mind to quit thinking about problems, at least temporarily.
- **Competition.** Similarly, many people enjoy some level of competition, whether it's a friendly recreational tennis group or a highly competitive age-group sports contest. Competition motivates clients to train and provides a great diversion from life's stress, unless of course the competition itself creates too much anxiety and stress! Highly competitive activities may be counterproductive for clients reporting problems with stress or anxiety.
- **Vigorous exercise.** Healthy, fairly fit people may find that vigorous activity provides more enjoyment and greater stress relief than exercise of a more-moderate intensity. Clients may also see greater fitness gains with more-intense exercise. Vigorous exercise delivers its conditioning stimulus in a shorter period of time than exercise of lower intensity, a plus for clients whose schedules are packed. Health and fitness professionals can urge such clients to step up the pace a bit. Caution: be sure vigorous exercise is appropriate for the client before recommending high-intensity exercise.
- **Mind–body activities, such as yoga and tai chi** (Fig. 8-9). In these disciplines, physical activity is a vehicle through which the participant strives for emotional balance. These activities are usually appropriate for a wide range of fitness levels and ages, and many people find these activities to be a nice change of pace.
- **Rhythmic breathing.** Rhythmic breathing is often a component of mind–body activities and may be partly responsible for the relaxed, meditative mental state experienced during these activities. Other activities, such as swimming and running, may offer rhythmic breathing as well.
- **Recreational activities.** Just about any activity perceived as fun has psychological benefits. Nothing beats having a good time or building a sense of accomplishment. Many dance activities, such as folk dancing, contra dancing, square dancing, and even ballroom dancing, can be quite vigorous as well as a lot of fun.
- **Activities with a purpose.** Psychologists have observed that people who successfully incorporate physical activity into their lives do so because activity has a purpose (Morgan, 2001). People may bike or walk for transportation or

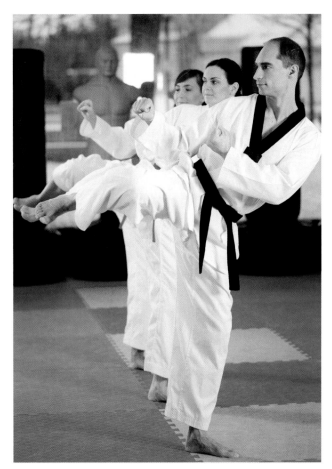

Figure 8-9. **Mind–body balance.** © Thinkstock

garden in order to have beautiful flowers or fresh vegetables.

- **Meaning.** Perhaps the greatest psychological benefit of physical activity is finding meaning—in the best case meaning in life, but meaning in the activity is also beneficial. For example, many people connect with nature while hiking. Others train for physical activities that involve fundraising for meaningful charities. Physical activity may provide a vehicle for strengthening an important relationship with a family member or friend. Mind–body activities may involve a search for emotional balance and philosophical understanding.

Exercise Partners

Some clients may enjoy exercising with a friend or family member. Exercise partners enhance exercise adherence in many ways. While some people enjoy solitary exercise, others find the social connection of exercising with another person motivational. Some of the ways an exercise partner can enhance exercise adherence include the following.

- **Exercise partners provide gentle coercion and limit negative self-talk.** One of the most-common reasons people fail to stick to their exercise programs is that they talk themselves out of exercising. This is most likely to happen when people feel fatigued or are experiencing a negative mood. When people are feeling stressed, they may begin thinking about all the things they have to do and how little energy they have. The exercise partner short-circuits the mental meanderings that might lead to the decision to skip exercising.

- **Exercise partners promote a positive mood and reduce feelings of stress.** Good exercise partners help make fitness fun. At best, they provide a positive emotional connection that helps people look forward to their exercise sessions. Conversation and good company help pass the time, if people find exercise boring. When exercise is pleasurable and provides a positive emotional experience, people are more likely to stick to their exercise programs.
- **Exercise partners enhance exercise self-efficacy.** Many forms of social support, including exercise partners, enhance exercise self-efficacy. This may be because exercise partners tend to cheer each other on and provide positive feedback.
- **Social support aids planning.** Because exercising with another person requires coordinating schedules, exercisers must plan. Planning increases exercise adherence.
- **Exercise can become a way to spend time with family members or close friends.** Busy people often like the idea of accomplishing two goals at once when they exercise. They may be able to find activities that include family members or friends with whom they would like to spend more time. Parents may wish to use activity time as quality time with their children or teens. Some parents report they get more conversation out of their sons and daughters when they are doing something active than when they ask at dinnertime, "How was school?" Many parents are eager to increase the activity level of their children, and they stick to an exercise program to set a positive example.
- **Animal lovers know that no discussion of exercise partners would be complete without a mention of their beloved pets.** Dogs especially encourage a great deal of physical activity, since they need daily walks to stay healthy and because they can sometimes cajole their owners into active play.

Health and fitness professionals can encourage clients to think about asking a coworker, neighbor, friend, or family member to exercise with them and discuss the qualities of a good exercise partner. The partner should be someone with whom the client wishes to spend time. Both exercise partners must enjoy the exercise activity and be able to work at a good pace. This means that they should be able to perform the target activity, such as walking, cycling, and so on at a similar pace or to work out on adjacent machines that allow them to individualize exercise

intensity. Scheduling can often be a major hurdle: clients will need to find partners who are available at the right times.

Exercise partners are not easy to find. Clients may need to think creatively. They may wish to invite a variety of people to try different activities with them in the beginning and then see who will actually follow through consistently. Clients should also think of alternatives for days when the exercise partner is unavailable. If exercising with a partner makes exercise less convenient or more time consuming, clients will have more excuses than ever to drop out of the exercise program. A partner should make exercise easier, not harder.

Injury Prevention

Injury from exercise is one of the leading causes of exercise dropout. Sometimes injury is caused by simple bad luck. People miss a step and sprain an ankle, or a racquetball partner inadvertently collides with competition. But some factors that increase injury risk are influenced by exercise program design and other lifestyle factors. These factors include the following.

Sports Equipment and Footwear
Exercise machines must be safe and maintained regularly. People should use good safety equipment recommended for their sport: eye protection for racquet sports, helmets for cycling, and so forth (Fig. 8-10). Equipment should be of good quality, fit well, and be maintained in good condition. Equipment should be replaced as necessary. Good sport-specific footwear prevents injury as well. Shoes should fit well and accommodate sport demands.

Exercise Environment
Fitness centers should be careful to maintain a safe exercise environment and minimize conditions that could lead to falls and injury (Tharrett & Peterson, 2012). People should avoid or be careful on slippery or sticky playing surfaces. Altitude and hot environments require acclimation. Weather may present challenges in the form of heat, humidity, cold, or lightning.

Exercise Training Overload
Exercise programs must walk the fine line between effective conditioning and overtraining. A well-designed exercise program stimulates the training effect and improves fitness. But it is easy to overtrain, which leads to a decline in performance and increases risk of overuse injury (Fig. 8-11). Exercise workload must be increased slowly and gradually over time to allow the body sufficient opportunity to accommodate new demands.

Injury Prevention Training Programs
Many athletes follow specialized training procedures that help prevent injury. For example, core-training exercises prevent back injuries by strengthening the muscles that stabilize the torso.

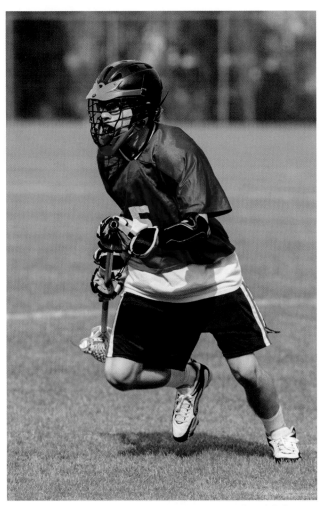

Figure 8-10. Proper exercise equipment reduces injury risk. © Thinkstock

Education Regarding Injury Warning Signs

People often ignore early aches and pains that indicate the development of overuse injuries. Overuse injuries tend to come on gradually, and by heeding early warning signs, people can prevent more troublesome injuries from developing. Early signs of overuse injury include pain at night that goes away during activity, as well as daytime pain, joint swelling, muscle fatigue, numbness, and tingling (Johnson, Haskvitz, & Brehm, 2009). People can often continue to exercise by switching to a different form of physical activity that allows overuse injuries to heal.

Adequate Rest and Recovery

Rest and recovery are essential components of well-designed sports-training programs. The body needs rest to respond to a training stimulus and become stronger. Inadequate recovery hurts performance and increases risk of injury.

Stress

Feeling overwhelmed by stress increases injury risk in several ways (Johnson & Ivarsson, 2011). Under stress, peripheral vision narrows, so people are less aware of

what's going on around them (Rogers & Landers, 2005). Stress also increases unnecessary muscle tension, especially in the postural muscles of the back, neck, and shoulders, increasing injury risk to these areas. Stress interferes with good decision-making and distraction inhibits concentration; mistakes can lead to injury.

Behavior-Change Skills

Behavior-change skills (discussed in Chapter 4) are strongly associated with successful behavior change. Behavior-change skills include a variety of self-management techniques that people use to support their behavior-change efforts. Self-management refers to managing one's thoughts, feelings, and behaviors. Behavior-change skills are especially important in the implementation and maintenance of behavior-change programs. The behavior-change skills most strongly related to long-term exercise adherence include the following.

Making Specific Plans and Schedules

Discussed above in the section on effective exercise program design, specific plans are clearly spelled out and easy to follow. People should schedule their exercise sessions into their calendars just as they would important meetings.

Creating Systems for Self-Monitoring

With regard to exercise adherence, self-monitoring usually takes the form of a daily written record of completed exercise sessions. Most people prefer an exercise log that is fairly small, portable, and easy to complete (Fig. 8-12). Logs should contain enough room for a complete record of each workout. Clients may wish to use a workout card for strength-training sessions. In a typical log, people record time, calories expended, exercise heart rate, or other variables for cardiovascular exercise. Some clients may simply wish to record the type of activity and the number of minutes spent performing that activity. Details that might indicate improvement can be motivational, such as intensity level, weight lifted, or minutes of exercise, so clients may be willing to record these for each workout. Interestingly, the increased self-awareness that is associated with the act of recording seems to be more important than any particular method used for recording, so individual variation in exercise log procedures is fine (Foreyt & Carlos Poston, 1998).

Self-monitoring may increase exercise adherence for several reasons. Exercise logs testify to a person's adherence and achievement of attendance goals. Reaching such goals is motivational. In addition, the exercise log can serve as a foundation for conversations with a health and fitness professional about the factors that interfered with attendance and lead to helpful problem-solving discussions. The exercise log provides a fairly objective adherence record. While people may be thinking they are doing pretty well with getting to the

Training vs Overtraining

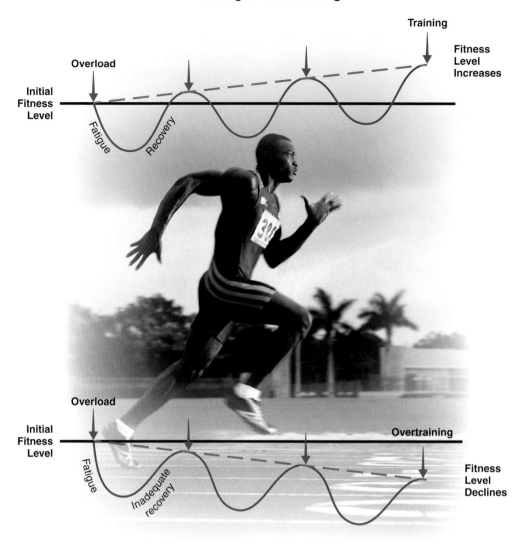

Figure 8-11. Training vs. overtraining. Photograph © Thinkstock

gym, two weeks of blank days tell them in objective terms where they stand on exercise program attendance. Self-monitoring systems increase people's vigilance regarding exercise adherence.

Finding Positive Reinforcement

When behaviors are rewarded, they are more likely to occur again. Intrinsic motivation often evolves from positive reinforcement, when pleasure or enjoyment is found during physical activity. Finding immediate emotional health rewards is positively reinforcing. If people feel less irritable and stressed on days they exercise, these good feelings can provide positive reinforcement.

Some programs provide extrinsic reinforcements for exercise participation: free t-shirts or water bottles, reduced insurance premiums, and so forth. Although long-term adherence is more strongly linked to intrinsic motivation, extrinsic reinforcement can also increase exercise adherence in the short run. Exercising for some sort of reward might at least give people time to establish an exercise habit or to discover that they enjoy exercising.

Solving Problems

Self-monitoring systems can provide information helpful for solving problems. If plans to walk on the weekend rarely come to fruition, perhaps people can identify what barriers prevent weekend activity or simply schedule more activity on weekdays. Problem-solving techniques have been categorized in several ways. Some of the most applicable to working with exercise behavior include stimulus control and counterconditioning. These techniques come from behavior-modification programs as well as cognitive-behavioral therapy. They are both also listed as processes of change in the Transtheoretical model.

Stimulus control techniques are based on the observation that for each person, certain factors trigger automatic responses. Once these associations are understood, people can think of ways to change or avoid the stimulus. For example, if a person finds that he cannot summon the energy to get out of the house to take a walk after he has a beer, he could eliminate the stimulus (the beer), or at least drink it after his walk rather than before.

Date	2/7	2/8	2/9	2/11	2/12	2/14	2/15					
Exercise	wts/reps											
Warmup	Bike 20		Bike 20		Bike 20							
Squats	20/8		20/8		20/10							
Shoulder press	20/10		20/10		20/10							
Row	40/10		40/12		40/12							
Chest press	30/12		30/12		30/12							
Leg extension	50/8		50/10		50/10							
Chest fly	30/12		30/12		30/12							
Leg curl	50/8		50/8		50/10							
Back extension	8		8		8							
Abdominal series	✓		✓		✓							
Cardiovascular ex			Tread mill—20		TM—20							
Other			Yoga class—90 min		Yoga class—90 min	Hike—2 hrs						

Figure 8-12. Exercise log.

With counterconditioning, people plan a new response to a problematic stimulus. For example, a person might find that bad weather always leads to a decision to skip a scheduled walk. It's often too cold, too hot, too rainy, or too something to exercise. Instead of deciding not to exercise, that person could decide to exercise indoors, perhaps joining a fitness center and exercising in climate-controlled conditions. Or that person could try new types of apparel to achieve better comfort during exercise. The new response (counterconditioning) would be dressing better for exercise.

MOTIVATING CHANGE: Incorporating Behavior-Change Skills Into Work With Clients

How do clients learn behavior-change skills? While some clients may practice these skills intuitively, or from prior training, many clients appreciate the opportunity to work on these skills with a health and fitness professional. Fortunately, many self-management skills seem logical, and their application to exercise adherence is easily taught (although not necessarily easily practiced). In particular, health and fitness professionals should help clients set up effective exercise logs to record workouts and factors related to adherence. Health and fitness professionals can also anticipate and discuss the problematic situations that may interfere with clients' exercise programs and help clients make plans to prevent these from causing relapse. Be sure to let clients take the lead in devising solutions to their adherence problems. Ask them questions to get their ideas on what might work in their lives.

Motor Skill Acquisition

Sometimes exercise programs require learning new activities. Or people may include improving activity or sport skills as a training goal. Some will want to learn to use new fitness equipment. Others will wish to improve their golf or tennis games. Some people want to learn a new activity, such as scuba diving, swimming, or squash. The process of learning new motor skills or developing and improving existing skill levels can provide a stimulating and enjoyable experience. Or the experience may be overwhelming and frustrating and ultimately short-circuit good intentions. Feeling frustrated during motor-skill learning decreases feelings of competence and self-efficacy and leads to feelings of stress and negative emotions. Sometimes these frustrations are strong enough to motivate people to *avoid* exercise.

Motor learning is the process of acquiring and improving motor skills. People vary widely in the way that they learn and master motor skills. Anyone who has ever observed a children's physical education class has no doubt noted the variation in the ways children learn new skills. Some quickly master the task and others take much longer. Some learn by watching, while others listen carefully to instructions. And some are embarrassed by their perceived lack of coordination, cannot focus, and sit on the sidelines. Adults are not so different, except that they tend to learn more slowly and are able to avoid the activities for which they believe they have no aptitude. Health and fitness professionals with a strong background in physical education and sports are often surprised at the lack of motor ability they see in many adult clients.

Physical education researchers have found that many people tend to believe that good coordination and athletic ability are things that a person is born with (Rink, 2004). While ability in the motor-skills domain certainly varies from person to person, motor skills are more strongly related to practice and experience than to natural ability alone. People new to physical activity need to understand that motor-skill improvement takes a great deal of practice; the people they see in exercise classes have often been performing similar movement patterns, choreography, or exercise progressions for years. The same holds true for athletes in every sport.

One of the biggest barriers to learning is self-consciousness and embarrassment, which leads to difficulty focusing on the task at hand. Many people new to exercise feel self-conscious attending a new exercise class, participating in a personal training session, or taking a sport lesson. They may feel out of place, awkward, or clumsy. Even people with athletic experience may feel awkward when learning new motor skills. Such people may believe they should pick up new motor skills quickly, remembering how good they were at sports when they were young. They may become frustrated if motor learning does not come quickly and easily. When teaching new skills to clients, health and fitness professionals should try to help clients feel at home in the exercise environment and help new learners understand that most of the people they see working out have been performing these types of activities for months, years, and, often, decades. When possible, professionals should try to teach nervous learners in a setting where they are less likely to feel watched. Clients should try to relax and focus on the task at hand. If they are having difficulty focusing, health and fitness professionals should move to a simpler task that is easier to master. People generally enjoy learning most and learn best when the following guidelines are followed.

Introduce New Skills Slowly and Clearly

The introduction of a new skill should begin with a very short explanation of what is being taught and why. Explanations should be concise and clear. Learners are limited in how much information they can take in at one time. Safety information should be emphasized, including guidelines for injury prevention. A skill should be explained in terms of what it is accomplishing or why it is important, so learners can link the skill to the big picture of the activity or sport.

Keep Focus on Movement Goals

In general, people learn more quickly when the instructor focuses on the goal of the movement rather than on distracting details about limb position (Marchant, Clough, & Cramshaw, 2005). For example, personal trainers would not teach clients to use an elliptical trainer by describing when to bend and straighten the knees. Instead, they would emphasize moving the pedals around in a smooth, steady motion and then demonstrate the skill giving clients time to watch.

Obviously, describing limb position is important in many situations, so the above is a general guideline only. For example, when teaching squats, an instructor might ask clients to focus on keeping the knees from bending past a certain angle. Such descriptions are most helpful when kept brief and simple.

Accommodate Learning Style

Variations in the way people process and retain new information have been called learning style differences. Some people like a lot of explanation and ask many questions (verbal learning style). Others learn by watching and appreciate longer demonstrations with less talking (visual learning style), and still others learn by doing, needing to feel the movement before catching on (kinesthetic learning style). Good instructors working with a group provide verbal, visual, and kinesthetic learning opportunities. Health and fitness professionals who work over time with given individuals sometimes figure out which teaching style works best.

Provide Adequate Time for Focused Practice

People need plenty of time to practice new skills without being distracted by talking or listening. Most instructors tend to give too many corrections too soon. Often initial attempts at a skill improve if a person has time to practice (Renshaw, Chow, Davids, & Hammond, 2010).

Give Helpful and Motivational Feedback

After people have tried new skills a few times, feedback can be useful. Helpful feedback accomplishes three things:

- Provides reinforcement for what was done well
- Corrects errors
- Motivates people to continue practicing and improving

Most people feel better if corrections, which are usually seen as the more "negative" points, are sandwiched between reinforcement and motivation. An example might be, "Your breathing and timing were just right on the first four lifts. Remember to keep breathing, even as the exercise starts to feel harder. You'll find the work easier now that you are learning how to breathe correctly."

Feedback should be limited to a few simple points, so instructors must decide which errors are the most helpful to correct. Most important errors typically include those that involve safety, occur earliest in the movement sequence, or are fundamental in some other way (Bryant & Green, 2010). People generally respond better to corrections phrased in a positive fashion: "Remember to breathe," rather than "Don't hold your breath." Feedback given after positive efforts appears to improve motor learning more quickly than feedback given as corrections to poorer performance. Telling clients they are doing better than average leads to more improvement than telling them they are performing below average (Lewthwaite & Wulf, 2010).

FROM ACTION TO MAINTENANCE:
Maintaining Long-Term Exercise Adherence

Deciding to begin an exercise program and starting to exercise are not easy, but developing a habit of physical activity that lasts for more than 6 months may be even harder. About half of all adults who begin an exercise program drop out during the first 6 months (Dishman & Buckworth, 1996). Researchers have suggested that the psychological variables predicting long-term exercise adherence differ somewhat from those that describe forming an intention to become active and beginning an exercise program (Nigg, Borrelli, Maddock, & Dishman, 2008). Of course, many of the variables involved in forming a decision to exercise and starting an exercise program remain important and will motivate the problem-solving and stress-management behaviors that are critical for maintaining an exercise program. Some of the most important variables associated with maintaining long-term participation in regular physical activity include the following.

Satisfaction With Physical Activity Experiences and Outcomes

People are more likely to continue exercising if they are finding value in their exercise programs. If people began exercising to help with a specific health or fitness goal, and they continue to value that goal, they will be motivated by progress toward their goal. Even if people do not necessarily enjoy physical activity, when they find that it is helping them reach important goals, physical activity can become an integrated part of their self-regulation.

People who find physical activity a positive experience in and of itself will be more likely to continue exercising (Papandonatos et al., 2012). Positive emotions reduce feelings of stress and create self-control energy. Intrinsic motivation activates people to cope with difficulties and maintain physical activity.

Ability to Anticipate and Cope With High-Risk Situations

Individuals who can anticipate problems and devise coping strategies, or at least plan a return to exercise, are more likely to become long-term exercisers. Exercise maintainers have strong self-efficacy for dealing with exercise barriers and skills for coping with disruptions. This type of problem-solving was described in the previous section on behavior-change skills. Behavior-change

psychologists have found that many of the exercise barriers that arise during the first 6 months of an exercise program and frequently lead to exercise dropout come in the form of high-risk situations.

The most-common high-risk situations result in a disruption of the exercise routine. Once people set a behavior-change plan in motion, they rely on the routine they have developed to reach their goals. Anything that disrupts that routine can lead to nonadherence and ultimately to quitting an exercise program. Most people's lives are filled with disruptions: changes in schedule, unforeseen events, visitors, travel, holidays, and illness are a few. Injuries, bad weather, and loss of an exercise partner are other common reasons that people quit exercising.

Health and fitness professionals can help clients learn from disruptions that have occurred in the past and use their problem-solving skills to plan for future disruptions. What will they do when they get sick? Travel? Must stay home with the children on a snow day? What happens when it starts to get dark early? Accommodation for disruption must somehow be built into every exercise program.

Effective Ways to Cope With Stress and Negative Emotions

Feelings of stress and negative emotions such as depression, anger, and anxiety reduce motivation. Regular physical activity may no longer feel like a priority; reducing emotional distress becomes the priority. When life feels out of control, exercise may no longer seem very important. Stress and negative emotions may cause people to seek emotional relief in old behaviors that they are trying to change, such as overeating.

Some research suggests that one of the interesting characteristics of people who are long-term exercisers is that when feeling stressed, they may exercise more frequently, and non–long-term exercisers tend to exercise less frequently in similar circumstances (What's the Evidence? 8-1; Lutz, Stults-Kolehmainen, & Bartholomew, 2010). Perhaps long-term exercisers recognize that regular exercise helps them manage stress and helps them feel better and more able to address sources of stress.

It is appropriate for health and fitness professionals to ask clients what they currently do to manage stress and to encourage those coping behaviors that seem healthy. No matter what type of behavior clients are attempting to change, regular physical activity should be part of the behavior-change program since exercise reduces feelings of stress and increases self-confidence. For example, regular exercise increases the likelihood of success in smoking-cessation programs. Of course, if stress or negative emotions seem to be significantly interfering with daily life, health and fitness professionals should refer clients for professional counseling.

WHAT'S THE EVIDENCE? 8-1

The Stress–Exercise Adherence Relationship

Lutz, R. S., Stults-Kolehmainen, M. A., & Bartholomew, J. B. (2010). Exercise caution when stressed: Stages of change and the stress–exercise participation relationship. *Psychology of Sport and Exercise, 11*: 560-567.

■ PURPOSE

Many researchers as well as health and fitness professionals have observed that people solidly in the maintenance phase of behavior change for physical activity differ from those for whom exercise behavior is difficult to maintain. One of the factors most frequently associated with relapse from behavior-change programs is perceived stress. Some studies have found that people generally reduce their physical-activity levels when faced with stressful events or when they perceive higher levels of stress. But other studies have not found this association.

■ STUDY

Lutz and colleagues knew that some people find that regular physical activity reduces feelings of stress. Some people even turn to exercise to cope with feelings of stress. Thinking about these observations, Lutz and colleagues hypothesized that stage of change may mediate the relationship between perceived stress and physical-activity levels. They hypothesized the following:

> First, exercisers at lower stages of change may experience exercise engagement with more negative feelings in comparison with those at more-advanced stages of change, thus making it more aversive during stressful times. Less-frequent exercisers may respond to stress with more inactivity, as it would help them avoid negative feelings during exercise. Frequent exercisers may exercise more during stressful episodes as exercise *promotes* positive feelings *after exercise*. Second, as there appear to be regulatory differences between frequent and infrequent exercisers, and because research supports the notion that stress can deplete regulatory resources . . . we might expect infrequent exercisers' relatively weaker regulatory effort in this area to lead to more inactivity (561).

To test their hypotheses, Lutz and colleagues recruited 95 female participants from undergraduate psychology courses at their university in Texas. Students completed questionnaires regarding exercise levels and stage of change for physical activity. They also recorded their exercise participation over the course of 6 weeks as well as measures of stress events and stress intensity. When the data were analyzed, a clear relationship emerged and verified the researchers' original hypotheses. The researchers found different relationships between stress events and minutes of exercise per day for students in maintenance versus students in other stages of change. At higher intensities of stress, students in maintenance achieved *more* minutes of exercise, while students in other stages achieved less, with exercise levels approaching zero at the highest levels of stress events. Similar relationships were found between stress events and days of exercise per week: people in the maintenance stage exercised more as the number of stressful events in their lives increased, while everyone else exercised less as they experienced more stress events in their lives.

The researchers suggest that people in maintenance have learned how to use exercise to reduce feelings of stress. People in maintenance feel better when they exercise, so they may be even more conscientious about exercising regularly when they feel stressed. People who do not exercise or have a newly developed exercise program may not enjoy exercise, or they may not be in the habit of exercising. When feelings of stress increase, they may perceive the demand of getting their exercise session completed as one more source of stress. Therefore, they exercise less when feeling more stress.

■ IMPLICATIONS

Stress is a leading cause of relapse from exercise programs. Any behavior-change program must address this issue and prepare clients for coping with stress. It may be possible for some clients to learn to enjoy exercise and to observe that they feel better after a workout or when they are exercising regularly. If clients can establish the connection between exercise and stress reduction, they are more likely to exercise in the face of stress. If an exercise program is perceived as a problem or a stressor, clients are likely to drop out, or at least attend less regularly during high-stress periods.

Ability to Cope With Lapses and Setbacks

- Just as successful exercisers have learned to make plans for dealing with high-risk situations, so too have they learned to view days or weeks with no exercise as lapses or setbacks from which they can recover, rather than reasons or opportunities to quit exercising (Behavior Change in Action 8-3). Rather than seeing exercise adherence as an all-or-nothing proposition, they are able to respond more flexibly to disruptions and persist in their efforts to get back into an exercise routine.

BEHAVIOR CHANGE IN ACTION 8-3

Dealing With Lapses

■ CHALLENGE

How do I help clients reengage with their exercise programs after lapses in exercise adherence?

■ PLAN

Teaching yourself and your clients to view a lapse as a learning experience can enhance the effectiveness of exercise program design and help clients overcome a sense of failure and return anew to the fitness center.

Don't take it personally. Before you initiate discussions with your falling-by-the-wayside clients, you must get over any emotional response you may be having to your clients' difficulties. Getting frustrated, irritated, and angry won't coax your clients back. Maintain your interested, sympathetic, and professional attitude.

Avoid negative emotions. If clients feel embarrassed about skipping exercise sessions, it may seem easier to them not to face you. They may associate the fitness center with feelings of failure and low self-esteem. Try to help these clients develop a more-positive and realistic attitude toward exercise. Start by stating your understanding that life can get complicated and acknowledging that your clients have other commitments in their lives besides their exercise programs. While urging clients to make their health and fitness a priority, admit that this can even be a struggle for you and other clients with whom you have worked. If possible, show that you appreciate them as people, even as you remind them of the importance of their resolutions to exercise.

Help clients view lapses as learning experiences. When opportunity arises, help clients explore setbacks in more depth. Ask about these experiences. Be a good listener and work with clients to figure out how to use this knowledge to improve their chances of success. Take the word "relapse" out of your vocabulary when talking with your clients. Help your clients learn from their difficulties. This learning can increase the likelihood of success in future behavior-change efforts. Help your clients see prior "failures" as learning opportunities, rather than indicators of limited potential or personal weakness.

Coach clients to imagine a return to exercise. Encourage clients to imagine that in the future something may force them to temporarily abandon their exercise plans. Sample questions include:

- Can you envision something that might disrupt your exercise plan?
- What will it feel like?
- And how will you get back into exercising regularly?

Help clients realize that skipping a workout can happen and should not be construed as failure. Advise clients that when they miss a workout, the best thing is to think about how they will get to their next exercise session. Clients must also learn not to let negative feelings of failure get in the way of their continuing commitment to their exercise program.

Relapse means returning to behavior patterns, such as being sedentary or overeating, that one has attempted to change. How do lapses turn into relapse? Health and fitness professionals as well as their clients often behave as though exercise nonadherence means one thing: failure—on the part of the helping professional and on the part of the client. Because failure tends to feel embarrassing and shameful, people don't want to talk about it very much. It's no wonder their clients end up seeing poor attendance as an indication that an exercise program isn't going to work.

Such thinking is unproductive and leads to missed opportunities. It blocks creative problem-solving and hurts self-esteem, and thus it undermines success in the future. While it is natural for people to feel disappointed when they fail to achieve important goals, professionals and clients alike must learn to view behavior change as a lifelong process that requires patience, understanding, and compassion.

Jessica is pleased when Sheila arrives 4 days later for her third personal training session. Jessica's focus today is to *continue to build Sheila's self-efficacy for strength-training exercise. Jessica observes Sheila perform the exercises that they worked on at the last session. Sheila has forgotten much of what they covered, but she remembers quickly after Jessica gives her a few reminders. Jessica tries not to talk too much as Sheila performs her workout. She answers Sheila's questions and praises her progress. At the end of the session, Jessica takes Sheila through some stretching exercises. Sheila is pleased with herself and is excited about making progress on her strength-training resolutions.*

"I think you will really like working out here," Jessica assures Sheila. "Pretty soon, you are going to look like one of the regulars." Sheila is less worried now about how she looks but thinks maybe she won't mind working out at the fitness center after all. If it prevents future fractures from weak bones, it will definitely be worth the effort. ■

KEY TERMS

epiphanies

expectancies

expectations

green exercise

learning style differences

mastery experience

motor learning

self-management

CRITICAL THINKING QUESTIONS

1. Self-Determination Theory states that people look for autonomy, competence, and connection in their lives. How can personal trainers apply Self-Determination Theory in their work with clients?

2. Apply the ecological model to factors that promote and discourage physical activity in your own life. Draw a diagram like that of Fig. 8-1, listing not only barriers to physical activity but also helpful factors at each level as well.

3. Imagine you are opening your own fitness center. What factors would you consider as you design your policies for medical clearance and fitness testing? Would fitness testing be mandatory for all clients? What tests and measures would you include?

4. As part of your new fitness center policy, you offer new clients a free personal training session. You are in charge of training the personal trainers who work at your center. What would you advise them to do during this free session with new clients? How could that time best be spent?

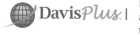 For additional resources log in to Davis*Plus* (**http://davisplus.fadavis.com/** keyword "Brehm") and click on the Premium tab. (Don't have a *Plus*Code to access Premium Resources? Just click the Purchase Access button on the book's Davis*Plus* page.)

REFERENCES

Bandura, A. (1977). Self-efficacy: toward a unifying theory of behavioral change. *Psychological Review, 84*(2), 191-215.

Bandura, A. (1997). *Self-efficacy: The Exercise of Control.* New York: Freeman.

Baumeister, R. F., Gailliot, M., DeWall, C. N., & Oaten, M. (2006). Self-regulation and personality: how interventions increase regulatory success, and how depletion moderates the effects of traits on behavior. *Journal of Personality, 74*(6), 1773-1802.

Bennie, J. A., Timperio, A. F., Crawford, D. A., Dunstan, D.W., & Salmon, J. L. (2011). Associations between social ecological factors and self-reported short physical activity breaks during work hours among desk-based employees. *Preventive Medicine: An International Journal Devoted to Practice and Theory, 53*(1-2), 44-47.

Brehm, B. A. (2004). *Successful Fitness Motivation Strategies.* Champaign, IL: Human Kinetics.

Bryant, C. X., & Green, D. J. (2010). *ACE Personal Trainer Manual.* San Diego, CA: American Council on Exercise.

Bryant, C. X., Franklin, B. A., & Newton-Merrill, S. (2007). *ACE's Guide to Exercise Testing and Program Design: A Fitness Professional's Handbook.* Monterey, CA: Healthy Learning.

Canadian Society for Exercise Physiology. (2002). *Par Q & You: Physical Activity Readiness Questionnaire.* www.csep.ca/cmfiles/publications/parq/par-q.pdf. Accessed 12/12/12.

Caperchione, C. M., Kolt, G. S., & Mummery, W. K. (2009). Physical activity in culturally and linguistically diverse migrant groups to Western society: a review of barriers, enablers and experiences. *Sports Medicine, 39*(3), 167-177.

Cerin, E., Leslie, E., Sugiyama, T., & Owen, N. (2010). Perceived barriers to leisure-time physical activity in adults: an ecological perspective. *Journal of Physical Activity & Health, 7*(4), 451-459.

Cox, A. E., Ullrich-French, S., Madonia, J., & Witty, K. (2011). Social physique anxiety in physical education: social contextual factors and links to motivation and behavior. *Psychology of Sport and Exercise, 12*, 555-562.

Cramp, A. G., & Bray, S. R. (2011). Understanding exercise self-efficacy and barriers to leisure-time physical activity among postnatal women. *Maternal and Child Health Journal, 15*(5), 642-651.

Deci, E. L., & Ryan, R. M. (2008). Facilitating optimal motivation and psychological well-being across life's domains. *Canadian Psychology, 49*(1), 14-23.

DiBartolo, P. M., Lin, L., Montoya, S., Neal, H., & Shaffer, C. (2007). Are there "healthy" and "unhealthy" reasons for exercise? Examining individual differences in exercise motivation using the Function of Exercise Scale. *Journal of Clinical Sports Psychology, 1*(2), 93-120.

Dishman, R. K., & Buckworth, J. (1996). Increasing physical activity: a quantitative analysis. *Medicine and Science in Sports and Exercise, 28*, 706-719.

Dunton, G. F., Intille, S. S., Wolch, J., & Pentz, M. A. (2012). Children's perceptions of physical activity environments captured through ecological momentary assessment: a validation study. *Preventative Medicine: An International Journal Devoted to Practice and Theory, 55*(2), 119-121.

Foreyt, J. P., & Carlos Poston II, W. S. (1998). What is the role of cognitive-behavior therapy in patient management? *Obesity Research, 6*(S1), 18S-22S.

Gammage, K. L., & Klentrou, P. (2012). Predicting osteoporosis prevention behaviors: Health beliefs and knowledge. *American Journal of Health Behavior, 35*(3), 371-382.

Garber, C. E., Allsworth, J. E., Marcus, B. H., Hesser, J., Lapane, K. L. (2008). Correlates of the stages of change for physical activity in a population survey. *American Journal of Public Health, 98*(5), 897-904.

Gaston, A., Cramp, A., & Propavessis, H. (2012). Enhancing self-efficacy and exercise readiness in pregnant women. *Psychology of Sport and Exercise, 13*(5), 550-557.

Golden, S. D., & Earp, J. A. L. (2012). Social ecological approaches to individuals and their contexts: twenty years of Health Education & Behavior health promotion interventions. *Health Education and Behavior, 39*(3), 364-372.

Gonzalez, R. C. S., & Jirovec, M. M. (2001). Elderly Mexican women's perceptions of exercise and conflicting role responsibilities. *International Journal of Nursing Studies, 38*, 45-49.

Greenlund, K. J., Giles, W. H., Keenan, N. L., Croft, J.B., & Mensah, G.A. (2002). Physician advice, patient actions, and health-related quality of life in secondary prevention of stroke through diet and exercise. *Stroke, 33*, 565-571.

Haas, S., & Nigg, C. R. (2009). Construct validation of the stages of change with strenuous, moderate, and mild physical activity and sedentary behaviour among children. *Journal of Science and Medicine in Sport, 12*(5), 586-591.

Hart, E. A., Leary, M. R., & Rejeski, W. J. (1989). The measurement of social physique anxiety. *Journal of Sport & Exercise Psychology, 11*, 94-104.

Hayes, A. M., Laurenceau, J.-P., Feldman, G., Strauss, J.L., Cardaciotto, L. (2007). Change is not always linear: the study of nonlinear and discontinuous patterns of change in psychotherapy. *Clinical Psychology Review, 27*, 715-723.

Husebo, A. M. L., Dyrstad, S. M., Soreide, J. A., & Bru, E. (2013). Predicting exercise adherence in cancer patients and survivors: a systematic review and meta-analysis of motivational and behavioural factors. *Journal of Clinical Nursing, 22*(1-2), 4-21.

Johnson, J. H., Haskvitz, E. M., & Brehm, B. A. (2009). *Applied Sports Medicine for Coaches.* Philadelphia: Wolters-Kluwer.

Johnson, U., & Ivarsson, A. (2011). Psychological predictors of sport injuries among junior soccer players. *Scandinavian Journal of Medicine & Science in Sports, 21*(1), 129-136.

Jones, F., Harris, P., Waller, H., & Coggins, A. (2005). Adherence to an exercise prescription scheme: the role of expectations, self-efficacy, stage of change and psychological well-being. *British Journal of Health Psychology, 10*(3), 359-378.

Karavirta, L., Hakkinen, K., Kauhanen, A., Arija-Blázquez, A., Sillanpää, E., Rinkinen, N., & Häkkinen, A. (2011). Individual responses to combined endurance and strength training in older adults. *Medicine and Science in Sports and Exercise, 43*(3), 484-490.

Kotecki, J. E. (2011). *Physical Activities and Health: Activities and Assessment Manual.* Sudbury, MA: Jones & Bartlett.

Lewthwaite, R., & Wulf, G. (2010). Social-comparative feedback affects motor skill learning. *The Quarterly Journal of Experimental Psychology, 63*(4), 738-749.

Li, K., Seo, D. -C., Torabi, M. R., Peng, C. Y., Kay, N. S., & Kolbe, L. J. (2012). Social-ecological factors of leisure-time physical activity in Black adults. *American Journal of Health Behavior, 36*(6), 797-810.

Livneh, H. (2009). Denial of chronic illness and disability. Part I: theoretical, functional, and dynamic perspectives. *Rehabilitation Counseling Bulletin, 52*(4), 225-236.

Lopez, I. A., Bryant, C. A., & McDermott, R. J. (2008). Influences on physical activity participation among Latinas: an ecological perspective. *American Journal of Health Behavior, 32*(6), 627-639.

Lovallo, D., & Kahneman, D. (2003). Delusions of success: how optimism undermines executives' decisions. *Harvard Business Review, 81*(7), 56-63.

Lucove, J. C., Huston, S. L., & Evenson, K. R. (2007). Workers' perceptions about worksite policies and environments and their association with leisure-time physical activity. *American Journal of Health Promotion, 21*(3), 196-200.

Luszczynska, A., Schwarzer, R., Lippke, S., & Mazurkiewicz, M. (2011). Self-efficacy as a moderator of the planning-behavior relationship in interventions designed to promote physical activity. *Psychology & Health, 26*(2), 151-166.

Lutz, R. S., Stults-Kolehmainen, M. A., & Bartholomew, J. B. (2010). Exercise caution when stressed: stages of change and the stress-exercise participation relationship. *Psychology of Sport and Exercise, 11*(6), 560-567.

Marchant, D., Clough, P., & Cramshaw, M. (2005). Influence of attentional focusing strategies during practice and performance of a motor skill. *Journal of Sports Sciences, 23*(11-12), 1258-1259.

Marcus, B. H., Williams, D. M., Dubbert, P. M., Sallis, J.F., King, A.C., Yancey, A.K., . . . Interdisciplinary Working Group on Quality of Care and Outcomes Research (2006). Physical activity intervention studies: what we know and what we need to know—a scientific statement from the American Heart Association Council on Nutrition, Physical Activity, and Metabolism (Subcommittee on Physical Activity; Council on Cardiovascular Disease in the Young; and the Interdisciplinary Working Group on Quality of Care and Outcomes Research). *Circulation, 114*, 2739-2752.

McLachlan, S., & Hagger, M. S. (2011). The influence of chronically accessible autonomous and controlling motives on physical activity within an extended theory of planned behavior. *Journal of Applied Social Psychology, 41*(2), 445-470.

Morgan, W. P. (2001). Prescription of physical activity: a paradigm shift? *Quest, 53*(3), 366-382.

Muraven, M. (2010). Building self-control strength: practicing self-control leads to improved self-control performance. *Journal of Experimental Social Psychology, 46*(2), 465-468.

Nigg, C. R., Borrelli, B., Maddock, J., & Dishman, R. K. (2008). A theory of physical activity maintenance. *Journal of Applied Psychology, 57*(4), 544-560.

O'Connor, J., Alfrey, L., & Payne, P. (2012). Beyond games and sports: a socio-ecological approach to physical education. *Sport, Education and Society, 17*(3), 365-380.

Ogden, J., & Hills, L. (2008). Understanding sustained behavior change: the role of life crises and the process of reinvention. *Health (London), 12*(4), 419-437.

Papandonatos, G. D., Williams, D. M., Jennings, E. G., Napolitano, M. A., Bock, B. C., Dunsiger, S., & Marcus, B. H. (2012). Mediators of physical activity behavior change: findings from a 12-month randomized controlled trial. *Health Psychology, 31*(4), 512-520.

Parschau, L., Richert, J., Koring, M., Ernsting, A., Lippke, S., & Schwarzer, R. (2012). Changes in social-cognitive variables are associated with stage transitions in physical activity. *Health Education Research, 27*(1), 129-140.

Perry, C. K., Garside, H., Morones, S., & Hayman, L. L. (2012). Physical activity interventions for adolescents: an ecological model. *Journal of Primary Prevention, 33*, 111-135.

Pfeffer, I., & Alfermann, D. (2008). Initiation of physical exercise: an intervention study based on the transtheoretical model. *International Journal of Sports Psychology, 39*(1), 41-58.

Plotnikoff, R. C., Lippke, S., Johnson, S. T., & Courneya, K. S. (2010). Physical activity and stages of change: a longitudinal test in types 1 and 2 diabetes samples. *Annals of Behavioral Medicine, 40*(2), 138-149.

Pretty, J., Peacock, J., Sellens, M., & Griffin, M. (2005). The mental and physical health outcomes of green exercise. *International Journal of Environmental Health Research, 15* (5), 319-337.

Prochaska, J. O., & Marcus, B. H. (1994). The transtheoretical model: applications to exercise. In: Dishman, R. K. (ed.). *Advances in Exercise Adherence*. Champaign, IL: Human Kinetics.

Reed, G. R. (1999). Adherence to exercise and the transtheoretical model of behavior change. In: Bull, S. J. (ed.). *Adherence Issues in Sport and Exercise*. Chichester, West Sussex: John Wiley & Sons.

Renshaw, I., Chow, J. Y., Davids, K., & Hammond, J. (2010). A constraints-led perspective to understanding skill acquisition and game play: a basis for integration of motor learning theory and physical education praxis? *Physical Education and Sport Pedagogy, 15*(2), 117-137.

Resnicow, K., & Page, S. E. (2008). Embracing chaos and complexity: a quantum change for public health. *American Journal of Public Health, 98*(8), 1382-1389.

Rink, J. E. (2004). It's okay to be a beginner: teach a motor skill, and the skill may be learned. *Journal of Physical Education, Recreation, and Dance, 75*(6), 31-35.

Rogers, T. J., & Landers, D. M. (2005). Mediating effects of peripheral vision in the life event stress/athletic injury relationship. *Journal of Sport & Exercise Psychology, 27*(3), 271-288.

Rothman, A. J., Baldwin A., & Hertel, A. (2004). Self-regulation and behavior change: Disentangling behavioral initiation and behavioral maintenance. In: Vohs, K. D., & Baumeister, R. F. (eds.). *Handbook of Self-regulation*, 130-148. New York: Guilford.

Rothman, A. J., Bartels, R. D., Wlaschin, J., & Salovey, P. (2006). The strategic use of gain- and loss-framed messages to promote healthy behavior: how theory can inform practice. *Journal of Communication, 56*(S1), S202-S220.

Sears, S. R., & Stanton, A. L. (2001). Expectancy-value constructs and expectancy violation as predictors of exercise adherence in previously sedentary women. *Health Psychology, 20*(5), 326-333.

Schmeichel, B. J., & Vohs, K. (2009). Self-affirmation and self-control: affirming core values counteracts ego depletion. *Journal of Personality and Social Psychology, 96*(4), 770-782.

Smith, L. H., & Holm, L. (2011). Obesity in a life-course perspective: an exploration of lay explanations of weight gain. *Scandinavian Journal of Public Health, 39*, 396-402.

Speer, E. M., Reddy, S., Lommel, T. S., Fischer, J. G., Heather, S., Park, S., & Johnson, M. A. (2008). Diabetes self-management behaviors and A1c improved following a community-based intervention in older adults in Georgia Senior Centers. *Journal of Nutrition for the Elderly, 27*(1-2), 179-200.

Tamers, S. L., Beresford, S. A. A., Cheadle, A. D., Zheng, Y., Bishop, S. K., & Thompson, B. (2011). The association between worksite social support, diet, physical activity, and body mass index. *Preventive Medicine, 53*, 53-56.

Thaler, R. H., & Sunstein, C. R. (2008). *Nudge: Improving Decisions About Health, Wealth, and Happiness*. New York: Penguin.

Tharrett, S. J., & Peterson, J. A., eds. (2012). *ACSM's Health/Fitness Facility Standards and Guidelines*. Champaign, IL: Human Kinetics.

Timmons, J. A. (2011). Variability in training-induced skeletal muscle adaptation. *Journal of Applied Physiology, 110*(3), 846-853.

Trottier, K., Polivy, J., & Herman, C. P. (2009). Effects of resolving to change one's own behavior: expectations vs. experience. *Behavior Therapy, 40*(2), 164-170.

Vohs, K. D., Baumeister, R. F., Schmeichel, B. J., Twenge, J. M., Nelson, N. M., & Tice, D. M. (2008). Making choices impairs subsequent self-control: a limited-resource account of decision making, self-regulation, and active initiative. *Journal of Personality and Social Psychology, 94*(5), 883-898.

Webb, T. L., & Sheeran, P. (2006). Does changing behavioral intentions engender behavior change? A meta-analysis of the experimental evidence. *Psychological Bulletin, 132*(2), 249-268.

White, K. M., Smith, J. R., Terru, D. J., Greenslade, J. H., & McKimmie, B. M. (2009). Social influence in the theory of planned behavior: the role of descriptive, injunctive, and in-group norms. *British Journal of Social Psychology, 48*(1), 135-158.

Williams, D. M., Anderson, E. S., & Winett, R. A. (2005). A review of the outcome expectancy construct in physical activity research. *Annals of Behavioral Medicine, 29*(1), 70-79.

Woolf, S. H., Dekker, M. M., Byrne, F. R., & Miller, W. D. (2011). Citizen-centered health promotion: building collaborations to facilitate healthy living. *American Journal of Preventive Medicine, 40*(1 Suppl 1), S38-S47.

Zhang, R., Solmon, M. A., Gao, A., & Kosma, M. (2012). Promoting school students' physical activity: a social ecological perspective. *Journal of Applied Sport Psychology, 24*(1), 92-105.

CHAPTER OUTLINE

LEARNING OBJECTIVES

After reading this chapter, you will be able to:

1. Understand your scope of practice in terms of giving nutrition advice to clients and deciding when to refer clients to licensed nutrition professionals or health-care providers.

2. Describe several health concerns that may prompt clients to seek advice on changing eating behaviors.

3. Discuss the six basic nutrient groups and common health concerns related to them.

4. Educate clients about public-health dietary guidelines and where to find sound nutrition information.

5. Answer clients' questions about common eating behavior issues, encouraging a positive, mindful attitude toward food and eating.

6. Analyze the many factors influencing a client's eating behaviors, using an ecological perspective.

7. Apply the Health Belief Model and Theory of Planned Behavior with clients in the early stages of change to help them shift decisional balance toward a decision to change.

8. Target behavior-change interventions to a client's stage of change for specific eating behaviors.

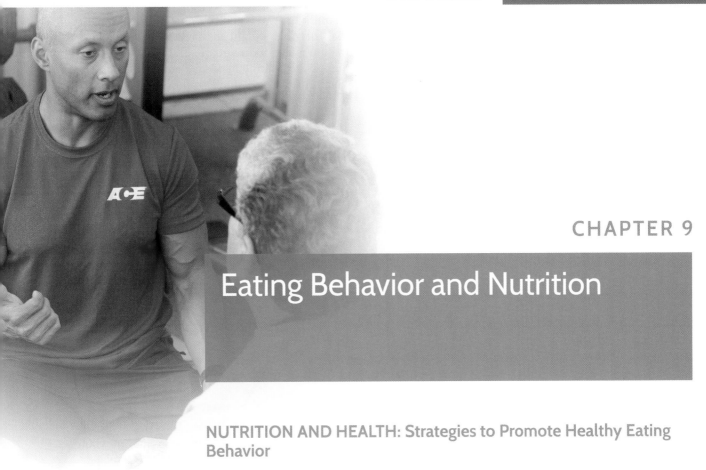

Eating Behavior and Nutrition

NUTRITION AND HEALTH: Strategies to Promote Healthy Eating Behavior

Jackson has recently begun a new job at a health and wellness retreat center. Clients typically stay at the center for a week, although some come only for a weekend; others stay the whole month. The center offers comprehensive spa services, fitness assessments, a variety of physical activity and stress-management options, personalized nutrition counseling with the staff dietitian, and evening lectures by well-known speakers who are informative and inspirational. The food served at the center is delicious and made from fresh, often-local ingredients. Jackson has been hired to teach and lead outdoor activities, including kayaking and hiking in the summer and cross-country skiing and snowshoeing in the winter months. He also conducts orientation sessions for the climbing wall and helps with fitness testing.

Jackson's job is not only to teach these outdoor activities but also to make his sessions fun, uplifting, and compelling. Jackson enjoyed the new instructor orientation program and agrees with the center's philosophy on the importance of a healthy lifestyle. The only area in which he feels he needs more preparation is modeling healthy eating behaviors and talking intelligently about food. After a few weeks on the job, he sees that the clients seem to be light years ahead of him in nutrition knowledge, and they bring up nutrition questions and issues to which he can't respond. He is getting tired of saying, "Let me check on that," and "What do you think?" While he enjoys most of the clients, he does wonder if some of them are crazy when they talk about fasting, eating only raw foods, or trying various "cleanses." Jackson decides to learn more about nutrition and health so that he can discuss food and nutrition issues more intelligently with his clients. ■

Nutrition refers to the process of nourishing the body with food. The science of nutrition studies everything related to this process, including how people decide what to eat; the biochemistry of consuming, digesting, absorbing, and metabolizing food substances; and the relationship between eating behavior and health. People who study nutrition are sometimes also concerned with systems of food production, distribution, and availability; the manufacture of food products; or the special nutritional needs of people with health problems.

People seek nutrition advice and advice on changing eating behaviors from health and fitness professionals for many reasons. Some clients' doctors have asked them to modify their eating habits for reasons related to health. They may have received a diagnosis of hypertension, type 2 diabetes, heart disease, or other health problems that can improve with better eating habits. Other clients want to have more energy throughout the day and come to health and fitness professionals for advice on how to structure meals in ways that improve mood and energy level. Many clients seek health and nutrition advice because they want to lose weight or improve appearance.

Weight loss is one of the most-common reasons that people say they are changing their eating habits, and Chapter 10 is devoted to working with clients whose goals involve weight management. The focus of this chapter is nutrition and health since clients attempt to change their eating habits for many reasons other than weight loss (Box 9-1)

This chapter provides information about nutrition and eating behaviors that will help health and fitness professionals give appropriate, supportive guidance to clients seeking to modify their eating habits in healthy ways. The first section in this chapter presents general guidelines regarding the scope of practice for most health and fitness professionals in terms of giving dietary advice, spelling out what types of advice may be given and to whom. The second section provides a brief overview of nutrition and health and summarizes basic healthy eating guidelines. The next section addresses common nutrition issues and questions that arise for health and fitness professionals in their work with clients. The last section focuses more closely on changing eating behaviors, applying the behavior-change models and information presented in Chapters 4 and 5.

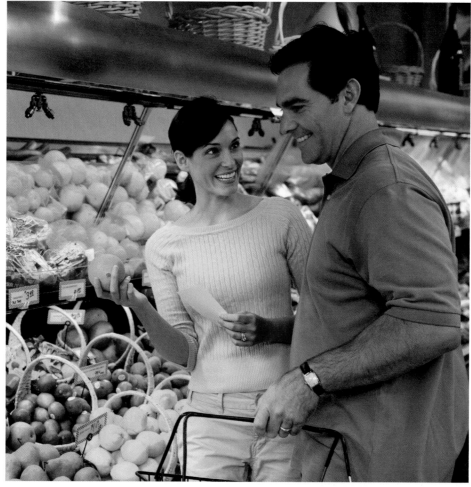

© Thinkstock

Box 9-1. Issues That May Motivate Eating Behavior Change

People think about changing their eating behavior for many reasons. Health and fitness professionals may work with clients who are trying to change their eating habits for the reasons listed below. These clients should be referred to a dietitian for meal-planning advice in all such situations. Health and fitness professionals can reinforce the dietitian's advice and support clients in their eating behavior-change work.

- Food allergies or intolerances
- Type 1 or type 2 diabetes
- Pregnancy
- Pregnancy-related problems, such as gestational diabetes
- Heart disease or artery disease
- Digestive system problems, such as irritable bowel syndrome, ulcers, chronic constipation
- Osteoporosis and/or sarcopenia—clients wanting to build muscle and bone and slow the age-related loss of both
- Cancer
- Obesity
- Weight loss
- Weight gain

NUTRITION ADVICE

Many people today worry about food and eating, and they approach health and fitness professionals with many questions. Which foods are good to eat and which foods should one avoid? Is sugar bad for you? How about meat? People are concerned about fats, carbohydrates, and proteins. What are the best sources of these nutrients? How much of each should be consumed and when? Clients are worried about additives, pesticides, agricultural practices, dietary supplements, and obesity. Parents want information on feeding their children, shopping and preparing meals on a budget, and eating on the run. Many clients have read a great deal about food and thought extensively about food choices. Many empathize with author and journalist Michael Pollan, who describes the difficulty of eating well in the United States when feeling overwhelmed with food products and nutrition information, but with few cultural guidelines and supports for making good choices (Pollan, 2009). Should one choose local food to conserve resources (Kingsolver, 2007) or organic food from across the ocean that might provide less cancer risk to eaters and farmers? Should one purchase the cheapest product or make an effort to look for food produced by sustainable farming practices? Nutrition information is everywhere, and much of it is alarming and contradictory. It is natural for clients to turn to health and fitness professionals for answers to their questions about food, nutrition, and health.

Scope of Practice

Many health and fitness professionals have quite a bit of training in nutrition and are comfortable discussing the general nutrition questions asked by clients. Other professionals are less informed regarding nutrition and are uncomfortable discussing eating habits or food. Because nutrition is such a common and significant topic that arises in work with clients, it is important for all health and fitness professionals to understand basic nutrition principles and general dietary guidelines. It is also important for health and fitness professionals to stay within their scope of practice when giving nutrition advice and discussing eating behaviors with clients. Several guidelines can help health and fitness professionals as they consider their scope of practice with regard to giving nutrition advice.

Consult Employer and Certifying Organizations

Health and fitness professionals' scope of practice, which describes the activities that they are allowed to do in their profession, is proscribed by several different institutions, including professionals' employers and their licensing and/or certification organizations.

- **Employer:** Employers may set limits on how much nutrition advice health and fitness professionals can give. Professionals should understand these policies and get answers to their questions. Some employers may restrict certain practices, even though the professional may feel qualified to provide these services. Sometimes this is because of state regulations. Individual states govern the licensure of nutrition professionals. Some states, such as Ohio and Florida, mandate that only licensed professionals, such as registered dietitians (R.D.s), may provide nutrition advice for monetary gain. Employers may be worried about a variety of liability issues if employees give nutrition information.
- **Certification and licensure organizations:** Most of these also provide guidance regarding scope of practice. Many fitness certification organizations, such as the American Council on Exercise, the American College of Sports Medicine, and the National Strength and Conditioning Association, include some basic sports nutrition information in many of their certification programs, and they allow people with certain certifications to provide basic nutrition information to clients. Athletic trainers are qualified to discuss many dietary issues with their patients. Health and fitness professionals should consult their organizations for more information.
- **Academic institutions and sport-governing bodies:** People who teach physical education classes or coach a sport are similarly limited in

how much nutrition information they may give their athletes. For example, most coaches may encourage athletes to drink plenty of fluids and replenish fuel stores with carbohydrates and proteins following workouts. However, coaches should not provide specialized diet plans to individual athletes with medical conditions such as diabetes or hypertension, for example. Teachers and coaches should check with their departments and sport-governing bodies for more information.

Stick to Scientifically Sound Advice

Health and fitness professionals should deliver mainstream, scientifically endorsed advice. In general, health and fitness professionals may give their clients nutrition recommendations that are backed by established public-health organizations, particularly their national government. In the United States, for example, health and fitness professionals may promote the basic nutrition information posted by the Food and Nutrition Information Center, U.S. Department of Agriculture (USDA) (http://fnic.nal.usda.gov). A wide variety of nutrition information is available on this website, and health and fitness professionals may endorse this information for healthy clients. For example, they can urge clients to consume less salt and more fruits and vegetables. Health Canada has a helpful website full of nutrition information (www.hc-sc.gc.ca/fn-an/food-guide-aliment/index-eng.php). Organizations such as the American Council on Exercise (Muth, 2009) and the American College of Sports Medicine (Rodriguez, Di Marco, & Langley, 2009) have excellent nutrition information available in their publications and on their websites.

Educate Clients About Healthy Eating

Health and fitness professionals may educate clients about healthy eating in many ways, following the guidelines described above. For example, it is fine for professionals to provide cooking demonstrations, teach clients how to read food labels, give grocery store tours, or provide guidelines for eating in local restaurants (Fig. 9-1). They may discuss how nutrient needs vary with life stage and provide statistics regarding how eating behaviors and nutrition are related to chronic illness (Muth, 2009).

MOTIVATING CHANGE: Model a Positive Attitude
One of the most-important things that health and fitness professionals can do is to model positive attitudes toward eating. This may be difficult for many professionals, especially for those who struggle with eating and food, which is pretty common in the health and fitness fields. It is important for health and fitness professionals to make peace with food, to see food as fuel and as a friend, and to model these attitudes for clients.

Nutrition discussions can easily turn into "don't eat this," along with complicated recommendations that become negative, confusing, and discouraging. Rather than focusing only on what to avoid, keep recommendations upbeat and positive (eat more vegetables). Encourage clients to eat well for positive outcomes, that is, to be healthier now and in the future and to feel more energetic. Health and fitness professionals who are passionate about healthy lifestyles for positive reasons can be motivational and inspirational.

Support Clients Following Personal Dietary Recommendations

Health and fitness professionals may find themselves working with clients who have consulted their healthcare providers and/or dietitians for individualized dietary recommendations. Professionals can help these clients as they work to implement the recommendations. For example, a client may have received recommendations for a diet to reduce hypertension. Typically, the client's dietitian will have designed meal plans that increase fruits, vegetables, and low-fat dairy products and reduce foods high in salt. At this point, the client should know what to do; the health and fitness professional can support the client's behavior-change program efforts. The professional can help the client monitor eating habits, such as recording the number of servings of vegetables each day. The health and fitness professional does not prescribe a particular diet but can assist clients in implementing specific dietary recommendations from an R.D.

Avoid Interventions That Could Be Problematic

Health and fitness professionals should never diagnose health problems or prescribe treatments, including dietary supplements. They should not design or prescribe individual nutrition plans (Sass, Eickhoff-Shemeck, Manore, & Kruskall, 2007), nor act as psychotherapists in situations where clients have problems with food.

Health and fitness professionals should be ready to refer clients to a licensed nutritionist, dietitian, or other health-care provider if clients:

• Show symptoms of disordered eating or exercise behavior

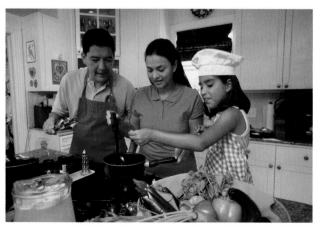
Figure 9-1. **Cooking demonstration.** © Thinkstock

Chapter 9: Eating Behavior and Nutrition

297

- Have a lot of questions about diet that go beyond "general information"
- Have a medical condition, such as diabetes, heart disease, or cancer
- Want to follow a very-restrictive diet, such as a low-carbohydrate diet
- Want specific daily meal plans

The Dietitian's Role

Registered dietitians are licensed professionals who specialize in nutrition and health. In the United States, R.D.s have completed a baccalaureate degree program approved by their licensing organization, the Academy of Nutrition and Dietetics (formerly the American Dietetic Association). In order to earn a license, R.D.s also complete a supervised internship of at least 900 hours and pass a licensing exam. In order to maintain their license, they participate regularly in continuing education programs. In Canada, licensure procedures are similar and are overseen by the Dietitians of Canada.

Dietitians work in a wide variety of settings, from hospital food services to worksite wellness programs. People diagnosed with health problems who could benefit from advice on improving eating behaviors are often referred to a dietitian; some health insurance plans help to cover the cost of these consultations. Dietitians meet with patients, sometimes including in the meeting the patient's family members who participate in food shopping and preparation. They educate patients about target eating behaviors and give specific recommendations on what to eat at each meal. They calculate patients' nutrient requirements and structure eating plans to meet those needs. Good dietitians will listen carefully to patients' descriptions of their current eating habits and structure meal plans in ways that accommodate their cultural practices and food preferences.

Designing eating plans is just one step in the behavior-change process. Just as exercise recommendations are useless if not followed, dietary recommendations similarly yield no results unless people can incorporate them into their daily lives. Health and fitness professionals may work with clients who have seen a dietitian a few times and started improving their eating habits. If clients still have questions about their eating plans, they should ask their dietitians. If they are clear about dietary recommendations, they can work with various health and fitness professionals to use the best behavior-change strategies to shape lifelong, sustainable eating habits that will maximize the benefits of a healthy lifestyle. Many dietitians use motivational interviewing and similar behavior counseling methods to help motivate their patients to improve eating behaviors. Dietitians often join forces with a health-care team that includes other health and fitness professionals to offer clients comprehensive behavior-change support.

■ *Jackson asks Alana, the staff dietitian, if she can give him a reading list to get him up to speed with the nutrition philosophy of the retreat center and feel more secure discussing nutrition issues with clients. Alana gives Jackson a list of good websites to check out and a few articles to read, and she offers to meet with him to answer any questions. Jackson ploughs through the material, making a list of questions as he goes. Some of the information is pretty complicated, but most of it makes good sense. Jackson doesn't see anything in the readings about fasting or cleanses. He makes an appointment to talk to Alana about some of the topics clients ask about that are not addressed in the readings.*

Alana discusses the retreat center's nutrition philosophy with Jackson and clarifies her role as primary dietary consultant. She also explains to Jackson what he should be able to answer or discuss and when he should refer clients to make an appointment with her. Alana also explains that the retreat center does offer fasting and cleansing programs but that frankly, these can promote disordered eating behaviors in vulnerable clients. "I never say that to the clients, of course," Alana explains. "But just send them to me if they want to talk about these. I try to be sure that these programs are done safely and for the right reasons." ■

NUTRITION AND HEALTH

Nutrition influences people's health and wellness on many levels. On a daily basis, eating poorly, skipping meals, or overeating can contribute to suboptimal energy levels and fatigue. Over weeks, months, and years, food choices and eating behavior play an important role in the prevention or development of many chronic health problems. For example, hypertension, diabetes, artery disease, osteoporosis, and obesity all have strong links to dietary practices. So do disorders of the gastrointestinal (GI) tract, such as colon cancer and irritable bowel syndrome. Nutrition is important for peak performance in athletics and for recovery from exercise (Rodriguez, Di Marco, & Langley, 2009).

Nutrition Basics

Health and fitness professionals need to understand some basic nutrition vocabulary and concepts in order to discuss healthy eating behavior with their clients and to help clients work with dietary recommendations they have received from their dietitians or health-care providers. Knowledge of the basic nutrient groups and general healthy eating guidelines allow health and fitness professionals to discuss eating behavior change in a productive fashion with clients. However, professionals who work frequently with clients on eating behavior change would benefit from a course or further training in nutrition and health.

Food provides the nutrients needed by the body for all life processes. Nutrients are the substances in food that provide raw material for growth and maintenance of the body and the chemical bonds that supply the energy captured and used by the cells for fuel. Nutrients are classified into six categories based on their chemical composition: carbohydrates, proteins, fats, vitamins, minerals, and water. The following sections will briefly describe these six nutrient groups and highlight health applications involving them.

Carbohydrates: Energy and Fiber

Three classes of nutrients provide energy. The most-plentiful sources of energy for most people are carbohydrates. Carbohydrates are a large group of organic molecules that include starches, sugars, cellulose, and other types of fibers. Plants make carbohydrates from carbon dioxide and water, using energy from the sun. Sugars, or simple carbohydrates, are relatively small molecules of carbohydrate found naturally in fruits and vegetables as well as milk. They are especially concentrated in sweeteners such as table sugar (usually made from sugar beets or sugar cane), honey, molasses, and maple syrup. Corn syrup is a sweetener made from the sugar in corn. Many food products contain added sweeteners.

Simple carbohydrates contain two small sugar units and are called disaccharides (Fig. 9-2). Each disaccharide is comprised of two monosaccharides. The molecules glucose and fructose are examples of monosaccharides. Table sugar, for example, is comprised mainly of the disaccharide sucrose, which consists of one glucose molecule bonded with one fructose molecule. During digestion, simple sugars are broken down into monosaccharides that are transported into the bloodstream. The liver converts fructose and other monosaccharides into glucose or other molecules, including large chains of glucose called glycogen. Monosaccharides can also be converted into fats.

Complex carbohydrates are larger molecules of carbohydrate and include starches and some types of dietary fibers. Starches are composed of over two glucose units, and can be hundreds of glucose units strung together in various formations (Fig. 9-3). Foods high in starch include grains and grain products; root vegetables such as potatoes, carrots, beets, and cassava; and vegetables that are the seeds of plants, such as corn, peas, and beans are high in starch. During digestion, starches are broken down into glucose units.

Glycogen is a form of starch manufactured by animals. Humans manufacture and store glycogen primarily

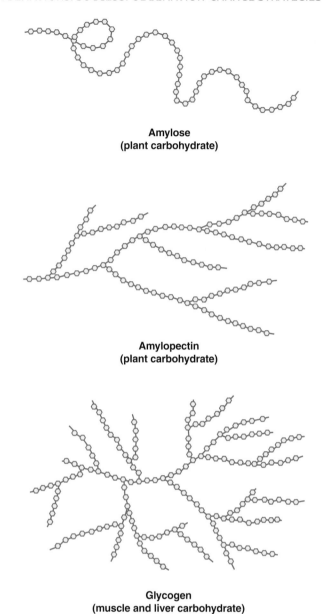

Amylose
(plant carbohydrate)

Amylopectin
(plant carbohydrate)

Glycogen
(muscle and liver carbohydrate)

Figure 9-3. Basic structure of complex carbohydrates.

in the liver and in skeletal muscles. Glycogen serves as a source of glucose when the body needs fuel. Liver glycogen is converted to glucose and released into the bloodstream when blood glucose levels fall too low. Skeletal muscles use glucose liberated from glycogen to fuel muscle contraction. Many athletes are careful to consume adequate amounts of carbohydrate to maximize glycogen stores so that they have adequate energy for training and performance. Athletes preparing for important endurance events may even consume extra-high amounts of carbohydrate for a few days prior to an event to maximize glycogen stores. (Glycogen stores will also be more likely to be at maximal levels if athletes taper training—reduce training volume—for several days before their event.)

Dietary fiber refers to structures that are not broken down by the digestive system. Dietary fiber comes primarily from plants. Some types of dietary fiber, such as cellulose, are composed of carbohydrates. Humans lack

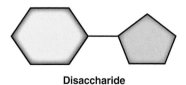

Disaccharide
Figure 9-2. Basic structure of simple carbohydrates.

the necessary digestive enzymes for breaking down these structures, so they pass through the digestive system, adding bulk to the stools. Adequate intake of dietary fiber contributes to good health. There are many kinds of dietary fiber. Dietary fibers are classified as water soluble and water insoluble, and both groups have beneficial effects on health (Anderson et al., 2009). Most dietary guidelines encourage people to consume adequate amounts of vegetables, fruits, legumes, and whole grains to promote a healthy intake of dietary fiber.

All types of fiber increase food volume without adding a significant number of calories. High-fiber meals generally provide feelings of satiety with fewer calories than low-fiber meals. A high-fiber diet may promote colon health by providing an environment inside the GI tract that favors the growth of beneficial bacteria, the probiotics (Fuller & Gibson, 2008).

Water-soluble fiber attracts water and forms a gel-like mix in the digestive system. This mixture slows stomach emptying, helping eaters feel full longer. Delayed stomach emptying also means that glucose is absorbed from the digestive mass more slowly, thus preventing a rapid rise in blood glucose, which can lead to high blood insulin levels. Water-soluble fiber tends to bind bile acids in the small intestine. Bile acids are high in cholesterol. When the bile acids are bound to the fibrous mixture, their cholesterol is not available for reabsorption; thus, soluble fiber is thought to be beneficial for people trying to reduce blood cholesterol levels (Anderson et al., 2009).

Water-insoluble fiber provides bulk to the feces and speeds their passage through the GI tract. Water-insoluble fiber reduces risk of constipation. Like most dietary components, too much soluble or insoluble fiber can be problematic, causing diarrhea and intestinal discomfort. People trying to increase their fiber intake are advised to do so gradually so that their bodies have time to adjust to the new levels.

Blood Sugar Regulation and Diabetes

The term blood sugar refers to blood glucose levels. The body regulates blood glucose levels very carefully, since blood glucose is an important source of energy, especially for the central nervous system (CNS) (Fig. 9-4). When blood glucose levels fall too low or rise too high, people experience symptoms of CNS dysfunction: dizziness, disorientation, confusion, unconsciousness, and, in extreme cases, even death. Blood glucose levels are controlled by two important hormones produced by the pancreas. The pancreas releases insulin when blood glucose levels get too high. Insulin binds with receptors on cell membranes that encourage cells to take up glucose from the blood, thus reducing blood glucose levels. The cells either use the glucose for energy, if energy is needed, or store it for future use. Liver and muscle cells may convert glucose to glycogen. If glycogen stores are full, then the glucose may be converted to triglycerides and stored as fat. Fat is stored in adipose tissue but can also be stored in muscles and in the liver. Fatty liver is a harmful condition that can result when energy intake exceeds energy needs over time. (Fatty liver can also develop from excessive alcohol intake.)

If blood glucose levels fall too low, the pancreas releases the hormone glucagon. Glucagon signals the liver to break down glycogen and release glucose into the bloodstream. As the liver releases glucose into the blood, blood glucose rises, meeting the body's immediate energy needs. The liver can also produce glucose from other precursors such as amino acids.

Knowledge of blood glucose regulation helps health and fitness professionals understand the difficulties presented by conditions that disrupt this process. In people with type 1 diabetes mellitus, the pancreas loses the ability to produce insulin due to the destruction of insulin-producing cells, the beta cells in specialized tissue in the pancreas called the islets of Langerhans. (Alpha cells in the islets of Langerhans produce glucagon.) Without insulin, blood glucose levels rise

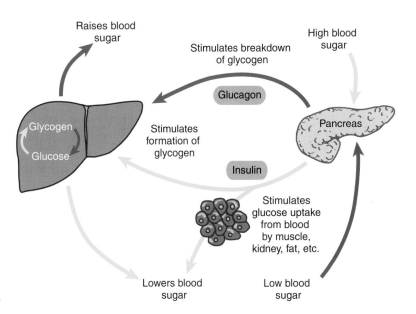

Figure 9-4. **Blood glucose regulation.**

after food consumption, yet the glucose is unable to enter the cells. People with type 1 diabetes are able to give themselves insulin. They must time its administration to achieve good control of blood sugar levels. People with type 1 diabetes develop a schedule of insulin administration, meals, and physical activity that tries to mimic nature's intended insulin response, making sure that insulin is available when nutrients are being absorbed from meals and that blood sugar does not dip too low during physical activity. Health and fitness professionals who work with clients who have type 1 diabetes should discuss clients' diabetes-management plans, and receive directions on how they should help if clients appear to be having a blood sugar emergency. Clients whose blood sugar is poorly controlled will need medical advice if they are changing physical activity level.

People with type 2 diabetes mellitus usually produce adequate insulin (until later stages of the illness), but the insulin receptors on the cell membranes do not respond well to insulin. People with this condition are said to be insulin resistant, meaning that their insulin receptors "resist" the action of insulin. Although insulin is present in adequate concentrations in the blood, blood glucose remains high because the cell membrane receptors for insulin are not responding and allowing the cells to take up glucose from the blood (Fig. 9-5). As discussed in Chapter 1, insulin resistance and type 2 diabetes are components of the metabolic syndrome, usually associated with visceral obesity and low levels of physical activity.

Glycemic Index and Glycemic Load

The digestive system breaks down carbohydrates in foods and transports the resulting monosaccharides into the bloodstream. After a meal, blood sugar rises. The speed of the rise depends on many factors, including the amount of simple carbohydrates versus complex carbohydrates in the food and the composition of other foods consumed at the same time as the carbohydrate food. Dietary fiber, especially water-soluble fiber, and fats slow down the digestion and absorption of carbohydrates. Food stays in the stomach longer, and digestion of carbohydrates occurs more slowly.

The glycemic index of a food is a measure of how quickly the carbohydrate in that food is digested and absorbed into the bloodstream as glucose. Specifically, glycemic index is a measure of how quickly glucose appears in the blood after a standard amount (such as 50 or 100 grams) of carbohydrate from a given food is

Insulin Resistant Cell

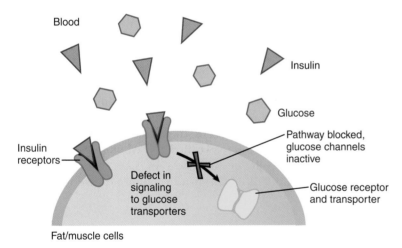

Normal Cell

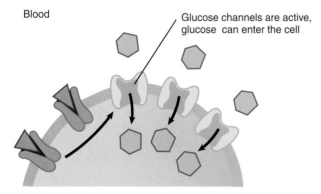

Figure 9-5. Insulin resistance.

consumed, relative to the same amount of a standard such as white sugar. This means that GI is simply a relative value rather than a precise number. In general, a GI of 55 or less is considered low; 56-69 medium; 70 or more high. Foods like sugar, white bread, and instant white rice have a high glycemic index. The sugars and starches in those foods are digested quickly, since they contain very little or no fat or fiber. Foods such as whole-grain breads, oatmeal, and berries have a lower glycemic index, since these foods are higher in fiber.

Some researchers suggest that the glycemic index of a particular food is not as important as a variable called glycemic load, which represents the glycemic index multiplied by the grams of carbohydrate in the food, divided by 100 (Bao, Atkinson, Petocz, Willett, & Brand-Miller, 2011). So while GI is measured for a standard amount of carbohydrate, GL reflects the typical serving size of foods, and better represents what people actually eat. For example, cooked beets have a relatively high glycemic index (64) but a fairly small amount of carbohydrate per serving, and thus, a low GL (4). Macaroni has lower glycemic index (45) but quite a bit of carbohydrate per serving, and thus a high GL (22). (In general, a GL of 10 and under is considered low; 11-19, medium; and 20 or greater high.) Studies suggest that people consuming a relatively high-glycemic-load diet throughout their lives tend to have higher rates of chronic disease, especially heart disease (Baer et al., 2011; Barclay et al., 2008). A high glycemic load is correlated with higher blood glucose levels after meals, which appear to be related to higher risk of disease progression, perhaps through higher levels of insulin and obesity.

Athletes sometimes speak of low- and high-glycemic-index foods as slow and fast carbohydrates. Tables listing food's glycemic index can be found at www.glycemicindex.com. Applications include the following:

- Athletes (and all people) who experience hypoglycemia (low blood sugar) need a snack that can bring blood sugar quickly up to normal. High-glycemic-index foods are best in this situation: sports drinks, fruit juice, or dried fruit, for example.
- People with diabetes may strive to minimize spikes in blood glucose levels. Consuming carbohydrate foods with protein, fat, and fiber can slow carbohydrate absorption.
- Athletes participating in multiple contests or practices during the day need to replenish muscle glycogen stores quickly between sessions. High-glycemic-index foods are helpful in this situation.
- Athletes often want to avoid a rapid rise in blood sugar immediately before exercise, since that can be followed by a release of insulin and then a rapid drop in blood sugar, causing fatigue. Low-glycemic foods and meals are often preferred for pre-event meals: pasta dishes, smoothies (yogurt-fruit drinks), or bananas, for example (Johnson, Haskvitz, & Brehm, 2009).

Protein

Proteins are composed of smaller units called amino acids. The body uses amino acids to build its own proteins. Protein is found throughout the body, in structures such as muscle and bone; the immune cells that fight infection; the red blood cells that carry oxygen to all parts of the body; neurochemicals and hormones such as serotonin and epinephrine; and the enzymes that regulate biochemical processes such as digestion and energy production. The body can also break down some amino acids to produce energy, especially during long or heavy bouts of physical activity or when glycogen stores are depleted.

Experts often liken amino acids to letters and proteins to words spelled with those letters. To spell a given word, one must have all letters available. The human body needs about 20 different amino acids to make all proteins required for life. If humans have an adequate intake of protein in general, they can make 11 of these in sufficient quantities. The other nine must be obtained from the diet on a daily basis. Amino acids that people must obtain from the diet are called essential amino acids. Amino acids that the body can manufacture are called nonessential amino acids. (Of course, these amino acids are still "essential" to life, just not an essential part of the diet.)

The human body can store only a limited quantity of amino acids, which is why one must consume foods containing proteins every day. Foods that contain all nine essential amino acids are called complete proteins. These foods include eggs, dairy products, animal flesh (chicken, fish, beef, etc.), animal organs (liver, kidneys, etc.), soybeans, and a few other plant foods. Animal foods more closely match the amino acid profile needed by humans, which is logical since humans are animals, so their composition is similar. However, it is not difficult to consume adequate amino acids if one eats a variety of plant sources, as the amino acids that are generally low in grains, for example, are more plentiful in legumes, and vice versa. Combining incomplete proteins (proteins lacking one or more essential amino acids) usually results in an adequate intake of protein (Fig. 9-6). The U.S. Department of Agriculture recommends 0.8 grams of protein per kilogram of body weight (or 0.36 g/lb). People who are significantly overweight (in the form of excess body fat) should base their protein intake calculations on a weight that would be healthier for them.

Conditions Requiring Extra Dietary Protein

Several conditions call for extra protein in the diet. Whenever more tissue is being built, more protein is required. Pregnancy, bodybuilding, strength training, and adolescent growth spurts place high demands for amino acids on the body. Lactating mothers may be producing a quart or more of milk per day and thus need a higher-than-normal protein intake. People, especially athletes, restricting calories force the body to consume protein for fuel, depleting valuable amino

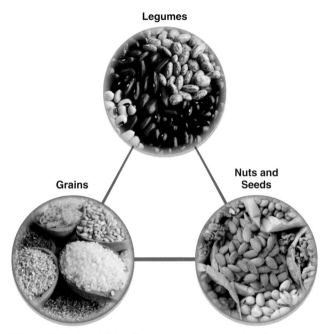

Figure 9-6. Combining incomplete protein foods.
Photograph © Thinkstock

acid stores, and must consume more protein to make up for the loss of other food groups in the diet. (These athletes should also add some carbohydrate to their diet.) Endurance athletes usually burn a certain amount of protein for fuel and need higher protein intakes than sedentary people. Vegetarian athletes, especially vegans (consuming no animal products), will require somewhat higher protein intakes than athletes who are omnivores (eating all kinds of foods of both plant and animal sources), since much of their protein will be incomplete (Craig, Mangels, & American Dietetic Association, 2009). Any combination of the above (such as vegan, pregnant, teenage, dieting, endurance athletes) will need more dietary protein, up to 2 g/kg body weight (Colombani & Mettler, 2011).

Fats and Cholesterol

Clients often have many questions about fat and cholesterol. Fats and cholesterol play important roles in the body's biochemical processes. They are also found in the diet, but dietary intake does not necessarily correlate directly with the levels of these chemicals in the body or with their behavior in the body. To make matters more complex, there are many types of fat in the diet. Some appear to be healthy, whereas others may exert negative effects on health, at least when intake or body fat reaches a certain level.

Dietary fat provides a concentrated source of energy, with 9 kilocalories (kcal)/gram, compared with 4 kcals/g for carbohydrates and proteins. (Alcohol has 7 kcal/g.) This is usually why people trying to limit calories generally attempt to limit fat intake. Some fat in the diet is important, however. Fat gives food flavor and slows gastric emptying and the rise of blood sugar following a meal. Some types of fatty acids (a component of dietary fats) must come from the diet. These are called essential fatty

acids, and they include alpha-linolenic acid (ALA) and linoleic acid.

The names of fatty acids reflect their chemical composition. Saturated fatty acids refer to fatty acids in which the bonds between carbon atoms are all single (Fig. 9-7). Single carbon–carbon bonds are more stable than double bonds and affect the behavior of these fatty acids. For example, saturated fats tend to be more stable at higher temperatures. This explains why butter (higher in saturated fatty acids) is solid at room temperature, and plant oils are not (lower in saturated fatty acids).

Trans fatty acids (trans fats, or TFAs) are usually created by hydrogenation, a process used by food product manufacturers to make fatty acids in foods more saturated, and thus more stable and with a longer shelf life. While TFAs have a carbon–carbon double bond, the arrangement of other atoms around the bond lead to a shape of the fatty acid that is similar to saturated fatty acids (Fig. 9-7). Greater intake of trans fats in the diet has been linked to higher rates of artery disease. Trans fats may increase this risk through effects on blood lipid levels (raising LDL cholesterol levels and lowering HDL cholesterol levels), artery lining function, and making the blood more likely to form blood clots (Oh, Hu, Manson, Stampfer, & Willett, 2005) (Game Changers 9-1).

Unsaturated fatty acids have at least one carbon–carbon double bond. Monounsaturated fatty acids have one carbon–carbon double bond, whereas polyunsaturated fatty acids have more than one. The location of this carbon–carbon double bond helps to name the fatty acid and affects the fatty acid's structure and behavior in the body. Omega-3 fatty acids have the carbon–carbon double bond at the third carbon from the end of the fatty acid. Dietary sources of omega-3s include fish oils and some plant and nut oils. Fish oils contain special long-chain omega-3 fatty acids, including

Saturated fatty acid

Trans fatty acid

Unsaturated fatty acid

Figure 9-7. Basic fatty acid structures.

Game Changers 9-1. Walter Willett, Nutrition, and Health

Walter C. Willett, M.D., Dr. P.H., is professor of epidemiology and nutrition, chair of the Department of Nutrition at the Harvard School of Public Health, and professor of medicine at the Harvard University Medical School. Willett has been a guiding force in some of the largest and most highly regarded epidemiological studies on lifestyle and health, especially nutrition and health. These landmark studies include the following.

- The Nurses' Health Study began in 1976 under the direction of Frank Speizer, collecting data on lifestyle behaviors and health of 121,700 women. Willett joined the research team soon thereafter. This study was one of the first to examine lifestyle and health in women.
- The Nurses' Health Study II, established by Willett and colleagues in 1989. This study is gathering data on 116,000 younger women.
- The Health Professionals' Follow-up Study was organized by Willett and colleagues in 1986 to examine data from 52,000 male medical professionals.
- The Growing Up Today Study began in 1996 and is looking at 16,000 children of women participating in the Nurses' Health Study II.

Willett and his research teams have published hundreds of research papers over the years, eventually overturning several important theories while building new models explaining the associations between many lifestyle and medical risk factors and health. For example, his research found no relationship between total fat intake and breast cancer, positive associations between animal fat and red meat intake and colon cancer risk, and no association between egg consumption and heart disease risk. In this way, Willett and colleagues have changed many fundamental assumptions regarding the links between nutrition and health.

Research by Willett and colleagues helped to bring trans fats into the research and public-health arenas. Research published by this group in 1997 showed that higher trans fat intake was associated with greater risk for heart disease (Hu et al., 1997). This was a surprise, since at that time people had been encouraged to switch from butter, because it was high in saturated fat and cholesterol, to margarine in order to reduce heart disease risk. Willett brought to scientific and public attention the fact that margarines were manufactured using hydrogenation to make them solid at room temperature, that this process of hydrogenation created products high in trans fats, and that these fats increased heart disease risk. This work eventually influenced the FDA to require trans fat labeling on the nutrition facts panel of food products.

Willett's was one of the early voices to question USDA public-health dietary guidelines. His work demonstrated that the simple advice of the 1990s to eat less fat and more carbohydrates was not sound. According to his research, high-glycemic-load diets carry a higher risk of heart disease than diets high in unsaturated fats. Statistical analyses of data from the Nurses' Health Study suggest that replacing saturated fats with unsaturated fats lowered heart disease risk, whereas replacing unsaturated fats with carbohydrates actually increased risk (Hu, Manson, & Willett, 2001).

Willett continues to criticize the U.S. Dietary Guidelines, MyPlate recommendations, and the process that creates them (Willett & Ludwig, 2011). He has made many suggestions for improving this process, including the recommendation to move the job of developing the guidelines from the USDA to the Centers for Disease Control and Prevention or Institute of Medicine, since the USDA has a conflict of interest in promoting commodities such as meat and dairy products.

Hu, F. B., Manson, J. E., & Willett, W. C. (2001). Types of dietary fat and risk of coronary heart disease: a critical review. *Journal of the American College of Nutrition, 20*(1), 5-19; Hu, F. B., Stampfer, M. J., Manson, J. E., Rimm, E., Colditz, G.A., Rosner, B.A., . . . Willett, W.C. (1997). Dietary fat intake and risk of coronary heart disease in women. *New England Journal of Medicine, 337,* 1491-1499; Willett, W.C., & Ludwig, D. S. (2011). The 2010 Dietary Guidelines—best recipe for health? *New England Journal of Medicine, 365*(17), 1563-1565.

docosahexaenoic acid (DHA) and eicosapentaenoic acid (EPA). DHA and EPA have been associated with beneficial health effects, including reduced levels of inflammation and slower rates of blood clotting. This is why many public-health recommendations suggest that people increase their consumption of fish (Lichtenstein et al., 2006). Oily fish such as salmon, tuna, sardines, mackerel, and herring have the highest concentrations of these fatty acids. In some studies, fish oil supplements have also been associated with reductions in symptoms of depression, although results have not been consistent (Soh, Walter, Baur, & Collins, 2009). ALA is another type of omega-3, although its effects on the health variables mentioned above do not appear to be as strong as those of DHA and EPA. On the other hand, omega-6 fatty acids, found primarily in plant oils, have been associated with higher levels of inflammation and increased rates of blood clotting.

Cholesterol is a waxy substance that does not dissolve in water. In the diet, cholesterol is only found in animal products. Many people confuse cholesterol with dietary fat. In fact, much of dietary cholesterol is found in animal cell structures, so even very-lean meats, such as shrimp and chicken, still have cholesterol. Cholesterol is also found in milk and eggs.

Most of the cholesterol in the body is manufactured by the liver. Cholesterol is not an essential nutrient for this reason. Cholesterol is an important precursor for all steroid hormones, including vitamin D, the sex hormones (including testosterone, estrogen, and progesterone), and the glucocorticoids (such as cortisol) and mineralocorticoids (including aldosterone), which participate in the stress response.

Diet, Blood Lipids, and Heart Disease

High levels of blood cholesterol, especially LDL cholesterol, have been associated with increased risk for artery disease, as explained in Chapter 1. However, the effect of dietary cholesterol on blood LDL levels and the role of dietary cholesterol in the progression of artery disease are not clear. Epidemiological studies suggest that except for people with abnormalities in blood lipid regulation, dietary cholesterol levels are not strongly correlated with artery disease risk. Nevertheless, since a few studies have found a negative effect of high cholesterol consumption in people with diabetes, a low (less than 200–300 mg/day) level of cholesterol intake is recommended by the American Heart Association and the USDA (Box 9-2; Eckel, 2008; Lichtenstein et al., 2006).

It is likely that the most-common driver of high LDL cholesterol levels is excess calorie intake, including excess carbohydrate intake. Overeating may stimulate the liver to manufacture triglycerides, which are created as a vehicle for storing extra calories. Triglycerides need lipoprotein carriers to travel in the bloodstream to reach adipocytes and other storage locations, so the liver creates more lipoproteins to shuttle the fat around. Many nondietary factors affect blood lipid concentrations as well, including genetics, gender, activity level, and body mass index (BMI) (Siri-Tarino, Sun, Hu, & Krauss, 2010).

Vitamins and Minerals

Vitamins and minerals are needed by the body in relatively small amounts, compared with carbohydrate, protein, and fat. Vitamins are fairly complex organic molecules created by plants and animals, whereas minerals are elements found in nature. Minerals are absorbed by plants from the soil and by animals from food. People do not obtain energy directly from the chemical bonds in vitamins or minerals. But vitamins and minerals play thousands of important roles in the physiological functioning of the body, from helping enzymes speed chemical reactions to providing components for stomach acid, joints, bones, and teeth.

People require 13 vitamins: A, C, D, E, K, and the family of eight B vitamins (thiamine, riboflavin, niacin, pantothenic acid, biotin, vitamin B_6, vitamin B_{12}, and folate). People can usually get plenty of vitamins from the foods they eat. People can also make vitamin D (from exposure to the sun) and vitamin K (made by helpful bacteria in the GI tract). Vegetarians may need to take a vitamin B_{12} supplement, since this vitamin is only found in foods of animal origin.

Minerals needed by people include the macrominerals calcium, phosphorus, magnesium, sodium, potassium, chloride, and sulfur. Macrominerals are needed in larger amounts than the other minerals, known as trace minerals, which are needed in small amounts. Trace minerals are equally as important as macrominerals. Trace minerals essential for humans include iron, manganese, copper, iodine, zinc, cobalt, fluoride, and selenium. The best way to obtain the wide variety of vitamins and minerals needed for good health is to consume a variety of foods, making good choices from all food groups.

Antioxidants and Health

A variety of vitamins, minerals, and other substances in food serve antioxidant functions in the body. Antioxidants neutralize harmful chemicals that are produced as a byproduct of energy metabolism or from the intake of pollutants. Fortunately, plants and

---

Box 9-2. Diet Recommendations From the American Heart Association for the Prevention of Cardiovascular Disease

1. Consume an overall healthy diet.
2. Try to maintain or reach a healthy body weight by balancing calorie intake with physical activity.
3. Consume a diet rich in vegetables and fruits.
4. Consume a diet rich in whole-grain, high-fiber foods.
5. Eat fish, especially oily fish such as salmon and mackerel, two or more times a week.
6. Limit consumption of saturated fats to less than 7% of total daily calories.
7. Limit consumption of trans fats to less than 1% of total daily calories.
8. Limit consumption of cholesterol to less than 300 mg/day.
9. Minimize intake of beverages and foods with added sugars.
10. Limit consumption of salt.
11. If alcohol is consumed, use in moderation.

Lichtenstein, A. H., Appel, L. J., Brands, M., Carnethon, M., Daniels, S., Franch, H.A., . . . Wylie-Rosett, J. (2006). Diet and lifestyle recommendations revision 2006: a scientific statement from the American Heart Association Nutrition Committee. *Circulation, 114*, 82-96.

animals, including humans, have evolved complex antioxidant systems. At one time, it was hoped that supplements made from antioxidant nutrients would provide health benefits, especially reducing the processes of artery disease, some cancers, and even aging, all thought to be associated with oxidative damage. A meta-analysis published in 2007 examined 385 peer-reviewed publications that came out of 68 randomized trials involving 232,606 participants that examined the effect of various antioxidant supplements (Bjelakovic, Nikolova, Gluud, Simonetti, & Gluud, 2007). The analysis found no significant positive effect for any of the supplements and in fact found an increase in mortality rate for subjects receiving beta-carotene, vitamin A, or vitamin E. Researchers have noted that food provides a complex mixture of hundreds of different antioxidants that work together to promote health (Van Horn et al., 2008; Van Horn, 2011). It is possible that high intakes of single antioxidants may throw the mixture out of balance, perhaps limiting the absorption or utilization of other important substances or altering the biochemical processes in which they are involved.

Rather than trying to attain a good intake of antioxidants from supplements, people are generally better off consuming a wide variety of foods (Fig. 9-8).

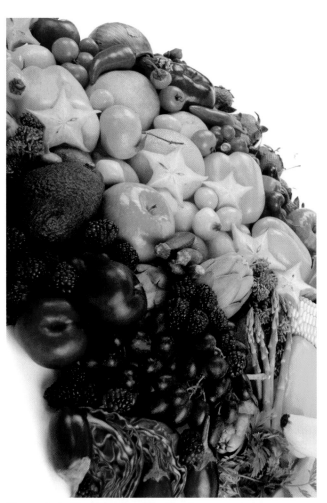

Figure 9-8. Choosing healthy foods. © Thinkstock

Some of the antioxidants that health and fitness professionals (and clients) may be familiar with include:

- **Anthocyanins:** found in red and purple fruits such as eggplant, blueberries, and raspberries
- **Astaxanthin:** found in red algae and animals who eat red algae, including salmon and some shellfish
- **Carotenoids:** found in yellow and orange fruits and vegetables, such as carrots, cantaloupe, and winter squashes
- **Lutein:** found in spinach and red peppers
- **Lycopene:** found in red tomatoes and watermelon
- **Zeaxanthin:** found in corn

One exception to the supplement picture appears to be eye health. Studies suggest that supplements containing antioxidants, especially lutein and zeaxanthin, and zinc may delay the progression of macular degeneration, an eye condition involving progressive damage to the retina, which results in a loss of vision in the center of the visual field (what a person sees) (Olson, Erie, & Bakri, 2011). People with macular degeneration eventually lose the ability to read the letters on a page or to see faces when they look directly at a person. In addition to special antioxidant and zinc supplements, diets high in DHA and EPA and low in glycemic load may help to prevent or delay the progression of macular degeneration (Chiu, Klein, Milton, Gensler, & Taylor, 2009). Because antioxidant supplements may be harmful to some, only those at risk for macular degeneration should take them as indicated by their eye doctors. Risk factors include older age, Caucasian ethnicity, smoking, high blood pressure, high serum LDL cholesterol level, and family history of macular degeneration.

Diet and Bone Health

Bone health is influenced by many lifestyle factors, especially diet and physical activity patterns. Many dietary components appear to influence bone health. Since bones contain a large amount of calcium and phosphorus, a great deal of attention has been paid to attaining adequate levels of these in the diet, especially calcium, since intake of calcium is considerably lower than intake of phosphorus for most North Americans. However, studies linking the intake of calcium supplements to artery disease suggest that calcium supplementation may slightly increase risk for heart disease and other cardiovascular diseases, especially for older adults (Bolland, Grey, Avenell, Gamble, & Reid, 2011). Calcium naturally found in foods, such as dairy products and vegetables, has not been associated with cardiovascular risk. While the increased risk associated with calcium supplements is small, such studies nevertheless suggest that simply popping several calcium supplements each day is not the best strategy for preventing osteoporosis. Calcium supplements have not been shown to increase bone density in early postmenopausal women (less than 5 years after menopause); however, calcium and vitamin D supplements may be helpful in older women, especially those with low calcium intakes (Heaney & Layman, 2008).

Other nutrients important for bone health include vitamins D and K (Lanham-New, 2008). Vitamin D can be made by the body, given adequate sunlight. Medical professionals often recommend supplements of vitamin D_3 for people who do not or cannot obtain adequate sun exposure. Vitamin K is manufactured by bacteria in the GI tract but may also be obtained from many vegetable sources, including spinach, kale, and brussels sprouts.

The Western diet, with its rich supply of meat and grain, may increase risk for osteoporosis through a variable known as net endogenous acid production (NEAP). NEAP does not reflect the acidity of foods eaten but how digestion of these foods affects the body's acid–base balance. In general, protein foods and grains cause a relatively high production of acid, whereas fruits and vegetables reduce NEAP. So even lemon juice, which is itself quite acidic, actually has an alkalizing effect on the body after its digestion and absorption. Fruits and vegetables contain potassium and magnesium, which have an alkalizing effect on the body. Higher levels of NEAP have been associated with lower bone density in several studies (Wynn, Krieg, Lanham-New, & Burckhardt, 2010). NEAP levels are especially of concern as people age and kidney function declines. How does NEAP affect bone health? When the body becomes too acidic, bone tissue releases minerals to buffer the excess acids. Over time, a slow-but-steady loss of bone mineral can result in low bone density. Years of low-grade metabolic acidosis may help to explain why osteoporosis rates are so high in cultures consuming a lot of meat and grains and low levels of fruits and vegetables. Researchers have shown that an adequate intake of protein in the later years is important for the maintenance of muscle and bone, and they suggest that rather than decreasing protein, it is more important for people to increase intake of vegetables and fruits (Heaney & Layman, 2008).

Water

Many people take water for granted, but it is the most-essential nutrient. People can only survive for a short time without water. A lean, adult body is about 60% water by weight. Water is found in every cell of the body, in the fluid between cells, in the blood, and in the fluids produced by the body, including the cerebrospinal fluid that bathes the spinal cord and brain, the synovial fluid found in joints, and the digestive juices produced by the digestive system. All of the physiological processes in the body work best with optimal hydration. Water is lost throughout the day through urination, bowel movements, sweat, and breathing, so people should drink four to eight glasses of water a day (or the equivalent in other beverages) and more if water loss increases for any reason.

Thirst is not a reliable indicator of a need for water, especially in children and older adults. People often forget to drink when they are busy. Dehydration can increase feelings of fatigue and hunger, so drinking adequate water has many benefits. Health and fitness professionals should encourage clients to reach for water, rather than sugary drinks or even sports drinks, unless they are dehydrated. Sports beverages can be very helpful for preventing and treating dehydration. Health and fitness professionals who work with people training for long periods of time in hot conditions should be especially careful about helping clients prevent dehydration.

Public-Health Dietary Guidelines

Public-health dietary guidelines can provide helpful general advice on eating for good health. When devising these guidelines, the goal of nutrition educators and public policy specialists is to take the mountains of nutrition research available and synthesize the most-important points into easy-to-understand, universally applicable advice that will do the most good and the least harm. For most people, simple, concrete advice is easiest to understand and follow. As with advice on physical activity, simple advice will not always apply to every single person, but at least it can help a large percentage of people make a few steps in the right direction.

The dietary advice posted by the USDA's Center for Food Policy and Promotion is helpful, easy to understand and easy to follow (www.choosemyplate.gov). Canada's Food Guide materials are similarly easy for health and fitness professionals to access and promote (www .hc-sc.gc.ca/fn-an/foog-guide-ailiment/index-eng.php). Professionals may educate clients using these guidelines in a general educational fashion, as long as they refrain from activities (prescribing meal plans or diagnosing health problems) outside their scope of practice, as described earlier. Some of the advice found on the USDA website includes the following.

MyPlate

The "MyPlate" icon (Fig. 9-9) replaces the older food pyramid icon as a visual guide to making better food choices. The move to a plate (rather than a pyramid) was calculated to encourage people to build healthier meals, one meal at a time, rather than to think about food choices throughout an entire day, as the nutrition information in the pyramid was designed to do. The main thrust of the nutrition advice included in the MyPlate materials is to help people eat well to prevent chronic illness, especially obesity and obesity-related health problems.

The MyPlate icon divides foods into five groups. On the plate are vegetables, fruits, grains, and protein, pictured in the approximate proportions in which they should be consumed. A circle with the word "dairy" represents the fifth food group. Of course, no simple image can capture the entire range of nutrition advice people need. People must make good choices within the various food groups. They must consider how to

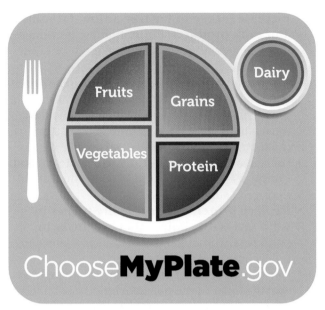

Figure 9-9. MyPlate icon. (Courtesy of ChooseMyPlate.gov)

add treats wisely and how to adapt the advice to their food preferences and eating schedule. Many people are lactose intolerant and must find nondairy sources of calcium. Vegetarians must use nonmeat sources of protein. A person's meal may not be divided into food group "sections." For example, it might actually be a nutritious casserole that combines vegetables, grains, and protein foods, and eaters must calculate what needs to be added to their plates to make a good meal.

■ *Jackson becomes curious about his own diet. He hasn't thought about what he eats too much and often grabs whatever is close at hand and not too expensive. He uses the dietary analysis program on the MyPlate website, entering the foods he eats for one day. His results look pretty good, except that his sodium intake is way too high and his potassium intake too low. His intake of vitamin E also falls short. He doesn't quite make the number of vegetable servings recommended either. Jackson figures his diet is probably better than it used to be since he gets lunch as part of his job at the retreat center, and they serve really good meals. And since Jackson knows some of the clients may be watching what he eats, he is careful to always put some vegetables on his plate and to only eat one helping (the largest piece he can find) of dessert.*

Jackson shows his results to Alana and asks if he should start taking vitamin E. She cautions him to take the results of a 1-day analysis with a grain of salt, or perhaps something healthier since his sodium is too high. She agrees that adding more vegetables would be beneficial but cautions against taking vitamin E supplements and instead suggests adding more nuts and seeds to his diet. Alana shows Jackson various nuts and seeds at the salad bar and suggests

using these liberally. She also suggests adding wheat germ to his cereal at breakfast, as wheat germ is high in many important nutrients, including vitamin E. ■

Additional MyPlate Advice
The MyPlate website is full of easy-to-follow advice to which health and fitness professionals can refer their clients. Under the MyPlate icon on the website's home page is a short list of advice to guide food choices. This list encourages people to enjoy their food but limit the consumption of excess calories; consume more fruits, vegetables, whole grains, and low-fat dairy products; and limit intake of salt and added sugars, especially sugary beverages.

Also on the MyPlate website are links to a variety of helpful nutrition-education materials. The "10 Tips" series features excellent advice that health and fitness professionals can download and distribute to their clients in educational settings. "10 Tips to a Great Plate" offers advice that goes into a little more depth than the simple list of advice that goes with the icon. Other handouts in the "10 Tips" series offer concrete suggestions on a variety of topics health and fitness professionals frequently address. For example, "Make Half Your Grains Whole" spells out what this phrase means and guides consumers in interpreting this guideline. "Healthy Eating for Vegetarians" is especially helpful for clients new to vegetarian eating. "With Protein Foods, Variety Is Key" explains that the protein group is more than a hunk of meat on the plate and also includes eggs, bean dishes, soups, and soy foods as well as seafood and poultry. Clients often seek advice on incorporating more vegetables and fruits into their diets and improving children's diets, and the "10 Tips" series has information on these topics.

Dietary Guidelines for Americans
The U.S. Dietary Guidelines for Americans was created by the Departments of Agriculture and Health and Human Services to guide nutrition policy in the U.S. It is revised every 5 years. These guidelines sound similar to the MyPlate advice but go into more depth on each recommendation. Recommendations from the Dietary Guidelines include the following (www.cnpp.usda.gov/dietaryguidelines.htm):

Balance calories to manage weight
This guideline encourages people to balance calorie intake with expenditure throughout all the life stages. It encourages people to increase physical activity and reduce sedentary behaviors. Emphasis in this section is on achieving and sustaining a healthy weight.

Consume nutrient-dense foods and beverages
Nutrient density refers to the nutritive value per calorie of a given food. If one food has a higher nutrient density than another, it means it has more nutrition per calorie. For example, milk has a higher nutrient density than soda, since milk contains more protein, vitamins, and minerals than soda. The dietary guidelines emphasize the observation that people get too

many of their calories from solid fats (TFAs and saturated fatty acids), added sugars, and refined grains. These ingredients add calories but little helpful nutrition. Foods and beverages high in these ingredients are often said to be "empty-calorie" foods, meaning that the calories contribute little toward a person's nutritional needs. The guidelines urge readers to avoid empty-calorie foods and make good food and beverage choices by looking for foods that contribute positively to one's nutritional needs.

Foods and food components to reduce

This section of the Dietary Guidelines goes into more depth than the MyPlate recommendations on several issues. Much of this advice is difficult to translate into food intake and is thus confusing for clients. Nevertheless, some clients are familiar with this advice, so health and fitness professionals may be asked about it and should understand these recommendations. The issues addressed include:

- **Sodium:** The guidelines recommend that sodium intake be reduced to less than 2,300 mg per day for healthy young people. The guidelines suggest an even lower limit, 1,500 mg, for about half of the population, including people over 50, all African Americans (who have a higher risk of hypertension), and anyone with hypertension, diabetes, or kidney disease.
- **Saturated fatty acids:** The guidelines recommend reducing these to less than 10% of total daily calories, replacing them with unsaturated fats.
- **Cholesterol:** The guidelines recommend less than 300 mg per day.
- **Trans fatty acids:** The guidelines recommend keeping these as low as possible by limiting consumption of products with hydrogenated oils.
- **Refined grains:** The guidelines suggest limiting food with refined grains, especially those with added sugars, sodium, and solid fats. Solid fats refer to saturated fats and TFAs.
- **Alcohol:** The guidelines suggest limiting alcoholic beverages to one per day for women and two per day for men, if alcohol is consumed.

Foods and nutrients to increase

Individuals are cautioned to stay within their calorie needs as they increase these foods:

- **Increase vegetable and fruit intake:** Health and fitness professionals have been pleased to see this advice take center stage in both the MyPlate and the U.S. Dietary Guidelines.
- **Eat a variety of vegetables:** This guideline encourages consumers to expand their vegetable choices and to include dark-green, red, and orange vegetables in their diet as well as beans and peas.
- **Consume at least half of all grains as whole grains:** This guideline encourages people to replace refined grains with whole grains. For example, the guidelines advise people to replace white rice with brown rice, and use whole-wheat products in place of those made with white flour.

- **Increase intake of fat-free or low-fat milk and milk products:** Consumers are encouraged to look for non- or low-fat dairy products such as milk, yogurt, and cheese.
- **Choose a variety of protein foods:** The protein food group is no longer called the "meat" group. Sources of protein include seafood, lean meat and poultry, eggs, beans and peas, soy products, and unsalted nuts and seeds.
- **Increase the amount and variety of seafood:** Consumers are encouraged to consume seafood in place of some other meats.
- **Replace protein foods that are higher in solid fats with choices that are lower in solid fats:** This guideline encourages people to reduce intake of saturated fat.
- **Use oils to replace solid fats:** This guideline's goal is similar to the one above.
- **Choose foods that provide more potassium, dietary fiber, calcium, and vitamin D:** These nutrients are likely to be low in the average diet. The guideline urges consumers to increase consumption of vegetables, fruits, whole grains, milk, and milk products.

Mindful Eating

One of the most-effective ways to improve eating behavior is to eat mindfully. Mindful eating refers to a present-moment, nonjudgmental awareness of the physical and emotional experience of eating. Mindful eating means paying attention to the appearance, smell, textures, and tastes of food (Health Psychology in Your Life 9-1). Mindful awareness during food consumption may enhance people's ability to tune into their physiological feelings of hunger and satiety (feeling like one has had enough to eat). If nothing else, mindful awareness can enhance the pleasure of eating, so that people enjoy their food more, as they focus on eating rather than distractions such as working, reading, or watching television. MyPlate urges people to enjoy their food but eat less. Studies suggest that eating mindfully may be related to eating less. For example, one study divided 29 female college students into three groups, which consumed a standard meal under three conditions (Higgs & Donohoe, 2011). In the first condition, subjects ate while listening to a recording that guided them to focus on the sensory characteristics of the food they were eating and the process of eating. The second group read a newspaper article about food. Subjects in the third group were simply asked to eat their meal with no other direction. Later in the afternoon, subjects were presented with three plates of cookies and allowed to eat as many as they wished. The study found that subjects who ate mindfully chose significantly fewer cookies later in the day. They also had more-vivid memories of their lunch foods than subjects in the other two groups. The authors suggest that memory of previous meals may influence food intake later in the day and that eating mindfully

HEALTH PSYCHOLOGY IN YOUR LIFE 9-1
Mindful Eating Exercise

This exercise asks you to focus mindfully on eating, trying to keep your attention focused on the food and the act of eating. Mindfulness means simply observing with awareness your sensations, feelings, and thoughts in the present moment. Try to observe your experience without judging or analyzing it. You may wish to try this with a friend, so that one of you can read the instructions aloud while the other does the exercise. This exercise should last for at least 1 minute.

Begin by taking a raisin or other small piece of food you enjoy. (If you don't like raisins, try a piece of chocolate or a piece of an apple or other fruit.) Hold the raisin in your hand and notice its appearance. Sense the weight of the raisin and raise the raisin to your nose to smell it. After observing the raisin, place it in your mouth. Observe any sensations associated with this action, such as the weight of the raisin on your tongue or the release of saliva into your mouth. Begin to slowly chew the raisin, observing its taste and texture and the feeling of chewing. Note the impulse to swallow and as you swallow, focus on the sensations of swallowing the raisin and the way that your mouth feels after you swallow.

Variation: Try eating an entire meal in this same mindful fashion, focusing on the food and the process of eating. Do not read, talk, or watch TV while eating your meal. Chew each bite thoroughly and pay attention to your levels of hunger and fullness. When your mind starts to wander, simply bring your focus back to your food and how it tastes. Stop eating when you feel like you have had enough food.

enhances memory (Higgs & Donohoe, 2011). Eating when distracted may lead to more eating later in the day. For example, one study found that women who watched television during a meal ate larger afternoon snacks than women who did not watch television during a meal (Higgs & Woodward, 2009).

Mindful awareness, when eating or in other settings, can reduce feelings of stress and enhance relaxation. Relaxation allows the parasympathetic nervous system, which facilitates digestion, to perform its functions and reduces incidence of stress-related GI tract disorders. Clients may find that listening to the signals of hunger and satiety helps them eat the right amount of food, without the need to count calories or grams. People trying to gain weight and increase calorie consumption may also benefit from mindful eating, as they may be able to consume more food when feeling relaxed.

COMMON NUTRITION AND EATING BEHAVIOR ISSUES

Health and fitness professionals commonly encounter nutrition and eating behavior questions in their work with clients. The ones presented here are some of the most-common issues clients bring up, and their answers allow professionals to educate clients and encourage healthy eating. Obesity and weight control are discussed in Chapter 10, and eating disorders are discussed in Chapter 11.

Orthorexia: Struggling to Achieve the Perfect Diet

Sometimes health and fitness professionals encounter clients who are struggling to make good food choices, appear to be unhappy with their diets, and worry a great deal about nutrition. When does a healthy concern about eating behavior turn into an obsession? If concerns about correct eating begin to exert a negative effect on a person's life, this person is sometimes said to have orthorexia. Orthorexia is not a medical diagnosis but simply a term describing people overly concerned with dietary perfection (Korinth, Schiess, & Wentenhoefer, 2010; Vandereycken, 2011). Health and fitness professionals who sense they are getting too many questions about the "perfect" diet from clients who seem obsessed with nutrition should refer these clients to a dietitian. Clients who feel that their concerns about nutrition and eating behaviors are interfering with their daily lives or causing feelings of distress should be referred to a mental health professional who can help clients put food in perspective.

One of the dangers of working with clients to improve food intake is the possibility that advice from a health and fitness professional might encourage a developing disordered eating pattern or an obsession with food. This is a good reason for health and fitness professionals to focus on the positive and to encourage clients to see food as nourishment and fuel, rather than an endless source of concern and worry (Health Psychology at Work 9-1).

Many people designate foods and eating behaviors as "good" and "bad." This is unfortunate, because they then also label themselves as "good" or "bad" depending upon how they have eaten that day. Some people push back against advice that places certain foods in a "forbidden" category and find themselves consuming more, rather than less, of those foods (Carr, 2011; Chesler, Harris, & Oestreicher, 2009).

Do Nutrient Needs Change With Increased Levels of Physical Activity?

Health and fitness professionals often work with clients who are trying to increase their physical activity levels and have questions about the effect of activity level on nutrient needs. In general, very few nutrient needs

HEALTH PSYCHOLOGY AT WORK 9-1: Healthy Attitude More Important Than "Perfect Diet"

Brent Bode, M.S., C.S.C.S. has his master's degree in exercise and sport studies and has also studied nutrition extensively. Brent has worked in a variety of settings, including teaching strength-training classes for college students, working with athletic trainers in an orthopedic sports-medicine clinic, and working as a personal trainer in a health and fitness center. He is currently coaching competitive youth and adult recreational rowers for Community Rowing, Inc. in Boston. In high school, Brent was a competitive junior category 2 cyclist and mountain biker. At Dowling College, he was a medalist varsity lightweight rower. After that, Brent became interested in nutrition during his 3 years as a formula-car racing driver as a way to optimize his driving performance.

"Questions about food come up all the time, whether you are a coach, exercise instructor, or personal trainer. Exercise and eating go together for many of the goals clients are pursuing.

"Many clients think there is some perfect diet out there. They say to me, 'Give me a list of foods I should eat.' My reply is, 'The food itself is not as important as the behavior underlying your choices.' Healthy eating is about your lifestyle around, and relationship with, your food. Clients start out looking for a simple solution and the optimal diet and are disappointed to realize that eating is about making choices meal after meal, day after day, and that diets are never 'perfect.' On top of this, our culture makes eating healthily quite difficult; there is no simple, easy way. It takes effort to eat well, but with practice healthier choices become habitual. You have to experiment with eating habits that may work for you. You can try a new breakfast cereal, for example, and allow yourself time to adjust. Gradually you figure out how to shop, cook, select, and enjoy foods in ways that nourish your body and spirit. I've tried all kinds of training diets myself. I understand it's difficult to make permanent behavior changes. When you go through challenges in your own life, you have more compassion and empathy for your clients.

"One of my strengths is my enthusiasm for the people I am working with. When people have questions about training, including eating a balanced diet, I take time to find out about each person, their environments, family backgrounds, and daily routines. I encourage them to make healthy changes that personally work for them. I listen carefully and try to empower people to make healthy choices. I might find them reputable articles that address their questions, for example, so they get the information they need to consider changing. I never tell someone what to do or not to do. A 'self-directed' approach allows the client to be part of the process of behavior change.

"There isn't one right way. Instead, there are many ways to reach optimal performance, fitness, and health. With my personal experiences as my compass, I try to be supportive and not punishing. It's best to get people away from dichotomous thinking like I was good or I was bad. This kind of thinking sets you up for internal struggle and 'yo-yo' type behavior. For example, someone might tell me, 'I was bad—I went to a birthday party and ate some cake.' They are thinking, 'Cake is bad; therefore, I am bad.' I would reply, 'No! You're not bad. You were simply celebrating someone's birthday as we all do! Birthday celebrations are fun and don't happen every day!' People have to work with the life they live—their culture, family traditions, and food preferences; they have to enjoy eating and enjoy life."

increase with physical activity (Genton, Melzer, & Pichard, 2010; Rodriguez et al., 2009). People increasing activity up to about an hour per day will have greater energy and water needs (Box 9-3), but their increased needs for other nutrients are very small. Most people will feel a little hungrier if they are more active and thus naturally consume more calories and nutrients.

MOTIVATING CHANGE: Can Clients Change Exercise and Eating Behaviors at the Same Time?

If clients have begun exercising because they have new health concerns or simply an interest in improving lifestyle to stay healthy and get in shape, health and fitness professionals can take advantage of this motivation to give interested clients good information about diet. While it might sound like too much change at once to some people, others are ready to do what is necessary to improve their health. Such clients might be ready to consume more vegetables or drink less soda. They might be ready to give vegetable juice a try or increase seafood intake. Even a few simple but symbolic changes may feel good to clients. As usual, health and fitness professionals should try to get the client to take the lead and decide how much change is realistic. Most fitness professionals would advocate starting with exercise, if doing both at once is not realistic and if there is no medical reason to address diet first. Hopefully, physical activity will reduce stress and improve mood, which will make other changes easier.

Box 9-3. Fluid Requirements With Physical Activity

Many people have questions about how much water and other fluids they should drink, especially as they increase their levels of physical activity. Most people are aware that higher levels of physical activity demand an increased fluid intake. Water loss during exercise in the heat is obvious: clients get hot, sweaty, and thirsty. But fluid needs also increase when exercising in a cold environment, as water vapor is lost with respiration. It is important to give clients good advice on fluid replacement in every season.

A lean, adult body is about 60% water by weight. All physiological processes, including energy metabolism, muscular contraction, and temperature regulation, work best with adequate hydration. A water loss of even 1% or 2% can cause a decrease in physical performance. Any factor that increases fluid loss increases fluid requirements. For example, exercise increases water loss through extra sweating and breathing. Blood loss, vomiting, and diarrhea cause extra fluid losses as well. Athletes who use diuretics (water pills) to lose weight increase their risk of dehydration.

Dehydration Hurts Performance

Explaining the physiological effects of dehydration shows clients why adequate hydration is important. When water loss exceeds replenishment, water is lost from all areas of the body. Water levels decline in both the intracellular and extracellular fluid, which can interfere with electrolyte concentrations and optimal performance.

Blood volume also declines as dehydration occurs. The decrease in blood volume hurts physical performance, since it decreases the amount of blood that the heart can pump per beat. One of the early signs of dehydration is an increased heart rate (beyond one's normal heart rate at rest or for a given amount of work). If blood volume continues to decline, cardiac output may decline as well. Muscles need oxygen and fuel to work, so performance decreases as cardiac output is reduced.

Since there is not enough blood for every system, the body tries to maintain blood volume to the muscles by constricting vessels in the skin. Blood flowing near the skin allows heat to escape from the body, which is very helpful during vigorous exercise. A reduction in skin blood flow means less heat is lost and body temperature rises. To make matters worse, the body decreases sweat production when not enough water is available, so the body has even more difficulty getting rid of heat. This explains why dehydration can lead to heat illness.

Exercise in the Cold Increases Fluid Needs, Too

While dehydration is more likely when exercising in hot weather, dehydration is a concern in cold weather as well. Cold air contains less moisture. When this cold air leaves the lungs, it is fully humidified and warmed. Vigorous exercise for a prolonged period is therefore accompanied by significant fluid loss via respiration.

In a cold environment (water or air), the body attempts to conserve its heat by reducing circulation to the skin. An increased core blood volume stimulates the kidneys to produce more urine to reduce blood volume. However, as exercise progresses and one warms up, the body now opens circulation to the skin to get rid of heat. People need a higher blood volume, so they must replenish those lost fluids.

Water is also lost as sweat when people exercise in the cold, although not usually to the same extent as in the heat. Wearing too much clothing can increase heat and sweating, so cold weather exercisers must learn to shed layers as they warm up so they don't get too hot.

How Much Is Enough?

Most people should try to drink about 8 cups of fluids per day. Recreational exercisers can generally tell if they are drinking enough by checking the color of their urine, which should be pale yellow if adequately hydrated. Some vitamin supplements (containing riboflavin) will make the urine a bright yellow; these do not indicate dehydration. It is not possible to recommend an exact amount of water that a person should drink based on exercise time because this amount varies widely with a person's size and with environmental conditions. People exercising in the heat can gauge water loss by their weight loss during exercise. They should replace each pound of weight loss with about 2 cups of fluids.

Sport Beverages

Sports beverages can be helpful for preventing and treating dehydration. The wide array of product choices in the sport beverage market mean that consumers must read labels to be sure they are getting the ingredients they are looking for and not others. Some beverages primarily replenish electrolytes, and others also add carbohydrates for rebuilding glycogen stores. Athletes who use sport beverages must use a process of trial and error to determine which work best for them and not try a new product before or during competition, as some products might result in gastric distress.

Food, Energy, and Mood

Sometimes clients have questions about eating to maximize feelings of energy or to improve mood, which tend to be the same thing. As discussed in Chapter 3, most people equate feeling good with feeling energetic yet calm and focused. For clients with questions about energy or fatigue, health and fitness professionals should explore the many variables that influence fatigue level, including sleeping patterns, stress, and physical activity as well as diet.

Can certain foods or eating patterns give people more energy? This complicated question appears to have a different answer for each person. Some people seem fairly bulletproof when it comes to food and energy: they have plenty of energy and feel good no matter how they eat. Other people report feelings of fatigue if they consume a heavy meal or skip breakfast. Health and fitness professionals can encourage clients to be aware of their energy levels and their food consumption and to observe whether the two are related. In general, people feel better when they are consuming a healthy diet with plenty of vegetables and more tired when eating a lot of empty-calorie snack foods. Health and fitness professionals can help clients improve their energy levels and good health by promoting a balanced diet. Eating regular meals and snacks helps to prevent hunger and fatigue, which can lead to negative mood.

Some research suggests that low-glycemic-load diets may be associated with better mood. In one study, 42 healthy overweight adults (age 35±5 years) followed either low-glycemic-load or high-glycemic-load eating plans for 6 months. Subjects on the high-glycemic-load diets reported worsening mood over time, compared with the other group (Cheatham et al., 2009). Although this was a small study, professionals whose clients consume many processed foods should urge them to eat better by reducing their glycemic load.

On the other hand, reducing carbohydrate intake too much may be experienced as stressful and result in a more-negative mood. In some people, a negative emotional state seems to increase the consumption of "comfort foods," often high in fat and carbohydrate (Parylak, Koob, & Zorrilla, 2011). Research suggests that some level of carbohydrate consumption helps people feel relaxed. One interesting study of 686 college students found that people who ate breakfast on the sample day reported feeling happier and more relaxed during the morning (Benton & Brock, 2010). In male volunteers, carbohydrate content of breakfast was related to increased feelings of happiness and relaxation during the morning. The researchers suggested that females probably respond similarly to the presence of some carbohydrate in breakfast, but that in general, because they ate less than the men, this relationship did not show up in their study.

An interesting study of 80,000 people in the U.K. found that higher intake of fruits and vegetables a day was linearly associated with level of happiness and mental health (Blanchflower, Oswald, & Stewart-Brown, 2012). In other words, feelings of well-being increased in a dose–response fashion with the number of produce servings, peaking at about seven servings per day.

Another common suggestion for sustained energy is to consume some protein with meals and snacks. This is part of the MyPlate guideline. As clients eat more healthy meals and snacks, they may find they have more energy. Intriguing evidence suggests that ingestion of omega-3 fatty acid supplements may reduce depression symptoms, although the results of studies on this topic are mixed (Hegarty & Parker, 2011; Soh, Walter, Baur, & Collins, 2009).

Just as there is no "best" time to exercise, there is no one "best" time to eat. Clients must figure out how to make time for meals around their other commitments. For example, some people just cannot look at food first thing in the morning and prefer to eat a "breakfast" after they have been awake a few hours. Clients must learn to work with their hunger, energy levels, and food preferences to build meals that work well for them.

People generally feel best if they spread their food consumption out over the day, rather than skipping breakfast and lunch and then overindulging in the evening. To this end, health and fitness professionals should encourage clients to consume three or four balanced meals or snacks over the day, beginning with a good breakfast. Daily breakfast consumption is associated with a number of positive health benefits (Smith et al., 2010). In addition, a good breakfast, with several food groups including protein, may help prevent hunger and overeating later in the day (Jakubowicz, Froy, Wainstein, & Boaz, 2012).

What Is the Best Way to Gain Weight?

When clients ask this question, they usually mean that they want to get bigger and look good, not just get fatter, although some clients may also want more body fat. Some clients may seek advice on gaining weight for aesthetic reasons. Thin men, especially teens and young adults, may wish to become more muscular. Some women also perceive themselves to be too thin and may ask for advice on gaining weight. When thinness is characterized by a loss of lean body mass, as often occurs with aging, frailty can be the result. Becoming frail in one's later years predisposes a person to falls that can lead to fracture and other disabilities. Frailty is associated with a lower quality of life as the activities of daily living become more difficult.

To guide healthy weight gain, health and fitness professionals should first refer clients to their health-care providers to be sure that the low body weight is not indicative of a health problem. These clients should also meet with a dietitian to get specific advice on meal planning. Most clients seeking weight gain will want to build muscle mass, so they should participate in a strength-training program. The foundation of weight gain is good strength training combined with increasing intake of high-quality calories.

Some clients have low levels of hunger and small appetites and have trouble eating a lot at meals. Presuming that they are healthy, they may find that greater amounts of exercise will increase appetite and help them enjoy eating more. They will also need to eat more often throughout the day to increase calorie consumption. Some suggestions for healthy weight gain include:

- **Assess current lifestyle and solve any problems that prevent adequate food intake and regular strength training.** Are clients skipping meals? Grabbing meals that are too small? A little organization and planning may help clients have access to the foods they want to eat and make more time for eating.
- **Reduce feelings of stress, if stress interferes with appetite.** Encourage clients to eat more mindfully and in a relaxing environment.
- **Increase strength training.** Resistance training triggers muscle building, so clients should include a good amount of lifting in their exercise programs (Fig. 9-10). Clients new to strength training should start slowly and build gradually. Guidance from a personal trainer or other qualified fitness professional can help clients prevent injury and maximize muscle building. Some people worry that exercise will make them thinner, but, as long as they increase their calorie intake, this will not occur. Exercise can reduce feelings of stress, stimulate appetite, and help clients eat more as they build muscle.
- **Have a good snack after exercise.** Strength training stimulates muscle repair and growth. During recovery, the body replenishes muscle glycogen stores and rebuilds muscle fibers to make them bigger and stronger. Consuming some protein within 30 minutes of exercising allows recovery metabolism to work in high gear (Cermak, Res, de Groot, Saris, & van Loon, 2012). Most people are not very hungry immediately after exercise, so cool beverages such as smoothies and shakes may work best.
- **Allow muscles at least 48 hours of recovery time to optimize muscle building.** If clients strength train almost every day, the health and fitness professional must structure workouts to alternate muscle groups and include at least one rest day each week.
- **Eat more food.** Clients should add more meals and snacks to their day, thinking of snacks as small meals. Clients will probably need to plan ahead to be sure that good food choices are available when they need to eat. Encourage clients to choose calorie-dense foods as much as possible. For example, they should choose chili or split pea soup rather than broth-based soups. Granola has more calories per bowl than puffy cereal. Beverages such as smoothies are a great way to add calories.
- **Consume some protein foods with each meal or snack.** This recommendation is especially important for frail elders, who build muscle much more slowly.

Today Jackson is working with a new guest, Neil, showing him the ropes at the climbing wall. Neil is 32 and has a sedentary office job that demands over 60 hours of work a week, leaving little time for recreation or exercise. Neil catches on quickly and enjoys following the trail up the wall. Several other guests are climbing as well. At closing time, Neil lingers as Jackson puts away the gear. He asks Jackson if he can recommend a protein supplement to improve muscle definition. Jackson knows Alana does recommend protein supplements to some people who have a poor appetite and don't eat enough, especially her older clients. But Neil looks like he is carrying about 30 or 40 extra pounds. Jackson asks Neil about his exercise program, especially how much time he spends strength training. Neil admits he only gets around to lifting once or twice a week. Jackson wonders, "How do you tell a guy that when you are carrying 30 extra pounds, your muscle definition is going to suffer? And he's only lifting once or twice a week? I guess it's easier to drink a protein shake than work out." Jackson suggests that Neil speak to the dietitian to be sure he is consuming adequate protein and eating a balanced diet. Jackson also suggests that Neil work with one of the personal trainers to set up a strength-training workout. "That will do more for you than adding more protein (and calories) to your diet."

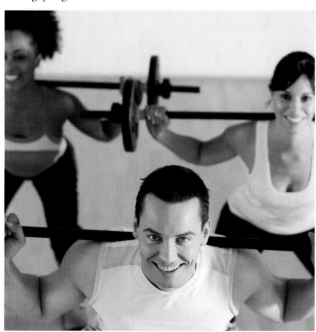

Figure 9-10. Strength training stimulates muscle growth.
© Thinkstock

Dietary Supplements

Many clients want to discuss supplements with health and fitness professionals. Dietary supplements are a multibillion-dollar-a-year industry, with new formulations appearing on the market daily. The mailbox and Internet overflow with advertisements for new products promising to help users slim down, bulk up, or improve performance. The ads are often very sophisticated, and the products mimic pharmaceutical preparations. To understand the dietary supplement industry, it is important to understand how these products are regulated.

In the United States, this industry is regulated by the Food and Drug Administration (FDA), a division of the Department of Health and Human Services. The Center for Food Safety and Applied Nutrition (CFSAN) is the branch of the FDA that works with food and dietary supplements. Good information on supplements and their regulation is available on the FDA website, www.fda.gov/Food/default.htm.

The regulation of dietary supplements is described in the Dietary Supplement Health and Education Act (DSHEA), which was enacted by Congress in 1994. This Act allows manufacturers to market many products as "dietary supplements" rather than as drugs. To qualify as a "dietary supplement," the product must contain one or more of the following substances: "a vitamin; a mineral; an herb or other botanical; an amino acid; a dietary substance for use by man to supplement the diet by increasing the total dietary intake (e.g., enzymes or tissues from organs or glands); or a concentrate, metabolite, constituent, or extract" of the above (U.S. Food and Drug Administration, 2009).

The DSHEA mandates that manufacturers of dietary supplements ensure the safety of their products before selling them. However, supplements do not need approval before being sold, nor do manufacturers need to submit any studies to the FDA before marketing a new product. Products sometimes contain substances, such as caffeine, that are not listed. The FDA does not need to look at a product unless it receives a minimum number of complaints about it. When the FDA becomes aware of a questionable dietary supplement, it must show that product is unsafe before the agency can take it off the market. An example of such action occurred in 2004, when the FDA declared that ephedrine could no longer be used in dietary supplements. The FDA ruling followed the heat stroke death of Baltimore Orioles pitcher Steve Bechler, a death attributed to ephedrine. (Ephedrine may still be a component of over-the-counter medicines, which are regulated more strictly).

The DSHEA does not mandate that dietary supplements be effective. If a product is shown to be ineffective, the FDA need not require that the product be removed. However, if many complaints are received, the Federal Trade Commission (FTC) may take action by investigating fraudulent advertising (www.ftc.gov; click on Consumer Protection, then File a Complaint).

Some sports-nutrition and weight-loss products, such as sports drinks and bars, fall into the category of food, not supplements. Both foods and supplements are subject to labeling requirements of the Nutrition Labeling Education Act of 1990 (NLEA). The NLEA prohibits labels from claiming that a product or its ingredients help to treat or prevent disease, except for certain health claims allowed by the FDA. Since sports performance is not a disease, statements claiming to improve sport performance are allowable without proof that the claim is true. Many experts have urged reform to require better regulation of dietary supplements (Denham, 2011).

Health and fitness professionals will find that many clients are using supplements, since about half of the U.S. population, and approximately 70% of adults over 71 take them (Bailey et al., 2011). About a third of U.S. adults take a multivitamin mineral supplement (Bailey et al., 2011). People often take such supplements just in case their diets are lacking. Many clients (as well as health and fitness professionals) feel confused about whether supplements can be helpful, as some studies support their use and others do not. Some researchers question the benefits of dietary supplements for healthy people eating healthy diets and suggest that studies do not support this practice. In fact, some studies have actually associated supplements with a very slight increase in risk of premature mortality (Mursu, Robien, Harnack, Park, & Jacobs, 2011). One study found that women using multivitamins showed a slightly higher incidence of breast cancer (Larsson, Akesson, Bergkvist, & Wolk, 2010). On the other hand, a meta-analysis looking at multivitamin use and breast cancer did not show an association (Chan, Leung, & Wang, 2011). The studies finding harmful multivitamin effects have been criticized because they included people who may have started taking supplements because of the development of health problems, confounding the effect of supplements for preventing health problems (Li, Kaaks, Linseisen, & Rohrmann, 2012). Other research has found benefits for people taking a daily multivitamin/mineral supplement (Haskell et al., 2010; Li et al., 2012).

Clients may be taking supplements on the advice of their health-care providers; that is fine. For example, people at risk of osteoporosis may be taking vitamin D and calcium. Supplements to slow the progress of macular degeneration appear to be supported by good research. People with heart disease may be taking fish oils. The Dietary Guidelines for Americans recommend foods fortified with folate for women during their childbearing years and vitamin B_{12} supplementation for people over 50. Clients with iron-deficiency anemia may be taking iron. However, professionals should refrain from giving advice in this area and stick to the standard recommendations to obtain nutrients from a good diet. Recommending supplements to clients is outside the scope of practice for most health and fitness professionals, unless they are R.D.s.

ECOLOGICAL PERSPECTIVES: Factors Affecting Eating Behavior

Most health and fitness professionals need look no further than their own lives to understand that many factors influence eating behavior. Because people cannot live without eating, except in the extreme case of tube feeding, food consumption generally occurs several times a day. Strong biological drives to eat have ensured the survival of animals since the beginning of their history. Every culture, society, and family follows basic written and unwritten rules about food and eating. Eating is a significant part of daily life for most people.

The complexity of eating behavior makes behavior change in this area especially challenging. While people can increase physical activity by adding a workout once a day, they must make decisions about eating several times throughout the day. Although overcoming addiction is difficult, people can quit smoking and using substances. But people who have difficulty with food can't just quit eating. Changing eating behavior often means making several changes, eating less of some things and more of others.

When working with clients who are attempting to change eating behaviors, an ecological approach is often helpful for understanding the many factors that may be influencing the way they eat. When working with groups, ecological approaches also help reveal a picture of the many forces that shape eating behaviors. Once professionals understand the factors affecting eating behaviors, they can design more-effective interventions to influence dietary choices.

Intrapersonal Level

People's food choices are strongly influenced by intrapersonal factors. Biological factors, such as feelings of hunger, taste preferences, and individual energy needs influence what and how much people eat. Other intrapersonal variables include whether the individual has food allergies or intolerances, enjoys cooking and/or eating, and values time spent shopping for and preparing meals. People have been eating all their lives and have developed personal beliefs, knowledge, and attitudes regarding eating behaviors and food. They may have emotional associations with certain foods and specific eating habits that are woven into the fabric of daily life.

Interpersonal Level

Eating is often social behavior and is shaped by family members and peer groups. Family shopping, cooking, and eating patterns may determine food availability for family members not involved in food preparation. Peer groups usually evolve certain behaviors that include food: college student friends may order late-night pizza for a study break (Fig. 9-11). Coworkers may share dessert every day at lunch. Friends may gather for

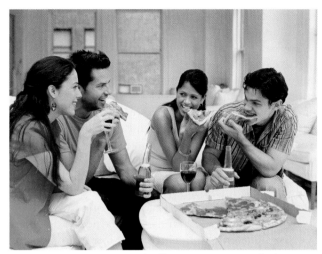

Figure 9-11. Interpersonal influences on eating behaviors. © Thinkstock

drinks after work. Family members may enjoy a snack together as they watch their favorite TV shows in the evening.

Organizational Level

Eating behavior is influenced by organizations in which people spend time. For example, members of a church congregation may gather for coffee hour after a service. Clubs often have snacks at meetings. Children are guided in food selection at school by the meals available there. Workplaces may have meals served at certain meetings or cafeterias from which employees choose foods.

Community Level

People's food choices are often limited by community resources, especially the restaurants and grocery stores to which they have access. Some communities have opportunities for gardening or offer farmers' markets where local growers sell their wares. In communities known as "food deserts," people may only have access to liquor stores and convenience stores for food shopping, with larger grocery stores too far away or unreachable with transportation options. Restaurant options in food deserts may be primarily cheap fast-food operations.

Societal and Cultural Level

Food and eating are integral parts of society and culture. While families transmit many social and cultural traditions, these traditions are shaped by the larger forces of the society and cultures themselves. Religious traditions may prohibit or recommend certain foods and the manner in which they are consumed. Public policy shapes legislation that promotes certain agricultural practices, supporting certain farming methods and discouraging others, and influencing the price of food. Public policy shapes governmental recommendations, school lunch programs, and nutrition-education curricula in public schools. Government and private efforts may create food-donation programs for low-income residents.

Looking at eating behavior from an ecological perspective can help health and fitness professionals devise culturally sensitive and appropriate interventions that encourage good food choices. For example, consumption of fruits and vegetables is associated with better health. Low-income groups tend to be the least likely to meet the USDA recommendations for consumption of these nutritious foods. One interesting research project looked at 12 studies that had examined the fruit and vegetable intake of low-income African Americans (Robinson, 2008). Tanya Robinson combined the information from the 12 studies into an ecological perspective to determine the important factors influencing fruit and vegetable consumption (or lack of consumption). She found that factors at all levels of her ecological perspective influenced produce consumption. For example, personal preference to consume foods other than vegetables often guided food choices. Family and peer group eating patterns often included few fruits and vegetables. Availability of quality produce was often low in the areas studied. Robinson suggested that comprehensive behavior-change efforts be aimed simultaneously at several levels of the ecological perspective; she believed this approach to be more beneficial than simply educating individuals to make better choices.

Research manipulating food options has demonstrated that changing the food environment may change consumption patterns. For example, in New York City, researchers Di Noia and Contento (2010) examined the food choices of 156 low-income African American children aged 10 to14 enrolled in a summer camp program. The camp offered three servings of fruits, fruit juice, and vegetables at each meal for 3 days. During this period, the children consumed an average of 5.41 daily servings of these foods, which was much higher than the national average consumption for youths of similar ages, about 3.6 servings daily (Di Noia & Contento, 2010).

STAGES OF CHANGE: Understanding Dietary Behavior Change

Dietary change can take many forms. Some people may simply want to increase the number of vegetable servings that they consume each day, perhaps adding a glass of vegetable juice each afternoon and an additional serving of vegetables at dinner. People newly diagnosed with a gluten allergy may be learning to eliminate all gluten-containing foods from their diets. Other people may have a low-quality diet along with a medical diagnosis such as diabetes and need to implement a number of challenging changes.

The Transtheoretical Model's Stages of Change Theory was originally derived from studies of behavioral

change for addictions such as alcoholism and cigarette smoking. Studies suggest that this model is also useful for describing dietary behavior change (Di Noia & Prochaska, 2010a; Hildebrand & Betts, 2009; What's the Evidence? 9-1). Research applying the Stages of Change Theory have studied the following changes:

- Reducing intake of fats
- Implementing weight-control recommendations
- Increasing consumption of dairy products
- Increasing intake of whole grains
- Increasing intake of fruits and vegetables

While other dietary changes have been studied less, it is likely that people go through the stages of change as they move from considering change, to deciding to change, to implementing new eating behaviors.

It is important to remember that individual clients may be ready to change some dietary behaviors but not others. For example, research by Plotnikoff and colleagues (2009) looked at stages of change for reducing dietary fat in 1216 adults in Ontario, Canada. Randomly selected adults who agreed to participate completed questionnaires to evaluate a large number of variables, including stage of change for four different fat-consumption statements, including the following (Plotnikoff et al., 2009):

- Consistently avoiding eating high-fat foods
- Cooking meals using techniques to reduce fat
- Choosing low-fat products
- Preparing food at the table in ways that reduce fat

About 65% to 70% of subjects reported being in the action stage for each behavior. However, only 32% reported being in the action stage for all four behaviors. Although the primary purpose of this study focused on the applicability of the Transtheoretical Model to dietary change, the results of this study underscore the observation that stage of change may vary for related behaviors.

MOTIVATING CHANGE: The Complexity of Dietary Change

Because dietary change can be complex, health and fitness professionals should ensure that they and their clients are talking about the same behaviors as they work together. Professionals should use their client-centered guiding skills to figure out which behaviors clients are ready to change. "Are you ready to make some changes in your diet?" is fine to start the conversation, especially if clients have already mentioned that dietary change is one of their behavior-change goals. As clients clarify their goals and specify dietary changes that they wish to implement, the health and fitness professional can try to encourage a short list of these and sense readiness to change for each. It is probably best to begin with those behaviors the client is most ready to change. If clients are still assessing the pros and cons of certain behaviors, it is better to shift to a more-educational approach on these issues.

WHAT'S THE EVIDENCE? 9-1

Does the Transtheoretical Model Describe Behavior Change for Low-Income Parents Increasing Family Servings of Fruits and Vegetables?

Hildebrand, D. A., & Betts, N. M. (2009). Assessment of stage of change, decisional balance, self-efficacy, and use of processes of change of low-income parents for increasing servings of fruits and vegetables to preschool aged children. *Journal of Nutrition Education and Behavior, 41*(2), 110-119.

■ PURPOSE

The purpose of this study was to examine application of the Transtheoretical Model to a group of low-income parents and primary caregivers (PPCs) enrolled in government-sponsored, nutrition-education programs in the southwestern U.S. The researchers wanted to examine the stages of change, the processes of change, decisional balance, and self-efficacy for serving at least five servings of fruits and vegetables daily to household children aged 1 to 5 years.

■ STUDY

The researchers recruited 238 PPCs to complete a survey. Questions on the survey assessed stage of change for serving fruits and vegetables as well as other constructs of the Transtheoretical Model. The researchers found that PPCs were in the whole range of stages, including precontemplation (10%), contemplation (33%), preparation (29%), action (3%), and maintenance (25%). Examining the transtheoretical constructs for PPCs in these different stages led the researchers to observe that the Transtheoretical Model fit this group fairly well. Observations fitting the Transtheoretical Model included the following:

- Cons were stronger than pros for changing for PPCs in precontemplation and contemplation.
- PPCs in preparation, action, and maintenance still listed cons but had developed stronger pros for serving fruits and vegetables to young children.
- Subjects in preparation, action, and maintenance used more cognitive and behavioral processes of change and had higher self-efficacy scores than subjects in precontemplation and contemplation stages.

■ IMPLICATIONS

The researchers felt that since the PPCs in this study demonstrated a good fit for the Transtheoretical Model constructs, tailoring nutrition-education programs to stage of change is probably a good idea. For example, interventions for precontemplation and contemplation participants might provide education regarding meal planning with more fruits and vegetables, to reduce perceptions of cons, which typically focus on the difficulties of serving more of these foods. PPCs in preparation might benefit from skill building for convenient and affordable serving ideas for fruits and vegetables, discussion of the importance of PPCs as models of good eating behavior, and goal setting and planning exercises. Helping PPCs engage in the processes of change might be useful for increasing self-efficacy and serving of fruits and vegetables for children in these low-income households.

Precontemplation

People in the precontemplation stage are not thinking about changing their eating behavior. As discussed previously, precontemplators may be divided into two groups, depending upon their beliefs about the value of dietary change as well as their abilities to change their eating behavior.

Precontemplation Nonbelievers

Precontemplation nonbelievers may not realize that some of their eating behaviors are problematic. Although information on healthy eating is everywhere, advice is often confusing and contradictory and leads some people to quit believing any of it. Nonbelievers may have reached the conclusion that diet just doesn't matter that much. For some, denial of the importance of diet may be a defense mechanism, to justify why they are not trying to change.

Precontemplation Believers

Precontemplation believers might believe a healthy diet is a reasonable goal, but change is not something they are currently considering. Over time, they may have decided changing is not worth the considerable effort required, so they have stopped thinking about it. Precontemplation believers may feel unable to change. Certainly many people have repeatedly tried to change their eating behaviors, only to find themselves unable to stick to a (commonly unrealistic) plan. Experiences such as this may lead people to feel they do not have enough willpower to change eating behavior.

The Health Belief Model and Dietary Change

People start thinking about their eating habits for many reasons. The Health Belief Model highlights several factors that influence people's decisions to start thinking about changing eating behavior. If people see dietary behavior as a way to address an important health issue, they may be moved to consider changing. According to the Health Belief Model, factors that motivate the decision to change include:

- **Perceived susceptibility to and seriousness of a health problem:** People are more likely to decide to change behavior when they perceive that they are susceptible to a particular health problem or issue. Serious health problems make more of an effect than health problems that seem minor, unless the problem is frightening and appears to be untreatable. Health problems most likely to prompt dietary change include heart disease, diabetes, hypertension, obesity, osteoporosis, or food allergies. People most commonly feel susceptible because they are diagnosed with a health problem. But their perceptions of susceptibility may also increase due to diagnosis of a friend or family member, a public-health campaign, or for other reasons.

- **Perceived benefits of dietary change:** A great deal of research supports the efficacy of dietary change for treating many health issues. Unfortunately, health-care providers often do not emphasize strongly enough the potential benefits of a healthy diet. Unless providers have made a strong case for the importance of dietary change and referred clients to a dietitian to make a plan, dietary changes are often overlooked. Advice on diet is complex, and it is much easier for providers to say, "Take one of these pills twice a day." This is very frustrating for health and fitness professionals and very unfortunate for patients who could really benefit from making a few changes in their diet. If the provider has not emphasized dietary change, and if patients have not received good guidance on changing their diets to treat/prevent illness, it is hard for health and fitness professionals to give much specific advice. They can still give general advice, reinforce the importance of diet for good health, and recommend a referral to a dietitian who specializes in the client's particular health issues. Research shows that people trying to change dietary habits because of a type 2 diabetes diagnosis were more likely to decide to change eating behavior if dietary change was believed to be effective and if diabetes was perceived to be a serious problem (Harvey & Lawson, 2009).

- **Perceived barriers to dietary change:** Because dietary recommendations can be so complex and affect clients' lives in so many ways, clients' perceived barriers to dietary change are many. Clients must have access to the foods they want to eat more of and be able to afford these foods. They may need to reorganize their days and their households to make time to shop, plan meals, learn new recipes, cook, eat, and clean up. Dietary advice must be tailored to clients'

abilities, energy levels, resources, and schedules. Eating advice that is simple, affordable, easy, and quick to implement is best.

- **Cues to action:** Precontemplators may perceive cues to action in the advice of a health-care provider or a health and fitness professional. Precontemplators are often moved to action by an urge to change appearance, as they prepare for an important event, such as a class reunion or wedding. Clothes becoming too tight or remarks from friends may push precontemplators into the contemplation stage. Sometimes beginning an exercise program motivates people to improve eating habits.

MOTIVATING CHANGE: Processes of Change for Precontemplators

Consciousness raising and emotional relief can help turn precontemplators into contemplators (Di Noia & Prochaska, 2010b). When working with precontemplators, health and fitness professionals should use their client-centered communication skills to find out what is important in clients' lives. Consciousness raising to increase awareness of the importance of dietary change will have the greatest effect if such change is personally relevant. If clients can decide that maintaining health is a priority that will allow them to reach important goals or perform priority tasks, perhaps they will also see dietary change as a priority.

If clients are asked to change their diet to address health problems, they may feel relieved to know that dietary change makes a difference and that the health and fitness professional can help them structure effective goals and behavior-change plans.

Contemplation

People in contemplation are thinking about making changes in their eating behavior, weighing the pros and cons of changing. They may be wondering if they should make some changes but are ambivalent about the importance of changing and their abilities to change. When working with clients in the contemplation stage of change, health and fitness professionals should help clients shift their decisional balance by reinforcing change talk and by strengthening clients' perceptions of the benefits of dietary change and reducing the perceived barriers to change. In addition, professionals should help clients build confidence in their abilities to make improvements in eating behaviors.

The Theory of Planned Behavior and Dietary Change

The Theory of Planned Behavior highlights several variables important in helping people form a decision or intention to change and has shown some promise in moving people to consider changing eating behaviors

(Baranowski, Cullen, Nicklas, Thompson, & Baranowski, 2003). As discussed in previous chapters, intentions may (Blanchard et al., 2009; Blue, 2007) or may not (Sniehotta, 2009) result in actual behavior change, but behavior change usually requires a conscious decision to change, along with subsequent planning. Health and fitness professionals may be able to guide discussions of these variables with clients in the contemplation stage:

- **Attitudes toward nutrition, food, and eating behaviors:** Health and fitness professionals should discuss with clients how they think and feel about the eating behaviors they are considering changing. These attitudes are often very complex. If potential changes involve giving up beloved comfort foods, consuming foods considered unpalatable, or making changes that will be financially costly or time consuming, barriers to change increase. People's expectations of what change will be like must be associated with anticipation of positive, valued outcomes, or the energy for overcoming barriers will be low. People's attitudes and expectations about the results of making dietary change are often unrealistic. While the potentially positive outcomes (better health, weight loss) are highly valued, clients may expect too much change too quickly and become frustrated when change is not immediate. Health and fitness professionals should guide clients to hope for positive but realistic outcomes from dietary change.
- **Subjective norms regarding eating behavior and nutrition:** Because eating often occurs with others, subjective norms can translate into social pressure to consume or not consume certain foods. If everyone else at the table is enjoying a delicious dessert, it may be hard for clients to decline. Subjective norms may reinforce notions such as "It's cool to be a vegetarian," or "It is really weird to be a vegetarian." Subjective norms can support behavior change. For example, in a study of people diagnosed with type 2 diabetes, subjective norms contributed to people's intentions to eat a healthy diet (Blue, 2007).
- **Perceived behavioral control or self-efficacy:** Perceived behavioral control or self-efficacy (from social cognitive theory) contributes to behavior-change success in every realm, and dietary change is no exception. It is important to remember that self-efficacy is situation specific, so health and fitness professionals should explore with clients ideas about what changes will be relatively easy to implement (from the client's point of view) and what changes will be difficult. For example, clients may feel like breakfast and lunch are easy to plan but that dinner is harder to organize into a healthy meal. It may feel easy to add another vegetable with dinner but not with other meals. As clients weigh the pros and cons, high self-efficacy will make the cons seem less problematic.

Self-Determination Theory and Processes of Change for Contemplators

Autonomous motivation is essential for eating behavior change. Unfortunately, many clients may begin changing eating behaviors because they feel pushed or bullied into change by health-care providers, friends, family, or society at large. Internal conflict over changing eating behavior can lead to a great deal of negative emotion, stress, and ultimately failure, as anger, hunger, or exhaustion win out over good intentions.

Health and fitness professionals should remember the three basic needs that underlie motivation: autonomy, competence, and connection. When discussing eating behavior change, professionals should encourage clients to change because they want the benefits of better eating habits for themselves and not just to please someone else. If eating behavior change is not intrinsically enjoyable, clients must at least incorporate healthy diet goals as personally meaningful and a path that will help them achieve good health. (This is the integrated and identified self-regulation discussed in Chapter 5.)

Competence echoes self-efficacy, described previously. Health and fitness professionals should help clients design realistic dietary changes they feel able to achieve. Connection with others often supports behavior-change efforts. Clients may be more successful if family members are included in the goal setting and planning processes. Health and fitness professionals may encourage groups of clients with similar goals to work on eating behavior changes together, meeting periodically to support one another.

Several of the Transtheoretical Model's processes of change can support autonomous motivation in clients changing eating behaviors. Social support is similar to connection, discussed above. Self-reevaluation often moves contemplators into the preparation stage of dietary behavior change, as people begin to see themselves in new ways. A medical diagnosis, new health information, or other consciousness-raising processes may lead to self-reevaluation. Similarly, as clients begin to see themselves and their eating habits in a new light, they may begin to notice things in their environment they overlooked before (social liberation). They may notice that other people like themselves are eating vegetables in a restaurant or choosing a salad at a fast-food establishment. They may become aware of the variety of vegetables in their local markets or notice new recipes lower in sugar or other things related to their behavior-change ideas. These new ideas may help contemplators see behavior change as more within their abilities.

Preparation

People preparing to change their eating behaviors may be gathering information from books, articles, websites, and health professionals. They may be meeting with dietitians and health-care providers to get dietary advice. People in the preparation stage may be talking to health and fitness professionals with whom they work to get some guidance on eating behavior change. Clients may be cleaning up their eating environments: giving away the chips and sodas in their kitchens or the candy in their offices. They may be trying new recipes and foods or talking to their friends and families about changes they are thinking of making.

Setting Goals and Making Plans

Health and fitness professionals who are not licensed nutrition professionals should refer clients with health problems to dietitians for help with actual meal planning and dietary-change recommendations. Hopefully, clients' dietitians have guided them in positive, motivating ways and have been clear about dietary recommendations. If clients still seem confused about what to eat or not eat, they should meet again with their dietitians to have their questions answered. Health and fitness professionals who often work with clients changing eating behaviors should network with dietitians in their location and cultivate a good referral network, finding dietitians who are most effective at giving clear advice and motivating behavior change.

Once clients have specific recommendations, health and fitness professionals can help them implement the prescribed eating behavior changes. Clients may be guided to devise S.M.A.R.T. goals, as discussed in Chapter 5. One of the most-common dietary behavior-change goals is to consume more vegetables. To turn this vague goal into a more-useful goal, the health and fitness professional could use good guiding skills to help clients make this goal fit the S.M.A.R.T. criteria. For example:

- **Specific:** Consume five servings of vegetables a day, incorporating a wide range of choices.
- **Measurable:** Consume two servings of vegetables with lunch, a cup of vegetable juice around 4 p.m., and two servings of vegetables with dinner.
- **Attainable:** Clients should try to be realistic about their abilities to attain the above, adjusting as necessary.
- **Relevant:** Professionals should listen to clients as they discuss goals and verify that the goals address health concerns.
- **Time-bound:** Clients should spell out a time frame for achieving this goal. While some clients who are already consuming three or four servings of vegetables per day may be comfortable jumping to five servings right away, others may find that it is more realistic to begin with three and then the following week move to four, then five.

Clients may form similar goals for decreasing intake of refined sugars and grains, drinking less coffee, reducing soda intake, drinking more water, consuming less food in the evening, and other common dietary goals.

Once clients clarify their eating behavior goals, they are well on the road to making specific plans for achieving them. Using the five vegetable servings example above, clients can plan ways to fit two vegetables into lunch. What does lunch usually look like? Where do they eat? What are the choices? Will they need to bring along food from home (if they don't eat at home)? How can they be sure that they have these foods on hand? Similar specific planning should occur for the vegetable juice snack and dinner vegetable servings.

Self-Control and Eating Behavior

The notion that people have limited self-control has enormous implications for eating behavior change (Behavior Change in Action 9-1). Behavior-change goals and plans that look great on paper will fail if they exceed a client's self-regulatory skills. Challenges to eating behavior change occur throughout the day, as clients make decisions about meals and snacks. Given that self-control is very limited (Baumeister & Tierney, 2011), health and fitness professionals should guide clients to make simple changes that become habits as quickly as possible, limiting the need to make decisions. Suggestions for minimizing the self-control needed for eating behavior change include:

- Set reasonable goals that feel attainable to clients. Don't expect unlimited self-control.
- Manipulate eating environments to promote desired behaviors. Reduce foods that lead to unwanted eating at home and work and urge clients to have healthy foods for meals and snacks readily available.
- Help clients set up grocery shopping lists and meal plans. Try to make healthy eating as simple, convenient, and affordable as possible.
- Urge clients to prevent hunger by eating delicious, nourishing, well-balanced meals and snacks. Hunger is stressful for most people, and distress depletes self-control energy. Plus, the brain uses blood glucose in its efforts to exert self-control (Baumeister & Tierney, 2011). Hunger is also a powerful drive in its own right and can easily overwhelm self-control efforts.
- Encourage clients to get adequate sleep, manage stress, and exercise. Self-control energy increases with these behaviors.

Build on Success

Many clients will have stories of past failures and successes. As with any behavior-change plan, health and fitness professionals should keep track of these stories and use past successes to figure out which elements to incorporate into new programs. Likewise, professionals should try to avoid or reduce elements that led to failure. Positive thinking and expectations are essential for behavior-change success. Past successes build self-efficacy and promote positive thinking. Health and fitness professionals should remind clients of these positive stories when appropriate to boost self-confidence and energy for behavior change.

BEHAVIOR CHANGE IN ACTION 9-1

Organization Supports New Eating Behaviors

■ CHALLENGE

Establishing new eating behaviors often demands new organizational skills from clients who already feel some-what stressed out by the prospect of changing eating behaviors. How do I help clients become better organizers in a client-centered fashion, without lecturing and making them feel more stressed?

■ PLAN

Use your OARS communication skills to clarify clients' goals and to help them make an action plan for achieving them. Get a sense of clients' perceptions of barriers to change and the many issues that may arise on a daily basis as new plans are put into place. Clients will probably realize that their food shopping, meal preparation, and dining out habits will need to change. Elicit their ideas regarding these changes and remind them that a little organization can make change easier. Depending on a client's situation, the strategies listed below may be helpful. Select the ones appropriate for individual clients. Start with one suggestion, rather than overwhelming clients with too much information or too many ideas.

Acknowledge that getting organized takes time and energy but is worth it. If clients expect change to be simple and easy, they become frustrated when the day-to-day work of eating better is not so simple. Express your confidence in clients' abilities to reach their goals but sympathize that change can feel difficult at times. Show your support and remind them that eating well will help them have more energy, feel better, and be healthier.

Encourage clients to keep meal plans simple and limit choices. Making choices depletes self-control energy and creates opportunities for the breakdown of new eating habits and the resumption of old habits. On the other hand, people like to feel as though they have some choice, so plans should be flexible. Some people are fine with two or three standard breakfast meals that allow them to go on automatic pilot in the morning. Help clients evaluate and improve these plans if necessary. Do the same for lunch options, looking for simple changes. Can salad replace chips and salty snacks? Can water replace sodas? Many clients will put forward these simple suggestions themselves.

Consider a weekly dinner meal plan. Many clients like to minimize time spent worrying about dinner, especially if they are preparing meals for a household. A routine that rotates weekly reduces stress, especially for cooks in a hurry. For example, maybe Monday is soup and salad (with leftover soup from the weekend); Tuesday is pasta, sauce, and salad. Wednesday is a chicken dish, stir-fry with vegetables and rice; Thursday is Chinese take-out; and so forth. Take-out can be featured on longer workdays, and cooking can occur on easier days; or take-out can occur every day, if that works best, as long as most of the food choices are healthy.

Prepare extra and save for later. Making extra food when cooking can translate into lunch the next day and dinner a day or two later. Superorganized cooks sometimes make very large batches of soup, stew, or other items that freeze well and put away meal-sized portions to defrost and serve weeks later. This suggestion may not work for people who tend to overeat, if preparing more tonight means second and third helpings rather than lunch the next day.

Help clients make a plan for food shopping. Try to tailor this plan to clients' lives. When can they fit shopping in? Some clients like buying fresh produce on the way home from work each day, whereas others may prefer to do one large shopping trip a week. Remind clients to take a list and to avoid shopping when tired or hungry, that is, when willpower may be low. Some health and fitness professionals not only help clients make a shopping list but also take clients, either individually or in groups, on tours of local markets to teach good shopping skills. If clients have a weekly dinner meal plan, items needed for meals can be included on the shopping list.

Help clients find good recipes. Some clients love to cook and enjoy spending time finding new, delicious recipes. Steer them away from too many high-fat and sugary desserts and toward healthy dishes featuring fruits, vegetables, fish, legumes, and whole grains. If you have several clients who like to cook, they might like to share recipes. Some groups, including workplaces and other organizations, enjoy compiling members' recipes into cookbooks.

Encourage positive eating experiences. Food should be nutritious but also delicious. Encourage clients to eat mindfully and savor their meals. Keep a positive focus. Help clients to see these new ways of organizing and eating as beneficial, healthy, and important, rather than as deprivation and a chore.

Action

People in the action stage of change have decided to change certain eating behaviors and are at least attempting to stick to this decision. Because eating behavior is so complex, a person may look like action in the morning, contemplation in the afternoon, and even precontemplation in the evening, if the day really falls apart. During the action stage, some parts of the new eating plan may be working while others are not. For this reason, it can be hard to tell if people are really in the action stage or not. Psychologically, many people in the action stage still feel ambivalent about dietary change and may have low self-efficacy for making their planned changes. Clients who appear to be following their plan may still feel pretty shaky and uncertain. Health and fitness professionals should teach behavior-change skills that will help clients develop new eating behaviors that can become habits, replacing less-helpful behaviors (Michie et al., 2009). Some of the most-useful behavior-change skills for clients changing eating behaviors include:

Self-Monitoring

Self-monitoring is a very effective tool for helping people change eating behavior (Michie, Whittington, McAteer, McAteer, Gupta, 2009). Depending upon the behavior-change goal, people may benefit from very simple to fairly extensive self-monitoring systems. For example, people trying to consume more fruits and vegetables may simply record servings of those foods (Fig. 9-12). People making more-extensive changes may record food consumed, time of day, reasons for eating, hunger level, and activities occurring during the meal or snack (Fig. 9-13). Recording these details may help to uncover productive or unproductive eating patterns and behavior chains.

Keeping a record of food consumed and eating behaviors can feel time consuming and burdensome at first, since eating occurs throughout the day. Once clients develop some sort of habit, with an easily accessible system, keeping track of meals is less challenging. Nevertheless, many people prefer not to track eating every day. Depending on the situation, clients might benefit from self-monitoring for 3 to 7 days at the beginning of a behavior-change program, to get a baseline picture of current patterns. Once clients identify important issues and begin trying to change, self-monitoring is once again helpful to see how things are going. Many clients find self-monitoring very motivational and are

Fruit and Vegetable Serving Record

Sunday	Monday	Tuesday	Wednesday	Thursday	Friday	Saturday
B = Breakfast L = Lunch D = Dinner S = Snack				**1** B ____ L ____ D ____ S ____ Total ____	**2** B ____ L ____ D ____ S ____ Total ____	**3** B ____ L ____ D ____ S ____ Total ____
4 B ____ L ____ D ____ S ____ Total ____	**5** B ____ L ____ D ____ S ____ Total ____	**6** B ____ L ____ D ____ S ____ Total ____	**7** B ____ L ____ D ____ S ____ Total ____	**8** B ____ L ____ D ____ S ____ Total ____	**9** B ____ L ____ D ____ S ____ Total ____	**10** B ____ L ____ D ____ S ____ Total ____

Figure 9-12. Simple self-monitoring form for tracking intake of fruits and vegetables.

DAILY FOOD RECORD

Date ________

Time	Place	Food/Beverage	Amount	Where Consumed	Reason for Eating

Figure 9-13. More-comprehensive form for recording food intake and eating behaviors.

much more careful about food choices when they are recording dietary intake. Warning: people in recovery from eating disorders are often asked to *not* record food intake, as they may be hypervigilant and even obsessed with monitoring food intake.

Problem-Solving

As clients record eating behavior, they may become aware of patterns related to eating. Some patterns may support desired behaviors, whereas others interfere with behavior-change plans. Health and fitness professionals can discuss the behavior chains uncovered in the self-monitoring process and guide clients in devising workable strategies that will reduce unwanted eating and reinforce new behaviors. For example, clients may find they do not have enough vegetables on hand to prepare two servings every evening for dinner. They may complain that shopping is too time consuming or that the vegetables spoil when they are out of town. Rather than suggesting a quick solution, allow clients to mull the situations over and come up with their own solutions.

Coping Planning

If certain factors routinely interfere with behavior-change plans, clients may benefit from coping planning. For example, holidays often disrupt eating behavior-change plans. Clients often have experience with these routine factors and can draw on past experience to make future plans. When the holidays are approaching, clients can plan ahead of time to enjoy them and still follow through on their behavior-change plans. Clients may wish to plan for travel, vacations, eating out, illness, or any other events that tend to be disruptive.

Stress Management

Some clients may find that stress strongly influences eating behaviors. If stress-induced eating appears in the self-monitoring process, discuss how clients might better manage stress. For example, clients trying to consume less salt in efforts to reduce hypertension may be fine following their eating plan except when feeling stressed, and then they may reach for a bag of salty chips. Health and fitness professionals can work with clients to help them sense when a "stress-eating attack" may be coming and to be ready with alternate strategies. When stress is a problem, doing something active is often the answer, such as taking a walk or going out with friends. Clients may be able to identify emotions that trigger poor eating, such as anger, boredom, loneliness, irritability, and sadness. Health and fitness professionals can reinforce the observation that regular physical activity is helpful for reducing negative emotions and feelings of stress.

Cognitive Restructuring

Sometimes clients find that they have unhelpful thought patterns that interfere with eating behavior change. Most common is dichotomous thinking, where clients feel like they are either totally successful or a total failure. Eating behavior is rarely perfect. Clients often benefit from practicing mindful eating and learning to enjoy their food, savoring its flavors and textures. Many clients have spent years seeing food as "the enemy." Health and fitness professionals should encourage clients to see food as fuel and even as delicious and nutritious.

Some clients are constrained by unproductive thoughts and feelings about certain foods, such as "I hate vegetables." Health and fitness professionals can encourage creative problem-solving to explore new recipes, behaviors, and thoughts. Some clients need help coping with setbacks and lapses. Professionals may be able to help clients cultivate a more-flexible attitude and way of thinking about eating behavior, so they don't see lapses as the end of trying.

Maintenance

People are in the maintenance stage if they have stuck to their new eating behaviors for 6 months or more. The longer they sustain their new eating behaviors, the more likely it is they will continue. For any given individual, some behaviors may become habits that last for long periods of time (e.g., rarely eating breaded and fried foods). In contrast, some behaviors are more difficult to achieve every day (such as striving to eat five to nine servings of fruits and vegetables each day; while the striving may continue, the person may not reach this target every single day).

People in the maintenance stage for one group of eating behaviors may be in precontemplation for others. For example, people may have decreased their salt intake following a hypertension diagnosis but still have a low consumption of fruits and vegetables. Many people (including health and fitness professionals) find that dietary change is a lifelong process, with new habits evolving as health concerns change, nutrition science discovers new information, or concern for the environment leads consumers to look for more local eating options.

■ *Vanessa, the head of corporate sales for the retreat center, has asked Jackson to meet with her. She would like Jackson to lead a 2-hour hike for a group of 20 people who are attending the retreat center as part of a workplace staff-development program. The goal of the hike is to allow participants to experience the stress-reduction benefits of recreating in the great outdoors and to have them discuss a short list of topics as they walk. "One of the topics is developing a positive eating plan to maximize daily energy and productivity," she tells Jackson. "Alana tells me that you have developed some expertise in this area and have a good foundation in healthy eating advice. She said you would do a good job of helping clients keep this conversation on track with a positive focus.*

You'll also be guiding a discussion of physical activity for stress management. How does that sound?" Jackson smiles, thinking how this request would surely have intimidated him just 2 months ago. He thanks Vanessa for the opportunity to work with the group and is already thinking about some questions to guide the discussions. ■

KEY TERMS

amino acids

antioxidants

blood sugar

carbohydrates

cholesterol

complete proteins

complex carbohydrates

dietary fiber

disaccharides

docosahexaenoic acid

eicosapentaenoic acid

essential amino acids

essential fatty acids

fructose

glucagon

glucose

glycemic index

glycemic load

glycogen

hydrogenation

incomplete proteins

insulin

insulin resistant

islets of Langerhans

macrominerals

mindful eating

monounsaturated fatty acids

monosaccharides

net endogenous acid production

nonessential amino acids

nutrient

nutrient density

nutrition

omega-3 fatty acids

omega-6 fatty acids

orthorexia

polyunsaturated fatty acids

probiotics

proteins

registered dietitian

saturated fatty acids

simple carbohydrates

sucrose

trace minerals

trans fatty acids

unsaturated fatty acids

vegan

water-insoluble fiber

water-soluble fiber

CRITICAL THINKING QUESTIONS

1. You are a personal trainer, and your new client says he wants to lose 10 pounds and get in shape. You are trying to decide whether he needs a referral to a dietitian for meal planning. What questions might you ask him? What information would make you decide to refer?

2. Your friend teaches a physical conditioning class at your college. You have agreed to come to her class and give a 30-minute talk on nutrition and health. How would you shape your talk, using information on the MyPlate website? List 10 main points you would like to make.

3. Your client has recently been diagnosed with type 2 diabetes, has met with a dietitian, and has decided to consume less soda. He has been drinking four cans a day. He seems prepared to make changes in this behavior. What are some questions you might ask the client to elicit ideas for behavior-change strategies? What are some strategies you might suggest?

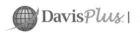 For additional resources log in to Davis*Plus* (http://davisplus.fadavis.com/ keyword "Brehm") and click on the Premium tab. (Don't have a *Plus*Code to access Premium Resources? Just click the Purchase Access button on the book's Davis*Plus* page.)

REFERENCES

Anderson, J. W., Baird, P., Davis, R. H., Jr., Ferreri, S., Knudtson, M., Koraym, A., . . . Williams, C. L. (2009). Health benefits of dietary fiber. *Nutrition Reviews, 67*(4), 188-205.

Baer, H. J., Glynn, R. J., Hu, F. B., Hankinson, S. E., Willett, W. C., Colditz, G. A., . . . Rosner, B. (2011). Risk factors for mortality in the Nurses' Health Study: a competing risks analysis. *American Journal of Epidemiology, 173*(3), 319-329.

Bailey, R. L., Gahche, J. J., Lentino, C. V., Dwyer, J. T., Engel, J. S., Thomas, P. R., . . . Picciano, M. F. (2011). Dietary supplement use in the United States, 2003-2006. *Journal of Nutrition, 141*(2), 261-266.

Bao, J., Atkinson, F., Petocz, P., Willett, W. C., & Brand-Miller, J. C. (2011). Prediction of postprandial glycemia and insulinemia in lean, young, healthy adults: glycemic load compared with carbohydrate content alone. *American Journal of Clinical Nutrition, 93*(5), 984-996.

Baranowski, T., Cullen, K. W., Nicklas, T., Thompson, D., & Baranowski, J. (2003). Are current health behavioral change models helpful in guiding prevention of weight gain efforts? *Obesity Research, 11*(S10), 23S-43S.

Barclay, A. W., Petocz, P., McMillan-Price, J., Flood, V. M., Prvan, T., Mitchell, P., & Brand-Miller, J. C. (2008). Glycemic index, glycemic load, and chronic disease risk: a meta-analysis of observational studies. *American Journal of Clinical Nutrition, 87*(3), 627-637.

Baumeister, R. F., & Tierney, J. (2011). *Willpower: Rediscovering the Greatest Human Strength.* New York: Penguin.

Benton, D., & Brock, H. (2010). Mood and the macro-nutrient composition of breakfast and the mid-day meal. *Appetite, 55,* 436-440.

Bjelakovic, G., Nikolova, D., Gluud, L. L., Simonetti, R. G., & Gluud, C. (2007). Mortality in randomized trials of antioxidant supplements for primary and secondary prevention: systematic review and meta-analysis. *Journal of the American Medical Association, 297*(8), 842-857.

Blanchard, C. M., Fisher, J., Sparling, P. B., Shanks, T. H., Nehl, E., Rhodes, R. E., . . . Baker, F. (2009). Understanding adherence to 5 servings of fruits and vegetables per day: a theory of planned behavior perspective. *Journal of Nutrition Education and Behavior, 41*(1), 3-10.

Blanchflower, D. G., Oswald, A. J., & Stewart-Brown, S. (2012). Is psychological well-being linked to the consumption of fruits and vegetables? *Social Indicators Research,* http://link.springer.com/article/10.1007%2Fs11205-012-0173-y. Accessed 12/12/12.

Blue, C. L. (2007). Does the theory of planned behavior identify diabetes-related cognitions for intention to be physically active and eat a healthy diet? *Public Health Nursing, 24*(2), 141-150.

Bolland, M. J., Grey, A., Avenell, A., Gamble, G. D., & Reid, I. R. (2011). Calcium supplements with or without vitamin D and risk of cardiovascular events: reanalysis of the Women's Health Initiative limited access dataset and meta-analysis. *British Medical Journal, 342,* d2040.

Carr, K. D. (2011). Food scarcity, neuroadaptations, and the pathogenic potential of dieting in an unnatural ecology: binge eating and drug abuse. *Physiology & Behavior, 104*(1), 162-167.

Cermak, N. M., Res, P. T., de Groot, L. C., Saris, W. H., & van Loon, L. J. (2012). Protein supplementation augments the adaptive response of skeletal muscle to resistance-type exercise training: a meta-analysis. *American Journal of Clinical Nutrition, 96*(6), 1454-1464.

Chan, A. L., Leung, H. W., & Wang, S. F. (2011). Multivitamin supplement use and risk of breast cancer: a meta-analysis. *Annals of Pharmacotherapy, 45*(4), 476-484.

Cheatham, R. A., Roberts, S. B., Das, S. K., Gilhooly, C. H., Golden, J. K., Hyatt, R., . . . Lieberman, H.R. (2009). Long-term effects of provided low and high glycemic load low energy diets on mood and cognition. *Physiology and Behavior, 98*(3), 374-379.

Chesler, B. E., Harris, B. G., & Oestreicher, P. H. (2009). Implications of emotional eating beliefs and reactance to dietary advice for the treatment of emotional eating and outcome following Roux-en-Y gastric bypass: A case report. *Clinical Case Studies, 8*(4), 277-295.

Chiu, C. -J., Klein, R., Milton, R. C., Gensler, G., & Taylor, A. (2009). Does eating particular diets alter the risk of age-related macular degeneration in users of the Age-Related Eye Disease Study supplements? *British Journal of Ophthalmology, 93*(9), 1241-1246.

Colombani, P. C., & Mettler, S. (2011). Role of dietary proteins in sports. *International Journal for Vitamin and Nutrition Research, 81*(2-3), 120-124.

Craig, W. J., Mangels, A. R., & American Dietetic Association. (2009). Position of the American Dietetic Association: vegetarian diets. *Journal of the American Dietetic Association, 109*(7), 1266-1282.

Denham, B. E. (2011). Dietary supplements: regulatory issues and implications for public health. *Journal of the American Medical Association, 306*(4), 428-429.

Di Noia, J., & Contento, I. R. (2010). Fruit and vegetable availability enables adolescent consumption that exceeds national average. *Nutrition Research, 30*(6), 396-402.

Di Noia, J., & Prochaska, J. O. (2010a). Dietary stages of change and decisional balance: a meta-analytic review. *American Journal of Health Behavior, 34*(5), 618-632.

Di Noia, J., & Prochaska, J. O. (2010b). Mediating variables in a transtheoretical model dietary intervention program. *Health Education and Behavior, 37*(5), 753-762.

Eckel, R. H. (2008). Egg consumption in relation to cardiovascular disease and mortality: the story gets more complex. *American Journal of Clinical Nutrition, 87*(4), 799-800.

Fuller, R., & Gibson, G. R. (2008). Probiotics and prebiotics: microflora management for improved gut health. *Clinical Microbiology and Infection, 4*(9), 477-480.

Genton, L., Melzer, K., & Pichard, C. (2010). Energy and macronutrient requirements for physical fitness in exercising subjects. *Clinical Nutrition, 29*(4), 413-423.

Harvey, J. N., & Lawson, V. L. (2009). The importance of health belief models in determining self-care behaviour in diabetes. *Diabetic Medicine, 26*(1), 5-13.

Haskell, C. F., Robertson, B., Jones, E., Forster, J., Jones, R., Wilde, A., . . . Kennedy, D. O. (2010). Effects of a multivitamin/mineral supplement on cognitive function and fatigue during extended multi-tasking. *Human Psychopharmacology: Clinical & Experimental, 25*(6), 448-461.

Heaney, R. P., & Layman, D. K. (2008). Amount and type of protein influences bone health. *American Journal of Clinical Nutrition, 87*(5), 1567S-1570S.

Hegarty, B. D., & Parker, G. B. (2011). Marine omega-3 fatty acids and mood disorders—linking the sea and the soul. *Acta Psychiatrica Scandinavica, 124*(1), 42-51.

Higgs, S., & Donohoe, J. E. (2011). Focusing on food during lunch enhances lunch memory and decreases later snack intake. *Appetite, 57*(1), 202-206.

Higgs, S., & Woodward, M. (2009). Television watching during lunch increases afternoon snack intake of young women. *Appetite, 52,* 39-43.

Hu, F. B., Manson, J. E., & Willett, W. C. (2001). Types of dietary fat and risk of coronary heart disease: a critical review. *Journal of the American College of Nutrition, 20*(1), 5-19.

Hu, F. B., Stampfer, M. J., Manson, J. E., Rimm, E., Colditz, G. A., Rosner, B. A., . . . Willett, W. C. (1997). Dietary fat intake and risk of coronary heart disease in women. *New England Journal of Medicine, 337,* 1491-1499.

Jakubowicz, D., Froy, O., Wainstein, J., & Boaz, M. (2102). Meal timing and composition influence ghrelin levels, appetite scores and weight loss maintenance in overweight and obese adults. *Steroids, 77*(4), 323-331.

Johnson, J. H., Haskvitz, E. M., & Brehm, B. A. (2009). *Applied Sports Medicine for Coaches.* Philadelphia: Lippincott, Williams, & Wilkins.

Kingsolver, B., with Hopp, S. L., & Kingsolver, C. (2007). *Animal, Vegetable, Miracle.* New York: HarperCollins.

Korinth, A., Schiess, S., & Wentenhoefer, J. (2010). Eating behaviour and eating disorders in students of nutrition sciences. *Public Health Nutrition, 13*(1), 32-37.

Lanham-New, S. A. (2008). Importance of calcium, vitamin D and vitamin K for osteoporosis prevention and treatment. *Proceedings of the Nutrition Society, 67,* 163-176.

Larsson, S. C., Akesson, A., Bergkvist, L., & Wolk, A. (2010). Multivitamin use and breast cancer incidence in a prospective cohort of Swedish women. *American Journal of Clinical Nutrition, 91*(5), 1268-1272.

Li, K., Kaaks, R., Linseisen, J., & Rohrmann, S. (2012). Vitamin/mineral supplementation and cancer, cardiovascular, and all-cause mortality in a German prospective cohort (EPIC-Heidelberg). *European Journal of Nutrition, 51*(4), 407-413.

Lichtenstein, A. H., Appel, L. J., Brands, M., Carnethon, M., Daniels, S., Franch, H. A., . . . Wylie-Rosett, J. (2006). Diet and lifestyle recommendations revision 2006: a scientific statement from the American Heart Association Nutrition Committee. *Circulation, 114*:82-96.

Michie, S. A., Whittington, C., McAteer, C., McAteer, J., Gupta, S. (2009). Effective techniques in healthy eating and physical activity interventions: a meta-regression. *Health Psychology, 28*(6), 690-701.

Muth, N. D. (2009). Nutritional considerations for an active lifestyle. In: Bryant, C. X., & Green, D. J. (eds.). *ACE Advanced Health & Fitness Specialist Manual*. San Diego, CA: American Council on Exercise.

Mursu, J., Robien, K., Harnack, L. J., Park, K. & Jacobs, D. R., Jr. (2011). Dietary supplements and mortality rate in older women: the Iowa Women's Health Study. *Archives of Internal Medicine, 171*(18), 1625-1633.

Oh, K., Hu, F. B., Manson, J. E., Stampfer, M.J., & Willett, W. C. (2005). Dietary fat intake and risk of coronary heart disease in women: 20 years of follow-up of the Nurses' Health Study. *American Journal of Epidemiology, 161*(7), 672-679.

Olson, J. H., Erie, J. C., & Bakri, S. J. (2011). Nutritional supplementation and age-related macular degeneration. *Seminars in Ophthalmology, 26*(3), 131-136.

Parylak, S. L., Koob, G. F., & Zorrilla, E. P. (2011). The dark side of food addiction. *Physiology and Behavior, 104*, 149-156.

Plotnikoff, R. C., Lippke, S., Johnson, S. T., Hotz, S. B., Birkett, N. J., & Rossi, S. R. (2009). Applying the stages of change to multiple low-fat dietary behavioral contexts: an examination of stage occupation and discontinuity. *Appetite, 53*(3), 345-353.

Pollan, M. (2009). *Food Rules: An Eater's Manual*. New York: Penguin Books.

Robinson, T. (2008). Applying the socio-ecological model to improving fruit and vegetable intake among low-income African Americans. *Journal of Community Health, 33*(6), 395-406.

Rodriguez, N. R., Di Marco, N. M., & Langley, S. (2009). American College of Sports Medicine position stand: nutrition and athletic performance. *Medicine and Science in Sports and Exercise, 41*(3), 709-731.

Sass, C., Eickhoff-Shemeck, J. M., Manore, M. M., & Kruskall, L. T. (2007). Crossing the line: understanding the scope of practice between registered dieticians and health/fitness professionals. *ACSM's Health & Fitness Journal, 11*(3), 12-19.

Siri-Tarino, P. W., Sun, Q., Hu, F. B., & Krauss, R. M. (2010). Saturated fat, carbohydrate, and cardiovascular disease. *American Journal of Clinical Nutrition, 91*(3), 502-509.

Smith, K. J., Gall, S. L., McNaughton, S., Blizzard, L., Dwyer, T., & Venn, A. J. (2010). Skipping breakfast: Longitudinal associations with cardiometabolic risk factors in the Childhood Determinants of Adult Health Study. *American Journal of Clinical Nutrition, 92*(6), 1316-1325.

Sniehotta, F. F. (2009). Toward a theory of intentional behaviour change: plans, planning, and self-regulation. *British Journal of Health Psychology, 14*(2), 261-273.

Soh, N., Walter, G., Baur, L., & Collins, C. (2009). Nutrition, mood and behaviour: a review. *Acta Neuropsychiatrica, 21*, 214-227.

Thomson, C. A., & Ravia, J. (2011). A systematic review of behavioral interventions to promote intake of fruits and vegetables. *Journal of the American Dietetic Association, 111*(10), 1523-1535.

U. S. Food and Drug Administration. (2009). *Overview of Dietary Supplements*. www.fda.gov/Food/DietarySupplements/ConsumerInformation/ucm110417.htm. Accessed 11/11/11.

Van Horn, L. (2011). Enhancing adherence to produce consumption: health benefits abound. *Journal of the American Dietetic Association, 111*(10), 1451.

Van Horn, L., McCoin, M., Kris-Etherton, P. M., Burke, F., Carson, J. A., Champagne, C. M, . . . Sikand, G. (2008). The evidence for dietary prevention and treatment of cardiovascular disease. *Journal of the American Dietetic Association, 108*(2), 287-331.

Vandereycken, W. (2011). Media hype, diagnostic fad or genuine disorder? Professionals' opinion about night eating syndrome, orthorexia, muscle dysmorphia, and emetophobia. *Eating Disorders, 19*(3), 291-293.

Willett, W. C., & Ludwig, D. S. (2011). The 2010 Dietary Guidelines—the best recipe for health? *New England Journal of Medicine, 365*(17), 1563-1565.

Wynn, E., Krieg, M. A., Lanham-New, S. A., & Burckhardt, P. (2010). Postgraduate symposium: positive influence of nutritional alkalinity on bone health. *Proceedings of the Nutrition Society, 69*(1), 166-173.

CHAPTER OUTLINE

LEARNING OBJECTIVES

After reading this chapter, you will be able to:

1. Discuss the meaning of body composition, how it is measured, and when body-composition assessments might be helpful.

2. List the areas where fat is stored in the body and the functions of these different stores.

3. Summarize the reasons why obesity is often associated with negative health effects and explain how in some cases people are obese yet healthy.

4. Describe the factors that influence energy balance, including factors related to both energy intake and energy expenditure.

5. Apply an ecological perspective to analyze factors that prevent or contribute to overweight and obesity.

6. Explain how behavior-change theories can be applied to weight-management programs.

7. Outline the behaviors and psychological factors most commonly associated with long-term weight-loss maintenance.

8. Describe how behavior-change skills are incorporated into successful weight-management programs.

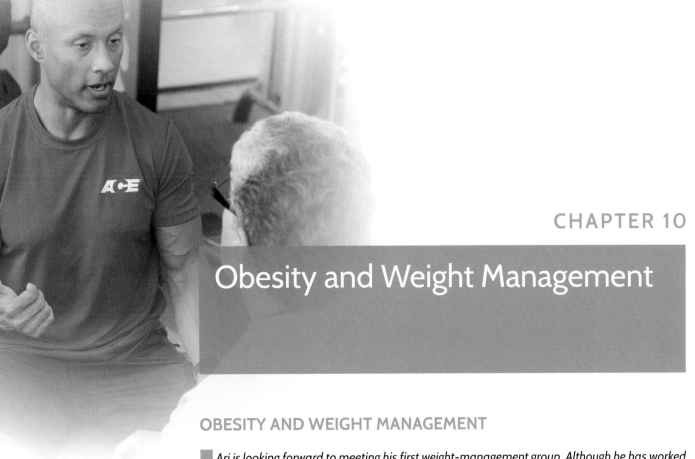

CHAPTER 10

Obesity and Weight Management

OBESITY AND WEIGHT MANAGEMENT

Ari is looking forward to meeting his first weight-management group. Although he has worked with clients trying to lose weight for several years, this is his first experience as a group leader. He has been hired by a local physicians' practice to run this group at the hospital's wellness center. All group participants have been referred by their providers and have been diagnosed with obesity and related health disorders such as hypertension or diabetes. They have also been referred to a dietitian who has helped them set up eating plans.

Ari himself lost about 30 lb several years ago through a combination of eating less and exercising more. He lost the weight on his own over a 2-year period and has kept it off, probably because his work as a fitness instructor and personal trainer get him to the gym every day. To prepare for this new work, he attended a weight-loss group for a few months, to see how the leader ran the groups and what kinds of issues tended to be discussed.

Ari is excited about his new work because he is making exercise the foundation of everyone's weight-management programs. Not only will all his clients attend the weekly group meeting, but they will also meet with Ari individually for five or six sessions to get started on a regular exercise program. Ari loves working out and hopes that people's positive exercise experiences plus the extra contact will lead to weight-loss success for his participants. ■

Lifestyle guidelines for good health are fairly clear in the area of weight control and obesity prevention: get regular physical activity, eat a balanced diet, and avoid overeating. But while some people have great success managing their body composition by adjusting food intake and activity levels, this sensible advice has failed to reverse the rising tide of overweight, obesity, and the chronic health problems that accompany disorders of excess body fat. With two-thirds of adults in the United States overweight or obese, it is imperative that health and fitness professionals improve their ability to work with this important demographic and develop the behavioral-counseling skills necessary to support healthy, lifelong weight management for their clients. Health and fitness professionals should expect to work with overweight and obese clients at some point in their careers. They should also understand the importance of helping clients develop the healthy lifestyles that may prevent obesity, which can develop gradually and unnoticeably over time.

This chapter begins with an introduction to the concepts of body composition and energy balance and then proceeds to explore the physiological, psychological, and sociological factors that contribute to obesity and associated health problems. Understanding what is causing excess weight or obesity in individual clients is the first step in developing effective behavior-change recommendations.

Research on the strategies used by people who successfully lose weight and maintain weight loss illustrates best practices for weight management. Such strategies are typically built on lifestyle change, and these will be explored in some depth in this chapter. Familiarity with evidence-based treatment recommendations for obesity will help health and fitness professionals work with clients to set reasonable behavior-change goals and develop intrinsic motivation for making positive lifestyle change.

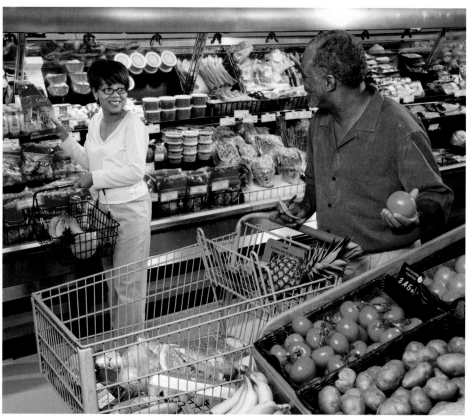

© Thinkstock

UNDERSTANDING BODY COMPOSITION

Health and fitness professionals should know that although clients and professionals alike talk a lot about "weight," often the amount, location, and activity of body fat is the underlying focus, especially when considering the health implications of obesity. Body composition refers to an estimate of how much of a person's mass is composed of fat. Body-composition estimates are sometimes helpful for planning weight-management strategies.

Body Composition versus Body Weight

In everyday conversation, the word *weight* generally refers to scale weight, the number that represents the gravitational effect on an object's mass. A person's body weight is easy to measure. Babies are weighed when they are born and regularly thereafter. Weight reflects a person's size and is often expressed in relation to one's height. Obviously, a taller person will usually have more mass and thus weigh more. One of the most-common weight-for-height measures of size is the body mass index, or BMI (Fig. 10-1). The higher the weight for a given height, the greater the BMI. A BMI of 25 or more is considered overweight, and a BMI of 30 or more is categorized as obese (Centers for Disease Control and Prevention, 2012a; Box 10-1). A BMI of 18.5 or less is considered underweight. Because information on weight and height is readily available, BMI is a very useful measure in epidemiological studies to describe variations in size among large groups of people. For example, the Centers for Disease Control

Body Mass Index

The body mass index (BMI) is used to determine who is overweight.

$$BMI = \frac{703 \times \text{weight in pounds}}{(\text{height in inches})^2} \quad OR \quad \frac{\text{weight in kilograms}}{(\text{height in meters})^2}$$

BMI score is at the intersection of height and weight.
A body mass index score of 25 or more is considered
overweight and 30 or more is considered obese.

Healthy weight   25 Overweight Limit   Overweight

Weight	100	105	110	115	120	125	130	135	140	145	150	155	160	165	170	175	180	185	190	195	200	205
Height																						
5-0	20	21	21	22	23	24	25	26	27	28	29	30	31	32	33	34	35	36	37	38	39	40
5-1	19	20	21	22	23	24	25	26	26	27	28	29	30	31	32	33	34	35	36	37	38	39
5-2	18	19	20	21	22	23	24	25	26	27	27	28	29	30	31	32	33	34	35	36	37	37
5-3	18	19	19	20	21	22	23	24	25	26	27	27	28	29	30	31	32	33	34	35	35	36
5-4	17	18	19	20	21	21	22	23	24	25	26	27	27	28	29	30	31	32	33	33	34	35
5-5	17	17	18	19	20	21	22	22	23	24	25	26	27	27	28	29	30	31	32	32	33	34
5-6	16	17	18	19	19	20	21	22	23	23	24	25	26	27	27	28	29	30	31	31	32	33
5-7	16	16	17	18	19	20	20	21	22	23	23	24	25	26	27	27	28	29	30	31	31	32
5-8	15	16	17	17	18	19	20	21	21	22	23	24	24	25	26	27	27	28	29	30	30	31
5-9	15	16	16	17	18	18	19	20	21	21	22	23	24	24	25	26	27	27	28	29	30	30
5-10	14	15	16	17	17	18	19	19	20	21	22	22	23	24	24	25	26	27	27	28	29	29
5-11	14	15	15	16	17	17	18	19	20	20	21	22	22	23	24	24	25	26	26	27	28	29
6-0	14	14	15	16	16	17	18	18	19	20	20	21	22	22	23	24	24	25	26	26	27	28
6-1	13	14	15	15	16	16	17	18	18	19	20	20	21	22	22	23	24	24	25	26	26	27
6-2	13	13	14	15	15	16	17	17	18	19	19	20	21	21	22	22	23	24	24	25	26	26
6-3	12	13	14	14	15	16	16	17	17	18	19	19	20	21	21	22	22	23	24	24	25	26
6-4	12	13	13	14	15	15	16	16	17	18	18	19	19	20	21	21	22	23	23	24	24	25

Figure 10-1. Body mass index.

Box 10-1. Overweight? Fat? What's in a Name?

This text uses the words *overweight* and *obese*, as these are the terms most commonly used by public health organizations around the world. Many people object to these terms, however, and for good reason. As previously noted, "overweight" is really a euphemism for overly fat, since excess fat is usually the problem. If the "extra" weight were bone or muscle, many people would be less concerned. Obese is a clinical term that medicalizes excess fatness. Not all obese clients are unhealthy, however, and resent the term.

The National Association for the Advancement of Fat Acceptance (NAAFA, www.naafa.org) prefers the term *fat* to overweight or obese. The mission of NAAFA is to fight size discrimination, which is rampant in North America and in most countries around the world. NAAFA suggests using the word fat to help people understand that people come in all shapes and sizes.

Should health and fitness professionals use these terms with clients? Most people prefer to not be labeled as overweight or obese, as both words have negative connotations. Nicer words might be heavyset, plump, or chubby, depending on the client's culture. It is usually best when working with clients to avoid labels entirely.

It should be noted that labels can be helpful in some settings if they encourage people to confront a situation they have been ignoring and motivate them to take action. For example, parents often deny the fact that their children are getting too fat. A doctor classifying them as "obese" and urging parents to improve family eating habits might lead to behavior change that could help slow the children's weight gain.

and Prevention collects weight and height data from samples in the United States every year to follow changes in obesity rates.

Although BMI provides some information about a person's size, it does not tell the whole story about the health or quality of that size (Box 10-2). Readers may be aware that large, muscular people, especially athletes, may have a high BMI but actually not be overweight in terms of being too fat. Similarly, people whose BMI is under 25 may actually be too fat because they have very little muscle mass and too much body fat (Romero-Corral et al., 2010). Nevertheless, BMI is the most commonly used indicator of underweight, overweight, and obesity. It is used by most physicians when evaluating patients and usually provides a good starting point for conversations about lifestyle and weight management.

In some cases, BMI (or weight) is all a health and fitness professional needs to monitor in clients adopting weight-control strategies. In other situations, measures of body composition can be helpful, if available. After all, health is more closely related to the volume and location of adipose tissue stores than weight per se (Cornier et al., 2011). Body-composition tests used in a health and fitness context typically divide body mass into fat mass (FM) and everything else, or fat-free mass (FFM). Some body-composition assessments also calculate bone mass. There are many ways to estimate body composition (Box 10-3). Some are used primarily in research and medical settings, whereas others are likely to be available in exercise physiology laboratories and in health and fitness facilities.

Box 10-2. Weight Can Be Misleading

Many health and fitness professionals have encountered clients who hold irrational beliefs about body weight. In fact, after years of regularly weighing themselves, some clients come to put more faith in what the scale says than what they can see in the mirror with their own eyes. Weight measurements carry much more weight (pun intended) than they should as people consider behavior-change goals.

Sometimes clients set an unrealistic goal weight, only to find they gain weight as they increase their exercise volume. It is not uncommon for such clients to quit exercising, even though the weight increase reflects a healthy increase in muscle size and strength, rather than an increase in fat tissue. Some clients may even experience their clothes fitting better, or getting looser, but are more concerned about the number on the scale than their actual size. Other clients, usually females, may stop exercising when they find clothes feeling tighter in the shoulders because they don't want to become more muscular.

Some people get excited when their scale weight drops following a single exercise session, even though this drop simply reflects a loss of body water and even a potentially unhealthy or dangerous level of dehydration. Similarly, clients may lose weight during an illness and several days of bed rest. Unfortunately, this weight loss probably represents muscle and bone loss and dehydration rather than an improvement in body composition.

A singular focus on weight sometimes drives people to practice harmful, or pathogenic, weight-control measures, discussed in more detail in the next chapter. These individuals will do anything to see a lower number as they step onto the scale, such as taking laxatives or diuretics or even vomiting after eating.

Day-to-day fluctuations in scale weight are common and often reflect changes in water volume. For example, it is common for women to gain a few pounds of water during the premenstrual phase. Many people weigh more the day after consuming a very salty meal. Health professionals usually recommend stepping on the scale once a week, rather than every day, and considering weight in the context of lifestyle change and body-composition measures. Weekly weigh-ins are important for people who have lost weight to be sure they are not gaining it back as they adjust calorie intake. But others who can't help weighing themselves 10 times a day may want to get rid of the bathroom scale and focus on lifestyle and how their clothes fit, rather than weight.

Box 10-3. Techniques for Estimating Body Composition

- **Hydrometry:** Hydrometry methods give an estimate of total body water (TBW), how much water is contained in a person's body. Because fat tissue contains very little water, finding out how much water is in a given body allows researchers to estimate fat mass and fat-free mass for a given body size. Subjects are given some form of tracer that diffuses into all water compartments. A sample of water, such as saliva, is taken and TBW is extrapolated from the tracer amount in the sample. Hydrometry procedures are expensive and used primarily for research and medical purposes.

Box 10-3. Techniques for Estimating Body Composition—cont'd

- **Dual-energy x-ray absorptiometry:** Dual-energy x-ray absorptiometry (DEXA) technology uses two x-ray energies to measure bone density and body composition. It is becoming common for older clients at risk for developing osteoporosis to receive DEXA scans to evaluate and monitor changes in bone density. DEXA technology is used to assess body composition primarily in research settings.
- **Medical imaging techniques:** Both magnetic resonance imaging (MRI) and computed tomography (CT) are used to assess body tissues and can be used to calculate body composition. MRIs and CT scans can also provide information on the location of adipose tissue stores. These techniques are used for research on body composition.
- **Hydrostatic weighing or underwater weighing:** For this test, a subject sits on a seat underwater. The seat is attached to a scale, which measures the person's weight. The heavier a person is in the water, the greater his or her density. Density refers to weight per volume. Two people with the same BMI may have different densities. A denser person has more FFM and less fat. By calculating density from water weight, a person's percentage of body fat can be estimated. Error can occur with this measure because the density of nonfat tissues, such as bone, varies from person to person, yet the test calculations rely on an average value. Similarly, body-composition prediction equations take into account the air remaining in the lungs after a complete exhalation. If this volume is estimated and not measured and/or if the person has difficulty exhaling and holding the breath underwater, body composition estimates will not be as accurate. Underwater weighing tanks are most likely to be found in research and academic settings, such as in kinesiology department facilities.
- **Air displacement:** Instruments such as the Bod Pod estimate body composition from air displacement. The heavier people are for a given size, the denser they are. As with underwater weighing, higher density means less fat tissue. Individual variations in tissue density reduce the accuracy of body-composition predictions. Air-displacement equipment is most commonly found in research and academic settings.

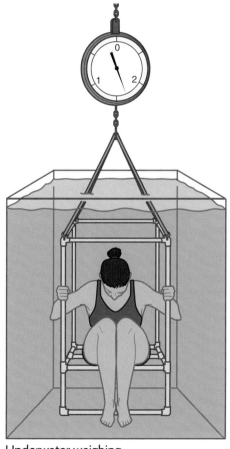

Underwater weighing.

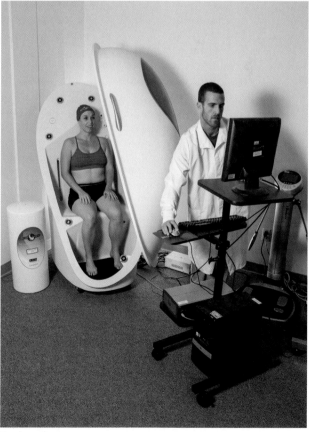

Bod pod.

Continued

Box 10-3. Techniques for Estimating Body Composition—cont'd

- **Bioelectrical impedance analysis (BIA):** BIA tests are based on the fact that fat tissue conducts electricity more slowly than nonfat tissue, which contains quite a bit of water. BIA equipment sends a weak electrical current through the body. The speed of the current reflects relative fatness. BIA measures assume a constant body water content for various tissues, so anything that alters hydration status or causes water retention will affect BIA body-composition estimates. Dehydration, premenstrual water retention, elevated muscle glycogen levels, and food in the stomach can interfere with the accuracy of BIA body-composition estimates. BIA equipment is found in many health and fitness facilities. Because equipment is quite portable and easy to use, BIA is often the technology of choice at health fairs.

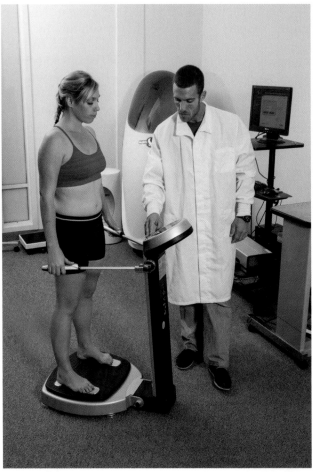

Bioelectrical impedance.

- Anthropometric measures: Anthropometry means "the measurement of human beings" and refers to measures that describe physical characteristics. The anthropometric measures used for estimating body composition include circumferences and skinfold thicknesses. Circumference in this context refers to the distance around a particular body part, such as the waist, hips, and upper arm. Circumferences are usually taken with a tape measure and then entered into an equation to predict body fat. Skinfold thickness is the thickness of the skin and layer of subcutaneous fat as it is pulled away from the underlying muscle. Skinfold thickness is measured with calipers at several standard anatomic sites. These measurements are then entered into prediction equations to predict body composition. Circumference and skinfold measures are most accurate when taken by an experienced test administrator. Even then, body-fat predictions based on these measures are often inaccurate, because the equations that are used are based on population averages and may not apply to a given individual. Some health and fitness professionals use circumferences and skinfolds as "stand-alone" measures. When taken over time, they can show changes in and of themselves, without predicting body composition from them. For example, if a person is losing fat, waist circumference may decrease. Anthropometric measures are the least-expensive but also the least-accurate means of estimating body composition.

Box 10-3. Techniques for Estimating Body Composition—cont'd

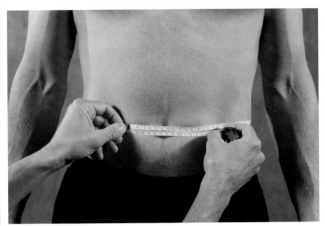

Measurement of body circumferences.

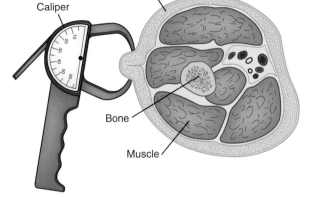

Skinfold measurement.

Researchers have a rough idea of the range of body fat percentiles that are normal and healthy for various population groups (Cornier et al., 2011; Heymsfield, Lohman, Wang, & Going, 2005), although less information is available for ethnic minorities. Unlike BMI-based definitions of overweight and obesity, no categorizations of obesity level have been established using body-composition measures (Ho-Pham, Campbell, & Nguyen, 2011). The healthy range for adult males can be anywhere from 6% to 24% and 14% to 31% for adult women, depending on the person's build and body type (Bryant, Green, & Merrill, 2013). Athletes tend to be leaner, although this varies by sport.

The most-accurate measures of body composition involve isotope turnover methods and nuclear imaging techniques, which are expensive and not readily available in most human-performance laboratories. In terms of accessible tests, bioelectrical impedance analysis (BIA) and air-displacement plethysmography appear to give the most-reliable results (Cornier et al., 2011).

Waist Circumference

Many health and fitness professionals now use waist circumference in addition to BMI to assess body fatness. Although waist circumference does not provide an estimate of body composition, it does provide information about torso mass. Excess fat stored in the abdominal region, especially inside the torso around body organs such as the liver and pancreas, exerts the greatest negative impact on health. The National Institutes of Health advise measuring the waist just above the iliac crests of the pelvis (the hipbones) (Cornier et al., 2011). Waist circumferences over 35 inches (88 cm) in women and 40 inches (102 cm) in men are associated with increased health risks, such as type 2 diabetes and hypertension.

When are Body-Composition Tests Helpful?

Body-composition tests are most helpful when used with other measures of fitness and presented as part of a larger picture. Body-composition tests can be helpful in several situations, including the following:

- An apparently lean person is gaining a little scale weight but appears to be getting more muscular, not fatter. Body-composition tests might assure lean or muscular people that they are not fat.
- A person has a normal BMI but lacks muscle size and strength. Such people may fall into the category of normal-weight obesity, which is associated with the same health risks as obesity (Romero-Corral et al., 2010). A body-composition test might help motivate these individuals to improve eating and exercise behaviors.
- An athlete is attempting to reach a specific weight category or weight minimum. Such athletes may find body-composition tests helpful to see if their weight goal is realistic.
- An individual has a high BMI but appears fairly muscular. A body-composition test can help reassure such people that they are not overly fat and should not focus on losing weight, unless other obesity-associated health risks indicate that some weight loss would be beneficial.

Can body-composition tests be helpful for clients engaged in weight-loss programs? Weight is usually a more-motivational measure, since it tends to change more quickly than body-composition measures. In fact, some of the weight lost when people shed pounds is often FFM, so body-composition measures may change very little (Cornier et al., 2011). This lack of change is very discouraging and misleading when people are making real progress. With obesity, weight loss is usually accompanied by many health benefits, even though body-composition measures do not show a big change.

If body composition is taken as part of the health and fitness assessment, it should not be the only or even the primary variable used to track improvement.

Body-composition tests are most accurate when performed by experienced professionals. If body-composition measures are taken over time, the same test should be used repeatedly and, if possible, the same professional should perform the test.

MOTIVATING CHANGE: Body-Composition Data and Motivation

Health and fitness professionals should think carefully before administering body-composition assessments. How will they contribute to client motivation? Body-composition tests are not helpful if they make clients feel bad and decrease self-efficacy. Skinfold and circumference measurements can be demoralizing. Many people, especially overweight people, do not like being measured in such a personal way. Having one's abdominal fat pulled or pinched by a technician can be embarrassing or demeaning.

The limited accuracy of most tests is also a problem. Although we tell clients we are "measuring" body composition, in reality these tests are only estimates. A client found to have 25% body fat may actually have anywhere from 21% to 29% body fat. Reinforce this point with clients, especially if they will be retested. Get them ready for the fact that this number may not change a great deal.

If you include body-composition assessment in your work, try to frame the results in ways that will increase client motivation. The Health Belief Model may be useful here. If body composition demonstrates obesity, this may help clients take their extra weight seriously. They may feel more susceptible to health problems associated with extra body fat. At the same time that you deliver this negative diagnosis, move to the good news: lifestyle changes can reduce these risks. Promote the psychological and physical health benefits of regular physical activity and healthy eating. Focus on the solution rather than the problem.

Adipose Tissue: Friend or Foe?

Many clients assume that all fat is bad fat. In fact, some adipocytes and adipose tissues are helpful. When discussing body composition with clients, health and fitness professionals should be able to help them understand that not all fat is created equal. There are various types of fat found in different areas of the body, including:

Essential Fat

A certain amount of body fat, called essential body fat, is required for even the leanest person. Fat is a component of bone marrow, nerves, the spinal cord, brain, and many other internal organs. Cell membranes are composed largely of fat. Pads of fat help cushion vital organs. Essential fat contributes about 3% to 5% of body mass.

Sex-Specific Fat

Females have an additional category of essential fat: sex-specific fat, found in the breasts, hips, and thighs. Sex-specific fat explains why the leanest of females is fatter than the leanest of males. A great deal of energy is required to run the menstrual cycle and to grow and nurse a baby; hence the extra energy stores. Sex-specific fat stores contribute about 5% to 9% of body mass in females.

Intramuscular Triglycerides

Some fat is found in muscle tissue, in the form of intramuscular triglycerides (IMTG). This fat stores energy and can be used to support muscular contraction during physical activity. In general, IMTG are most commonly used during submaximal exercise of medium intensity (Roepstorff, Vistisen, & Kiens, 2005). IMTG are also used along with muscle glycogen during resistance exercise (Harber et al., 2008). Research indicates that women use about twice as much IMTG as men during exercise (Roepstorff et al., 2005) and that exercise training improves skeletal muscle's ability to metabolize IMTG for fuel (Alsted et al., 2009). The ability to use IMTG for fuel may vary with glucose tolerance. For example, one study examined the use of IMTG in obese subjects with normal or impaired glucose tolerance, qualifying subjects for a diagnosis of prediabetes (Perreault, Bergman, Hunerdosse, Playdon, & Eckel, 2010). The average BMI of these men and women was about 31.5, and body composition was about 36% fat. The subjects were 45 to 70 years old and fairly sedentary. The researchers found that subjects with prediabetes had higher levels of IMTG and showed a lower rate of IMTG use at rest, compared with subjects with normal glucose tolerance. This research supports the observation that prediabetes has a wide range of effects upon energy-production systems and not just blood sugar regulation.

So are IMTG a good thing? Young, lean endurance athletes seek to maximize their utilization of IMTG stores to supply fuel for activities such as endurance running, cycling, and swimming. Trained muscles effectively draw on these stores, and IMTG stores contribute to performance. However, these stores are higher in older adults and not linked to improved performance. In fact, in older adults, while IMTG stores increase, the number of mitochondria decline. The triglycerides must get into mitochondria to be metabolized into energy. One study found that older men and women had more IMTG not in contact with mitochondria (Crane, Devries, Safdar, Hamadeh, & Tarnopolsky, 2010). Both old and young subjects had similar levels of daily physical activity, so the researchers concluded that muscle cells become less efficient at producing energy from IMTG with age. And, as noted above, obese individuals also have higher IMTG stores. So whether IMTG is good or bad depends upon the amount, as well as a person's age, training status, BMI, and glucose tolerance.

Subcutaneous Fat

Approximately a third of a person's body fat is stored under the skin. These fat stores are called subcutaneous fat. Some subcutaneous fat is helpful for insulation, which keeps heat within the body in cold weather. People who have observed (or remember being part of) a pool or lake full of children will recall the thinner ones having less tolerance for staying in cool water, whereas their heavier friends were comfortable for longer periods of time. On the other hand, people with extra subcutaneous fat lose heat less quickly in hot environments and are at greater risk of heat illness, especially during high-intensity and prolonged physical activity. Subcutaneous fat improves the appearance of the face, helping to support the skin. The faces of very thin people usually look older in later life than their heavier peers.

Brown Adipose Tissue

Brown adipose tissue (BAT) is a special type of fat that contains a higher density of capillaries and mitochondria than white fat. Brown fat cells generate heat and help mammals maintain body temperature in cool environments without shivering. Although most mitochondria produce adenosine triphosphate (ATP) to fuel metabolic processes, the mitochondria in BAT are "energy inefficient" for ATP production and produce *heat* from fuel precursors, such as glucose, instead of ATP. In addition to keeping people warm, BAT appears to help them get rid of extra calories by "burning them up" (turning them into heat) rather than storing them (Ravussin & Galgani, 2011). Researchers have speculated that the higher levels of BAT in lean compared with obese individuals may partly explain differences in body composition. Higher levels of BAT contribute to a higher resting metabolism and the ability to consume more calories without gaining weight. Once thought to be present in significant amounts only in infants, BAT has now been shown in adults through nuclear imaging techniques (Ravussin & Kozak, 2009).

Research suggests that regular exercise stimulates white adipocytes to become brown adipocytes (Bostrum et al., 2012). During exercise, a myokine dubbed irisin (named after the Greek messenger goddess Iris) is produced. Irisin moves from the muscle to the bloodstream and appears to communicate with white adipose tissue, "telling" it to develop into BAT, especially in the visceral area. Increasing irisin levels in the blood of mice results in an increase in energy expenditure, with no changes in physical activity level or food intake (Bostrum et al., 2012). Although exercise alone does not cause significant weight loss in most people, researchers speculate that stimulating the development of larger amounts of BAT may at least help prevent future weight gain and obesity-related disorders.

Visceral Adipose Tissue

Visceral adipose tissue (VAT) consists of fat stored around the abdominal organs, including the liver, stomach, intestines, and kidneys. Excess VAT appears to be the link between obesity and negative health effects such as artery disease, type 2 diabetes, hypertension, and inflammatory disorders (Cornier et al., 2011). Although waist circumference gives some information about central obesity (excess fat storage in the torso), it does not reveal whether the excess fat is subcutaneous or VAT. CT scans provide information on the volume of fat inside the abdomen, but, as previously noted, such tools are not yet commonly used for diagnosis. Symptoms such as the metabolic syndrome, with disorders of blood sugar and blood pressure regulation, indicate the need for lifestyle change to reduce VAT and restore normal metabolic functions.

Obesity and Health

Whether defined by BMI, body-composition assessments, or symptoms, obesity increases risk for several health problems. When people eat more calories than they burn, the body converts extra calories into triglycerides and packs the triglycerides into fat cells. Fat cells can grow larger as more fat is stored, but they cannot expand indefinitely. Weight gain and too much body fat interfere with normal metabolic processes in many ways that contribute to the chronic health problems that are more likely to arise with obesity.

Researchers believe that when people are gaining weight and their bodies are making extra triglycerides, expanding fat cells may become damaged, manufacture faulty proteins, or simply reach the end of their life expectancies when they get too full of fat (Iyer, Fairlie, Prins, Hammock, & Brown, 2010). It is possible that with obesity, adipocytes cannot keep up with the body's demand to store triglycerides. When this happens, immune cells called macrophages come in to help dispose of damaged and dead fat cells. The job of macrophages is to disarm potential attackers, like bacteria and viruses, by engulfing and digesting them. They try to attack triglycerides and dead fat cells in this manner but are often overwhelmed by the challenge. Macrophages, in turn, release cytokines, such as interleukins, that summon more white blood cells and lead to more inflammation (Fig. 10-2).

Another interesting messenger affected by adipose stores is adiponectin. Higher levels of body fat have been associated with lower levels of adiponectin (Liu et al., 2012). Adiponectin helps insulin do its job of getting sugar from the bloodstream into cells where it can be stored or burned for energy. This observation may help explain the insulin resistance that often develops with obesity (Liu et al., 2012). Adiponectin also helps regulate the metabolism of lipids. Adiponectin appears to have an anti-inflammatory effect on the cells that line the artery walls.

Inflammation is helpful for healing a wound, but chronic inflammation can interfere with a number of important biochemical processes in the body. Several of obesity's negative health effects are thought to be the

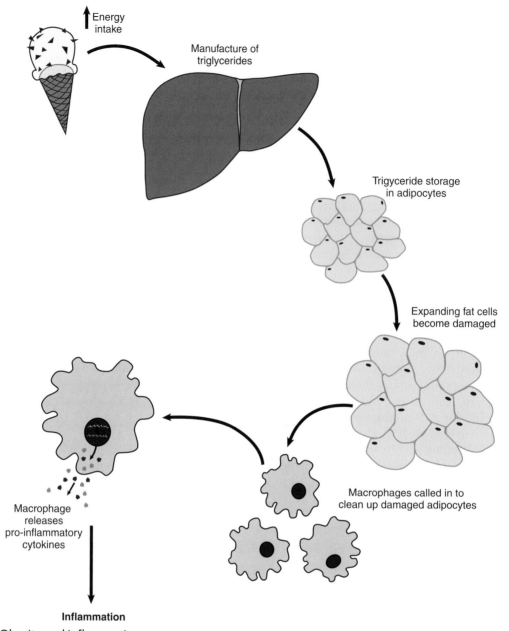

Figure 10-2. Obesity and inflammation.

result of inflammation in the fat tissue (Bliss, 2006). Other negative health effects may result from the extra weight imposed upon the musculoskeletal system. The most-common negative health effects of obesity include the following:

- **Type 2 diabetes and heart disease:** Diabetes may result when some of the chemicals produced by the macrophages interfere with blood sugar regulation. These chemical messengers prevent the body's cells from responding appropriately to the hormone insulin, which signals cells to take up sugar (glucose) from the blood. High blood sugar levels in turn cause more damage, including accelerated aging of the arteries, thus contributing to artery disease, the leading cause of heart disease and stroke. High blood sugar also causes damage to the eyes, kidneys, and nerves.

- **Hypertension:** High insulin levels create a stress response in the body, raising levels of stress hormones and activating the fight-or-flight response. This can contribute to hypertension.
- **Risky blood lipid levels and heart disease:** Excess triglyceride production (from excess calories) raises levels of blood fats, including blood triglycerides and low-density lipoprotein (LDL) cholesterol levels. These lipids contribute to the formation of arterial plaque and more inflammation, as macrophages attempt to deal with damaged arteries.
- **Other inflammatory disorders:** The inflammation caused by obesity may contribute to other disorders associated with inflammation, such as liver disease, pancreatitis, asthma, and rheumatoid arthritis. Obesity also increases risk for Alzheimer's disease (Juhasz, Foldi, & Penke, 2011).

- **Cancer:** Obesity is associated with increased risk for many types of cancers. Researchers have suggested that fat tissue may secrete chemicals that make people more susceptible to cancer. The inflammation associated with VAT may promote the transformation of precancerous cells into cancer cells, so that the immune system is aiding in cancer promotion rather than destroying dangerous cells (Balkwill, 2009; Stix, 2007). Adipose tissue may also promote existing cancers in other ways. For example, higher levels of adipose tissue increase estrogen levels, and estrogen promotes the growth of certain types of cancers, such as ovarian and breast cancer. In addition, excess subcutaneous fat may decrease the efficacy of cancer screenings, hiding cancer tumors. Health professionals emphasize, however, that this research is preliminary and advise that cancer patients not lose weight, as extra weight can be protective once cancer has already developed.
- **Nonalcoholic fatty liver disease:** Excess fat can be deposited in the liver. Excessive alcohol intake can also cause excess fat deposits, so nonalcoholic fatty liver disease is diagnosed when fatty liver develops in people who drink little or no alcohol. In severe cases, the fat that accumulates in the liver can cause inflammation and scarring.
- **Physical strain:** The physical strain of excess weight can overload weight-bearing joints such as the hips, knees, and feet, and accelerate development of the joint degeneration and pain associated with osteoarthritis. Excess weight in the belly can alter posture and cause back problems.

Fit and Fat: Is Obesity Always Risky?

Scientists have engaged in a heated debate about the health risks of obesity for decades. When does too much fat lead to the health risks discussed above? Is it too much fat that causes diabetes, hypertension, heart disease, and stroke? Or is it the sedentary lifestyle that tends to accompany obesity (Fig. 10-3)?

Research suggests that these diseases are probably caused by both (Gill, Baur, & King, 2010; Weiler, Stamatakis, & Blair, 2010). Overweight people with healthy lifestyles, including good eating habits and regular physical activity, have lower health risks and rates of premature mortality than their normal-weight but sedentary friends (McAuley & Blair, 2011). For example, a study done at the University of South Carolina followed 14,345 middle-aged men for 11 years (Lee et al., 2011). The researchers looked at changes in weight and fitness over that time, as well as causes of death for subjects who died during the study period. Subjects whose fitness improved during the study had a 44% lower rate of all-cause mortality than subjects whose fitness declined. Interestingly, this observation held regardless of whether the subjects' weight changed or not, and it held for normal-weight and overweight subjects. (The study included subjects who were overweight but not obese, as defined by BMI.) Similarly, subjects whose fitness stayed the same over the 11 years experienced a 30% percent lower rate of all-cause mortality than subjects whose fitness declined, independent of changes in body weight. The study did find that men who experienced an increase in BMI had a higher rate of cardiovascular events, such as heart attacks, than men who did not show an increase in weight.

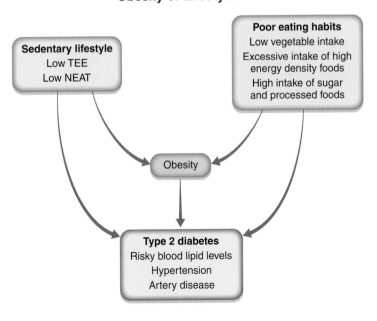

Negative Health Effects: Obesity or Lifestyle?

Figure 10-3. **Obesity or lifestyle?**

It is likely that the process of manufacturing and storing extra triglycerides explains part of the negative health effects associated with obesity. People actively gaining body fat may experience more obesity-related health problems than overweight and obese people who are in energy balance or actively losing body fat.

> **MOTIVATING CHANGE:** Obesity Treatment: Focus on Lifestyle
>
> Studies such as those discussed previously that find fitness and a healthy lifestyle reduce the health risks associated with obesity reinforce the importance of behavior change to achieve a healthy lifestyle rather than a specific scale weight. Many overweight and obese clients may never reach a BMI under 25. Knowing that physical fitness may reduce the negative health effects associated with obesity may help motivate clients to increase physical activity levels and eat a healthy diet. As clients develop a healthy lifestyle, they may even lose a little extra fat along the way.

ENERGY BALANCE AND BODY FAT

When trying to reduce fat stores by coaxing the body to use fat for energy, an understanding of how the body "decides" to use fat for energy is helpful. To stimulate the body's fat-utilization processes, people must create an energy deficit, or negative energy balance. Energy balance refers to the relationship between energy taken in (or eaten) and energy expended, or "burned." A negative energy balance means that more energy is expended than taken in (Fig. 10-4). Over time, a negative energy balance will result in pushing the body to use stored fat for energy, causing weight loss. A positive energy balance means that more energy is consumed, or eaten, than expended. Over time, a positive energy balance encourages the body to store energy as adipose tissue.

Creating the best conditions for fat loss is not as easy as it sounds, however. Many factors influence energy balance, so simply eating less does not always result in more fat loss. For example, sometimes the body compensates for reduced energy intake by conserving energy expenditure. Understanding the many factors that influence energy balance can help health and fitness professionals guide clients seeking to reduce body fat stores.

Energy Intake

Physiologists used to believe that all calories are equal. However, now an increased understanding of the way that foods and their nutrients behave in the body and the complex biochemical processes in which they participate has overturned this mechanistic view of calories. Some studies suggest that the metabolic effects among foods differ in ways that lead to variable effects on cardiovascular risk factors. For example, one interesting

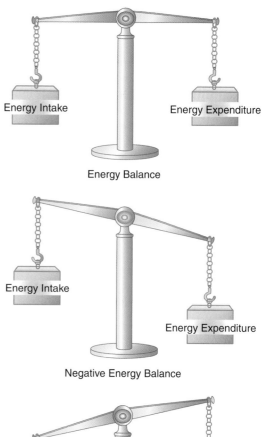

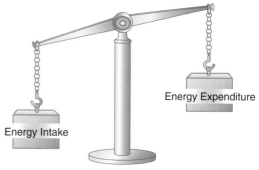

Figure 10-4. **Energy balance.**

study compared groups limiting calorie intake. One group included only whole-grain foods when consuming grains or grain products, and the other group was asked to avoid whole-grain foods (Katcher et al., 2008). Both groups consumed the same number of calories and lost the same amount of weight over the 12-week study. However, the whole-grain group lost more body fat from the abdominal region. At the end of the study, subjects in the whole-grains group also had greater decreases in C-reactive protein (CRP) level, a marker of inflammation, than subjects in the other group (Katcher et al., 2008).

An interesting meta-analysis examined a number of studies on the health effects of the consumption of sugar-sweetened beverages (SSBs), including sodas, sweetened fruit drinks, sports beverages, sweetened ice tea products, sweetened vitamin waters, and other sweetened beverages. The researchers found that higher consumption of SSBs was associated with higher risk of developing the metabolic syndrome and type 2 diabetes (Malik et al., 2010). Studies have also suggested that beverages sweetened with fructose may be more likely to contribute to obesity and obesity-related health disorders than those sweetened with glucose. One such study found that fructose-sweetened beverages increased visceral adiposity and blood lipids and decreased insulin sensitivity in overweight and obese people (Stanhope et al., 2009). Fructose is primarily metabolized in the liver to form triglycerides. This process is associated with an atherogenic blood lipid profile, including increased levels of blood triglycerides and LDL cholesterol and lower levels of HDL cholesterol (Bray, 2007).

The types of foods consumed throughout the day also have a major effect on people's level of hunger and feelings of well-being. Feelings of hunger can rise even though people have consumed "enough" calories if those calories have been stored and blood sugar falls. As discussed in Chapter 9, food choices can also influence mood and stress level, which in turn can influence eating behavior. People seeking to reduce food intake must devise eating strategies that help them feel nourished and nurtured, minimize feelings of hunger, and do not trigger the body's fat-storage pathways.

Energy Expenditure

Daily energy expenditure refers to the total amount of energy used in a 24-hour period and is commonly measured in calories. The body expends energy in many different ways. Metabolism refers to the entire collection of biochemical processes that occur in the body, many of which require energy. Most bodily functions require energy, from digesting food to contracting the muscles needed to walk down stairs. Metabolic rate is the energy expenditure required to sustain metabolism in a given time period, usually expressed per hour.

Most people are familiar with the terms "metabolic rate" and "metabolism" and generally use these words to mean how quickly the body consumes fuel, or burns calories. People often seek advice on how to get the most calorie-burning power from their workouts and lifestyle so that they can lose weight or eat more without gaining weight. People who gain weight easily or have difficulty losing weight often attribute their problems to a sluggish or slower-than-average metabolism, and they hope for tricks to speed up the metabolic machinery of their bodies. Metabolic rate at any given moment depends on activity level and the biochemical processes occurring in the body. Daily energy expenditure is often divided into several components, including the following.

Basal and Resting Metabolic Rate

Basal and resting metabolic rate are both terms that refer to the energy required just to stay alive in a resting state. Basal metabolic rate, or BMR, is measured when a person is awake but resting and lying down. Resting metabolic rate, or RMR, is taken in a seated position. RMR consumes well over half of the calories required in a 24-hour period.

The Thermic Effect of Food

The thermic effect of food (TEF) refers to the energy required for the processes of digestion and absorption. The term "thermic" refers to energy expenditure. This word is used because all of the body's energy expenditure processes generate heat; by measuring heat (calories), scientists can calculate energy use.

Why does eating take energy? Energy is required to chew food, contract the muscles of the gastrointestinal (GI) system, produce digestive enzymes and fluids, and absorb nutrients from the digestive system into the lymphatic system or bloodstream. TEF expends about 10% to 15% of people's daily caloric requirements.

The Thermic Effect of Exercise

By far, the most-significant effect on metabolic rate is achieved with exercise. The thermic effect of exercise (TEE) refers to the calories used during exercise. During moderately vigorous physical activity, metabolic rate increases by a factor of 10 or more, burning hundreds of extra calories. The more vigorous the exercise, the more calories expended. After vigorous activity, metabolic rate remains elevated for the time it takes for the body to return to resting level.

Nonexercise Activity Thermogenesis

The term nonexercise activity thermogenesis (NEAT) was coined by James Levine to describe activities that do not fall into the categories of sleeping, eating, or exercise (Levine, 2004). In this context, Levine uses the word exercise to refer to activity performed specifically for the purpose of playing sports or physical conditioning. NEAT includes all other activities such as taking the stairs, chewing gum, and jiggling around while seated, as well as the activities of daily living, such as grocery shopping, cooking, and cleaning. NEAT can expend hundreds of calories per day and exert a significant effect on energy balance. High levels of NEAT appear to have significant health benefits. On the other hand, research has found that long periods of sitting, even for people who exercise regularly, are associated with increased risk of obesity and metabolic syndrome (Healy et al., 2008).

What Factors Influence Metabolic Rate?

Many factors influence metabolic rate, so anything that affects these factors will influence the idle of the metabolic engine, both at rest and during activity. One of the most-significant factors is size, especially the amount of metabolically active tissue. Muscle is one of the most metabolically active tissues, so a large, muscular person will have a higher RMR than a small, obese person. This is why increasing muscle mass will increase RMR and why larger people can eat more than smaller people without gaining weight.

All sorts of chemicals affect RMR. Several hormones, including the catecholamines and the thyroid hormones, help regulate metabolic processes. The levels of these vary with genetic profile, age, stress level, and many other factors. Many drugs, such as nicotine, some diet pills, and stimulants such as caffeine, raise metabolic rate.

Dietary manipulations to increase TEF include eating several small meals at regular intervals, rather than one large meal, and consuming a high-protein diet (Farshchi, Taylor, & MacDonald, 2005; Lejeune, Westerterp, Adam, Luscombe-Marsh, & Westerterp-Plantenga, 2006). Proteins have a higher TEF than carbohydrates and fats. The cumulative effect of dietary manipulations is relatively small but may be helpful for some people, especially if dietary changes also reduce hunger and food cravings and lead to a lower calorie consumption each day.

On the other hand, severe calorie restriction reduces TEF and can also lead to physiological suppression of a variety of metabolic functions in an effort to conserve energy in the face of starvation. For example, body temperature may fall. Some women stop menstruating when calories are severely restricted. People may also experience fatigue and conserve energy by reducing NEAT.

RMR slows as people age, due partly to loss of muscle tissue, but partly to the aging process, which leads to changes in many physiological parameters, including various hormone levels.

The very best way to increase energy expenditure is to move (Box 10-4). Both NEAT and exercise have the capacity to expend a high number of calories throughout the day. Regular physical activity is an essential component of any weight-management program.

Box 10-4. Lifestyle Recommendations for Increasing Daily Energy Expenditure

The best strategy for increasing daily energy expenditure is to include a good amount of physical activity into one's day. Recommendations for increasing daily energy expenditure include the following.

Exercise
All types of physical activity require muscle contraction, which in turn requires energy. Exercise mode should match a person's fitness level and preferences. Those new to exercise should start slowly and build gradually. Activity recommendations should be safe and not cause injury.

Consider interval training
People who like high-intensity exercise and are in pretty good shape might try interval training, which allows one to exercise at very high intensities for short periods of time. These high-intensity periods are interspersed with bouts of lower-intensity work. High-intensity exercise requires a longer recovery, which means people burn a few extra calories during the post-exercise period. People new to exercise should build some strength and endurance before attempting interval training. People who don't really enjoy working out may still appreciate interval training because it requires less time than lower-intensity exercise.

Strength train regularly
Regular resistance training has many beneficial health and fitness effects, such as strengthening muscles, joints, and bones. It can also increase muscle mass somewhat, depending on a person's age, sex, and hormonal profile. More muscle mass means people burn a few more calories per hour even when resting. And, of course, people burn even more calories during strength-training workouts.

Get more daily activity
People increase daily energy expenditure when they take advantage of opportunities to be active throughout the day. They burn more calories taking the stairs than riding the elevator. People can try to walk to do their errands when possible, play with their kids, or take longer walks with their dogs. Screen time should be limited, since it can actually cause metabolic rate to drop below normal resting level (depending on what is viewed).

Consume protein with meals
It takes more calories to digest protein, and a high protein intake may also reduce hunger. People should replace high-carbohydrate, empty-calorie foods with proteins such as eggs, beans, soy products, fish, nonfat dairy products, and lean meats. People with kidney problems should only increase protein intake after checking with their physicians.

Get adequate sleep
One might think that since people burn more calories awake than asleep, getting less sleep would help someone lose weight. However, shorter sleep duration is associated with higher levels of ghrelin, feelings of hunger, and greater incidence of obesity. Daytime fatigue can also reduce daily energy expenditure.

> ## Box 10-4. Lifestyle Recommendations for Increasing Daily Energy Expenditure—cont'd
>
> **Avoid very-restrictive dieting**
> People trying to lose weight are often frustrated by the fact that as they diet, metabolic rate slows and weight loss stalls. Limiting calorie intake too severely can depress resting metabolic rate, a reaction known as the "starvation response." The body goes into energy-conservation mode to cope with a food shortage. Although one must decrease food intake to lose weight, experts usually recommend decreasing intake by only about 250 calories per day, if one's diet is fairly healthy to begin with, and consuming at least 1,200 to 1,600 calories daily.
>
> **Enjoy flavorful food and smaller portions**
> Delicious food pleases the appetite, so people are satisfied with less. Smaller portion sizes and high-fiber foods also help limit calorie intake. People who enjoy spicy foods may find that these decrease hunger and slightly increase resting metabolic rate.

■ *Ari's first group meeting gets off to a good start. What a talkative group! Several of the participants are old hands at dieting, but several in the group have never thought much about their lifestyles before. As soon as he talks for a few minutes about energy balance, the questions start. "Is there any way to increase my metabolic rate?" "Is it better to eat a few big meals or many small meals during the day?" "What are the best times of day to eat?" "Do some types of exercise stimulate metabolic rate more than others?" "Does it take more calories to digest grapefruit than the number of calories in the grapefruit itself?"*

Ari takes a deep breath and advises the group not to worry about pieces of advice that might help them burn a few extra calories here or there. "The real answer to increasing metabolic rate and energy expenditure is physical activity. Sure, you have to eat less, but getting more exercise will allow you to eat a normal amount of food; plus, you'll feel better and look better as well, as you build muscle and burn fat. You want to increase your metabolic rate? Get moving!"

Silence in the room. What is wrong? "Exercise takes too much work," one of the participants sighs. "It's boring," another chimes in. "You only burn a few hundred calories. That's hardly a piece of cheesecake!" a third bemoans. Ari wonders if maybe getting these folks hooked on exercise might be harder than he thinks. ■

Weight Control and Obesity Prevention: Energy Balance Requires Physical Activity

Although the big picture of weight control and obesity is complex and filled with many interacting variables, the bottom line is very simple, as stated at the beginning of this chapter. To reduce body fat stores and prevent obesity, people must eat less and exercise more. Most people are familiar with the advice to eat less, but some are still reluctant to accept the fact that regular physical activity is an essential component of energy balance.

Health and fitness professionals can already discuss the long list of physical and psychological benefits of regular physical activity. Exercise reduces risk of obesity-related disorders for those already overweight and obese. Especially important are the psychological benefits of physical activity. Too often, weight loss is a dreadful experience of restriction and denial: don't eat this, avoid that. Adding exercise can boost sagging determination and burn a few calories along the way.

Experts believe that sedentary people's daily energy expenditure has dropped so low that it is difficult for them to eat fewer calories than they burn. It may not be possible to compensate for such low energy expenditure with dietary change. Theoretically, even if people are expending very few calories, consuming even fewer calories should lead to a loss of body fat. And, indeed, weight loss does occur on low-calorie diets. This approach to obesity prevention and treatment has not been very successful over the long term, however. A vast majority regain the lost weight in a matter of months unless they add a significant amount of physical activity to their daily lives (Mitchell, Catenacci, Wyatt, & Hill, 2011). It is likely that very-low calorie intakes are unrealistic for most people to maintain over time. So, in order to eat a reasonable and nourishing amount of food, people must increase energy expenditure. As weight control and obesity treatment recommendations are discussed, health and fitness professionals will note that regular physical activity is assumed to be a component of every behavior-change program.

OBESITY AND ENERGY IMBALANCE: Ecological Perspectives

Health and fitness professionals are already familiar with many of the factors that contribute to a positive energy balance. Those preparing to help clients address weight issues should be able to use an ecological perspective to understand variables that contribute to positive energy balance in individuals and in groups. Understanding which factors may be changed and which factors may limit or interfere with behavior-change efforts can enable professionals to help clients design effective yet realistic weight-management programs.

Intrapersonal Level

People's genetic predisposition strongly influences how they respond to their environment. An individual's behaviors in turn interact with genetic predisposition to influence feelings of hunger, food choices, and engagement in physical activity.

Genetics

For centuries, scientists have observed enormous individual variation in body types, body composition, and the factors that contribute to energy balance. During the past three decades, studies of twins have led to the conclusion that genetic variation explains 40% to 75% of the variation in BMI among people (O'Rahilly & Sadaf Farooqi, 2008). Research in 5,092 twin pairs 8 to 11 years old found that genetics explained 77% of variation in waist circumference (Wardle, Carnell, Haworth, & Plomin, 2008). Researchers believe that a genetic predisposition to obesity allows an "obesogenic environment" to enable expression of obesity through long-term positive energy balance.

For some individuals and ethnic groups, genetic predisposition for obesity is especially strong. Their "thrifty" genes allow them to capture every calorie that they consume and efficiently store energy, primarily as fat, against future lean times. Unfortunately, in an environment where food is plentiful, these thrifty genes translate almost automatically into obesity.

Obesity genes may work in different ways for different people. They may influence the amount of brown adipose tissue that people develop and thus their ability to "waste" extra calories as heat. Genes may influence RMR and the rate at which certain energy-expending biochemical reactions occur in the body. People also vary in their tendencies to sit quietly for long periods of time or inability to sit still for more than a few minutes, and thus in NEAT. Genes also appear to influence individual experiences of hunger and satiety and preferences for certain foods.

Genes influence a person's size and shape. People usually look like others in their family. Everyone has noticed that some people are short and stocky with a tendency to be both muscular and heavy, whereas others are tall and slender, and many more are in between these types. The location of fat stores in the body also appears to be inherited. Some people may have lean upper bodies but heavy legs and thighs, or the other way around. Some women are busty and curvaceous, and others are not. Despite programs that promise "body sculpting," most of a person's shape is bequeathed by Mother Nature. Although some fat stores can be reduced with lifestyle-modification programs, it

is not possible to direct which fat stores will be drawn from first. Similarly, strength training can increase muscle size in some people, but they inherit the basic shape of their muscles.

Psychophysiological Signals: Hunger, Satiety, and Appetite

The psychophysiological signals that prompt eating and food choices vary greatly from person to person. Weight-management efforts are most effective when people work with their bodies. For example, the sensation of hunger is one of the strongest physiological drives. Behavior-change programs that ask people to ignore this important feeling may create stress and even lead to binge eating in response to hunger. Hunger is not meant to be ignored. Hunger is a healthy signal that prompts creatures to search for food and to eat. Since eating is essential for survival, Mother Nature has endowed animals with a strong urge to consume tasty food. Unfortunately, the physiological systems that may have worked well in the past can complicate people's efforts to avoid overeating today. People trying to alter eating behaviors must understand how to reduce feelings of hunger and the drive to overeat.

The term hunger refers to the biological drive to eat. Hunger's opposite, a feeling of having had enough to eat, is called satiety. Many different hormones and physiological systems influence feelings of hunger and satiety. For example, the hormone ghrelin is released by the stomach, and as ghrelin levels rise, hunger increases (Fig. 10-5). As one eats, these levels fall as the stomach senses the presence of food. Similarly, as food reaches the small intestine, it releases several neurochemicals, including cholecystokinin, which promote many digestive processes and tell the brain the body is no longer ravenous.

Another important chemical messenger is the hormone leptin. Leptin is manufactured in several places, including fat cells. Leptin levels help inform the body (including the brain) about total fat stores. It helps regulate other physiological functions as well, including reproduction and glucose metabolism. In general, higher leptin levels are associated with less hunger, although this relationship appears to be disrupted in people who are obese. Indeed, obesity is often associated with leptin resistance, where cellular receptors do not respond correctly to the presence of leptin. On the other hand, congenital leptin deficiency, where leptin

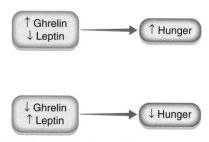

Figure 10-5. Ghrelin, leptin, and hunger.

levels are too low, has been associated with early-onset severe obesity in humans and laboratory animals. It is likely in these cases that excessive hunger, driven by low leptin levels, motivates people to overeat.

Appetite refers to a psychological desire to eat. Appetite is affected by hunger, of course; however, hunger refers to a strictly physical drive while appetite includes other physical and psychological drives. Appetite can prompt people to eat even in the absence of hunger. Who hasn't had the experience of finishing a large meal, feeling full or even stuffed, and still wanting the tasty dessert being served?

A "healthy appetite" encourages people to eat an assortment of foods with a variety of colors, flavors, and textures. This helps people consume adequate amounts of the more than 40 nutrients needed to stay healthy. Appetite makes eating pleasurable and helps people enjoy their food.

Although strong hunger and appetite signals encourage survival in a climate of scarcity, they cause people to overeat when food is abundant. People have a natural preference for the tastes of fat, salt, and sugar, which can lead to the consumption of too many processed, high-calorie foods.

But it gets worse. The modern lifestyle not only presents people with a wide array of delicious food. Several health behaviors can increase the drive to overeat, alter appetite, and interfere with the sensation of satiety, including the following:

- **Food choices:** One might think that a calorie is a calorie, but the body thinks differently. Some foods make the body think it has had a satisfying meal, while others don't seem to connect with hunger level the way they should. Foods high in fiber, such as fruits, vegetables, and whole grains, lead to more stomach fullness than foods high in fat and lower in volume. Warm broth-based soups and big delicious salads help eaters feel satisfied with fewer calories. Experts suggest that the stomach expects a certain volume of food and doesn't turn off the hunger signal until this is reached (Rolls, 2009). Many desserts and snack foods are high in calories but low in volume and are especially likely to lead to overeating.

  Beverages often add calories. Although increasing the water volume of a meal by adding more water in the form of vegetables decreases food intake (Rolls, 2009), the same is not true of beverages consumed with a meal. One study found that when caloric beverage portion increased at a meal, subjects did not adjust meal volume or calories and thus consumed more calories (Flood et al., 2006).

  Diet sodas seem to increase hunger and risk of obesity for many people. One interesting study followed a large number of middle-aged and older men and women over the course of 10 years (Nettleton et al., 2009). People who consumed at least one diet soda per day were more likely to have an increase in waist circumference and fasting blood glucose levels during that time period than other subjects. Could it be that people gaining weight might consume more diet sodas? In this study, diet soda consumption actually preceded the increase in waist circumference, so other factors must help explain this association. Researchers speculate that diet sodas may (1) increase people's desire for sweet foods, (2) interfere with the body's ability to estimate energy needs and energy intake, and/or (3) cause people to overestimate the number of calories "saved" by opting for diet soda and then consume more food as a result.

  Meals and snacks that lead to a sharp rise in blood sugar and a fast high-insulin response are typically followed by earlier hunger signals. Meals high in protein, fiber, and healthy fats lead to a lower rise in blood sugar and insulin and delay the return of hunger.

- **Sleep habits:** Even a single night of missed sleep is accompanied by a rise in ghrelin and a higher intake of calories (Knutson, Spiegel, Penev, & Van Cauter, 2007). Chronic sleep deprivation has become more common over the past several decades, and some researchers speculate that this is one of the reasons that obesity rates are rising in many countries (Knutson et al., 2007).

- **Chronic feelings of excess stress:** A lack of relaxation and chronic high levels of stress affect feelings of hunger and satiety as well as appetite. Although some people lose their desire to eat when feeling stressed, the majority of people tend to eat more than usual, perhaps turning to food for comfort (Roberts, 2008). Since food intake alters neurotransmitter levels and behavior in the central nervous system (CNS), food can indeed soothe. Stress may also leave people with less time to shop and plan healthy meals, so they grab whatever is near with less thought for nutritive value.

- **Emotional eating:** Research has demonstrated that food cues exert powerful effects on the CNS, especially in areas that integrate emotion, arousal, cognition, and energy balance (Blum, Liu, Shriner, & Gold, 2011). Food cues include food's appearance, taste, and smell, or even just thoughts about food. Studies have also found that food intake, independent of food cues, can affect emotion. In one study, volunteers received infusions of fat or saline directly into the stomach (Van Oudenhove et al., 2011). The infusion of fat, but not saline, was associated with less sadness in response to exposure to music and images that evoke sad emotions. The researchers believe that bodily signals, such as those from the digestive system, influence the brain as it regulates emotion. People can learn, on both conscious and subconscious levels, to use food to help them regulate emotions. Thus, people trying to lose weight should use comfort foods wisely and learn alternative coping skills.

- **Knowledge-based work:** Several intriguing studies have found that people eat more after performing demanding mental tasks than after sitting quietly (Chaput & Tremblay, 2007). People whose jobs involve challenging mental work (students take note!) may find themselves eating more. The brain uses glucose for energy, so perhaps the energy required by knowledge-based work lowers blood sugar level. In addition, the brain uses glucose when exerting self-control, which is often required for knowledge-based work.

- **Physical activity level:** Many people are afraid to exercise because they fear exercise will increase hunger. Ironically, people who engage in moderate exercise usually eat the same or only a few more calories than they do on days when they don't exercise (Elder and Roberts, 2007). In fact, appetite may even decrease with exercise for men, who are also more likely than women to see a decrease in fat stores with exercise alone (Hagobian & Braun, 2010). People often lose their appetites after a hard workout; even though they compensate later, they still come out ahead in that energy intake more closely matches their energy expenditure. In addition, exercise may reduce hunger for some people by improving sleep quality and reducing feelings of stress.

Health and fitness professionals can teach clients about the interactions among lifestyle, hunger, appetite, and satiety. They can help clients learn to tune into their feelings of hunger and satiety and work with their bodies to feel nourished and satisfied from their meals and snacks.

Portion Sizes Influence Individual Eating Behavior

The availability of food seems to motivate people to eat or continue eating even in the absence of hunger or the presence of satiety. Obesity researchers have proposed that larger portion sizes push people to overeat (Rolls, 2007). If extra food is on people's plates, they tend to eat more than they should (What's the Evidence? 10-1). In many fast-food restaurants, the more people order, the better the bargain. But the more people order, the more they eat. Portion sizes in many restaurants have increased over the years. Portion sizes of individual foods have also grown steadily. An average bagel weighed 2 to 3 ounces and contained 230 calories in the 1970s. Today, the average bagel is twice as large with about 550 calories. A serving of French fries in the 1970s contained about 30 fries and 450 calories. Today many establishments serve large orders of 50 fries and 790 calories. Interestingly, a serving of French fries, according to the USDA MyPlate guide, is only 10 fries, at 160 calories. Portions have also grown for soft drinks, candy bars, hamburgers, muffins, and many other food items.

WHAT'S THE EVIDENCE? 10-1

Large Portion Sizes Encourage Overeating

Rolls, B. J., Roe, L. A., & Meengs, J. S. (2007). The effect of large portion sizes on energy intake is sustained for 11 days. *Obesity, 15*(6), 1535-1543.

■ PURPOSE

Previous research had shown that increasing portion sizes was associated with increased food consumption at single meals and over the course of a few days. Rolls and colleagues wondered if people might compensate for a few days of overeating by spontaneously decreasing consumption during subsequent days, in order to maintain energy balance. The purpose of this study was to follow people presented with large portion sizes for 11 days to see if they would compensate for the first few days of overeating or continue to overeat during the entire study period.

■ STUDY

Volunteers consisted of 23 normal-weight and overweight people, including 10 women and 13 men. The researchers provided all foods and beverages for two different conditions. Each condition lasted 11 days, and conditions were separated by a 2-week interval. Volunteers received standard food and beverage portions during one period and portions that were 50% larger during the other period. The researchers recorded food and beverage intake.

During the 11 days with larger portions, both men and women increased daily calorie intake by about 423 kcal. The increase was sustained over the entire study period. A significant increase in consumption was observed for all meals and snacks and in all food categories except fruit as a snack and vegetables. The BMI of participants did not influence the effect of portion size on food intake.

■ IMPLICATIONS

This study supports the idea that larger portions lead to overeating and to weight gain. Health and fitness professionals should counsel weight-management clients on the importance of controlling portion sizes to prevent overeating.

People can develop new eating habits once they become aware of how large portions push overeating. When eating out, especially at fast-food restaurants, they can avoid bargains that promise better value if one orders more food. When restaurant portions are too large, people can split a meal with a friend or take the leftovers home for a meal the next day. People who can't resist cleaning their plates can order soup and salad. At home, people can serve small portions and eat slowly.

Interaction Between Lifestyle and Genetics
It is likely that lifestyle and genetics interact during the development of obesity. Research has demonstrated that dietary factors and excess body fat appear to be associated with damage to the hypothalamus, an area of the brain that helps regulate hunger and thirst. Studies in mice have found epigenetic changes associated with both high-fat diets and with leptin deficiencies. In one study, both high-fat diet and leptin-deficient states altered the expression of genes and then, through these changes, neuron behavior in the hypothalamus (McNay, Briancon, Kokoeva, Maratos-Flier, & Flier, 2012). Mice receiving a high-fat diet showed suppressed neurogenesis. Leptin-deficient mice also generated fewer new neurons and lost hypothalamic neural stem cells.

Research on both mice and humans has found an association between obesity and inflammatory damage with significant structural and functional changes in the hypothalamus (Thaler et al., 2012). Researchers speculate that poor dietary choices may contribute to obesity not only by adding empty calories but also by damaging the hypothalamus. Damage to the hypothalamus can lead to feelings of hunger even after having eaten enough. This could conceivably lead to a vicious cycle of increasing hunger driving poor eating behaviors, which in turn cause more damage to the hypothalamus and more hunger.

Gastrointestinal Microbiota
Intriguing research on the interaction of human cells with the organisms living in the GI tract suggest that these interactions have wide-ranging effects. These organisms, including bacteria, viruses, and other single-celled organisms, are called microbiota; the total collection is known as the microbiome. The number of microbiota cells inhabiting the body outnumber human cells 10 to 1. A majority of these, approximately 100 trillion organisms, inhabit the GI tract (Salzman, 2011). The bacteria in the digestive tract interact with components from the food passing through and with the cells lining the GI tract. Dietary components influence the type and activity of these bacteria, which in turn influence several variables related to health, including immune response and inflammation (Tilg, 2012).

Antibiotics exert strong effects on the composition of the microbiome, as these drugs kill bacteria indiscriminately. Interesting research has found that antibiotic administration may increase body fat levels. Indeed, livestock farmers have used this observation to their advantage; adding antibiotics to animal feed increases weight and fat gain, along with profits. In one study, when antibiotics were given to human subjects to eliminate the stomach bacteria H. pylori, thought to contribute in some cases to stomach ulcers, levels of the hormone ghrelin failed to fall after a meal, remaining six times higher than postmeal levels before antibiotic administration (Francois et al., 2011). Normally, ghrelin levels fall after a meal and hunger declines. Since higher ghrelin levels trigger hunger, this change may be one of the factors associated with increased obesity resulting from antibiotic administration. In fact, BMI increased in these subjects during the 18 months of the study.

Interesting studies in mice and humans suggest that certain types of bacteria are associated with obesity. In particular, a bacterial family known as Firmicutes appears to be good at extracting energy from the digestive mass in the gut and churning out small fatty-acid molecules that are easily absorbed by the human host (Kallus & Brandt, 2012). On the other hand, more bacteria from the family Bacteroidetes are associated with leanness. Obese mice and humans tend to have higher Firmicutes:Bacteroidetes ratios. This ratio may help explain why lean mice gain weight in the laboratory when researchers cause the intestines of the mice to become colonized by the bacteria from the obese mice (Turnbaugh et al., 2006).

It is not surprising that the activity of microbiota exert a strong influence on human physiology. The collective number of genes in the microbiome is approximately 100 times higher than the number of genes in a single human organism (Tsai & Coyle, 2009). That amounts to a great deal of cellular activity, as the microbiota respond to dietary components, substances produced by neighboring bacteria, and the biochemicals produced by human cells. In addition to generating more energy substrates for human absorption, the microbiota may also contribute to obesity by influencing levels of inflammation or promoting fat deposition (Tsai & Coyle, 2009).

A few studies have found that specific probiotic supplements can change body fat level (Kadooka et al., 2010). It is probably too early to begin recommending treatments based on these interesting studies, although including yogurt with a variety of cultures and probiotic supplements in the diet appear to be helpful for some. But these data reinforce the fact that scientists still have a long way to go in understanding the role of the microbiota and the many physiological factors that influence energy balance and body composition. These studies also reinforce the complexity of body composition and energy balance in any given individual. They may help explain why some people remain overweight even when restricting food intake and increasing physical activity levels.

Knowledge, Skills, Attitudes, and Habits
People bring a variety of knowledge, skills, and attitudes to their weight-management work. Those with positive

attitudes and skills for physical activity will have more success in this realm. Similarly, individuals familiar with food shopping and preparation may have a head start for changing eating behavior. People vary in their levels of self-efficacy for changing weight-management behaviors and their attitudes toward this work.

Habits accumulated throughout the years can settle in and strongly influence body weight. For example, mindless eating can cause overconsumption of food. Reading, watching media, and working while eating may interfere with a person's ability to respond appropriately to satiety signals. Sedentary habits may lead to an aversion to physical activity.

MOTIVATING CHANGE: Encourage Clients to Work With Their Bodies

In the process of following weight-loss diets, many clients may have quit trying to work with their bodies, or even listen to the physiological cues that guide eating behavior. Although the popular imagination paints overweight people as having little self-control, many in fact have exerted incredible self-control at various times in their lives, usually to follow a very-restrictive, low-calorie diet. Eating only according to rigid cognitive rules may decrease people's awareness of their own mind–body signals that guide eating behavior.

Health and fitness professionals should ask clients to become aware of feelings of hunger and satiety during the first few weeks working with them. They might wish to note and rate hunger and satiety levels at each meal or snack. Similarly, they might become aware of what kinds of food they feel like eating. Are they looking for something starchy and warm? Crunchy? Sweet? Salty? Many people have tried to tune out hunger, appetite, and satiety sensations and have difficulty listening to their bodies and minds. Eating in a quiet, mindful way is helpful for sensing body cues (Chapter 9).

People trying to lose weight may not be able to avoid hunger entirely. Many clients will need to live with some degree of hunger to lose weight. Can they learn to interpret a little hunger as a sign that their bodies are burning fat? Do they experience anxiety when they have hunger feelings? Does hunger lessen with a cup of tea or with physical activity? Does their eating schedule need adjustment?

What did clients learn? If they respond to this kind of work (some don't), encourage them to work with these cues. Help them come up with ways to eat that decrease hunger, such as eating at regular times throughout the day, including protein and healthy fats at each meal and snack, and so forth. When they start to feel full, maybe they can try to stop eating, even if there is still some food on the plate. Leftovers are great. Can they use their appetites to feel more nourished by their meals? They should try to eat foods they enjoy as much as possible, while still including enough vegetables.

Regular physical activity is essential for normalizing energy balance. Help clients become aware of the psychological benefits of activity, especially feelings of energy and positive mood, if not during exercise then hopefully after. Match exercise programs to client activity preferences and fitness level and avoid injury. Over time, clients may increase their self-confidence in listening to their bodies and using their innate mind-body communication to better regulate energy balance and enjoy life.

Interpersonal Level

Chapters 8 and 9 have reviewed the many ways interpersonal factors can influence physical activity and eating behaviors, and thus, energy balance. Friends, family, and other close relationships sway people to consume certain types of foods and participate in physical activity or to be inactive (Fig 10-6). Close relationships can prompt people to eat when they are not hungry, form positive associations with certain types of foods and eating rituals, and develop habits of physical activity.

In addition, studies suggest that when friends and family gain weight, obesity may become more acceptable to an individual. An interesting study examining weight changes in 12,067 participants in the Framingham Study found that risk of weight gain increases when a person's close friends and family members gain weight (Christakis & Fowler, 2007). Subjects in this study experienced a 57% increase in risk of gaining weight (above what would normally be predicted to occur over time) if a close friend gained weight. Risk increased by 40% if a sibling gained weight and by 37% if one's spouse gained weight. Although researchers could not pinpoint any particular causes for these associations, they ruled out shared environment as the strongest influence: the effect of close friends did not vary with proximity to the subject. In other words,

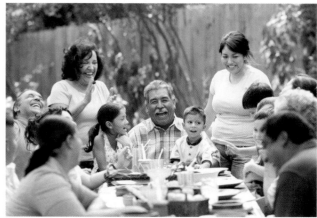

Figure 10-6. Interpersonal relationships influence physical activity and eating behaviors. © Thinkstock

whether best friends lived thousands of miles apart or in the same town, the effect was the same. Instead, the researchers proposed that friends and family affect each other's *perception* of fatness and change each other's ideas of what kind of body size is acceptable.

Organizational Level

Organizations such as workplaces, recreational groups, and health-care systems influence the many variables that contribute to body composition. For example, some work cultures value long hours at the job, which tends to be sedentary. Such cultures limit time for healthy activities such as exercise, grocery shopping, and cooking. High stress and not enough sleep translate into increased risk of obesity for many people.

On the other hand, as people have come to understand the high health costs of obesity, many organizations are trying to change their culture to promote more-healthy lifestyles, as discussed in previous chapters. Some health insurance groups adjust insurance premiums according to BMI. Many organizations offer incentives for participation in physical activity.

Community Level

The community level includes neighbors and the built environment, both of which can exert strong influences on physical activity and eating behaviors and, thus, on body weight. Of course, community often overlaps with interpersonal relationships and socioeconomic status. But an interesting study that randomly assigned participants to housing groups that varied in neighborhood conditions found that level of neighborhood poverty was associated with changes in body weight (Ludwig et al., 2011). These researchers followed 4,498 women with children living in public housing in high-poverty urban areas, where at least 40% of residents had incomes below the federal poverty threshold. The U.S. Department of Housing and Urban Development randomly assigned these women to one of three groups. The first group received vouchers for housing that were only valid if the women moved to an area with low poverty rates (less than 10% of residents with incomes below the poverty level), combined with counseling on moving. The second group received traditional vouchers and no counseling on moving. The third group received no vouchers or counseling. The subjects were followed for over 10 years. The first group, with subjects who moved to neighborhoods with less poverty, experienced small but significant reductions in the prevalence of extreme obesity (BMI > 35) and diabetes, while the other groups did not.

The researchers were unable to show which elements of lower-poverty neighborhoods might have caused a reduction in the rates of extreme obesity, but it is likely that many factors were involved. It is possible that single mothers felt less stressed in neighborhoods with less poverty or perhaps had more support from neighbors. Choices in places to shop for food may have exerted an influence on eating behaviors. School programs for the children may have affected behaviors in both children and their mothers. More options for physical activity may have been available. Whatever the reasons, this study at least suggests that neighborhood can make a difference in residents' body weight.

Many public-health experts are urging people to help their communities become healthier places to live. Miriam Nelson, well known for her excellent research on lifestyle and health, promotes healthy weight control along with community action (Nelson and Ackerman, 2011). While encouraging women to consume fewer added sugars and refined grains, the authors of *The Social Network Diet: Change Yourself, Change the World,* also urge readers to form Change Clubs and take on projects that will promote healthier lifestyles in their communities. Women are encouraged to select projects meaningful to them, such as improving school lunch options, promoting bike and walking trails, and forming supportive social networks.

College campuses provide an interesting example of communities that have a strong influence on the lifestyles of residents (Box 10-5; Health Psychology in Your Life 10-1). Students who commute to campus can also experience changes in weight because of erratic schedules, juggling work and classes, and a lack of time to shop for food or plan and prepare balanced meals.

Societal and Cultural Level

Societal forces can push people out of energy balance. Government policies, food production and distribution structures, and social and cultural norms regarding eating and exercise behavior, as well as acceptable body size, all influence the choices that people make on a daily basis. Economic forces drive consumer behavior. Social critic, author, and journalist Michael Pollan blames the U.S. obesity epidemic at least in part on farm subsidies from the federal government that push the production of too much corn, which becomes grain-fed meat and high-fructose corn syrup in too many supersized fast-food meals (Pollan, 2006).

Pollan also points out that Americans tend to have a fattening attitude about eating behavior. Instead of savoring small portions of delicious food, Americans prefer to consume the most calories for the lowest price. Researchers have remarked on the so-called French paradox, which refers to the observation that while French cuisine is high in fat and calories, the French have much lower rates of obesity and heart disease than people in the United States. How do the French not become obese on such rich food? They enjoy delicious meals, snack less frequently, and consume less sugar. The high fat content of the diet may lower hunger and decrease calorie intake. The French value a good meal, consume plentiful amounts of vegetables and fruits, and focus on dishes made with fresh, local, high-quality ingredients (Ferrieres, 2004).

Box 10-5. Does College Life Cause Weight Gain?

Many students do gain weight in college, although in general the average weight gain is well below the mythical "freshman 15." One study found that on average, college women gained just under 4 lb during their 4 years of college (Racette, Deusinger, & Strube, 2008). Yet this is still a concern if those few extra pounds represent the beginning of the gradual increase in body fat that tends to occur in adults in North America. And some students do gain 10 or 20 lb or even more, and plunge deeply into struggles with obesity and body image that may last several years or even a lifetime.

The change in body weight among college students is not always a bad thing. Some students are still growing, and weight gain merely represents normal growth. Other students began school underweight. And, of course, over the 4 years, some students lose weight, sometimes because of stress and a loss of appetite. However, sometimes they lose weight because they develop healthy eating and exercise habits that help promote a healthy body weight. Many factors influence how a student's body weight will respond to college life including:

- **College environment:** Students who leave home to go to college must adapt to a new environment. Life on a college campus is often marked by erratic schedules and regular opportunities to party. Some students adapt fairly quickly and establish a new routine that supports their ability to make the most of the academic and social challenges. Others have more difficulty settling in. Changes in weight usually reflect the lifestyle that a student develops. Some colleges do more than others to nurture healthy habits, but in the end it is usually up to the individual student to be sure he or she develops a healthy lifestyle.

- **Activity level:** Unless the student is an athlete or attends exercise classes, college life is a fairly sedentary one. Although students tend to walk from place to place, they also spend much of their time studying, reading, and writing—all sedentary activities. Students who do not sign up for an activity class of some sort, join a sports team, or participate regularly in campus recreation activities may get little exercise. This lack of activity contributes to weight gain and also to feelings of stress.

- **Stress:** Many students encounter emotional challenges during the college years. First-year students are especially likely to feel homesick and lonely, missing family and friends back home. The stress of difficult classes, roommate issues, and other problems that normally arise in life can make the college years even more challenging. Feelings of stress often cause changes in appetite and eating behavior. Food is familiar and can serve as a stand-in for missing family.

- **Fatigue:** Fatigue increases hunger, as higher ghrelin levels drive people to overeat. Students are notorious for skipping sleep and pulling all-nighters to complete assignments. Of course, a lack of time management and study skills, coupled with procrastination, are often the real culprits of sleep deprivation.

- **Knowledge-based work:** Knowledge-based work increases feelings of hunger and can drive excessive snacking. The boredom sometimes associated with completing homework assignments can also lead to snack attacks.

- **Dieting:** Ironically, students who try to lose weight by severely restricting food intake may end up gaining weight. Diets are often followed by periods of overeating as the dieter gives in to hunger and food cravings. Unfortunately, dieting behavior and more-serious disordered eating behaviors are very common on college campuses.

- **Social eating:** Most college social events involve food, from dining hall meals to campus parties. People are more likely to overeat in social settings, especially in all-you-can-eat dining halls where dessert is served at every meal. Parties encourage excess alcohol consumption and snacking.

Adapted from Johnson, J.H., Haskvitz, E.M., & Brehm, B.A. (2009). *Applied Sports Medicine for Coaches.* Baltimore: Lippincott Williams & Wilkins, p. 176. Used with permission.

HEALTH PSYCHOLOGY IN YOUR LIFE 10-1. An Ecological Perspective on Your College

Consider the factors mentioned in Box 10-5. Using an ecological perspective, outline the factors on your campus that influence eating and exercise behaviors as well as body weight. Consider both barriers and promoters of healthy-lifestyle behaviors.

Behavioral economists promote the idea of using economic theory to guide consumer behavior (Thaler & Sunstein, 2008). For example, governments can levy taxes to raise the price of undesirable behaviors (e.g., junk food) and subsidize healthy behaviors (fruits and vegetables). This approach has gradually made tobacco products more expensive in many countries and, hopefully, discouraged smoking. Perhaps this approach could help guide better food choices.

Many public-health efforts are under way to promote a better energy balance and a healthier lifestyle. The CDC (2012b) offers a variety of ideas for communities to implement in their efforts to reduce obesity. The website also has a legislative database that enables users to find state bills related to physical activity and nutrition.

By the third week, the 12 participants in Ari's group have learned each other's names, and only two people have been avoiding their personal training sessions with him. The conversations have been juicy, and sometimes Ari can hardly get a word in. Today's topic is environmental pressure to overeat. This seems to strike a chord with almost everyone. One of the participants, Janet, seems to have thought about this a great deal. "It's no wonder we are a nation of fatties," she complains. "Opportunities to eat are everywhere. And we love to eat! We eat while we have meetings, go shopping, watch television, go to the movies, and drive in the car. And on top of that we have three meals a day! When we eat in restaurants, a serving provides enough food for two people. When we go to a party and are overwhelmed with the variety of good food, we try a little of everything.

"How do thin people do it? I've lost weight lots of times, but it always comes back on within a year. I'm fine while I'm 'on the diet,' but when the diet's over, the endless temptations gradually call me back to my true self and what has become my true size. Is there any way I can learn to eat more carefully when everyone and everything around me seems to be telling me to eat more?"

Ari calls for suggestions from the group, and many thoughtful suggestions are given. Ari smiles as he listens to all of the good advice. "If I had just lectured for an hour on this advice, they would all be asleep by now." He is pleased that the participants have gotten into the spirit of group work so quickly.

BEHAVIOR-CHANGE THEORIES AND WEIGHT MANAGEMENT

A large percentage of people attempting to change physical activity, eating, and other lifestyle behaviors are also trying to change their weight. The behavior-change theories and their applications to physical activity and eating behaviors discussed in earlier chapters are helpful when weight management is the goal. This section will not repeat all of the information about behavior-change theories presented previously but will instead highlight important applications for weight management and obesity treatment.

The Transtheoretical Model and Stages of Change

Applying the Stages of Change Model to weight-management programs can be somewhat tricky, because it requires addressing several different behaviors simultaneously. Some changes come more easily than others, and people may be ready to change some behaviors but not others. For example, a client might already be entering the action stage in terms of reducing foods with added sugars but have doubts about his or her ability to stick to an exercise program. This scenario is common for people with a history of obesity. They may have avoided exercise because physical activity was embarrassing or difficult for them but may have had plenty of practice dieting. When working with clients who are trying to lose weight, health and fitness professionals may want to assess stage of change for diet and exercise separately and use appropriate intervention strategies according to readiness to change.

Is the Stages of Change Model helpful for people trying to lose weight? Research suggests that taking a stages of change approach can be moderately helpful compared with a "usual care" approach, according to one meta-analysis (Tuah et al., 2011). This analysis examined randomized controlled clinical trials that compared these two approaches for weight control in overweight or obese adults. Five studies met the criteria for inclusion in the analysis, with a total of 3,910 subjects. The five studies varied between 6 weeks and 24 months in length, and stages of change approaches yielded a slightly greater weight loss. In addition, a stage-based approach did tend to produce more diet and exercise behavior change, so health improvements other than weight loss may have occurred for many of these subjects; and more weight may have been lost if behaviors were maintained for longer time periods.

The Health Belief Model

The Health Belief Model highlights factors involved in forming a decision to change behavior. This model can provide topics of discussion for health and fitness professionals working with clients in the precontemplation and contemplation stages of change. This may be most likely in medical settings with people newly diagnosed with obesity-related disorders, such as type 2 diabetes or hypertension, where the Health Belief Model may be helpful. Educating clients about their health risks (susceptibility and severity) and the importance of behavior change (understanding the health behavior's benefits in terms of addressing the health risks) may help clients form a decision to change (Fig. 10-7). Discussions can help clients address barriers to performing the health behavior and their self-efficacy for performing target behaviors. Such information may not only help clients move toward a decision to change but will also help guide professionals in formulating recommendations to accommodate clients' readiness to change and self-efficacy for taking on specific behaviors. Research on people who have successfully maintained large weight losses has found that a majority of success stories began when people received specific medical information that motivated them to lose weight, thus supporting the Health Belief Model (Wing & Phelan, 2005).

The Theory of Planned Behavior

Similarly, the Theory of Planned Behavior provides directions for discussion (Fig. 10-8). Exploring people's

attitudes, both positive and negative, regarding possible behavior change can gently nudge clients still weighing the pros and cons of change. Through discussion, people can explore the reasons behind their attitudes. Discussing clients' perceptions of social norms regarding exercise and eating behaviors can uncover potential benefits and barriers. As health and fitness professionals explore these factors with their clients, clients may move toward forming an intention to change and thus a stronger likelihood of sticking to their behavior-change programs.

Self-Efficacy

Asking people about self-efficacy in terms of physical activity and dietary change can guide health and fitness professionals' expectations and recommendations. Like readiness to change, self-efficacy is behavior specific. Open questions and mindful listening usually allow health and fitness professionals to guide conversations to questions of self-efficacy for exercise behaviors, as

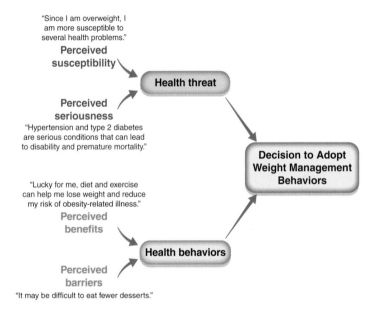

Figure 10-7. The Health Belief Model and weight management.

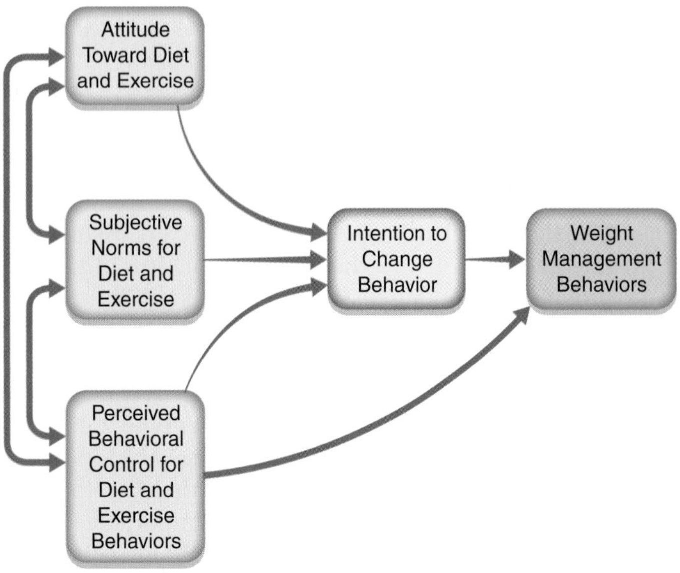

Figure 10-8. The Theory of Planned Behavior and weight management.

well as eating behaviors. Weight-management program behavior expectations should match clients' levels of self-efficacy. As clients are successful in following behavior-change recommendations, hopefully self-efficacy will grow stronger.

Self-Determination Theory and Motivation

Because societal and cultural forces can create great shame and low self-esteem for overweight people, many clients embark upon weight-management programs with mixed feelings and unrealistic ideas about what weight loss will help them achieve in life (Puhl & Heuer, 2010). For some, concepts of body size and personal body image have become tightly interwoven with feelings of self-worth and explanations for their present circumstances. Too often, weight becomes the reason for everything: problems in relationships, unrewarding work, financial difficulties, or global unhappiness. Many overweight people report postponing the pursuit of important personal goals until they lose weight. When weight is lost, people may be disappointed to find they are still themselves and that they have not been magically transformed. The same problems remain. The stigmatization of obesity is associated with increased rates of unhealthy eating, lower levels of physical activity, and psychological disorders such as anxiety and depression (Puhl & Heuer, 2010).

What does all of this have to do with motivation for weight loss? As discussed in Chapter 4, autonomous motivation for behavior change, motivation that grows out of a person's interests and meaningful goals, is most effective for generating the energy required to sustain behavior change. People who begin hiking because they love being outdoors (intrinsic motivation) will likely be more successful (and have more fun) than people who begin hiking because their spouse drags them along in an effort to make them lose weight (external or intro-jected regulation). Those who begin a fitness program because they want to have more energy and reduce the complications of their diabetes (integrated regulation) will probably fare better than those beginning a fitness program because a friend nags them to.

Self-Determination Theory reminds health and fitness professionals that people have three important drives. All three have great bearing on behavior-change work in weight management (Brehm, 2013):

- **Autonomy:** People seek autonomy. They want to feel like they have choices and that they are acting in accordance with their own wishes. Health and fitness professionals should use a guiding style when recommending behavior change in any situation, including behavior change for weight management. Professionals should support weight-management clients in shaping meaningful goals and rewarding lifestyles, rather than "telling clients what to do" and focusing solely on weight loss. Clients must develop intrinsic or at least integrated or identified motivation and positive reasons for changing behavior.
- **Competence:** People like to feel as though they have some skill in the activities in which they engage. They like to feel competent, or at least as if they are improving and doing fairly well. When people feel incompetent, they lose motivation to continue trying. Health and fitness professionals should uncover clients' strengths in the health behaviors that are the program focus. For example, if clients are good dancers, or love to dance, help them find fun dance-type exercise classes rather than forcing them onto an exercise machine. If clients love to cook, guide them toward sources of healthy recipes. Maybe they would like to develop a cookbook for your program, soliciting recipes from other participants.
- **Connection:** Relationships that generate positive feelings are motivational. Here is where many health and fitness professionals fall short, as their lifelong biases against overweight people, stereo-typical beliefs, or simply feeling superior to people who are overweight can interfere with authentic relationships (Box 10-6). People who have them-selves been overweight and successfully coped with many of the issues their clients are facing are often effective at establishing motivational rela-tionships with their weight-management clients (Health Psychology at Work 10-1).

An interesting qualitative study examined the factors associated with weight loss in obese patients' participation in counseling interventions that used mo-tivational interviewing and Self-Determination Theory (Hardcastle & Hagger, 2011). The study concluded that extensive contact and support were helpful for the obese patients. The patients responded positively to monitoring and support, finding that "you can't do it on your own" (Hardcastle & Hagger, 2011). Patients were most successful when they developed au-tonomous motivation, and they felt the listening sup-port of health and fitness professionals was helpful. The authors confirmed the notions from Self-Determination Theory that obese patients respond to having a choice of options and to professionals who acknowledge their feelings, experiences, and perspectives. Autonomous motivation increased the likelihood of the patients developing self-regulatory skills and addressing barri-ers. In this study, the men seemed just as likely to de-velop physical activity habits with or without social support, whereas the women were more likely to be active with social support. The women were also more likely to feel "sabotaged" if domestic partners did not support their physical-activity efforts.

Principle of Limited Self-Control

Clients seeking weight control often say, "If only I had more willpower." It takes effort to change one's lifestyle, exercise regularly, and change one's eating

Box 10-6. Weight-Management Work: Barriers to Connection

Health and fitness professionals new to working with weight-management programs sometimes experience surprise and frustration when their clients don't lose weight. As one young health and fitness professional once complained, "It's so frustrating! My client does well for a few weeks, eats well, exercises regularly, and loses a few pounds. These past few weeks she lost 8 lb. Then suddenly, something happened, and her weight went right back to where it was. All that progress lost. I just know she could lose weight if she would stick with her program. How can I get her to lose weight?"

A group of participants that gathered for a weight-control workshop at a fitness conference (Brehm, 2007) included several fitness professionals who had themselves lost significant amounts of weight. Several had lost over 50 lb, and one woman had lost over 100 lb. An interesting discussion evolved as conference participants questioned and listened to the fitness professionals with these significant weight-loss experiences. Some of the most important issues included:

Many obese clients have experienced discrimination and harassment.
People obsess about calories, fat grams, and muscle tone and judge others more by their appearance than by their character. Many overweight clients have stories of the cruelty they experienced when exercising in public (Puhl & Heuer, 2010).

"You can't do it for them."
Just as health and fitness professionals can't "make" someone exercise, so too are they unable to "make" someone lose weight. Changing one's exercise and eating behaviors takes enormous effort and willpower. There are no magical techniques for "making" clients stick to their weight-control resolutions. They must do the work and make the changes in their habits that will facilitate weight loss.

Health and fitness professionals can be supportive and understanding. They can use good communication techniques, including open questions and mindful listening. They can share their experience and expertise, but then they must let their clients do the work. They must maintain a professional, positive regard for each client, whether or not the client loses weight.

A focus on weight can be frustrating.
When weight loss is the goal, clients can become frustrated when weight loss slows, as it usually does after the first few weeks of a weight-control program. In addition, changes may be occurring in body composition and hydration so that in some weeks, the scale shows no change.

One participant described how she quit her weight-control group because of the weekly weigh-in. She felt like a failure the weeks she didn't lose any weight. But she eventually lost over 50 lb with diet and exercise. The process is a healthy lifestyle, which will hopefully lead to the product—weight loss. Experts don't agree on the health impact of obesity, but everyone agrees that a healthy lifestyle is important.

Sometimes people don't lose weight, even with exemplary lifestyles.
Sometimes the cause of obesity is unknown. This situation is very frustrating for clients and fitness professionals. Encouraging clients to develop a healthy lifestyle is the best advice a professional can give in this situation.

Some clients must overcome serious food issues to lose weight.
Some clients cope with negative emotions by overeating. They may need professional help to change firmly entrenched behavior patterns that have developed over a lifetime. Unless the health and fitness professional is a licensed psychotherapist, this is probably beyond his or her scope of practice.

On the other hand, it is important that health and fitness professionals not assume all overweight clients have "serious issues" above and beyond what most people deal with. It is normal to enjoy eating; to like the taste of foods high in sugar, fat, and salt; and to eat for reasons other than hunger. When excessive overeating for emotional rescue causes obesity, clients need help.

Environment matters.
Following a healthy lifestyle is like swimming upstream in cultures where access to a healthy lifestyle is limited. Fresh produce is more expensive than fast food, and active recreational opportunities may be nonexistent. Experts agree that lifestyle change is the only way to lose weight, but many people face insurmountable obstacles to lifestyle change. This is especially true for those who lack economic and social resources for following a healthy lifestyle.

HEALTH PSYCHOLOGY AT WORK 10-1. Listening and Understanding Improve Client Motivation

Kelly Coffey has worked as a personal trainer since 2006 and is certified by ACSM. Clients flock to Kelly because she herself has struggled with food addiction, weight, and body-image issues for most of her life, attending her first Weight Watchers meeting with her mom at the age of 5. Kelly watched her mother struggle with obesity, losing and regaining over 100 lb five times. Kelly graduated from college, an English major, a smoker, and weighing 300 lb, unable to walk more than 1/4 mile. Following bariatric surgery (and quitting smoking), Kelly lost a great deal of weight but felt sick and out of shape. She also watched her appetite grow quickly back to normal as her stomach stretched to accommodate the load. Realizing that lifestyle change was the only way to health, Kelly began exercising and developing healthy eating behaviors. Recently, Kelly gained 50 lb during her pregnancy, experiencing cravings for starchy comfort foods that she had given up years ago. ("My body felt like it had been upholstered.") But she successfully returned to her prepregnancy weight within a few months after her daughter was born. Her empathy, understanding, and appreciation for her clients, along with her emotional honesty and boundless sense of humor, fuel her clients' commitment to lasting lifestyle change. Learn more about Kelly at her website, www.strongcoffey.com.

"Most people think that the fitness professionals they see in the gym have perfect lifestyles. As someone once said, it's human nature to compare your insides with other people's outsides. Clients feel instantly inferior and even overwhelmed with this level of perfection they imagine in personal trainers; they feel like failures before they even begin training. My clients feel comfortable with me because they understand I am human and face the same challenges they do. I let them know I tend to gain weight easily, that I can go several days without exercising, but that I then get back on track. My clients appreciate the fact that they can be honest with me.

"How do I motivate clients? I ask them how I could be the best motivational tool. I ask them what has worked in the past. They tell me the best way to proceed. Some want to text or e-mail their daily food intake and exercise records; others check in between training sessions in other ways. I do whatever works best for them. My clients know I care about them. You have to let your clients into your heart. I love my clients, whether they succeed or fail. I feel blessed and honored to be the support person I am for them.

"I only give advice when asked. Telling people what to do doesn't work. It changes the dynamic. I go from being the support person to being the parent they want to rebel against. My clients know I am a wealth of knowledge and experience. All they have to do is ask.

"My advice for new professionals just getting started as health and fitness professionals? Get to know all kinds of people. Hang out with your parents' friends—these are your future clients. Go talk to them and see what makes them tick. Listen carefully and see what you learn. This will also develop your ability to listen. Listening is a priceless skill. It makes people feel comfortable with you and sets up a dynamic where people want to work with you."

---

habits. Previous chapters have discussed the implications of limited self-control for the design of behavior-change recommendations. Because weight-management programs often include a great deal of change, minimizing the need for self-control is especially important. Lifestyle-change recommendations should try to incorporate the following suggestions:

- Keep changes as simple as possible.
- Structure changes in ways that they can quickly become habits.
- Help clients develop practices to reduce and cope with stress, since stress depletes self-control energy.
- Recognize that self-control tends to decline throughout the day.

One type of self-control that has been extensively studied is dietary restraint. People who exert a great deal of self-control over their food intake, even though they are feeling hungry and unhappy about their diet, develop the ability to maintain dietary restraint. Although early research proposed that excessive dietary restraint might be linked to binge eating, other researchers have suggested that high dietary restraint may simply be a marker for people who have problems overeating (Johnson, Pratt, & Wardle, 2011). People wanting to lose weight must exercise dietary restraint. Some research suggests that people who develop dietary restraint have lower BMIs and are more successful in not overeating than "dieters," people temporarily following a food-restriction plan (Rideout & Barr, 2009). Health and fitness professionals must help clients devise realistic suggestions for modifying their lifestyles that will help build dietary restraint but do not require excessive levels of self-control. Clients can often guide dietary recommendations, using examples of their own prior experiences of successfully exerting restraint. Many people have some idea of how much self-control is realistic for them.

BEHAVIOR-CHANGE STRATEGIES FOR WEIGHT MANAGEMENT

People seek advice on weight control for many reasons. Some people may be seeking only a temporary weight loss. Athletes trying to make a weight class or lose a few pounds for their season fall into this category (Box 10-7). Most people, however, are hoping for long-term change, even though their initial motivation might be to lose a few pounds for a big event, such as a relative's wedding, an upcoming class reunion, or travels that require public appearance in a swimsuit.

Box 10-7. Weight Loss for Clients With Normal Weight

Although the bulk of this chapter has focused on weight management for people who are overweight, it is common for health and fitness professionals to also see clients who are already fairly lean, with a normal BMI, who are still seeking to lose additional weight or fat. Some of these people are athletes who want to improve performance in sports such as running or cycling, where less extra body fat can translate into faster times. Others want to achieve a lean physique to enhance their ratings in sports or professions where appearance is part of the evaluation, such as gymnastics, diving, dancing, figure skating, bodybuilding, or fashion modeling. Some may need to reach a specific weight to qualify for a certain activity, such as lightweight rowing or a lower weight class in wrestling. Some clients will want to lose the 5 lb that have slowly come on over the years. And some may just be obsessed with food and weight. Some considerations for working with the already lean include the following.

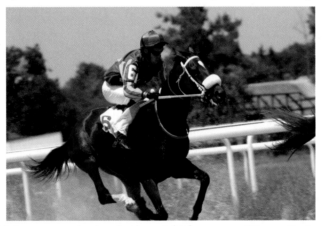

Athletes may seek a low body weight for competition. © Thinkstock

Are weight goals realistic?
Lean athletes may be able to lose a few pounds, depending on their body composition. Recognizing the error in body-composition scores, health and fitness professionals may wish to calculate a goal weight range, rather than a single number. If clients' goals seem unrealistically low, health and fitness professionals should tell them so. Is this weight one that the person has previously achieved as an adult? How long was it maintained? How difficult was it to maintain the goal weight? For women of childbearing age, did the low weight interfere with the menstrual cycle? Was the client healthy at this low weight?

Athletes should focus on performance and lose weight out of season.
If performance measures improve, athletes are succeeding. If performance starts to decline, the weight-loss program may be hurting rather than helping. Athletes may be overtraining, losing muscle tissue, and/or failing to maintain optimal glycogen stores. If weight loss becomes more important to athletes than sport performance, they may be developing a problem with food and weight or even an eating disorder. Fitness professionals should refer them to a health-care provider who can help them regain perspective.

To burn fat: eat a little less and exercise a little more.
Successful weight loss (fat loss) is most likely when people cut extra calories from the diet and increase exercise volume. Clients should cut out the least-nutritious foods (breads, grains, chips, desserts, etc.), while consuming plenty of lean proteins, vegetables, and fruits, maintaining a nutritious diet. They should add a little more calorie-burning exercise if they can. But if their exercise volume is already very high, adding more exercise may lead to overtraining. They should focus instead on dietary changes, continue their usual level of training, and consume enough carbohydrate foods to support exercise level.

Stay Healthy
If weight refuses to budge, perhaps muscle mass is increasing. Clients must not fight their bodies but accept the weight their bodies reach with a healthy lifestyle.

Behavioral-Learning Theory and cognitive-behavioral approaches form the heart of most weight-management programs. When overweight people change eating and physical activity behaviors, they usually lose weight. The challenge is maintaining the weight loss (Game Changers 10-1). Research shows that people can lose weight on just about any kind of plan that cuts calories, from nutritious, well-balanced diets that reduce portion sizes to fad diets that include limited food groups. Unfortunately, a majority of losers regain the weight within a year. This observation has led to the understanding that obesity is a chronic illness, meaning that it never really goes away. Although people may lose weight, they must maintain vigilance and healthy eating and exercise behaviors to avoid returning to their prior body-fat levels.

Research by Wing and colleagues has described which behaviors are most strongly associated with long-term weight-loss maintenance. Research from this group suggests that about 20% of people are successful in maintaining significant weight loss, almost all with lifestyle-modification approaches. Other research reinforces the importance of lifestyle modification as the primary approach for weight management (Wadden, 2011). This section addresses the nuts and bolts of applying Behavioral-Learning Theory and cognitive-behavioral approaches to weight-management programs.

 Game Changers 10-1. Rena Wing Champions Intensive Lifestyle Intervention to Treat Obesity and Type 2 Diabetes

Studies on weight-loss success are fairly dismal. The majority of people who lose weight regain the lost weight and sometimes more, within a few months of stopping their weight-control programs. But research by Rena Wing, Ph.D., and colleagues has shown that long-term weight management is possible and occurs more frequently than previous studies had supposed. Although her peers were busy seeing how fast they could make people lose weight, Wing changed the game by pointing out that most people regain the weight: the real issue is not how fast or how much weight can be lost but how can the lost weight *stay* off? Wing's decades of work have helped to determine the most-effective lifestyle interventions for obesity and obesity-related disorders. Wing has led both epidemiological research and randomized clinical trials to examine this issue.

One of Rena Wing's best-known research efforts is the founding, with James O. Hill, of the National Weight Control Registry (NWCR) in 1994. The NWCR solicits information from individuals who have lost at least 30 lb and kept the weight off for at least 1 year. Early studies from the center included 629 women and 155 men who had lost on average over 66 lb and kept the weight off for at least 5 years (Klem, Wing, McGuire, Seagle, & Hill, 1997). Since the early days, the sample has grown to over 10,000 people, 3,000 of whom have been in the Registry for over 10 years. For this 10-year group, the average weight-loss maintenance is 51 lb (maintained for 10 years) (www.nwcr.ws). How do people do it? A majority of Registry participants do the following (www.nwcr.ws; Wing & Phelan, 2005):

- Keep careful track of their daily food intake
- Count calories or fat grams
- Consume a low-calorie (about 1,800 kcal/day), low-fat (less than 30% of calories from fat) diet
- Eat breakfast almost every day
- Limit eating out, averaging dining away from home three times a week, consuming fast food less than once a week
- Develop regular eating habits, tending to consume similar foods every day, even on weekends and holidays
- Walk about an hour a day or expend the same calories with other exercise
- Watch less than 10 hours of TV a week
- Weigh themselves at least weekly

Registry members report many significant improvements in physical and psychological health, including improvements in energy level, physical mobility, general mood, and self-confidence (Klem et al., 1997).

One of Wing's most interesting clinical trials is the Look AHEAD Study. AHEAD is an acronym for Action for Health in Diabetes. This study recruited 5,145 overweight women and men who had been diagnosed with type 2 diabetes. Subjects were randomized to either an intensive lifestyle intervention (ILI) group with weekly group or individual meetings the first year, or a usual-care group that received diabetes education and met three times each year. Results showed good support for ILI, which encouraged subjects to make lifestyle changes (Table 10-1). Of the subjects in the ILI group who lost over 10% of initial weight the first year, 42.2% still maintained the weight loss at year 4. Participants who maintained the loss attended significantly more educational/support sessions and reported more-favorable eating and physical activity habits. These data demonstrate that comprehensive lifestyle change can lead to clinically important weight loss.

Continued

Game Changers 10-1. Rena Wing Champions Intensive Lifestyle Intervention to Treat Obesity and Type 2 Diabetes—cont'd

Table 10-1. Look AHEAD Study

	ILI GROUP	USUAL-CARE GROUP
Average weight loss	4.7% of initial weight	1.1% of initial weight
Percentage of group that lost >5% of initial weight	46%	25%
Percentage of group that lost >10% of initial weight	23%	10%

Source: Wadden, T. A., Neiberg, R. H., Wing, R. R., Clark, J. M., Delahanty, L. M., Hill, J. O., . . . Look AHEAD Research Group. (2011). Four-year weight losses in the Look AHEAD Study: factors associated with long-term success. *Obesity, 19*(10), 1987-1998.

Sources: Klem, M. L., Wing, R. R., McGuire, M. T., Seagle, H. M., & Hill, J. O. (1997). A descriptive study of individuals successful at long-term maintenance of substantial weight loss. *American Journal of Clinical Nutrition, 66*(2), 239-246; Wadden, T. A., Neiberg, R. H., Wing, R. R., Clark, J. M., Delahanty, L. M., Hill, J. O., . . . Look AHEAD Research Group. (2011). Four-year weight losses in the Look AHEAD Study: factors associated with long-term success. *Obesity, 19*(10), 1987-1998; Wing, R. R., & Phelan, S. (2005). Long-term weight loss maintenance. *American Journal of Clinical Nutrition, 82*(1), 222S-225S.

Realistic and Motivational Goals

Too often people begin a weight-management program, either alone or working with health and fitness professionals, by focusing solely on a particular goal weight. Professionals should encourage clients to broaden their goals to include improvements in psychological and physical health variables. They should also advise clients to include process goals, such as exercising 5 days a week and attending their weight-management group meetings. Using open questions, health and fitness professionals should explore clients' hopes and dreams and link health behaviors to these goals, if reasonable.

Nevertheless, clients often want a weight-loss goal as well. Setting weight-loss goals is a very tricky business, because many overweight people may never reach them and thus may become so discouraged they quit exercising and eating well. Studies have found that overweight people who lose only 5% to 10% of their initial body weight experience good improvements in many health variables, including blood pressure, blood sugar, and lipid levels. This amount of weight loss is also more likely to be achieved and maintained, the important and most difficult part. Although clients may come in with hopes of losing 25% or more of their body weight, health and fitness professionals should encourage them to think more realistically and to focus on lifestyle change rather than on dramatic but unrealistic weight loss.

■ *Ari greets Lily, who has finally arrived for her first personal training session, the last of the group to get around to this. As they review Lily's medical history, Ari acknowledges that Lily's* doctor has referred her to this program to help get her blood pressure down. "Yes," she replies, "but he also wants me to lose some weight. What is my ideal weight anyway?"

This is Ari's least-favorite question, but he has heard it so many times that he is ready with a helpful response. "We don't talk about ideal weight anymore, because no one can really say what ideal is. We do know that losing even 5% or 10% of your body weight, which for you would be about 8 to 15 lb, could help your health in many ways, hopefully even lowering your blood pressure. How about trying for about a 10-lb loss to start? Does that sound reasonable to you?"

Ari can see she feels a little disappointed that he hasn't promised her fast, effortless weight loss. "Hopefully, the more realistic goals we set together will help her feel more successful in the end and focus more on lifestyle than weight," he thinks. Lily perks up a bit as she starts walking on the treadmill. She is happy to see there is television for her to watch as she logs her miles. ■

Behavior-Change Skills

Basic behavior-change skills are the foundation of successful weight management. One of the first steps in creating weight-management recommendations is to try to figure out the causes of the extra weight. Clients often have some ideas about this. Some clients have been overweight all their lives and developed sedentary lifestyles and habits of overeating. Others may have gained weight during a particular time period, perhaps during a period of stress or a pregnancy. Many middle-aged clients simply gain weight slowly over time, often just a pound or two a year during winter and the holidays, which never quite comes off (Box 10-8).

Weight management through lifestyle modification is very simple in principle. First, people figure out which lifestyle habits and other behaviors are a problem. Second, they replace the problematic behaviors with new habits that will promote a healthier weight. Previous chapters have explored the processes of change, Behavioral-Learning Theory, and cognitive-behavioral approaches to behavior change in some depth. This section will focus on their applications to weight management.

Box 10-8. Winter Weight Gain

Many people gain weight during the winter months. Some people joke that they are eating and sleeping more because they are getting ready for hibernation. However, people do not get to crawl into a cozy hiding place and sleep the fat away. Some of those extra pounds acquired over the holidays may stay on year after year, eventually contributing to obesity and consequent health problems. People gain weight during the winter months for different reasons, including the following.

Seasonal Affective Disorder
Sometimes winter weight gain is a byproduct of seasonal depression. Seasonal depression ranges in severity from quite mild, as in the winter doldrums, to quite severe, a condition known appropriately as seasonal affective disorder, or SAD. SAD is a type of depression characterized by recurrent episodes of depression, sleeping more than usual, fatigue, increased appetite with carbohydrate cravings, and weight gain. These symptoms typically begin in September, when the days become shorter, and continue into March. Yearly appearances of winter symptoms and their disappearance in the summer months tend to confirm a SAD diagnosis. Research suggests that in general, about 1% to 10% of people experience SAD, while an even larger number have milder forms of winter depression (Howland, 2009).

Most adult clients with winter depression will probably have already observed the seasonal nature of their symptoms and will appreciate sympathy if this topic comes up in discussions of winter weight gain. If clients complain of depression, health and fitness professionals should urge them to seek treatment from their health-care providers as they work to set up a regular exercise program. Exercise helps reduce depressive symptoms, but many clients will need more than exercise to ameliorate winter depression. Clients' health-care providers may recommend special light treatments, which are effective for many people with SAD. Patients are commonly advised to sit under these bright lights for 30 minutes or more per day, usually in the morning.

Winter Lifestyles
The weight gain associated with the winter doldrums or with SAD is often made worse by winter lifestyles. Whether clients are depressed or not, winter can lead to a decline in weekly caloric expenditure, as darker days and inclement weather limit opportunities for physical activity. This is the perfect time for prospective clients to join a fitness center. Indoor options become more attractive when winter darkness sets in. However, getting outdoors can be beneficial for combating winter weight gain. Clients whose schedules let them get outdoor exercise, especially at midday, will get double benefits of exercise and light exposure. Clients with both indoor and outdoor exercise options have more ways to fight winter weight gain.

Holiday Excess
People who have a tendency to gain weight during the winter often find that the extra stress imposed by the holiday season, combined with extra exposure to high-calorie treats, turns that tendency into a reality. In addition to stress, there is usually less time to exercise and extra alcohol—a perfect recipe for weight gain.

People concerned with winter weight gain should plan a holiday survival (and enjoyment) strategy that makes health a priority. Regular physical activity should be the cornerstone of every plan since exercise not only burns calories but also reduces feelings of stress. Individuals should think about factors that have made holiday exercise difficult in the past: loneliness, travel, busyness, lack of childcare, and so on. Health and fitness professionals should help clients with active problem solving to come up with realistic plans for staying active through the holidays.

What about holiday eating? Again, a survival strategy is helpful. What treats are an essential part of the holidays? How can clients avoid munching and drinking just because "it's there"? Getting enough sleep, drinking plenty of water, and finding time for fun and relaxation can help reduce hunger by reducing feelings of fatigue and stress.

Self-Monitoring: A Lifestyle Reality Check

Behavior change for weight management begins with a look at a client's current lifestyle. Clients might begin by recording everything they eat for at least 3 days. They may wish to record foods and also the factors that influenced decisions to eat and food choices. Clients should also keep track of physical activity, including daily activities such as walking, taking the stairs, and doing housework and yard work.

Self-monitoring helps both clients and professionals assess which behaviors need to be changed. In some cases, self-monitoring helps people realize that they are eating more than they thought, such as nibbling as they cook dinner or snacking as they watch television. Self-monitoring acts as a kind of a mirror so people get a good look at their behavior.

Problem-Solving and Behavior Chains

Once people have recorded their eating and exercise behaviors for a few days, the self-monitoring records can be assessed. What is working well? Which behaviors are problems? In particular, which factors are causing the weight problem?

People who study behavior change and lifestyle modification look at both the causes and rewards of behavior. Are there certain things that seem to trigger problematic eating? If so, can the trigger be changed (stimulus control)? If not, can a new response to that trigger be learned (counterconditioning)?

For example, let's say that several times a week a person walks into a convenience store to get a cup of coffee, but he ends up buying a large candy bar, too. What can he do about this? To change the trigger, could he avoid the convenience store? Take coffee from home or buy it somewhere else? Give up the coffee? Or, could he change his response? Go ahead and buy the coffee but pass on the candy bar? Or buy a small piece of chocolate instead of the large candy bar?

People hold on to many unproductive behaviors because the behaviors provide a reward. They help people feel good or reduce feelings of stress. Changing these behaviors may be difficult if people are afraid of losing these rewards. They will need to develop negative associations with problematic behaviors (the greasy feeling on the roof of one's mouth after eating a donut) and find positive reinforcement from other activities and healthier foods.

MOTIVATING CHANGE: Let Clients Lead Behavior-Change Recommendations

Health and fitness professionals tend to get excited when clients can pinpoint situations that lead to overeating. This, after all, is the beginning of success. Once the problem is identified, solutions call out for attention. At this point, however, professionals must remember their open questions and reflective-listening skills to guide clients to devise solutions that are most likely to work in the context of clients' individual lives.

If clients get caught up in the planning fallacy, professionals should suggest they do a reality check as to the plan's feasibility. While maintaining a hopeful outlook, encourage realistic solutions. Express confidence in clients' abilities to perform the suggested solutions. Affirm their strengths, reminding them of past success stories relevant to the present situation. Health and fitness professionals should emphasize the rewards clients will experience from implementing this solution and how they look forward to hearing next week about how the clients' new options worked.

Weight-Management Advice and Scope of Practice

Chapter 9 explained the scope of practice limitations with regard to giving dietary advice. Weight-control clients who are new to meal planning should meet with a dietitian to plan a personalized weight-loss program. Health and fitness professionals can support client adherence to the prescribed diet guidelines and offer practical suggestions for following the advice. Patients who are receiving medications for weight loss, on special very-low-calorie eating plans, or undergoing or recovering from bariatric surgeries should be under continuous medical care.

What kind of diet is best for producing weight loss? Most dietitians will prescribe a well-balanced diet with plenty of vegetables, lean protein, and smaller portions of carbohydrate foods. Some people do well on a very-low-carbohydrate diet, while others have trouble sticking to this type of diet. Many clients will have had experience reducing calories and have good ideas about what works best for them. People trying to eat less must still be able to consume foods that they are familiar with and enjoy, while limiting empty calorie items. Meals should be structured in ways that quickly become routine, reducing the need for self-control and decision making.

Stress Management and Healthy Lifestyle

Dietary change should be seen as one part of a healthy lifestyle that supports emotional health and feelings of well-being. Health and fitness professionals should educate clients about the importance of adequate sleep and stress management. Regular physical activity should be the cornerstone of every weight-management program.

Social Support and Weight-Management Groups

Social support can take many forms and can help people stick to their weight-management programs. Health and fitness professionals with some skill and experience at working with groups might find that running weight-management groups is a rewarding experience. Professionals who have been part of similar groups themselves will have some good ideas about which techniques work to build group camaraderie. Weight-management groups typically meet weekly and discuss people's successes and challenges. The leader may invite guest speakers or prepare presentations on motivational or informational topics for the group. The group may even exercise together, or individuals may arrange their own physical activities. A good group can provide a feeling of social support to its members.

Health and fitness professionals can also encourage clients to develop social support by suggesting they recruit exercise partners or even form their own small groups. Some personal trainers are willing to work with pairs or small groups. Clients might build their own support systems, recruiting coworkers, friends, and family members to engage in similar lifestyle changes. They may all agree, for example, to walk several times a week together. They may all decide to quit drinking soft drinks or limit desserts together. Clients may have many good ideas about how they can most effectively create or strengthen social support for their weight-management programs.

Cognitive Restructuring

Significant changes in the way people think often accompany successful weight loss. An interesting meta-analysis of the psychological factors associated with weight-loss maintenance found that the following factors were associated with success (Ohsiek & Williams, 2011):

- **Ability to avoid dichotomous thinking:** Dichotomous thinking refers to an irrational thought pattern that offers only two possible categorizations. In terms of weight control, common dichotomous thinking that leads to failure is "I am either on the diet or not on the diet. I am either a success or a failure." In other words, people with dichotomous thinking are uncomfortable with shades of gray; things are either black or white. Successful losers are able to be more flexible in their thinking and view lapses as something they can recover from, rather than evidence that they are no longer with the program and therefore should abandon weight-loss efforts. This observation underscores the importance of helping clients view behavior change as a lifelong journey, filled with challenges and compromises.
- **Ability to avoid eating to regulate mood:** Successful losers are able to find alternative strategies for coping with negative moods.
- **Dietary restraint:** Higher levels of dietary restraint are associated with weight-loss maintenance. Dietary restraint helps people avoid disinhibited eating. Disinhibited eating refers to a lack of dietary restraint, where people feel unable to control how much they eat.

- **Perception that lifestyle-change benefits outweigh costs:** Successful losers have tipped the decisional balance in favor of lifestyle modification. Although they may sometimes face difficulties maintaining their eating and exercise behaviors, the pros outweigh the cons for them.
- **Lower or stable levels of depression:** Higher levels of depression predict relapse. Behavior change, maintaining dietary restraint, and exercise all take energy. Depression depletes self-control energy.
- **More-positive body image:** People with a more-positive body image may have positive associations with the results of their weight-loss programs. A more-positive body image may be one of the benefits that outweigh program costs.

Health and fitness professionals who have the opportunity to work with clients for extended periods of time may be able to help them identify psychological factors that may help or hinder weight loss and weight-loss-maintenance efforts. Members of weight-loss groups often point these things out to each other and encourage more-positive perspectives.

Dangers of Dieting

Many overweight clients have a long history of dieting. In fact, many blame their dieting history for their problems with weight and food. Very-restrictive eating can interfere with metabolism, hunger, appetite, and psychological relationships with food. Unsuccessful weight-loss attempts can lead to feelings of guilt, failure, food cravings, and, ironically, obesity, as food becomes too much of a focus in people's lives (Fig. 10-9). Instead of short-term, restrictive diets, health and fitness professionals should encourage lifestyle modification that people can live with for a lifetime.

Coping With Food Cravings

Many people experience food cravings, defined as an overwhelming desire to consume a particular kind of food. Cravings feel uncomfortable in that the craving

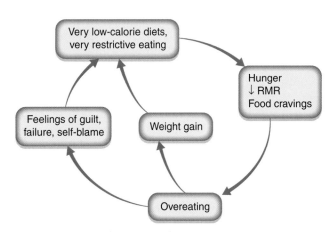

Figure 10-9. The dangers of dieting.

dominates a person's awareness until it is either satisfied or it passes. Research suggests that the brain reward circuitry response involved in food cravings is similar to that involved in drug cravings and addiction (Blum, Liu, Shriner, & Gold, 2011). Food cravings can interfere with concentration and distract people from other activities.

Food cravings are not necessarily a problem if the craved food is close at hand and if eating it has no negative repercussions. If a person would really like a little chocolate, she can eat a few small candies, and the craving is satisfied.

Food cravings become problematic for people who are trying to avoid overeating or who are restricting their food intake in order to lose weight. People tend to crave "forbidden" foods that are high in fat, sugar, and salt. When cravings call, they are hard to ignore. Giving in to a craving can mean the beginning of the end of a healthy eating plan, especially for people who have dichotomous thinking about dieting.

For some people, food cravings can trigger episodes of emotional overeating, a leading cause of obesity. Emotional overeating occurs when people eat in order to reduce emotional pain and relieve negative feelings. In some people, food cravings can even lead to binge eating and other disordered eating behaviors, which are covered in more detail in Chapter 11.

Researchers who have asked volunteers to record and analyze their food cravings believe that a craving typically begins with thoughts about a particular food, often triggered by seeing the food or remembering something about eating the food (Kessler, 2009). A person may then begin to focus on how good that food tastes or other positive associations with that food. Thinking leads to an emotional "need" for that food that then develops into an urge to obtain and eat that food. This explains why some people eat in response to viewing advertisements for food.

What determines which food is the object of a craving? There is little evidence to support the notion that people crave foods that supply a nutrient in which they are deficient. More likely, the food has been associated with positive feelings in some way. Chocolate, for example, has chemicals that make some people feel good. Similarly, carbohydrates help some people feel more relaxed. Cravings probably evolve from past experiences, both social and biochemical, with the consumption of specific foods.

Restrictive dieting may cause food cravings for several reasons. People are more likely to be drawn to foods categorized as "forbidden," because it seems to be human nature to want what one cannot have. This is one reason nutritionists encourage people to see that all types of food can be included in a diet, if the food is consumed in reasonable portions and in the context of an otherwise well-balanced diet.

Some research suggests that food cravings are more likely to develop when a person follows a restrictive diet, such as when certain food groups are eliminated (Pelchat, 2009). After following a bland diet for several days, for example, people often begin to crave more-flavorful foods, such as pizza.

People are also more likely to experience food cravings when they are hungry. The hunger signal can evolve into a focus on a particular food. Restrictive diets can also make people feel stressed, grumpy, anxious, and depressed. These are the very emotions that can trigger the need for comfort foods, a need that can turn into cravings that increase the risk of emotional overeating.

One interesting study suggests that exercise might help reduce cravings and consumption of craved foods, at least for chocolate (Oh & Taylor, 2011). Subjects were regular chocolate eaters who walked for 15 minutes or rested and were then given either a stressful task or an easier one. Throughout the tasks, chocolate was freely available. All volunteers had been deprived of chocolate for 2 days prior to the experiment, so cravings were presumably aroused. The subjects who exercised ate about half as much chocolate during the tasks as the subjects who did not.

Observations from alcohol addiction research may be applicable to food cravings. Researchers Ostafin and Marlatt encourage people in recovery and abstaining from alcohol to "surf the urge" (Ostafin & Marlatt, 2008). Many people fear that their feelings of craving will continue to rise, getting worse and more uncomfortable. According to Ostafin and Marlatt's research, experiences of cravings actually rise and fall. The feeling of craving grows and then diminishes. When people become anxious about the craving, it gets much worse. The researchers advise people to allow themselves to mindfully observe and experience the craving, noticing the events, feelings, and thoughts that occur with the craving. Being present to the experience can make it less anxiety provoking. People who "surf the urge" usually observe that the craving gradually becomes less intense. Over time, the intensity of cravings tends to diminish as well (Ostafin & Marlatt, 2008).

Emotional Eating

Emotional eating is so common that it is sometimes considered well within the range of normal behavior (Behavior Change in Action 10-1). Problems arise when emotional eating becomes excessive and interferes with a person's lifestyle and health. For emotional eaters, the drive to eat is often associated with unpleasant feelings such as boredom, loneliness, depression, anxiety, anger, or fatigue (Spoor, Bekker, Van Strien, & van Heck, 2007). Eating provides comfort and solace, numbing the pain and "feeding the hungry heart."

In extreme cases, people can become addicted to binge eating, and it's not so much that eating feels good as that not eating feels bad. Binge eaters have an eating disorder that causes them to consume large quantities of food and have no sense of control over their eating behavior. Food becomes an escape from negative emotions calling for

BEHAVIOR CHANGE IN ACTION 10-1

When Clients Are Consumed by Food

■ CHALLENGE

Some clients tend to overeat when experiencing difficulties and negative emotions.

■ PLAN

If clients are bothered by emotional eating, they may wish to seek help from a therapist with expertise in this area, as suggested above. Health and fitness professionals should support clients' wishes to deal with this problem in another setting. Even if clients have the support they need, they may also turn to you for help. Sensible directions you can take with emotional eaters include the following:

Reevaluate eating guidelines. Is the client consuming a balanced diet? Diets that are very low in calories or that restrict certain food groups are psychologically self-defeating, often leading to food cravings and too much focus on food and eating. Such diets also rarely lead to long-term weight control and good health. If clients are working with a dietitian, suggest that they make an appointment to reevaluate eating guidelines.

Encourage clients to make all food soul food. A weight-management diet should nourish body and soul. Food is supposed to be delicious and eating pleasurable. Clients should include "comfort foods" as appropriate. Nutrition knowledge can be harnessed to work with appetites to create a well-balanced and delicious diet.

Help clients enjoy regular physical activity. Exercise reduces stress, helps control appetite, increases energy, and improves sleep quality. All of these factors help reduce emotional eating. Could the client's exercise program recommendations be improved to make activity more enjoyable?

Suggest self-monitoring to increase self-awareness. If clients tend to overeat when stressed, self-monitoring may help change this behavior. Emotional eaters who monitor their eating behaviors often find that the drive to eat masks unpleasant feelings, such as anxiety, depression, loneliness, fatigue, boredom, and anger. They learn to differentiate between "mouth hunger" or emotional eating and "stomach hunger" or true physical hunger. They uncover situations and feelings that trigger emotional overeating.

Help clients to address emotional eating triggers. If stress triggers overeating, can clients address the sources of stress? Can they look for solutions to problems at hand, talk them over with a friend, or write in a journal? People must acknowledge and address feelings of depression, anger, or anxiety. They must also accept the fact that negative emotions are a part of life and, at the same time, engage in activities to address problems and feel better.

Most people find that overeating tends to occur in specific places and at specific times. A common time is at home during the evening. Possible solutions include engaging in a hobby that keeps mind and hands busy or getting out of the house.

Urge clients to get a life. At the same time that clients may benefit from becoming more self-aware, encouraging self-obsession can be counterproductive. Perhaps your client would be better off engaging in more activities, keeping busy, and having fun. Pets can create positive energy–how about a dog that needs daily walks? Would your clients enjoy volunteering for a cause that would enable them to use their skills to help others? Altruistic work is rewarding and can get one's mind off of one's own problems.

Encourage clients to make time to relax and have fun. Fatigue is one of the most-common causes of overeating. Getting plenty of rest and relaxation helps manage stress and reduce overeating. Some emotional eaters find that they overeat because eating is the only time they relax, enjoy life, and reward themselves. These people can learn to enlarge their repertoire of "healthy pleasures" so that they have other ways to nurture themselves besides eating.

their attention. Binge eaters say that stuffing oneself with food becomes a metaphor for stuffing down undesirable feelings so they won't come to the surface.

When should health and fitness professionals refer clients for psychological counseling? If clients express concern about an eating problem, it is appropriate to refer them to a therapist, especially someone trained in eating disorders. If the professional suspects binge eating disorder or bulimia, suggestions for referral should be very strong. Eating disorders can be very dangerous and even fatal. Early referral and treatment can save lives.

Coping Planning: Preventing Relapse

Most people experience lapses during their behavior-change efforts. Lifestyle-modification programs for weight loss can be especially difficult to maintain long term, as they involve modification of many different behaviors and habits. Health and fitness professionals can encourage clients to accept the difficulty of this work and anticipate factors that may contribute to both success and relapse. Professionals should help clients understand that it is human to make mistakes and that self-forgiveness is the correct response, followed by renewed efforts to resume a healthy lifestyle. A lapse need not be interpreted as a relapse. Some variables that can influence risk of relapse include the following:

- **Flexible attitude:** Lifelong behavior change requires a great deal of flexibility and adaptation. Flexibility helps people work around the roadblocks that inevitably arise to challenge plans and to make decent choices within the constraints of daily life. People must learn how to adapt accordingly to schedule interruptions and adjust food and exercise as best they can. Most important is the ability to recover from setbacks. Lapses in weight-control programs are universal: almost everyone has good days and bad days.

- **Coping planning for high-risk situations:** Many clients can describe situations that tend to be especially difficult for them. Parties, vacations, holidays, visitors, eating out, and travel may present circumstances that disrupt the normal routine or present irresistible temptation. Health and fitness professionals can encourage clients to anticipate challenges and plan effective coping strategies. Eventually, these plans themselves become habits.

- **Negative emotional states and food cravings:** Coping with stress and negative moods requires self-control energy, and spending energy on stress management depletes the self-control needed for behavior change. People with mood disorders such as depression and anxiety may have extra difficulty with behavior change if these changes increase feelings of stress. Clients should do what they can to manage stress and avoid negative emotional states. Cravings that arise when people are facing high-risk situations in a negative mood are difficult to resist.

- **Outcome expectancies:** Outcome expectancies refer to what people think will happen if they engage in a given behavior. If a client thinks eating a big meal will make him feel better, he will be more likely to indulge. If a person thinks exercise will make her feel tired, she'll skip her workout if she is already stressed and tired. Health and fitness professionals can help clients create positive expectancies for their new behaviors. For example, people might be able to learn that a moderate workout helps them feel more energetic and less irritable.

- **Abstinence violation effect:** The abstinence violation effect describes the behavior of people who resume a behavior that they are trying to avoid after a period of abstinence. People feel a loss of control and guilt when they violate a self-imposed rule, such as a rule about not overeating or a rule about following some sort of eating plan. Once they break their rule, they feel self-blame and a loss of control and reach for the behavior that they think will make them feel better, and they fall into relapse (Hendershot, Witkiewitz, Goerge, & Marlatt, 2011).

- **Close relationships:** Friends and family can either sabotage or support clients' behavior-change efforts. People are more likely to be successful in their weight-management efforts if they can cultivate a helpful and supportive social network.

■ *Today Ari is meeting with a representative of the practice that hired him to start the weight-management program. During the 3 months of the program thus far, many of the clients have lost several pounds and most are becoming more active. A few have joined the wellness center at the hospital, and several are walking regularly at home. Although Ari is pleased with his group, he knows that 3 months is nothing in the context of a lifetime and works hard to present this idea. He cites the research showing that continuing support leads to better long-term weight control. "A majority of these people have lost weight before," he explains, "but it comes back on. The medical problems continue. If you really want these folks to sustain their lifestyle changes, they will need more than 3 months of support." He describes some of the improvements he has seen in the group. The representative takes careful notes and promises to get back to Ari soon. The following week, Ari receives the go-ahead to continue the group for 3 more months. ■*

KEY TERMS

abstinence violation effect

adiponectin

anthropometry

appetite

basal metabolic rate (BMR)

bioelectrical impedance analysis (BIA)

body composition

brown adipose tissue (BAT)

central obesity

circumference

density

dichotomous thinking

dietary restraint

disinhibited eating

dual-energy x-ray absorptiometry

energy balance

essential body fat

fat-free mass (FFM)

fat mass (FM)

French paradox

ghrelin

hunger

hydrometry

hydrostatic weighing

intramuscular triglycerides (IMTG)

irisin

leptin

metabolic rate

metabolism

microbiome

microbiota

negative energy balance

nonalcoholic fatty liver disease

nonexercise activity thermogenesis (NEAT)

normal-weight obesity

outcome expectancies

pathogenic

positive energy balance

resting metabolic rate (RMR)

seasonal affective disorder

sex-specific fat

skinfold thickness

subcutaneous fat

satiety

thermic effect of exercise (TEE)

thermic effect of food (TEF)

total body water (TBW)

underwater weighing

visceral adipose tissue (VAT)

CRITICAL THINKING QUESTIONS

1. Imagine that you are working with a client with normal-weight obesity who also has been diagnosed with type 2 diabetes. The client argues that he does not need to exercise since he is not overweight. How might the results of a body-composition test help you use the Health Belief Model to motivate your client to become more active? What other information (besides the body-composition test results) might you give the client as you apply the Health Belief Model?

2. Visit a cafeteria, perhaps one at your school. Using the foods available at one meal, plan two meals, one that is high in energy density and one low in energy density. Describe why you chose the foods you did for each meal.

3. Your client, who wants (and needs) to lose 20 lb, prefers to lose the weight quickly with a 600-calorie-per-day liquid diet. She hates to exercise, has a very high-stress lifestyle, and only sleeps about 5 hours most nights. Would you support this approach to weight loss? Explain why or why not. What questions might you ask your client, using your OARS skills, to guide her in the direction of considering a more-comprehensive, lifestyle-modification approach to weight loss?

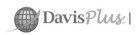 For additional resources log in to DavisPlus (http://davisplus.fadavis.com/ keyword "Brehm") and click on the Premium tab. (Don't have a PlusCode to access Premium Resources? Just click the Purchase Access button on the book's DavisPlus page.)

REFERENCES

Alsted, T. J., Nybo, L., Schweiger, M., Fledelius, C., Jacobsen, P., Zimmermann, R., . . . Kiens, B. (2009). Adipose triglyceride lipase in human skeletal muscle is upregulated by exercise training. *American Journal of Physiology: Endocrinology and Metabolism, 296*(3), E445-E453.

Balkwill, F. (2009). Tumor necrosis factor and cancer. *Nature Reviews, 9,* 361-368.

Bliss, R. M. (2006). Inflammatory news about fat cells: molecules that sequester dying fat cells also spread inflammation. *Agricultural Research, 54*(3), 4-7.

Blum, K., Liu, Y., Shriner, R., & Gold, M. S. (2011). Reward circuitry dopaminergic activation regulates food and drug craving behavior. *Current Pharmaceutical Design, 17*(12), 1158-1167.

Bostrum, P., Wu, J., Jedrychowski, M. P., Korde, A., Ye, L., Lo, J. C., . . . Spiegelman, B. M. (2012). A PCG1-alpha-dependent myokine that drives brown-fat-like development of white fat and thermogenesis. *Nature,* Published online 1/11/12, doi:10.1038/nature10777.

Bray, G. A. (2007). How bad is fructose? *American Journal of Clinical Nutrition, 86*(4), 895-896.

Brehm, B. A. (2007). Helping clients with weight control. Presentation for Canadian Fitness Professionals (Can-Fit-Pro) International Fitness and Club Business Conference and Trade Show, Toronto, August 17, 2007.

Brehm, B. A. (2013). Lifestyle modification and behavior change. In: Bryant, C. X., Green, D. J., & Merrill, S. (eds.), 385-408. *ACE Health Coach Manual.* San Diego, CA: American Council on Exercise.

Bryant, C. X., Green, D. J., & Merrill, S. (eds.). (2013). *ACE Health Coach Manual.* San Diego, CA: American Council on Exercise.

Centers for Disease Control and Prevention. (2012a). About BMI for adults. www.cdc.gov/healthyweight/assessing/bmi/adult_bmi/index.html. Accessed 12/23/12.

Centers for Disease Control and Prevention. (2012b). Communities putting prevention to work: resource center. www.cdc.gov/CommunitiesPuttingPreventiontoWork/resources/index.htm. Accessed 12/23/12.

Chaput, J. P., & Tremblay, A. (2007). Acute effects of knowledge-based work on feeding behavior and energy intake. *Physiology & Behavior, 90*(1), 66-72.

Christakis, N. A., & Fowler, J. H. (2007). The spread of obesity in a large social network over 32 years. *New England Journal of Medicine, 357*(4), 370-379.

Cornier, M.-A., Despres, J. -P., Davis, N., Grossniklaus, D. A., Klein, S., Lamarche, B., . . . Stroke Council. (2011). Assessing adiposity: a scientific statement from the American Heart Association. *Circulation, 124*(18), 1996-2019.

Crane, J. D., Devries, M. C., Safdar, A., Hamadeh, M. J., & Tarnopolsky, M. A. (2010). The effect of aging on human skeletal muscle mitochondrial and intramyocellular lipid ultrastructure. *Journal of Gerontology, Series A: Biological Sciences, 65*(2), 119-128.

Elder, S. J., & Roberts, S. B. (2007). The effects of exercise on food intake and body fatness: a summary of published studies. *Nutrition Reviews, 65*(1), 1-19.

Farshchi, J. R., Taylor, M. A., & MacDonald, I. A. (2005). Beneficial metabolic effects of regular meal frequency on dietary thermogenesis, insulin sensitivity, and fasting lipid profiles in healthy obese women. *American Journal of Clinical Nutrition, 81*, 16-24.

Ferrieres, J. (2004). The French paradox: lessons for other countries. *Heart, 90*(1), 107-111.

Flood, J., Roe, L., & Rolls, B. (2006). The effect of increased beverage portion size on energy intake at a meal. *Journal of the American Dietetics Association, 106*, 1984-1990.

Francois, F., Roper, J., Joseph, N., Pei, J., Chhada, A., Shak, J. R., . . . Blaser, M. J. (2011). The effect of *H. pylori* eradication on meal-associated changes in plasma ghrelin and leptin. *BioMed Central Gastroenterology, 11*, 37-46.

Gill, T. P., Baur, L. A., & King, L. A. (2010). Should health policy focus on physical activity rather than obesity? No. *British Medical Journal, 340*, c2602.

Hagobian, T. A., & Braun, B. (2010). Physical activity and hormonal regulation of appetite: sex differences and weight control. *Exercise and Sport Sciences Reviews, 38*(1), 25-30.

Harber, M. P., Crane, J. D., Douglass, M. D., Weindel, K. D., Trappe, T. A., Trappe, S. W., & Fink, W. F. (2008). Resistance exercise reduces muscular substrates in women. *International Journal of Sports Medicine, 29*(9), 719-725.

Hardcastle, S., & Hagger, M. S. (2011). "You can't do it on your own": experiences of a motivational interviewing intervention on physical activity and dietary behavior. *Psychology of Sport and Exercise, 12*(2), 314-323.

Healy, G. N., Dunstan, D. W., Salmon, J., Cerin, E., Shaw, J. E., Zimmet, P. Z., & Owen, N. (2008). Breaks in sedentary time: beneficial associations with metabolic risk. *Diabetes Care, 31*(4), 661-666.

Hendershot, C. S., Witkiewitz, K., Goerge, W. H., & Marlatt, G. A. (2011). Relapse prevention for addictive behaviors. *Substance Abuse Treatment, Prevention, and Policy, 6*, 17.

Heymsfield, S. B., Lohman, T. G., Wang, Z., & Going, S. B. (2005). *Human Body Composition*. Champaign, IL: Human Kinetics.

Ho-Pham, L. T., Campbell, L. V., & Nguyen, T. V. (2011). More on body fat cutoff points. *Mayo Clinic Proceedings, 86*(6), 584.

Howland, R. H. (2009). An overview of seasonal affective disorder. *The Physician and Sportsmedicine, 37*(4), 104-115.

Iyer, A., Fairlie, D. P., Prins, J. B., Hammock, B. D., & Brown, L. (2010). Inflammatory lipid mediators in adipocyte function and obesity. *Nature Reviews Endocrinology, 6*(2), 71-82.

Johnson, F., Pratt, M., & Wardle, J. (2011). Dietary restraint and self-regulation in eating behavior. *International Journal of Obesity (London), 36*(5):655-674.

Juhasz, G., Foldi, I., & Penke, B. (2011). Systems biology of Alzheimer's disease: how diverse molecular changes result in memory impairment in AD. *Neurochemistry International, 58*, 739-750.

Kadooka, Y., Sato, M., Imaizumi, K., Ogawa, A., Ikuyama, K., Akai, Y., . . . Tsuchida, T. (2010). Regulation of abdominal adiposity by probiotics (Lactobacillus gasseri SBT2055) in adults with obese tendencies in a randomized controlled trial. *European Journal of Clinical Nutrition, 64*(6), 636-643.

Kallus, S. J., & Brandt, L. J. (2012). The intestinal microbiota and obesity. *Journal of Clinical Gastroenterology, 46*(1), 16-24.

Katcher, H. I., Legro, R. S., Kunselman, A. R., Gillies, P. J., Demers, L. M., Bagshaw, D. M., & Kris-Etherton, P. M. (2008). The effects of a whole grain-enriched hypocaloric diet on cardiovascular disease risk factors in men and women with the metabolic syndrome. *American Journal of Clinical Nutrition, 87*(1), 79-90.

Kessler, D. (2009). *The End of Overeating*. New York: Rodale Books.

Klem, M. L., Wing, R. R., McGuire, M. T., Seagle, H. M., & Hill, J. O. (1997). A descriptive study of individuals successful at long-term maintenance of substantial weight loss. *American Journal of Clinical Nutrition, 66*(2), 239-246.

Knutson, K. L., Spiegel, K., Penev, P., & Van Cauter, E. (2007). The metabolic consequences of sleep deprivation. *Sleep Medicine Reviews, 11*(3), 163-178.

Lee, D. -C., Sui, X., Artero, E. G., Lee, I. M., Church, T. S., McAuley, P. A., & Blair, S. N. (2011). Long-term effects of changes in cardiorespiratory fitness and body mass index on all-cause and cardiovascular disease mortality in men. *Circulation, 124*(23), 2483-2490.

Lejeune, M. P. G. M., Westerterp, K. R., Adam, T. C. M., Luscombe-Marsh, N. D., & Westerterp-Plantenga, M. S. (2006). Ghrelin and glucagon-like peptide 1 concentrations, 24-h satiety, and energy and substrate metabolism during a high-protein diet and measured in a respiration chamber. *American Journal of Clinical Nutrition, 83*, 89-94.

Levine, J. (2004). Nonexercise activity thermogenesis (NEAT): environment and biology. *American Journal of Physiology; Endocrinology and Metabolism, 286*(5), E675-E685.

Liu, Y., Turdi, S., Park, T., Morris, N. J., Deshaies, Y., Xu, A., & Sweeney, G. (2012). Adiponectin corrects high-fat diet-induced disturbances in muscle metabolomic profile and whole-body glucose homeostasis. *Diabetes, 62*(3):743-752.

Ludwig, J, Sanbonmatsu, L., Gennetian, L., Adam, E., Duncan, G. J., Katz, L. F., . . . McDade, T. W. (2011). Neighborhoods, obesity, and diabetes—a randomized social experiment. *New England Journal of Medicine, 365*(16), 1509-1519.

Malik, V. S., Popkin, B. M., Bray, G. A., Després, J. P., Willett, W. C., & Hu, F. B. (2010). Sugar-sweetened beverages and risk of metabolic syndrome and type 2 diabetes: a meta-analysis. *Diabetes Care, 33*(11), 2477-2483.

McAuley, P., & Blair, S. N. (2011). Obesity paradoxes. *Journal of Sports Science, 29*(8), 773-782.

McNay, D. E. G., Briancon, N., Kokoeva, M. V., Maratos-Flier, E., & Flier, J. S. (2012). Remodeling of the arcuate nucleus energy-balance circuit is inhibited in obese mice. *Journal of Clinical Investigation, 122*(1), 142-152.

Mitchell, N. S., Catenacci, V. A., Wyatt, H. R., and Hill, J. O. (2011). Obesity: overview of an epidemic. *Psychiatric Clinics of North America, 34*(4), 717-732.

Nelson, M., & Ackerman, J. (2011). *The Social Network Diet: Change Yourself, Change the World*. Campbell, CA: FastPencil.

Nettleton, J. A., Lutsey, P., Wang, Y., Lima, J. A., Michos, E. D., & Jacobs, D. R. Jr. (2009). Diet soda intake and risk of incident metabolic syndrome and type 2 diabetes in the Multi-Ethnic Study of Atherosclerosis (MESA). *Diabetes Care, 32*(4), 688-694.

Oh, H., & Taylor, A. H. (2011). Brisk walking reduces ad libitum snacking in regular chocolate eaters during a workplace simulation. *Appetite, 58*(1), 387-392.

Ohsiek, S., & Williams, M. (2011). Psychological factors influencing weight loss maintenance: an integrative literature review. *Journal of the American Academy of Nurse Practitioners, 23*(11), 592-601.

O'Rahilly, S., & Sadaf Farooqi, I. (2008). Human obesity: a heritable neurobehavioral disorder that is highly sensitive to environmental conditions. *Diabetes, 57*(11), 2905-2910.

Ostafin, B. D., & Marlatt, G. A. (2008). Surfing the urge: experiential acceptance moderates the relation between automatic alcohol motivation and hazardous drinking. *Journal of Social and Clinical Psychology, 27*(4), 404-418.

Pelchat, M. L. (2009). Food addiction in humans. *Journal of Nutrition, 139*(3), 620-622.

Perreault, L., Bergman, B. C., Hunerdosse, D. M., Playdon, M. C., & Eckel, R. H. (2010). Inflexibility in intramuscular triglyceride fractional synthesis distinguishes prediabetes from obesity in humans. *Integrative Physiology, 18*(8), 1524-1531.

Pollan, M. (2006). *The Omnivore's Dilemma: A Natural History of Four Meals.* New York: Penguin Books.

Puhl, R. M., & Heuer, C. A. (2010). Obesity stigma: important considerations for public health. *American Journal of Public Health, 100*(6), 1019-1028.

Racette, S. B., Deusinger, S. S., & Strube, M. J. (2008). Changes in weight and health behaviors from freshman through senior year of college. *Journal of Nutrition Education and Behavior, 40*(1), 39-42.

Ravussin, E., & Galgani, J. E. (2011). The implication of brown adipose tissue for humans. *Annual Review of Nutrition, 31*, 33-47.

Ravussin, E., & Kozak, L. P. (2009). Have we entered the brown adipose tissue renaissance? *Obesity Reviews, 10*(3), 265-268.

Rideout, C. A., & Barr, S. I. (2009). "Restrained eating" vs "trying to lose weight": how are they associated with body weight and tendency to overeat among postmenopausal women? *Journal of the American Dietetic Association, 109*(5), 890-893.

Roberts, C. J. (2008). The effects of stress on food choice, mood and bodyweight in healthy women. *Nutrition Bulletin, 33*(1), 33-40.

Roepstorff, C., Vistisen, B., & Kiens, B. (2005). Intramuscular triacylglycerol in energy metabolism during exercise in humans. *Exercise and Sport Science Reviews, 33*(4), 182-188.

Rolls, B. J. (2007). The effect of large portion sizes on energy intake is sustained for 11 days. *Obesity, 15*(6), 1535-1543.

Rolls, B. J. (2009). The relationship between dietary energy density and energy intake. *Physiology and Behavior, 97*(5), 609-615.

Romero-Corral, A., Somers, V. K., Sierra-Johnson, J., Korenfeld, Y., Boarin, S., Korinek, J., . . . Lopez-Jimenez, F. (2010). Normal weight obesity: a risk factor for cardiometabolic dysregulation and cardiovascular mortality. *European Heart Journal, 31*(6), 737-746.

Salzman, N. H. (2011). Microbiota-immune system interaction: an uneasy alliance. *Current Opinion in Microbiology, 14*(1), 99-105.

Spoor, S. T. P., Bekker, M. H. J., Van Strien, T., & van Heck, G. L. (2007). Relations between negative affect, coping, and emotional eating. *Appetite 48*(3), 368-376.

Stanhope, K. L., Schwarz, J. M., Keim, N. L., Griffen, S. C., Bremer, A. A., Graham, J. L., . . . Havel, P. J. (2009). Consuming fructose-sweetened, not glucose-sweetened, beverages increases visceral adiposity and lipids and decreases insulin sensitivity in overweight/obese humans. *Journal of Clinical Investigation, 119*(5), 1322-1334.

Stix, G. (2007). A malignant flame: understanding chronic inflammation, which contributes to heart disease, Alzheimer's and a variety of other ailments, may be a key to unlocking the mysteries of cancer. *Scientific American, 297*(1), 60-67.

Thaler, J. P., Yi, C. -X., Schur, E. A., Guyenet, S. J., Hwang, B. H., Dietrich, M. O., . . . Schwartz, M. W. (2012). Obesity is associated with hypothalamic injury in rodents and humans. *Journal of Clinical Investigation, 122*(1), 153-159.

Thaler, R. H., & Sunstein, C. R. (2008). *Nudge: Improving Decisions About Health, Wealth, and Happiness.* New Haven, CT: Yale University Press.

Tilg, H. (2012). Diet and intestinal immunity. *New England Journal of Medicine, 366*(2), 181-184.

Tsai, F., & Coyle, W. J. (2009). The microbiome and obesity: is obesity linked to our gut flora? *Current Gastroenterology Reports, 11*(4), 307-313.

Tuah, N. A., Amiel, C., Qureshi, S., Car, J., Kaur, B., & Majeed, A. (2011). Transtheoretical model for dietary and physical exercise modification in weight loss management for overweight and obese adults. *Cochrane Database of Systematic Reviews,* 10, CD008066. doi: 10.1002/14651858.CD008066.pub2.

Turnbaugh, P. J., Ley, R. E., Mahowald, M. A., Magrini, V., Mardis, E. R., & Gordon, J. I. (2006). An obesity-associated gut microbiome with increased capacity for energy harvest. *Nature, 144*(7122), 1027-1031.

Van Oudenhove, L., McKie, S., Lassman, D., Uddin, B., Paine, P., Coen, S., . . . Aziz, Q. (2011). Fatty acid-induced gut-brain signaling attenuates neural and behavioral effects of sad emotion in humans. *Journal of Clinical Investigation, 121*(8), 3094-3099.

Wadden, T. A., Neiberg, R. H., Wing, R. R., Clark, J. M., Delahanty, L. M., Hill, J. O., . . . Look AHEAD Research Group. (2011). Four-year weight losses in the Look AHEAD Study: factors associated with long-term success. *Obesity, 19*(10), 1987-1998.

Wardle, J., Carnell, S., Haworth, C. M., & Plomin, R. (2008). Evidence for a strong genetic influence on childhood adiposity despite the force of the obesogenic environment. *American Journal of Clinical Nutrition, 82*(2), 398-404.

Weiler, R., Stamatakis, E., & Blair, S. (2010). Should health policy focus on physical activity rather than obesity? Yes. *British Medical Journal, 340*, c2603.

Wing, R. R., & Phelan, S. (2005). Long-term weight loss maintenance. *American Journal of Clinical Nutrition, 82*(1), 222S-225S.

CHAPTER OUTLINE

LEARNING OBJECTIVES

After reading this chapter, you will be able to:

1. Conceptualize negative behaviors as occurring on a continuum that ranges from no use through addiction.

2. List the four most-common characteristics of addiction.

3. Describe several of the criteria for the diagnosis of substance-use disorders.

4. Understand the basic structure and function of the brain's reward pathways and explain how these appear to be related to substance dependency and addictive behaviors.

5. Explain several biological, psychological, and social/environmental risk factors for the development of substance-use disorders and addictive behaviors.

6. Describe some of the ways that public-health efforts attempt to prevent and address negative health behaviors, such as tobacco use.

7. Discuss some of the factors one should consider when working with people trying to change negative health behaviors.

8. Summarize evidence-based approaches for changing negative health behaviors.

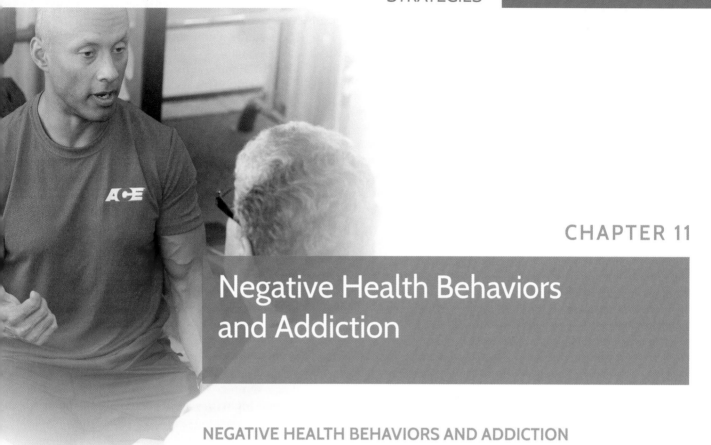

CHAPTER 11

Negative Health Behaviors and Addiction

NEGATIVE HEALTH BEHAVIORS AND ADDICTION

■ *Kim teaches group exercise classes, conducts personal training sessions, and is assistant manager of the fitness facility at a large community center. One evening, as she is preparing to lead her popular dance-exercise class, one of her longtime participants, Hope, arrives with a friend. Her friend, Eliza, looks like she has been crying, with her eyes red and a little swollen. She is smiling shyly at the moment, however. Hope explains that Eliza quit smoking two days ago and is a wreck. Eliza stops smiling and sighs, "I feel like I have lost my best friend." Hope explains that maybe getting out of the house and doing things in the evening will help Eliza get through the hard early days of quitting. Kim acknowledges that this is a great idea, and she gives Eliza a brochure featuring the variety of activities available at the community center. "Exercise doubles the success rate of people trying to quit smoking," Kim tells Eliza. Eliza picks up the steps quickly and manages to stay for the entire class. Kim praises her efforts and encourages her to sign up for the class. Eliza confesses that she is terrified of gaining weight and is hoping exercise will not only help her through nicotine withdrawal but also prevent weight gain as well. Kim asks Eliza to arrive 10 minutes early for the next class so that she can give her some materials on quitting smoking.* ■

Negative health behaviors are behaviors likely to cause harm. They may cause harm to a person's health, as when the use of tobacco products causes cancer, or when binge eating disorder leads to obesity and the litany of health problems linked to excess body fat. Negative health behaviors may also interfere with a person's life in other ways. For example, alcohol abuse may interfere with social relationships as well as academic and job performance. Illegal behavior, such as underage drinking, driving under the influence, or use of illegal substances, can result in punishments such as suspension from school, job termination, loss of one's driving privileges, or the imposition of fines and jail sentences. This chapter discusses several common negative health behaviors and behavior-change strategies useful for addressing them.

The first section of this chapter provides a context for evaluating negative health behaviors. It presents the psychophysiology of the most-difficult behaviors to change, including addictions and substance dependencies. Discussions of addiction, abuse, and use help develop the reader's understanding of the context of negative health behaviors. Negative health behaviors usually serve a purpose in a person's life. They may provide pleasure or a way to reduce negative emotions and cope with stress. Negative health behaviors might be an avenue for breaking out of old roles and family expectations. They may fuel creativity, become a part of a person's identity, or provide social connection and meaning in life. Negative health behaviors may even be a "life raft" that keeps a person afloat in a sea of despair. Changing behaviors central to a person's identity or ability to function in daily life is especially difficult. Negative health behaviors that include substance dependency and/or addiction can present special challenges, yet these are the health behaviors that are the most important to address.

Many behavior-change models, including The Transtheoretical Model (TTM) and its Stages of Change Model, were developed by researchers studying the process of changing negative health behaviors, including substance dependencies such as tobacco and alcohol use. The second section of this chapter provides an overview of behavior change theories, particularly what is different about the process of changing negative health behaviors. This section will review important factors that often influence the process of changing negative health behaviors and highlight suggestions for successful behavior-change strategies.

Chapter sections on alcohol, use of tobacco products, and harmful weight-control behaviors will apply behavior change theories to these important topics. Health and fitness professionals commonly encounter clients who may have disordered eating and exercise behaviors. These special forms of negative health behavior can be difficult to diagnose, as they can masquerade as "model behaviors," that is, dieting and exercising. This section will help readers better understand and work with clients showing symptoms of these negative health behaviors.

What is the role of the health and fitness professional when working with clients who have negative health behaviors? Sometimes people change negative health behaviors on their own as they adopt positive health behaviors. For example, some people curb emotional overeating behavior as they begin exercising and feeling stronger and healthier. Many people address negative health behaviors when motivated by a medical diagnosis or advice from a health-care provider. Health and fitness professionals can help clients recognize and address negative health behaviors as well. At some point in their careers, health and fitness professionals will probably find themselves working with people in recovery or in treatment for alcohol abuse, substance abuse, eating disorders, or other addictions. Some clients may be trying to quit smoking. While clients with substance dependencies

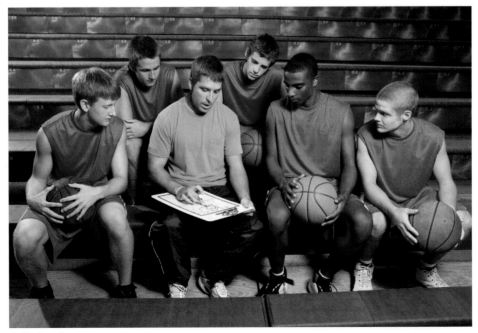

© Thinkstock

and addictions will need support beyond the health and fitness professional's scope of practice, these professionals sometimes work as part of a health-care team, and in this context they can help support clients with substance dependencies and other addictions as they try to develop healthier lifestyles. Understanding the nature of addiction allows professionals to move beyond a "blame the victim" attitude and work with people in treatment and recovery in ways most likely to motivate and support positive behavior change.

PLEASURE, ADDICTION, AND SUBSTANCE DEPENDENCE

People generally strive to feel good and try to cope with feeling bad. Sometimes this striving and coping takes the form of positive behaviors. People may discover they feel better when they get enough sleep, eat balanced meals, and avoid drinking too much coffee. Other times, seeking pleasure and coping with stress are associated with behaviors that may lead to positive feelings or help accomplish goals in the short run, but they cause harm or negative feelings in the long run. For example, frequently skipping sleep to complete assignments, grabbing whatever food is close at hand without regard for nutrition, and binge drinking may seem beneficial or harmless at the time, but these behaviors have negative physical and psychological consequences in the future.

Overview: Use, Abuse, or Addiction?

Addiction refers to the compulsive use of a substance or performance of an activity even though the person experiencing the addiction knows it is causing or is likely to cause harm. Addiction is also characterized by a loss of control over the substance use or performance of the activity as well as denial, since addicts do not accurately perceive the negative effects of the addictive behavior (Box 11-1).

People commonly use the word addiction with reference to substance abuse. Heroin addicts and alcoholics spring to mind as well as cigarette and caffeine habits. But people can also become addicted to unproductive relationships, food, gambling, work, using the Internet,

computer games, taking risks, exercise, and probably even to being a student. To become addicted is to devote or surrender oneself to something habitually or obsessively. It is ironic that the word addiction is derived from the Latin verb meaning "to give assent" since addicts become incapable of giving assent, having lost control of the habit in question. One of the characteristics of addiction is a reliance on something outside of oneself to cope with life and manage stress. Although people initially become addicted to something because it feels good, after a time, addictions may not provide pleasure so much as temporary relief, and addicted people may not feel good most of the time.

Addiction is not simply a function of the substance or activity in question, although some substances are especially likely to be addictive. The psychophysiology of substance dependence (compulsive use of chemicals such as drugs and alcohol) and addiction is discussed in more detail in the next section. Addiction is also not defined only by frequency or amount of use. Rather, whether use of a substance or performance of a behavior is categorized as an addiction depends on the reasons for and context of use or performance as well as the effect of the substance or activity on the user (Box 11-2). Addiction can be visualized as part of a continuum that extends from abstinence through use, abuse, and addiction (Fig. 11-1).

Figure 11-1 illustrates the continuum of a potentially addictive substance familiar to most readers: alcohol. At one end of the continuum is abstinence. Abstinence

Box 11-1. Basic Characteristics of Addiction

- Compulsive drive to use addictive substance or perform addictive activity
- Loss of control over the behavior
- Harmful consequences
- Distorted perceptions and denial concerning the addiction and its consequences

Box 11-2. Addiction Self-Assessment

The following questions can be applied to use of a substance, such as alcohol or marijuana, or to the performance of activities such as exercise, gambling, or use of social media. Even a single "yes" answer indicates that the behavior may become a problem and possibly an addiction.

1. Does the behavior provide the primary source of gratification in my life?
2. Does it provide the primary means of escape or avoidance of problems?
3. Does it decrease my self-esteem?
4. Am I developing a tolerance for the substance or activity, needing more than I did earlier to achieve the desired effect?
5. Do I need it to function?
6. Is it causing (or will it cause) the development of health problems?
7. Have others suggested I change or stop this behavior?
8. Does this behavior occur as a predictable, ritualistic, and compulsive activity?
9. Do I sometimes plan to decrease the behavior but then find I can't follow through on my plan, instead resuming previous levels of use?

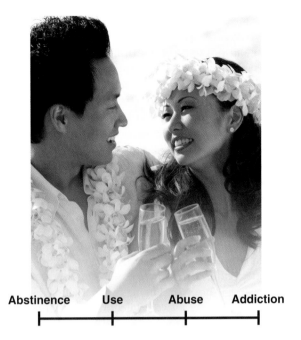

Abstinence   Use   Abuse   Addiction

Figure 11-1. Use, abuse, addiction continuum. Photograph © Thinkstock

refers to no use at all. A desire to avoid the devastating effects of alcoholism is one reason people abstain from imbibing. Underage people may abstain from using alcohol to avoid getting into trouble at school or in their communities. Many people believe that the health risks of alcohol outweigh any possible benefits; others shun alcohol because they have a strong family history of addiction. Some do not enjoy drinking or feel that alcohol calories could be better spent on something tastier. Many people do not use alcohol because its use is prohibited for religious reasons.

Of course, it is impossible to abstain from some potentially addictive substances or activities. For example, one cannot abstain from eating. Thus, people with eating disorders must learn to live with food. Treatment for eating disorders thus contrasts sharply with that for alcoholism, where a person addicted to alcohol has the option to just say no to alcohol. Similarly, it is not healthy to have no physical activity in one's day. People who exercise excessively must learn how to be active in ways that do not cause harm. Lastly, workaholics usually do not have the option to quit working, nor would they benefit from this. Instead, they must learn how to set limits on work involvement and broaden their participation in other activities to balance the energy they put into work and the degree to which their self-concept depends on working.

Not all potentially addictive substances or activities inevitably lead to addiction or harm for the user. To continue with the alcohol example, about 25% of adults in the United States develop alcohol-related problems (National Institute on Alcohol Abuse and Alcoholism, 2005). But the majority of users can learn to use alcohol in ways that are less likely to cause harm. They may drink appropriately in socially acceptable

settings. They use alcohol in moderation and for positive reasons, such as enjoying a glass of wine with a nice meal in the company of friends. The "use" point on Fig. 11-1 indicates this type of relationship to the substance or activity. Indeed, many potentially addictive substances or activities are a double-edged sword, with both potential benefits as well as risks. Exercise, food, Internet use, and work fit this description. In these cases, some level of use or performance can be safe and even beneficial. However, some substances, such as tobacco, have harmful effects and almost no benefit. Thus, even moderate "use" is harmful and should be discontinued.

Abuse occurs when use of the substance or performance of the behavior hurts or endangers the user or those around him or her. Alcohol abuse can occur in a single episode of drinking; driving while intoxicated is always considered alcohol abuse. Or alcohol abuse may consist of frequent heavy drinking that can lead to many health and behavioral problems. Going to class or work while intoxicated, getting into legal trouble as a result of drinking, experiencing blackouts, and getting injured while intoxicated are indicators of a drinking problem. Examples of abuse with other substances or behaviors are easy to spot because they are associated with causing harm. Gambling or shopping that involves losing or spending money a person cannot afford to lose or spend, consistently losing sleep because one cannot stop chatting with friends online, and failing to complete homework assignments because one tends to become distracted for hours while using the Internet are all examples of abuse. Abuse differs from addiction in that occasions of abuse are irregular in occurrence, without following a predictable pattern.

Addiction has developed when people lose the ability to control use of the substance or performance of the activity. While people who use alcohol in a controlled fashion may drink to relax at a social occasion and interact more easily with others, people with an addiction to alcohol may drink alone and forget all about going to the party. They may drink simply to cope. While controlled users of alcohol may enjoy the feeling of increased sociability that comes with a moderate amount of alcohol, addicts rely on alcohol to be able to socialize. They may feel incapable of social interaction without becoming intoxicated. When drunk, they may feel like "the life of the party." When sober, they may feel like they have nothing to say. The times when they drink may be the only times they do not feel bad.

Some people become addicted to substances or activities to escape from difficult issues. Instead of trying to solve a problem, they rely on the addiction to avoid the problem. The addiction may temporarily ease the hurt of painful emotions and provide a way to put off dealing with conflict. Eventually, the ability of addicts to tolerate uncertainty or anxiety may decline. New experiences and challenges cease to call forth innovative ideas and creative expression; they become simply an excuse to use the addictive substance or escape into the addictive behavior. Addicts are usually unable to perceive their own addictions accurately. They often deny the problem or make excuses that justify the continuation of the addiction behaviors.

Distinguishing habit from addiction is not always easy, especially for substances and behaviors condoned or encouraged by society. A good example is technology use. Many people compulsively check their cell phones and computers for messages several times an hour. They may frequently become distracted from work and from conversations with others physically present. Are people who text throughout the family dinner addicted? Or are they just developing a bad habit? If people are able to stop texting during meals with little difficulty, this was probably just a bad habit. If people decide to stop texting during meals but then surreptitiously continue to text under the table, have an inability to participate in meal-time conversation because they are too distracted worrying about what they are missing, or become anxious or depressed without the presence of technology every minute of the day and night, they may be addicted.

An important question is whether use or performance is causing or will be likely to cause harm. When people compulsively check their messages and communicate with others while they are "supposed" to be doing something else, this distraction detracts from the something else. An obvious example is texting while driving, an activity illegal in many states. Distraction reduces homework and work quality and productivity and the ability to be mentally present when spending time with others.

The use, abuse, addiction continuum represents the idea that people's relationships with potentially addictive substances and behaviors can be somewhat fluid (Health Psychology in Your Life 11-1). People's behavior may suggest different points on the continuum on different days. For example, some people will normally control their caffeine intake fairly well but occasionally overconsume and suffer anxiety and sleepless nights. The continuum also reinforces the observation that substance use and performance of potentially addictive behaviors are not dichotomous "good or bad" phenomena. While

negative health behaviors are negative (by definition), their negative outcomes are the issue; the behavior or substance itself is not always inherently negative, with a few exceptions.

The Psychophysiology of Pleasure, Addiction, and Substance Dependence

Pleasure, addiction, and substance dependence are mind–body phenomena. They are best understood using a biopsychosocial model, since biological, psychological, and sociological factors all play important roles in the perception of pleasure and the development of positive and negative health behaviors as well as addictions.

What causes pleasure and what is the function of pleasure? Psychologists have speculated that pleasure provides positive reinforcement for behaviors that help perpetuate life, such as eating, sex, caregiving behaviors, and finding physical comfort. The pleasure or reward pathways in the central nervous system help reinforce positive behaviors, such as physical activity. These pathways also reinforce negative and addictive behaviors.

Reward Pathways

The term reward pathway refers to the anatomic locations and biochemical events that make up the mind–body's experience of pleasure. To understand the basics of reward pathways, readers will need to recall the information presented in Chapter 2 about the nervous system, including its structure and function. The role and behavior of neurotransmitters are especially important, as they influence the nature of the thoughts, memories, and emotions produced in the brain. The areas of the brain activated also determine the nature of the mind–body experience that occurs.

One of the most-studied reward pathways involves the neurotransmitter dopamine (Ettinger, 2011). It is called the mesolimbic dopaminergic pathway. Mesolimbic refers to the location of some of the brain areas involved, in the central or middle portion of the limbic system. Dopaminergic relates to the hormone dopamine. Several areas of the brain participate in this reward pathway (Fig. 11-2). The ventral tegmental area (VTA) is found in the limbic area of the brain. Neurons originating in the VTA project to other areas of the brain, including a group of neurons in the limbic system known as the nucleus accumbens. Stimulation of the VTA in both laboratory animals and in humans causes feelings of pleasure. Neurons from these areas run to many other parts of the brain, including the amygdala, which helps process emotions, and the hippocampus, which is involved with memory. Neurons also connect these areas to the prefrontal cortex, an area of the brain important for making decisions and planning complex behaviors. This pathway illustrates the interconnectedness of various areas of the brain and the complex nature of pleasure and addiction

HEALTH PSYCHOLOGY IN YOUR LIFE 11-1.
Caffeine Use and Abuse

Draw the addiction continuum to illustrate caffeine use. Describe what abstinence, use, abuse, and addiction for caffeine use might look like. Where do your caffeine-use behaviors fall on the continuum? Interview a few friends or classmates about their caffeine-use behaviors and describe where you think they are on the addiction continuum. Explain your reasoning.

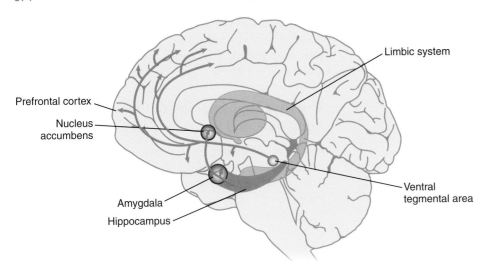

Figure 11-2. **The mesolimbic dopaminergic pathway.**

(Linden, 2011). The experience of pleasure is not simply a biochemical event but also involves learning, memory, and decision making. The mesolimbic dopaminergic pathway is thought to be involved with behaviors relating to reward and motivation, feelings of pleasure and euphoria, compulsive behavior, and perseverance.

Other reward pathways involve the neurotransmitter serotonin. Acetylcholine, norepinephrine, and epinephrine also make frequent appearances in discussion of neurotransmitters involved in experiences of pleasure and reward. Endorphins and anandamide, discussed in Chapter 3 in conjunction with exercise, are also involved in reward pathways. All pathways involve many regions of the brain and include sensory input; emotion; memory and learning; and thinking, planning, and decision-making functions (Ettinger, 2011).

A great deal of neuroscience research is exploring areas of the brain, such as the VTA and nucleus accumbens, that serve as hedonic hotspots, groups of neurons that when stimulated help produce sensations of pleasure (Berridge & Kringelbach, 2013). (Hedonic means relating to or characterized by pleasure.) Hedonic hotspots appear to exist in many areas of the brain. Hedonic hotspots are especially sensitive to specific types of neurotransmitters or chemicals. For example, some neurons in the nucleus accumbens have receptors for opioids but not cannabinoids, while some have both. Such research underscores the complexity of the central nervous system (CNS) and the psychophysiology of potentially pleasurable experiences and sensations.

Addiction research is also exploring how other areas of the brain interpret and respond to activation of these hedonic hotspots. For example, executive function areas of the brain, such as the prefrontal cortex, are intricately connected to the reward pathways. Executive function areas are involved in decision making, inhibiting impulsive behaviors, and evaluating the behaviors and substances involved in the reward pathways. Research suggests that executive function areas, such as the prefrontal cortex, may change in structure and function with addiction (Goldstein & Volkow, 2011). This makes

sense, since impulsivity often accompanies addiction behaviors.

Many things can activate reward pathways. For example, the ingestion of chocolate causes one of the largest food-related rises in dopamine (Goldstein, 2009). Many drugs lead to a rise in dopamine concentrations in the nucleus accumbens, including morphine, cocaine, and amphetamines. Thoughts and experiences as well as substances can cause biochemical changes in the CNS. Interestingly, just thinking about a rewarding behavior can lead to an increase in dopamine release (Goldstein, 2009). Research shows that charitable giving, exercise, meditation, and spiritual practices also activate the reward pathways (Linden, 2011).

Substance Dependency

Substance dependencies are especially likely to occur with addictive substances. Some substances, including nicotine, alcohol, and habit-forming drugs, appear to be particularly addictive. What does this mean? When a highly addictive substance, such as nicotine or morphine, activates a reward pathway, it changes the behavior of the affected neurons in some way. For example, in the dopaminergic pathway, under normal conditions, when a neuron receives a signal, it releases dopamine into the synapse. Some of the dopamine binds to receptors on the postsynaptic neuron. The rest of the dopamine is taken back up into the presynaptic neuron by dopamine transporter systems (Fig. 11-3).

Some drugs, such as cocaine and some amphetamines, affect the brain by blocking the dopamine reuptake transporter molecules in some of the neurons in the nucleus accumbens. This results in higher levels of dopamine in this area, which contributes to activation of this hedonic hotspot and feelings of pleasure. But over time, excessive levels of dopamine signal the neurons to produce less dopamine. This means the effect of the drug may be reduced, as less dopamine is released in response to it. Other drugs may alter neuron activity by inhibiting the release of certain neurotransmitters, thus suppressing the activity of certain neurons

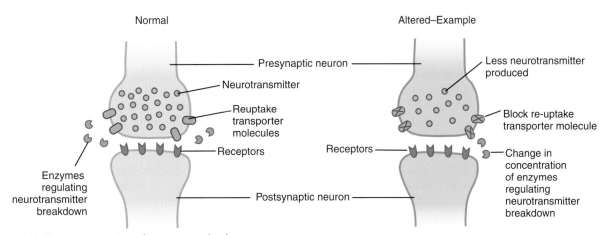

Figure 11-3. Neurotransmitter function and substance use.

or allowing prolonged activation of others. The nervous system responds by changing the amounts of neurotransmitters released or the concentration of enzymes regulating the breakdown of neurotransmitters in the synaptic cleft.

Adaptive mechanisms such as these are thought to explain the development of tolerance to addictive substances or behaviors. Tolerance means that it takes increasing amounts of the substance in question to produce a given effect. For example, people who use cocaine often find they need more of the drug to produce the high they used to feel when they first used cocaine. In some cases, people no longer achieve the same high but need greater amounts of the substance just to feel "normal." Similarly, as the nervous system adjusts to changes in neurotransmitter levels, feelings called cravings may develop. The term craving refers to a strong and usually uncomfortable drive to consume a given substance or participate in a given behavior. Cravings were discussed in the previous chapter in connection with eating and obesity. Cravings become troublesome when they are persistent and hard to ignore (DiFranza, Wellman, & Savageau, 2012). Cravings may develop when people need to use a particular substance to restore "normal" levels of neurotransmitter activity. In fact, one of the reasons addictions to substances such as nicotine and opiates are so difficult to overcome is that people feel so bad without the substance.

Withdrawal symptoms refer to signs and symptoms experienced by users when the substance to which they are addicted is not used. Withdrawal symptoms are somewhat specific to the substance of addiction. For example, nicotine withdrawal symptoms include irritability, difficulty sleeping, restlessness, impatience, and difficulty concentrating. Opiate withdrawal symptoms include anxiety, agitation, sweating, abdominal cramping, nausea, and vomiting.

Is there a difference between physical dependence and psychological dependence? Because thinking, planning, emotions, and moods include biochemical changes in the brain, with neurons communicating with each other via neurotransmitter release, it is impossible to neatly separate psychological and physical dependence. This explains why behavioral addictions such as gambling can be just as powerful as substance dependencies. For example, the excitement that gamblers feel as the event on which they place their bets unfolds is accompanied by strong physiological arousal and activation of reward pathways. While gambling is not a substance, the addiction process is still similar, and the dependence has physical and psychological components. However, physical withdrawal symptoms for behavioral addictions tend to be less severe than those for substances.

Substance-Related Disorders and Addiction

Until recently, psychologists considered the presence of tolerance and withdrawal symptoms part of the definition of addiction and thus part of the criteria for diagnosis and treatment. This definition was problematic for health professionals, since many people develop tolerance and withdrawal symptoms to medications or substances, such as caffeine and prescription drugs. Psychologists generally agree that more important than symptoms of tolerance and withdrawal is the issue of whether or not the substance or behavior is causing or likely to cause a problem. For example, both caffeine and cocaine users develop tolerance and withdrawal symptoms and experience cravings for the substances. But caffeine users can usually access their drug in convenient, legal ways for reasonable prices. While caffeine use can lead to health problems in some people (Box 11-3), especially if consumed in large quantities, the symptoms of tolerance and withdrawal alone are not adequate to diagnose a substance-use disorder. Cocaine use is quite a different story, as the substance is illegal and linked to serious health problems.

Health professionals also accept the fact that substances prescribed to treat medical conditions can be

Box 11-3. Caffeine: Friend or Foe?

Caffeine does not fall neatly into either the "dangerous drug" or the "safe and healthy food" categories. In fact, much of the research findings on caffeine contradict each other and leave consumers with feelings of confusion and ambivalence regarding their caffeine habits. Should people give it up, as they have done with cigarettes? Or should people drink more of certain caffeinated beverages, such as green tea, which contain helpful antioxidants? If individuals need many caffeinated beverages to get them through the day, should they be concerned about negative health effects in the near or distant future?

Caffeine is one of the most-studied drugs in the world. It has been consumed in some form for centuries by people in just about every culture of the world. Research examining the effect of the consumption of caffeine and caffeine-containing beverages on health suggests that in general, small doses do not appear to do too much harm to most people most of the time (Sunitha, Ramalakshmi, & Rao, 2008). Small-to-moderate amounts may even provide beneficial effects for some people. But caffeine does become harmful at higher doses, and some people are better off avoiding caffeine altogether.

Caffeine is similar in structure to the neurochemical adenosine, which slows brain activity. By blocking adenosine receptors, caffeine blocks adenosine's effects. This explains caffeine's positive effects, such as reducing feelings of fatigue, improving concentration, and enhancing mood. Caffeine's negative effects, including increased anxiety, irritability, nervousness, and insomnia, are also a result of blocking the action of adenosine in the brain.

As explained in Chapter 6, caffeine is considered a sympathomimetic drug, which means its effects mimic those of the sympathetic nervous system, the branch of the nervous system that produces the fight-or-flight stress response. Heart rate, blood pressure, and muscle tension temporarily increase as your body prepares to fight or flee in response to danger. Metabolic rate increases somewhat, and appetite may be reduced, which is why many weight-loss products contain caffeine.

Sensitivity to the effects of caffeine varies considerably from person to person. Smokers remove caffeine from their bodies twice as fast as nonsmokers and thus may be less sensitive to caffeine's effects. People who rarely consume caffeine are generally much more sensitive to caffeine's many effects, while people accustomed to caffeine experience less-pronounced reactions.

Most adults appear to self-regulate caffeine consumption fairly well. They learn, perhaps through trial and error, what amount of caffeine helps them feel alert and productive and when to stop before negative caffeine effects develop. Negative side effects, such as stomachaches, nausea, nervousness, insomnia, and anxiety, encourage most people to limit caffeine consumption.

However, some people develop negative symptoms with very small doses of caffeine and should avoid it entirely. The following factors suggest that it's time for people to take a closer look at their caffeine habits:

- **Irregular heartbeat.** Some people experience an irregular heartbeat when they consume caffeine. Their hearts feel like they are beating much too fast or are "skipping beats." For most of these people, any caffeine may be too much caffeine.
- **Feelings of stress and anxiety.** Many people experience feelings of stress and anxiety when they consume caffeine. And, to add insult to injury, people are more likely to overindulge in caffeine when stressed. And yet, because caffeine's effects mimic the stress response, it can leave people feeling more stressed than ever.
- **Insomnia.** If insomnia is a problem, giving up caffeine may be the answer. Some people find that even morning caffeine aggravates sleep problems that night.
- **High blood pressure.** Blood pressure rises for a fairly short time following caffeine ingestion. While this rise does not appear to be harmful for most people, those with hypertension may benefit by reducing caffeine intake.
- **High intakes.** High intakes of coffee and other caffeinated products have been associated with some health problems, such as increased risk for ovarian and pancreatic cancers. Risks usually are associated with over five cups of coffee per day (Lueth, Anderson, Harnack, Fulkerson, & Robien, 2008).
- **Concerns about bone density and osteoporosis.** Some studies have suggested a link between caffeine consumption and risk of osteoporosis in elderly women, although not in younger women who just drink a cup or two of caffeinated beverages a day (Cooper et al., 2009).
- **Reproductive concerns.** A high caffeine intake may interfere with fertility, so couples having difficulty conceiving should try reducing caffeine. High caffeine consumption during pregnancy is associated with birth defects in laboratory animals (Rivkees & Wendler, 2012) and miscarriage and low birth weight in humans, so only small amounts of caffeine (or none) should be consumed during pregnancy (Patel & Rizzolo, 2012). Caffeine gets into breast milk, and nursing moms who consume caffeine may end up with irritable, fussy babies who have trouble sleeping.

Box 11-3. Caffeine: Friend or Foe?—cont'd

- **Ulcers and heartburn.** Coffee, not caffeine, increases the production of stomach acids, so decaffeinated coffee is no solution. People with digestive complaints should reduce coffee intake or switch to tea.
- **High blood cholesterol levels.** A high intake of coffee may raise serum cholesterol levels. The chemicals in coffee thought to provoke higher cholesterol are caught by the filter papers in drip coffee makers, so coffee prepared in this fashion is the least risky (Bohn, Ward, Hodgson, & Croft, 2012). People with high cholesterol levels may wish to reduce or eliminate coffee and see if cholesterol goes down. Even small reductions in cholesterol decrease risk of heart disease.

---

associated with symptoms of tolerance and withdrawal. Thus, the use of narcotic pain medication is not considered a substance-related disorder when used within the bounds of medical treatment. Indeed, most health professionals agree that withholding narcotics from suffering patients would be unethical, even though patients may develop a chemical dependency. However, when use of medicinal narcotics extends beyond what is needed to treat the pain, the patient has likely developed a dependency.

Psychologists use the term **substance-related disorder** to refer to problems involving the use of substances, such as drugs, alcohol, and tobacco products, and associated difficulties such as coping with withdrawal symptoms or emotional health problems related to the substance (American Psychiatric Association, 2013). Psychologists use the term **substance-use disorder** (SUD) to refer to problems with substance dependence and abuse. (Substance-use disorder is one type of substance-related disorder.) Psychologists are more likely to use the term addiction to refer to nonsubstance involvements, such as gambling and overuse

of the Internet. Criteria for the diagnosis of SUDs are listed in Box 11-4.

Kim is pleased when Eliza arrives 10 minutes early for the next class. Kim has gotten a good self-help workbook for people trying to quit smoking and a link to the free website. She shares these materials with Eliza. Eliza looks exhausted and admits she is having a very hard time not smoking. Kim urges her to get nicotine patches or gum from her health-care provider to ease withdrawal symptoms and promises things will gradually get easier. She praises Eliza's ability to still not be smoking, even while having such strong symptoms. "You know, nicotine is even more addictive than heroin. That's why people get so addicted to it," Kim explains. "Are you having a hard time sleeping?" Eliza nods her head. "Maybe your doctor can give you some advice on that as well," Kim suggests. "Quitting smoking can be really hard, and there may be treatments that can help you."

Box 11-4. Substance-Use Disorder—Definition and Diagnostic Criteria

The American Psychiatric Association defines substance-use disorder as "a maladaptive pattern of substance use leading to clinically significant impairment or distress, as manifested by 2 (or more) of the following, occurring within a 12-month period":

1. Repeated substance use that results in a failure to fulfill major obligations, such as poor work performance or neglect of children.
2. Repeated hazardous use of the substance, such as driving under the influence of the substance.
3. Continued use of the substance despite the fact that it is causing social or interpersonal problems and even though the user acknowledges that these problems are the result of use.
4. Development of tolerance: needing more of the substance to produce the desired effect or experiencing less effect for a given dose.
5. Withdrawal symptoms.
6. Substance is taken in larger amounts or for longer periods than intended.
7. Efforts to reduce or eliminate use are unsuccessful.
8. A lot of time is spent procuring or using the substance or recovering from substance use.
9. Involvement in important activities is given up or reduced as a result of substance use.
10. Craving or a strong need to use the substance.

Source: American Psychiatric Association (2013). *The Diagnostic and Statistical Manual of Mental Disorders,* 5th ed. Washington, DC: American Psychiatric Association.

The Biopsychosocial Model of Negative Health Behaviors and Addiction

The neuroscience of addictive substances helps explain why people develop negative health behaviors and addictions. Yet the biochemistry of addiction is only a relatively small part of the addiction picture. In order to understand how people develop and have difficulty changing negative health behaviors, one must consider the many factors that can reinforce, influence, or even in some cases, prevent these behaviors (Fig. 11-4). Factors that influence the acquisition and development of negative health behaviors often occur in clusters and interact with one another. Factors may be classified as biological, psychological, or social/environmental, although these classifications are somewhat arbitrary since the factors related to them often overlap. For example, a mood disorder such as depression may have biological as well as psychological underpinnings. Some of the most important factors include the following.

Biological Factors

Biological factors include genetic heritage and physiological characteristics that interact with potentially addictive substances and behaviors.

Genetic Predisposition

A family history of addiction increases an individual's risk for developing an addiction. Studies in identical and fraternal twins suggest that genetics may account for about 40% to 60% of variation in risk for addiction (Linden, 2011). Some research indicates that genetic inheritance influences the number and type of dopamine receptors on neurons (Foll, Gallo, Strat, Lu, & Gorwood, 2009). Other genes and their effects are also under investigation (Blednov et al., 2012). It is clear that there is no single "addiction gene" that predisposes people to the development of addiction. Rather, the risk for developing an addiction is only partially influenced by genetics, and researchers agree that the relationship of genetics to addiction risk is fairly complex (Li & Burmeister, 2009).

Psychophysical Response to Substance or Behavior

People who experience improvement in mood, positive emotions, or euphoria in response to using a substance or performing a behavior will be more likely to want to repeat the experience than someone who has no response or a negative reaction. For example, alcohol causes nausea and vomiting in some people, with no pleasurable feelings at all, so these people would be unlikely to become addicted to this substance. People who experience euphoria during exercise will be more likely in the future to turn to exercise for mood improvement. They would also have a higher risk of becoming addicted to exercise than someone who experiences exercise as painful.

Adolescent Age

During adolescence, various areas of the brain mature at different rates. Of special concern is the observation that the limbic system, home of the reward pathway, develops earlier than the prefrontal reasoning and planning areas (Forbes et al., 2010). Such differences may help explain the higher levels of risky behaviors observed in many adolescents: the potential to have fun overrides ideas about reasonable action and inhibition of risky impulses. Of course, biological age interacts with family and other environmental factors to influence the development of negative health behaviors.

Early Exposure to Addictive Substances

Early exposure to addictive substances can occur in utero or early in a person's life. Developing fetuses, children, and adolescents are more vulnerable than adults to the effect of many substances. For example, a pregnant woman's use of cocaine appears to influence fetal development in a number of ways. Cocaine acts upon the fetus's developing nervous system and may cause epigenetic changes in important genes, altering their expression in the fetus, with effects lasting into childhood and adulthood (Lester & Padbury, 2009). Researchers have theorized that in-utero exposure to cocaine increases the fetus's exposure to stress hormones, the catecholamines

Biological	Psychological	Social/Environmental
• Genetic predisposition • Psychological response to substance or behavior • Adolescent age • Early exposure to addictive substances	• Attention deficit disorders • Mood disorders • PTSD • Less-effective coping skills • Hopelessness	• Access to substance or behavior • Childhood family and home environment • Social norms • Socioeconomic status • Social environment • Adverse childhood events

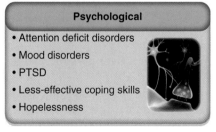
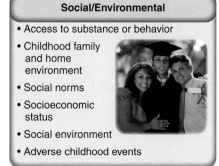

Figure 11-4. Factors that influence risk of developing negative health behaviors. Photograph © Thinkstock

and cortisol, which alters the activity of the hypothalamic-pituitary-adrenal axis. These alterations may set children up for brain activity changes leading to poor behavioral control and emotional regulation, which are risk factors for substance use in adolescence.

During adolescence, the brain undergoes many changes in its structure and function. Exposure to alcohol, marijuana, and other substances during adolescence appears to have significant and long-lasting effects on brain maturation. Both adult and adolescent brains respond to alcohol with increased dopamine concentrations in the nucleus accumbens and activation of the mesolimbic dopaminergic pathway. However, adolescent brains experience stronger effects in some areas than adult brains, probably because of developmental differences (Alfonso-Loeches & Guerri, 2011). Research shows that regular use of alcohol or marijuana during the teenage years is associated with reduced size of the hippocampus (important for memory) and prefrontal cortex areas (executive control). Regular and heavy users show less-efficient patterns of neural processing in response to a variety of tasks, which means the brain is less efficient in its functioning. Use of alcohol and marijuana is associated with decreased cognitive function, especially poorer performance in attention, visual and spatial functioning, the learning and retrieval (memory functions) of information, and planning and problem solving (Bava & Tapert, 2010). Unfortunately, such changes in brain structure and function may then increase the risk for continuing use of substances and more difficulty in regulating their use.

Psychological Factors

Many of the psychological factors associated with addiction risk have biological components, such as those described previously, and interact with other risk factors.

Attention Deficit Disorders

Addiction is marked by repeatedly using substances or performing behaviors despite the knowledge and experience of negative consequences. The prefrontal cortical areas of the brain are responsible for the executive functions that inhibit impulsive behavior, attend to tasks, plan, and think about consequences. Attention deficit disorders often indicate lower levels of executive function and higher levels of impulsivity. Studies suggest that people, especially adolescents, with attention deficit disorders are at higher risk for developing addictions (Crews & Boettiger, 2009), perhaps because of their lower ability to inhibit impulsive behaviors.

Mood Disorders and Post-Traumatic Stress Disorder

People with mood disorders such as anxiety and depression are more likely to develop substance-use disorders than people without mood disorders, although it is not easy to always know which came first: the substance use or the mood disorder (Hall, Degenhardt, & Teesson, 2009). Nevertheless, it is well documented that people with anxiety and other disorders sometimes use substances to reduce emotional distress, a practice known as self-medication (Bolton, Robinson, & Sareen, 2009).

Post-traumatic stress disorder (PTSD) is strongly associated with substance abuse disorders. Studies suggest that when treatment helps reduce the severity of PTSD symptoms, improvement in substance use patterns is likely to be seen as well (Hien et al., 2010).

Less-Effective Coping Skills

When people have better resources and abilities to cope with stress, they appear to be less likely to turn to substances for self-medication or to addictive behaviors for solace. Studies suggest that adolescents and adults can identify factors and situations that increase their risk of substance use and apply cognitive behavior therapy to learn better ways to cope with risky situations (Conrod, Castellanos-Ryan, & Strang, 2010).

Hopelessness

Hopelessness is often accompanied by feelings of helplessness and an external locus of control. Hopelessness generally restricts a person's feeling of choice and control, so that individuals perceive themselves as having fewer response options when facing a challenge. In addition, feelings of depression often accompany hopelessness, perhaps mediating the link between helplessness and external locus of control with negative health outcomes. Feelings of hopelessness lead to low self-efficacy and low drive to persist in coping with difficulties.

Social and Environmental Factors

People's social and built environments exert strong effects on their behavior, including risks of developing substance use and addiction disorders. A few of the more-powerful variables influencing risk include the following.

Access to Substance or Behavior

Access to a substance or behavior is obviously a prerequisite for development of substance use and addiction disorders. People tend to develop disorders for substances and behaviors more common in their environment, including in their social circles. Access may take the form of a substance being available, such as prescription drugs being sold by one's friends. It can also take the form of behaviors common in one's environment, such as gambling.

Childhood Family and Home Environment

Children are strongly influenced by their early home environment and their family members. Early environment shapes social norms and children's attitudes toward substances and behaviors. For example, an interesting study followed over 1,650 people for 20 years to explore risk factors for smoking (Paul, Blizzard, Patton, Dwyer, & Venn, 2008). The subjects were 9 to 15 years old at the beginning of the study. The researchers found that parental smoking increased the risk of children becoming smokers. In addition, the study found that childhood smoking experimentation also increased the risk of developing a smoking habit. Children who smoked 10 or more cigarettes per day at 13 to 14 years of age were more likely to become smokers as adults, compared with those who never smoked or smoked less.

Social Norms

Social norms regarding substance use and behavior exert a strong impact on an individual's perceptions. Social norms influence which substances an individual may decide to use and how use occurs. Similarly, social norms provide a context for behaviors that may become problematic, such as interpersonal dependence (being overly dependent on another person), gambling, work, and so forth. Peer group norms are especially strong. It is important to note that an individual's perception of social norms may be inaccurate, as when college students mistakenly believe "everyone is getting drunk on the weekend" or when athletes believe it is normal for people to exercise for many hours every day.

Socioeconomic Status and Social Environment

Socioeconomic status and social environment contribute strongly to people's stress levels, physical and emotional health, and risk of substance abuse. Stressors such as poverty and discrimination limit people's access to resources and behaviors that enhance likelihood of success in many life arenas, especially career and financial success. Sociologists have observed that stressors tend to proliferate: those with more challenges tend to continue to find themselves in challenging situations, while people who have the resources and abilities to cope effectively with stress tend to master challenges (Thoits, 2010). In addition, home and school environments usually reflect socioeconomic status and may expose and encourage adolescents to experiment with specific substances or behaviors, strengthening the effect of perceived peer norms.

Adverse Childhood Events

An abusive home environment and other adverse childhood events are associated with increased risk for the development of addiction. Studies suggest that such exposures may cause mood and anxiety disorders, which in turn increase risk for substance abuse and addiction because people seek to improve mood and reduce anxiety (Douglas et al., 2010). An abusive home environment may accompany other risk factors described previously.

MOTIVATING CHANGE: Use an Ecological Perspective to Understand Clients' Negative Health Behaviors

The above factors can be incorporated into an ecological perspective for negative health behaviors. Some factors are unchangeable but can enhance understanding of the target behavior. Other factors

will be irrelevant for a given client, while a few may help professionals and clients devise behavior-change strategies. For example, clients with a mood disorder such as depression should consider treatment for depression a critical component of their efforts to quit smoking or to change other negative health behaviors. Clients who use negative behavior to cope with stress would benefit from developing other strategies to reduce feelings of stress. Keep the factors mentioned in this chapter in mind as you listen to clients' stories about their negative health behaviors. The more you understand your client, the more effective your help will be.

As Kim had feared, Eliza does not appear the following week for the exercise class. Hope admits that Eliza has started smoking again and is too embarrassed to come to class. Kim assures Hope that most people have to try several times before quitting successfully and says she will e-mail Eliza. In her e-mail, Kim encourages Eliza to return to class and to join the smoking-cessation group at the community center, which will be starting in 2 weeks.

Kim is happy to see Eliza at the following class. After class, they talk for a bit. "So many of my friends smoke," Eliza tells Kim. "Plus my husband. But he said maybe he would quit with me. We want to have children soon, and everyone says I should quit smoking before I get pregnant." Kim figures this may be the key to Eliza's autonomous motivation. "That's wonderful!" she exclaims. "But definitely get your husband to quit with you. That will make things much easier." "I don't know," says Eliza. "If we both feel as bad as I felt last week, more likely we'll kill each other."

PREVENTING AND CHANGING NEGATIVE HEALTH BEHAVIORS

Understanding the neuroscience of the reward pathways and the many factors that predispose people to develop negative health behaviors and addictions can leave one with a sense of futility regarding the potential to help people change these behaviors. And yet, even people with the most serious addictions do change and overcome their addictions. The reward pathways can change in response to new lifestyle behaviors and learn new ways of experiencing pleasure. Health and fitness professionals working with clients to change negative health behaviors must not imply that negative behaviors are stronger than the clients are. Understanding how clients may be predisposed to developing negative health behaviors and addiction allows professionals to avoid a judgmental attitude that ruins all hope of working effectively with clients. But, at the same time that professionals can express understanding and support for clients, they must also encourage clients to take responsibility for lifestyle change. Health and fitness professionals can use behavior-change strategies to help strengthen clients' motivation for change and design effective behavior-change interventions, with appropriate support in the case of serious addictions.

This section provides an overview of the application of general behavior-change theory to negative health behaviors and addictions. Information on behavior change discussed thus far in this book applies to changing negative health behaviors and will not be reexamined in depth here. Instead, information especially applicable to changing negative behaviors will be the focus and will be integrated with the behavior-change theory and models already discussed.

Negative Health Behaviors: Importance of Prevention

With negative health behaviors, an ounce of prevention is worth a pound of cure. Any smoker who has had difficulty quitting can attest to the fact that never beginning to smoke is much easier than quitting. Once the reward pathways have been nurtured and have adapted to the negative behavior, they are upset when the behavior is withdrawn. It is better to never get these established. Prevention efforts can take many forms.

Health Education
Health education often focuses on preventing negative health behaviors by teaching people about the risks associated with the behavior. For example, health-education efforts may highlight the health risks of tobacco use, driving under the influence, or unsafe sexual practices. Health education may be targeted at any age group, and messages should be crafted for the specific audience. Public school health-education programs are often required to follow state guidelines regarding content and teaching methods. Health education at worksites typically targets behaviors that will offer the most benefit. For example, if workers have a high rate of cigarette smoking, a worksite might offer smoking-cessation programs to assist employees trying to quit.

Adolescent age groups tend to provide one of the most-difficult audiences for health-education efforts. Since emotional brain areas develop before the rational decision-making brain areas, adolescents may not connect with health information so much as with what appeals to them emotionally. Just learning the facts about substances and behaviors is usually not enough to discourage use. In fact, for some teens, learning about substances such as anabolic steroids may actually increase use. Similarly, vulnerable teens who learn about eating disorders sometimes adopt those behaviors. Instead, education must focus on empowering individuals to set goals and seek positive ways of achieving those goals. Schools, families, and communities must

help create ways for adolescents to develop positive behaviors that lead to good outcomes. Young people often benefit from participation in after-school activities including sports, arts, and community-service programs.

Preventive Cognitive Behavior Therapy
An interesting group of researchers has used targeted cognitive behavior therapy (CBT) interventions in adolescents (Conrod, Castellanos-Ryan & Strang, 2010). The London-based group has developed CBT sessions that target specific vulnerabilities that make adolescents prone to substance use. These interventions have been tested in several studies. In one study, the group gave adolescents in London schools a psychological assessment to determine those at greatest risk for developing habits of using alcohol, marijuana, and other drugs (Conrod et al., 2010). Students were considered "at risk" if they scored high on any of the following measures: hopelessness, anxiety sensitivity, impulsivity, and sensation seeking. In this study, 732 at-risk students aged 13 to 16 were randomly assigned to targeted CBT treatment or a placebo condition.

The students participated in two 90-minute group sessions conducted by counselors, teachers, and research assistants. The intervention began with goal setting and motivation for behavior-change exercises. The students then learned about their particular personality risk and problems associated with it, especially problematic coping strategies such as avoidance, aggression, interpersonal dependence, substance use, and other risky behaviors. Students were guided in the use of cognitive-behavioral strategies that would help them examine problematic thoughts and behaviors and learn new coping skills. As predicted, after 2 years more students in the intervention groups reported no drug use. This research is especially exciting because the intervention is brief and relatively easy to administer, since there are manuals that help group leaders conduct the workshops. Delaying adolescents' onset of drug and alcohol use even a few years significantly reduces the likelihood of them developing substance-use disorders.

Public-Health Campaigns Target Prevention and Promote Behavior Change

Public-health campaigns make use of a variety of strategies to change negative health behaviors, frequently targeting both prevention and behavior change. Public-health efforts frequently select an issue where the return, in terms of health improvement, is likely to be greatest for the resources devoted to the project. Two of the most-successful public-health campaigns have focused on reducing tobacco use and rates of driving under the influence of alcohol and drugs.

Stop-smoking campaigns have been some of the most successful in the history of public health. Since the 1960s, the rate of cigarette smoking in the United States has declined by 58% (National Research Council, 2007). Many public-health efforts use some form of media campaign, combined with other strategies. Media campaigns include public service advertising in a wide range of media, including television, print, the Internet, and social media. When media campaigns are successful, they can raise public awareness, increase the frequency and breadth of discussions about the behavior in question, and inspire other groups to take on the issue. They can also change people's perceptions of social norms in ways that reinforce motivation for behavior change. In the case of smoking, mass media campaigns have been associated with a decline in the number of young people starting smoking and with the number of adults who quit smoking (Wakefield, Loken, & Hornik, 2010). Over the past several decades, mass media campaigns have been combined with efforts from the medical, health-education, and legal communities. Some of the activities that have contributed to a reduction in tobacco use rates have included:

- Increased taxation on tobacco products, making them more expensive to consumers.
- More laws regulating allowable levels of second-hand smoke in the air of workplaces and public places. This led to prohibitions on smoking in many public venues, such as transportation centers and modalities, restaurants, offices, and schools.
- Laws regulating the advertisement of tobacco products.
- Legislation requiring health-risk warning labels on tobacco products (Fig. 11-5).
- Increased enforcement of penalties for businesses selling tobacco products to minors.
- Health-promotion programming at schools, workplaces, and community centers supporting people's efforts to quit smoking.
- Increased communication with medical and allied health professionals regarding the importance of advising patients to quit smoking and providing suggestions on how to help patients quit.
- Development of medical products, such as nicotine gum and other nicotine medications as well

as the electronic cigarette, to help people reduce tobacco use or to at least reduce some of the harmful effects of smoking.

Many public-health campaigns have been less successful in preventing and changing target behaviors. Some experts have even suggested that too much media attention to a behavior can have the effect of "normalizing" the behavior or making the target audience perceive the behavior to be more common than it actually is (Wakefield, Loken, & Hornik, 2010). For example, campaigns to change drug and alcohol use patterns among adolescents have been less successful. Health-education efforts to prevent eating disorders have similarly failed to reduce the increased rates of these disorders.

Behavior-Change Theory and Negative Health Behaviors

Psychologists have long been interested in how people change negative health behaviors, including substance-use disorders and addictions. All of the behavior-change theories and models help explain negative behaviors and addictions. Indeed, some were originally developed with a particular focus on negative health behaviors. For example, Prochaska's Stages of Change Theory was developed in the 1980s to understand the processes of change associated with changing addictive behaviors such as cigarette smoking (Prochaska & DiClemente, 1983). In many ways, changing negative health behaviors, such as quitting smoking, is no different from adopting positive behaviors, such as beginning an exercise program. The same factors are relevant. For example, in the Health Belief Model, a person who feels susceptible to a particular health problem and believes that behavior change will be helpful is predicted to be more motivated to make a decision to change. A diagnosis of alcoholic liver disease may motivate a patient to quit consuming alcohol. Learning that cigarette smoking is likely contributing to a person's high blood pressure might help that person decide to quit. Similarly, the factors of perceived behavioral control, attitudes about the behavior, and subjective norms, from the Theory of Planned Behavior, contribute to people's decisions to change negative health behaviors. In fact, there are only a few differences in either theory or behavior-change counseling applications for changing negative health behaviors, compared with those for adding positive health behaviors. Some of the differences are detailed below.

Settings for Behavior-Change Programs

Behavior-change efforts can occur in a variety of settings. The most-intensive forms of behavior-change treatment are more likely to be seen for negative health behaviors such as drug or alcohol addiction and eating disorders. When a negative health behavior has become a health problem, such as a substance-use disorder, treatment is likely to be more aggressive. For example, inpatient and residential treatment programs provide constant supervision for patients, along with a change

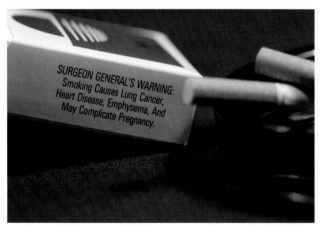

Figure 11-5. Warning label from cigarette pack. *(Courtesy of CDC/Deborah Cartagena.)*

of environment that can help remove people from the daily triggers that sustain a negative behavior. Sometimes such programs use an element of coercion, and patients may have to participate even though they don't want to (especially when it has been determined that their behavior is dangerous either to themselves, such as for people with eating disorders who are near starvation, or others, such as people committing crimes to support a drug addiction).

In some cases, behavior-change efforts for serious substance addictions begin with some sort of detoxification program. Detoxification refers to the initial stage of abstinence from an addictive substance, during which the person addicted may experience a number of physical and psychological withdrawal effects. This period may require medical supervision and treatment to reduce withdrawal symptoms and help patients adjust to a new normal.

Inpatient programs are very expensive, so they are usually reserved only for behaviors with the most-serious consequences and for people who can afford them. Inpatient programs usually offer options for cultivating a healthful lifestyle to help guide patients into new practices that will promote physical and psychological well-being.

Residential programs for positive health behaviors do exist. They are usually called spas, retreat centers, or something nice. These programs can help people jump-start new healthful behaviors, such as increasing physical activity, eating more healthfully, and managing stress more effectively. But, because of their expense, only a minority of people uses these programs.

Nonresidential behavior-change settings are less expensive and more common for programs in both positive and negative health behavior change. These programs may include everything from individual counseling and psychotherapy, to group therapy and support, to alternative and complementary medicine treatments such as acupuncture, hypnosis, and therapeutic yoga.

Executive Cognitive Functions

Another difference is that executive cognitive functions are more likely to be a problem, and therefore the therapeutic target, for behavior-change programs involving negative health behaviors and addiction. This is because lower levels of executive cognitive function (ECF) are associated with addiction (Blume & Marlatt, 2009; Goudriaan, Oosterlaan, de Beurs, & van den Brink, 2006). Executive cognitive functions include abilities that are critical for behavior change, including planning, organizing, problem-solving, and regulating one's behavior and emotions. Executive cognitive functions are essential for making the decision to change behaviors and to sustain one's motivation for change. It is likely that lower levels of ECF predispose people to addiction and substance-use disorders. In addition, addictions themselves appear to alter ECF.

Lower levels of ECF are associated with behaviors typically classified as denial and may be related to lower levels of self-awareness or awareness of the effect the addiction is having on others. Lower levels of ECF have also been related to lower self-efficacy for changing addiction behaviors (Bates, Pawlak, Tonigan, & Buckman, 2006). Less-effective coping skills and a lower capacity for delaying gratification and controlling impulses contribute to the difficulty that low-ECF people may experience when trying to change negative health behaviors.

Experts recommend that strategies to improve ECF be part of addiction treatment (Blume & Marlatt, 2009). For example, Blume and Marlatt have found that mindfulness meditation may help people with addictions become better aware of their thoughts and decision-making processes. Treatment recommendations should also take into account an individual's levels of ECF and self-efficacy for behavior change. For example, someone low in self-efficacy and ECF might do better in an abstinence-type treatment program than in a program with controlled use as its treatment goal. (The person needs to make fewer decisions in an abstinence-based program.) Such recommendations underscore the importance of individualizing treatment and referring people with addiction to trained professionals.

12-Step Programs

No discussion of behavior change would be complete without recognition of the important role that 12-step programs have played in the lives of many people in overcoming difficult addictions. The original 12-step program was designed by Alcoholics Anonymous (AA), which published its method of overcoming addiction in 1939 in the book *Alcoholics Anonymous: The Story of How More Than One Hundred Men Have Recovered from Alcoholism* (Alcoholics Anonymous, www.aa.org/timeline). Twelve-step programs generally endorse abstinence from the substance causing the addiction problem, such as alcohol, believing that any amount can trigger relapse. The original AA 12-step program is deeply rooted in spiritual practice, with participants guided to receive strength from the support of a higher power for relapse prevention. The program also endorses moral action, taking responsibility for one's life, and a strong network of social support. Members who have completed all 12 steps become sponsors of new members, guiding them through the 12-step process. Groups meet regularly to support one another in their efforts to maintain sobriety. More information on Alcoholics Anonymous is available in its manual, *The Big Book* (www.aa.org/bigbookonline).

Critics of Alcoholics Anonymous and other 12-step programs question several components of these programs. Some question whether abstinence from the substance or behavior is always necessary. Others have trouble with the higher power concept and the emphasis on the notion that if one has an addiction, one is an "addict for life," meaning that full recovery is never possible. However, research generally supports the effectiveness of 12-step programs for people who chose to participate, with success rates similar to those for other types of programs (Gross, 2010). Certainly, several elements of 12-step programs appear in behavior-change theory, especially social support for forming the intention to change and for sustaining behavior change. Twelve-step programs usually make special efforts to help participants overcome tendencies toward denial of addictive behaviors and the problems associated with the addiction.

Cravings

Strong cravings pose a significant challenge for people trying to change many negative health behaviors. People with addictions to substances or behaviors often experience strong urges to resume the behavior or substance use as they are trying to make positive changes. This makes changing negative health behaviors different in emotional tone from trying to add positive behaviors or to change behaviors that are not as habit forming. Food cravings were discussed in the previous chapter, as they often interfere with changes in eating behavior. Cravings can vary in intensity, and people have trouble coping with extremely strong cravings. People trying to change a negative behavior may focus extensively on strategies and treatments to help reduce cravings and the drive to resume the behavior they are trying to overcome. For example, people trying to quit smoking might try a variety of alternative and complementary medical therapies, such as acupuncture, hypnosis, and relaxation strategies. A variety of medications is also available to help reduce cravings for people in treatment programs. Coping skills for dealing with cravings are usually an important component of recommendations for changing negative health behaviors.

Stress Management

Strengthening clients' stress-management skills is important in every behavior-change setting but is especially critical for those changing negative health behaviors. Not only does changing the negative behavior create stress, but the behavior itself is often the client's preferred method for coping with stress. A good example of this is people who turn to alcohol to cope with feelings of stress. If they are trying to cut back on or eliminate alcohol consumption, they may feel stressed by this change. If drinking used to provide their most-reliable (in their perception) way to reduce feelings of stress, the drive to drink will be very strong. Staying sober under these conditions will require new ways of interpreting and responding to stressors and feelings of stress. These individuals might learn to use exercise to reduce stress arousal and improve mood or try new social activities to replace the socialization and pleasure experienced with drinking.

Co-occurring Mood Disorders

Research suggests that substance-use disorders frequently occur alongside mood disorders, such as depression and anxiety. This increases the complexity of designing successful behavior-change programs for negative health behaviors and addictions. For example, one study found that about a third of people diagnosed with major depressive disorder also had symptoms of a substance-use disorder (Davis, Uezato, Newell, & Frazier, 2008). Psychologists have noted that qualities such as stress vulnerability and ruminative thinking occur in both SUDs and mood disorders. Dysfunctional cognitive control patterns may be part of the problem in both types of disorders. Substance use may also be a way people with mood disorders attempt to self-medicate.

Many behavior-change efforts can benefit both SUDs and mood disorders simultaneously. For example, regular physical activity may improve mood, which in turn can strengthen feelings of self-efficacy for behavior-change efforts. If substance use and addictive behaviors serve as important ways that people cope with a mood disorder, then addressing the mood disorder itself must be part of addiction treatment efforts, as discussed previously in this chapter.

Perceptions of Social Control and Reactance Theory

Another difference between negative and positive health behavior–change programs is that many negative health behaviors have an associated stigma, and people who engage in these behaviors may feel a sense of shame. They may be embarrassed about their inability to control their smoking, gambling, eating, or other negative behavior. Feelings of embarrassment and shame may motivate people to hide negative behaviors, deny or downplay their importance, or avoid dealing with problems associated with them.

People in a close relationship with a person who has negative health behaviors often seek to motivate that person to change. In fact, the most-common social support for change (often viewed as nagging) comes from spouses, parents, and friends (Logic, Okun, & Publiese, 2009). Efforts to motivate other people to change their behavior are known as social control. Social control can be positive or negative. Positive social control offers help and strives to generate positive emotions and feelings of support. Negative social control is more likely to take the form of criticism and judgment and to generate negative emotions. Studies suggest that positive social control is more likely to lead to behavior change (Logic, Okun, & Publiese, 2009).

People in helping relationships, such as health and fitness professionals, sometimes try to exert social control when they help their clients. Of course, if the client has sought help, he or she is more likely to respond positively. However, if a client has come to the professional for one reason, perhaps to get advice on starting an exercise program, but the professional starts talking to the client about his smoking, then his emotional response is likely to be negative.

When social-control efforts, whether from close relationships, helping professionals, or others, are associated with a negative client reaction and with negative feelings such as anger and resentment, the result may be a phenomenon psychologists called "reactance." Reactance is doing the very thing a person has been told not to do. Reactance comes from "an impulse to restore behavioral freedoms that are perceived to have been threatened or lost" (Brehm, 2000). Psychologists and novelists throughout time have observed that forbidden fruit is sweeter; simply telling people they cannot have (chocolate, alcohol, sex, fill in the blank) makes that thing more desirable.

Because negative health behaviors are more likely to fall into this realm of "don't do this," health and fitness professionals need to be extra careful to suspend judgment and to let clients take the lead in discussions of negative health behaviors. If professionals decide to raise issues regarding the negative behavior, they should make every effort to frame these in a manner likely to be interpreted as supportive. Chapter 5 explained the research from positive psychology, which has demonstrated that behavior change proceeds best from a position of strength and positive emotions.

Harm-Reduction Programs

Harm-reduction programs have been promoted by many experts to help people at least suffer fewer harmful consequences from negative health behaviors. For some negative health behaviors, abstinence is the ideal goal. People who have trouble regulating alcohol intake may find it too difficult to just have a drink or two and will be better off not drinking at all. Underage drinking is against the law and can lead to negative consequences; abstinence from drinking would best prevent these consequences. Abstinence from sex provides the best protection from sexually transmitted infections. The health risks associated with tobacco use suggest abstinence from tobacco use is the most-prudent goal.

In many cases, abstinence is unlikely to occur in the near future. In these cases, psychologists recommend an approach known as harm reduction. **Harm reduction** means acknowledging that total abstinence may be an unrealistic goal at the present time. While helping professionals may still promote abstinence, in the meantime they also take immediate steps to at least reduce the level of harm associated with a given behavior. Some people oppose harm-reduction strategies, believing that they enable or allow the very behavior that needs to be extinguished. Harm-reduction proponents argue that harm-reduction efforts help keep clients "alive, healthy, and more motivated to make further habit changes," whereas an abstinence-only treatment model leaves many clients believing that they have failed and thus are more likely to drop out of treatment (Marlatt & Witkiewitz, 2010).

A good example of a harm-reduction effort is a needle-exchange program for intravenous (IV) drug users. The best possible outcome of a program addressing the high rates of infections such as hepatitis C and HIV among IV drug users would be to have everyone stop using these drugs (unless medically prescribed). Harm-reduction

approaches acknowledge the difficulty of helping people overcome addictions and look at the big picture of IV drug use. Reusing needles to inject drugs is the actual vector for blood-borne pathogens. Therefore, a helpful harm-reduction effort is teaching users how to clean needles effectively if they are reusing them or providing them with clean needles.

Harm-reduction efforts regarding sexual activity focus on "safer sex" for people who do not choose abstinence. Harm-reduction education for alcohol teaches people who will not abstain from using alcohol how to drink in ways that will not raise blood alcohol to dangerous levels or lead to risky behaviors such as drinking and driving. Harm reduction may teach community members the signs of alcohol poisoning so that friends and bystanders can get help for the victim as soon as possible.

Eliza continues coming to class. She and Kim count down the days until Eliza and her husband begin the smoking-cessation class. "We have nicotine patches from our doctor and something to help us sleep if we need it," Eliza says. "We have also been using the workbook you gave us to think about ways to avoid the things that make us want to smoke. It is really making a difference for me that Louis is going to quit, too." Kim encourages them to make use of community center activities, such as the exercise classes. "Don't forget exercise will help prevent weight gain, reduce feelings of stress, and help you sleep. Does Louis like basketball? There is a group that plays twice a week in the evening, same time as this class. Exercise can help you both stay busy. Plus nobody is allowed to smoke here!"

Positive Approaches for Changing Negative Health Behaviors

Health and fitness professionals who work with clients who have been advised to change a negative health behavior, or who are considering changing a negative health behavior, should use the guidelines presented in Chapter 5. Here are the most-important strategies.

Use of OARS Communication Skills

Because clients with negative health behaviors may quickly become defensive when others criticize them, professionals must be especially good listeners and try to engage clients in supportive, helpful ways. Client resistance is one of the greatest barriers to success in cognitive behavioral-change programs for addiction (Amodeo et al., 2011). Behavior-change theories such as the Health Belief Model and the Theory of Planned Behavior can provide professionals with important variables to address in discussions to help motivate a decision to change.

Tailoring Approach to Stage of Change

Open-ended questions and careful listening can help the professional determine the client's approximate stage of change and adjust behavioral-counseling approaches accordingly. Professionals can employ guiding discussions of the pros and cons for change with clients in precontemplation and contemplation stages to help them form the intention to change. Those with some training in motivational interviewing (MI) will find this approach helpful (Game Changers 11-1). Health and fitness professionals can affirm clients' statements and efforts that move them toward positive change, help them strengthen their reasons for changing, and address barriers to change. They can also guide clients to see the importance of change and build their motivation for changing by helping them link behavior change with important personal goals.

Health and fitness professionals can help clients in preparation and action stages implement helpful behavior-change strategies. Professionals must remember that the stage of change for a given client can fluctuate and be open to meeting clients wherever they may be without assuming that the journey through the stages of change will be linear or progressive.

Game Changers 11-1. William Miller and Stephen Rollnick: Motivational Interviewing Builds Autonomous Motivation

William R. Miller and Stephen Rollnick are best known for creating a client-centered approach to behavior change known as motivational interviewing (MI). While MI techniques were originally developed in the context of addiction treatment, they have been implemented and scientifically evaluated in many other health contexts and have become the basis for most evidence-based behavioral counseling today. Miller, Rollnick, and colleagues helped to radically change the way addiction was viewed and the way therapists and health and fitness professionals work with clients trying to change addictions and negative health behaviors.

The game-changing nature of Miller and Rollnick's work can best be appreciated in the historical context of addiction treatment. In the early 1900s, a variety of addiction treatments were available, from snake oil magic potions to AA groups to psychotherapy. AA meeting styles tended to be supportive, viewing alcoholism as a disease and alcoholics as people needing help and guidance to overcome their addiction. Similarly, psychotherapy techniques of the time were generally discussion based, encouraging clients to explore and resolve deep-seated reasons for the addiction (White & Miller, 2007).

However, during the middle of the 20th century in the United States, addiction-treatment programs developed aggressive and confrontational practices, and people with addictions came to be viewed as having a personality disorder marked by an immature and defensive character. Passive and empathetic counseling practices were seen as ineffective, and therefore the belief grew that the only way to get through to people with addictions was by force. In fact, people were even incarcerated for drug addiction. The goal of these practices was to "break 'em down to build 'em up," based on the idea that addicts had to reach rock bottom to overcome their denial and resistance to dealing with their addictions (White & Miller, 2007). Professionals believed that addicts needed to be confronted with the total picture of their problem, including an understanding of their deep personality flaws, in order to surrender to the therapeutic process of reconstructing a new personality. "Therapeutic" techniques for breaking addicts' resistance and denial included "frank feedback, profanity-laden indictments, screamed denunciations of character, challenges and ultimatums, intense argumentation, ridicule, and purposeful humiliation" (White & Miller, 2007). The theory was that if people felt bad enough, they would change (White & Miller, 2007).

Miller and Rollnick attribute their roots in the development of MI to Carl Rogers, who introduced an empathic, client-centered style of psychotherapy in the late 1950s (Rogers, 1959) and who continued to study and develop his approaches in the following decades (Rogers, 1980). Miller began developing the MI counseling methods in the late 1970s. As he was studying behavior therapy for problem drinking, he noticed in his results the powerful influence of the counselor conducting the therapy. Later studies confirmed the observation that the effect of the therapist was much greater than the effect of the different behavioral treatments being compared (Miller & Rose, 2009).

Miller continued to develop MI techniques, examining their effects scientifically. Research supported their effectiveness. For example, in several clinical trials, subjects were randomly assigned to receive or not receive a single MI counseling session at the beginning of behavioral treatment programs for problem drinking. Subjects receiving just one session of MI showed twice the rate of abstinence 3 to 6 months after treatment (Miller & Rose, 2009). In 1989, Miller met Stephen Rollnick while on sabbatical in Australia. Rollnick was familiar with MI and similar techniques being developed in the U.K., and together they coauthored a book on MI (Miller & Rollnick, 1991). While the first edition of the book focused on changing addictive behavior, the second edition expanded its focus to include all types of health behavior change (Miller & Rollnick, 2002).

Miller and Rollnick believe that the harsh, confrontational methods formerly used to treat addiction in the United States actually strengthened, rather than broke through, clients' denial. In their words, "Defensiveness

Game Changers 11-1. William Miller and Stephen Rollnick: Motivational Interviewing Builds Autonomous Motivation–cont'd

is a normal human response when one is accused, demeaned, labeled, disrespected, or threatened" (White & Miller, 2007). Counselors themselves can push resistance up or down, depending upon how they communicate. Counselors who employ MI work carefully to understand and empathize with clients, creating a supportive therapeutic relationship that reduces client resistance and denial. MI practices empower counselors to help clients voice and strengthen their reasons to change, increase their commitment to changing, and uncover autonomous motivation to change.

Sources: Miller, W. R., & Rollnick, S. (1991). *Motivational Interviewing: Preparing People to Change Addictive Behavior.* New York: Guilford Press; Miller, W. R., & Rollnick, S. (2013). *Motivational Interviewing: Preparing People to Change, 3rd ed.* New York: Guilford Press; Miller, W. R., & Rose, G. R. (2009). Toward a theory of motivational interviewing. *American Psychologist, 64*(6), 527-537; Rogers, C. R. (1959). A theory of therapy, personality, and interpersonal relationships as developed in the client-centered framework. In: Koch, S. (ed.). *Psychology: The Study of a Science. Vol. 3. Formulations of the Person and the Social Contexts*, 184-256. New York: McGraw-Hill; Rogers, C. R. (1980). *A Way of Being.* Boston, MA: Houghton Mifflin; White, W., & Miller, W. (2007). The use of confrontation in addiction treatment: history, science, and time for change. *Counselor, 8*(4), 12-30.

Applying the Principles of Self-Determination Theory

Principles of SDT should guide behavior-change efforts, including efforts to change negative health behaviors. According to Self-Determination Theory (SDT), people need to feel autonomous in their behavior, connected to others, and competent in the activities they undertake. Health and fitness professionals should keep all three of these in mind as they work with their clients.

People may be pushed to change behavior by concerned close friends and family members, so they may not yet have developed more-autonomous motivations to change. Professionals can explore reasons for change and help clients discover their own motivations for changing. People need to feel that they have choices in terms of their behavior, which gives them some feeling of control (Leotti, Iyengar, & Ochsner, 2010).

Helping clients develop autonomous motivation for changing negative health behaviors is critical. Motivation is strongest when it is connected to individuals' goals and values. If people find that addictive behaviors are interfering with their ability to achieve important goals, they may find and strengthen autonomous motivation to change their behaviors (Peele, 2004).

SDT also reinforces the importance of helping clients build social support for change to feel connected to others in this process. Additionally, clients need to feel competent in the measures that they are using to change their behavior and in their environment at large.

Building Self-Efficacy for Change

Low self-efficacy for changing negative health behaviors is often part of a learned helplessness pattern. People who have repeatedly failed at behavior change may develop the idea they do not have the wherewithal to change. As discussed in previous chapters, health and fitness professionals can help build clients' self-efficacy

by helping them set small, achievable behavior-change goals and then to perceive that they have achieved these goals. Professionals can expose clients to helpful role models and encourage clients to strengthen social support networks. Classes and group programs focused on behavior change often help increase clients' self-efficacy for behavior change.

Behavioral Therapies for Changing Negative Health Behaviors

For clients who have made the decision to change, the most-successful strategies for changing negative health behaviors incorporate principles of behavior learning theory and cognitive behavioral approaches. Some of the most-common and most-successful behavioral therapies include the following (Witkiewitz & Marlatt, 2010):

- **Coping skills training:** Coping skills training teaches cognitive and behavioral skills to improve individuals' abilities to cope with situations in which the negative health behavior is likely to occur. People learn new responses to the stimuli that provoke the negative behaviors.
- **Cognitive behavioral therapy:** CBT helps individuals become aware of thought and behavior patterns that promote the negative health behavior. People learn to use new ways of thinking and responding to high-risk situations. CBT typically addresses immediate behavior change as well as long-term relapse prevention.
- **Contingency management therapies:** Contingency management therapies use operant conditioning principles to shape behavior, usually through the use of rewards that clients can achieve by exhibiting desirable behaviors (such as abstaining from alcohol or drug use).
- **Family therapies:** Family therapies are especially helpful when negative health behaviors

involve family dynamics, as when family members cover up for an individual's alcohol-use disorder, unintentionally enabling the individual to persist in addictive behaviors. Disorders occurring in minors may also respond well to family therapies.

- **Brief behavioral interventions:** Some individuals succeed in changing negative behaviors with only a few sessions of help from physicians, health educators, or other providers who typically use some form of behavioral counseling or MI.
- **Self-help programs:** Many people change with support from books, online materials, or other media that teach goal-setting, self-monitoring, and other behavior-change skills.

Studies suggest that there is no one type of treatment program which stands out above all others in terms of changing negative health behaviors (Witkiewitz & Marlatt, 2010). Many individuals successfully change negative behaviors on their own, although some studies suggest that people who do not seek formal treatment may tend to have fewer serious risk factors and emotional health problems than those who seek treatment (Schutte, Brennan, & Moos, 2009). Researchers have identified important components common to successful behavior-change programs. These include the following:

- Social support
- Structure and goal setting
- Rewards, including rewarding activities that reinforce positive behaviors
- Normative models for behavior-change success
- Improvement in self-efficacy for behavior change
- Development of coping skills

MOTIVATING CHANGE: Individualize Your Approach and Connect With Clients' Goals

Health and fitness professionals who work with clients to change negative health behaviors should individualize the strategies that they employ with each client. Professionals should begin with an effort to discern where the client appears to be in terms of the stages of change, listening carefully and reflectively to assess how committed the client is to changing. Discussions can address the pros and cons of behavior change, guiding clients to see the difference between their desired goals and lifestyle and their current behavior. What do clients need to do to reach their goal? Once clients are ready to change, professionals can help them develop skills and new habits.

Discussions can reveal how helpful the clients' social support networks are and provide some idea about clients' levels of self-efficacy for changing the negative behavior. Health and fitness professionals can help clients identify both strengths and weaknesses. Most important is continuing to link behavior-change efforts with clients' values and important goals, so clients proceed with autonomous motivation for their behavior-change work.

Lifestyle Support for Changing Negative Health Behaviors

Can developing positive health behaviors help people overcome bad habits? Anecdotal reports suggest that good nutrition and regular physical activity can help bolster resolve for change. However, research evidence is fairly sparse. Researchers propose that exercise in particular can help people coping with addictions and negative health behaviors for the following reasons (Zangeneh, Ala-leppilampi, Barmaki, & Peric, 2007):

- Physical activity activates CNS reward pathways, so it could potentially serve as a source of pleasurable experience to replace the negative behavior.
- Regular physical activity is associated with improvement in symptoms of anxiety and depression, which motivate negative health behaviors for many people.
- Regular physical activity decreases stress reactivity and may offer a positive way to cope with feelings of stress.
- Physical activity venues may offer opportunities for social support. Exercise classes, community activities, walking groups, dance classes, and other group exercise programs bring people together. They generally provide environments lower in use of substances such as tobacco and alcohol.
- Sticking to a program of regular physical activity may help build people's self-efficacy for self-control and behavior change.

Exercise is no magic bullet, unfortunately, but it can be part of the process of developing a healthful lifestyle. A healthful lifestyle in turn provides support for people as they work to achieve personally meaningful goals and pursue important activities.

BEHAVIOR-CHANGE APPLICATIONS FOR NEGATIVE HEALTH BEHAVIORS

Health and fitness professionals are behavior-change experts. Not only do they help clients improve physical activity and dietary habits, they also help people with bad habits transform their lifestyles. Clients often approach health and fitness professionals with questions about alcohol use, quitting smoking, and harmful weight-control behaviors. The previous sections in this chapter have provided general background on negative health behaviors. This section will present behavior-change issues and applications for the most-common negative health behaviors that health and fitness professionals are likely to encounter in their work, including alcohol and tobacco use, harmful weight-control practices, eating disorders, and excessive exercise.

Alcohol

Alcohol use is embedded in many cultures and perceived as socially normal by a majority of North Americans.

About 70% of U.S. adults drink alcohol, at least occasionally, and most do so in a responsible fashion. However, 25% of U.S. adults report having alcohol-related problems or have behaviors that put them at risk for developing problems (National Institute on Alcohol Abuse and Alcoholism, 2005). This translates into a very large number of people for whom alcohol poses a problem.

Most people have heard that a little alcohol bestows health benefits. Indeed, some have been advised by their physicians to have one drink daily to prevent heart disease. Unfortunately, the fact that alcohol can be beneficial and at the same time harmful muddies the waters for many when people are trying to weigh the benefits and risks of alcohol consumption. Because alcohol is legal (for adults) and widely consumed, it can be hard for users and their friends and family to distinguish the line between use and abuse.

Health Effects

Health and fitness professionals often field questions about the health benefits and risks of alcohol. Some of the more-salient benefits and risks include:

- **Cardiovascular Health:** Moderate drinking, which means about one drink per day for women or one to two drinks per day for men, confers some benefit on the circulatory system (Mochly-Rosen & Zakhari, 2010). Figure 11-6 illustrates drink equivalents for various types of alcoholic beverages. Drinking at this level reduces risk for coronary artery disease (CAD). Physiological mechanisms for this effect include improvement in serum lipoprotein levels, with increases in HDL cholesterol levels and reductions in LDL cholesterol levels; and a reduction in blood clotting rate, thus reducing risk of clots forming inside the arteries. Moderate drinking not only reduces risk of CAD but also improves prognosis for people who have already suffered a heart attack. On the other hand, heavier drinking can cause hypertension, damage to the heart muscle, and heart failure (Mochly-Rosen & Zakhari, 2010).

- **Liver Disease:** Alcohol consumption is associated with a wide range of liver diseases (Fig. 11-7). Alcohol and its toxic metabolites (breakdown products of alcohol metabolism) damage liver cells. A large majority of heavy drinkers (over five drinks per day) develop steatosis, or fatty liver. Fatty liver describes the disease: fat deposits accumulate in the liver, and the liver becomes enlarged. Fatty liver is reversible with abstinence from alcohol. If steatosis is accompanied by inflammation and other damage to liver cells, it progresses to alcoholic hepatitis, or steatohepatitis. This condition is somewhat reversible, at least in earlier stages. Liver cirrhosis is diagnosed when collagen scar tissue replaces healthy liver tissue, thus leading to a decline in liver function. Cirrhosis is a very-serious illness and the 12th leading cause of death in the United States (Szabo & Mandrekar, 2010). Cirrhosis can also set the stage for the development of liver cancer, hepatocellular carcinoma.

- **Cancers:** Alcohol and its metabolites can initiate cancers in other areas of the body as well. Alcohol intake, even at relatively low levels, is associated with increased risk of cancers of the respiratory system; breast cancer; and cancers of the gastrointestinal (GI) tract, including the mouth, esophagus, stomach, colon, and rectum (Seitz & Becker, 2007).

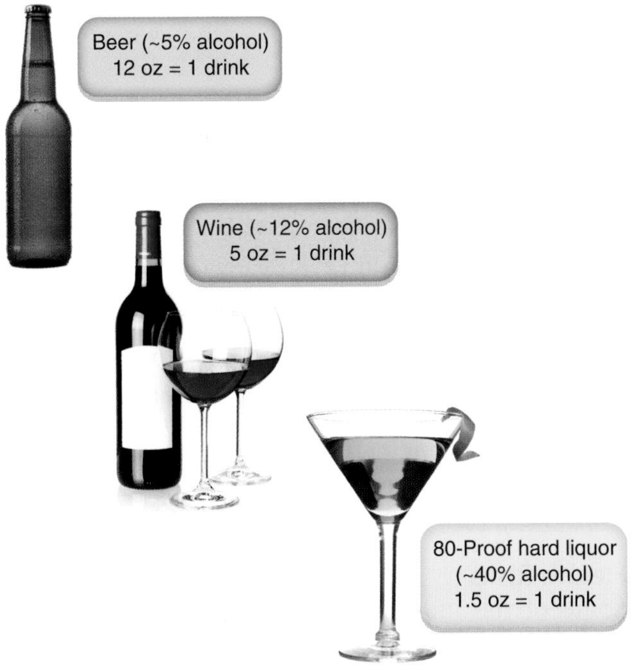

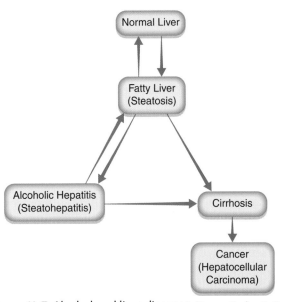

Figure 11-6. Drink equivalents for alcoholic beverages. Photograph © Thinkstock

Figure 11-7. Alcohol and liver diseases. (Source: Szabo, G., & Mandrekar, P. (2010). Focus on: alcohol and the liver. Alcohol Research & Health 33(1-2), 87-96.)

- **Pancreatitis:** Excessive alcohol intake is the primary cause of pancreatitis, chronic inflammation of the pancreas (Vonlaufen, Wilson, Pirola, & Apte, 2007).
- **Immune System Damage:** Acute and chronic alcohol abuse appears to interfere with many aspects of immune response, leading to a higher risk of all kinds of infections. Alcohol abuse is also associated with behaviors that increase the transmission of infectious diseases, which can exacerbate alcohol's negative effects on immune function. Especially harmful are the increased rates of pneumonia, tuberculosis, hepatitis C infections, and HIV infections associated with alcohol abuse (Molina, Happel, Zhang, Kolls, & Nelson, 2010).
- **Changes in Brain Structure and Function:** Alcohol abuse is associated with damage to several brain areas and symptoms of poorer brain function (Sullivan, Harris, & Pfefferbaum, 2010). Memory, decision-making, motor coordination, and other functions can decline with alcohol abuse.
- **Fetal Alcohol Spectrum Disorders:** Scientists have long known that alcohol can be a teratogen, a substance that disrupts fetal development, causing irreversible damage. Fetal alcohol spectrum disorders include a wide range of physical, behavioral, and cognitive abnormalities, caused by exposure to alcohol during fetal development. Not all babies exposed in utero to alcohol develop alcohol-related disorders, and scientists continue to look for the biological mechanisms behind alcohol's effects on fetal development (Thomas, Warren, & Hewitt, 2010). Because researchers have not been able to define a "safe" level of alcohol intake that poses no risk to a developing fetus, they recommend that pregnant women avoid alcohol.
- **Harmful Behaviors:** Alcohol abuse is strongly associated with a plethora of harmful behaviors, including accidental death and injury due to motor vehicle accidents, drowning, burns, and firearm accidents. Alcohol abuse is linked to domestic violence as well as to other forms of violence, including homicide and suicide (National Institute on Alcohol Abuse and Alcoholism, 2010). Poor decision making under the influence can result in unwanted, unplanned, and/or unprotected sexual activity and other relationship problems.

Individual response to alcohol varies greatly. On average, women appear to be more susceptible to the effects of alcohol. This is due partly to differences in size and body composition; women are generally smaller than men with a higher percentage of body fat for a given size. Alcohol diffuses primarily into lean tissue. This means a given amount of alcohol tends to be more concentrated in the lean body mass of women. In addition, differences in the rate of alcohol metabolism appear to differ between the sexes. Women's stomachs produce lower amounts of a key enzyme responsible for breaking down alcohol, alcohol dehydrogenase. Women thus generally break alcohol down more slowly, so blood alcohol levels remain high longer. These observations help explain why women develop alcohol-related disorders at lower alcohol intakes than men do.

Should health and fitness professionals promote the consumption of alcoholic beverages for good health? Experts believe that people should take a good look at their personal risks for the health issues presented above, along with their personal risk for alcoholism, and make prudent choices regarding their use of alcohol. Because such a high proportion of the population has difficulty using alcohol safely, health and fitness professionals should never advise people who don't drink to develop a drinking habit. In general, young people cannot rationalize drinking for health reasons, as the risks outweigh the benefits. People most likely to benefit from alcohol consumption are older adults at risk for heart disease, especially those who have already suffered a heart attack and are not prone to alcohol-use disorders.

Support Abstinence or Moderation

How should health and fitness professionals respond when clients express interest in changing their alcohol use behaviors? People who say they are concerned about their drinking behavior usually need to reduce consumption. Professionals should express support and help clients explore reasons for changing. They should also refer clients to substance-use professionals if they suspect a substance-use disorder (Health Psychology at Work 11-1). But, for the client who simply wants to limit alcohol to one to two drinks per day and rarely drinks too much, standard behavior-change strategies can be implemented, as described earlier in this chapter. The National Institute for Alcohol Abuse and Alcoholism has a helpful website with information and tools to assist people in evaluating and changing their alcohol-use patterns. The section of their website called "Rethinking Drinking" is especially helpful (http://rethinkingdrinking.niaaa.nih.gov/).

Tobacco Use

Unlike alcohol, tobacco use has only risks and no long-term health benefits. Smokers do describe experiencing increased alertness, pleasure, social connection, and weight-management benefits from their tobacco-use habit. However, these fleeting benefits do not result in improved health, because they are overshadowed by the very-powerful negative effects of tobacco use. As described in Chapter 1, tobacco use is number one on the list of actual causes of death in high-income countries (Mokdad, Marks, Stroup, & Gerberding, 2004).

Health Risks

Some of the most-serious health risks with which tobacco use has been linked include:

- **Cardiovascular Disease:** Chemicals in tobacco products act as sympathomimetic drugs, speeding

HEALTH PSYCHOLOGY AT WORK 11-1. Motivating Healthy Choices About Alcohol Use

Mike Durham, L.S.W., L.I.C.D.C., is a substance abuse counselor and educator. He works with students at the Kenyon College Counseling Center and teaches a course on drug abuse and treatment for the Social Work Department at North Central State College in Ohio. The initials after his name stand for licensed social worker and licensed independent chemical dependency counselor. Mike has more than 20 years of experience in drug abuse treatment and prevention, relapse prevention, and education. Motivating young people in the precontemplation and contemplation stages of change to address drinking and drug-use behavior is not easy work. Mike often works with students who don't even want to see him, so it is a testament to his patience, compassion, and communication skills that by and large the students think he is pretty cool. (Maybe that is partly because he rides a motorcycle, even though he only has one arm. Or maybe they have seen him working at a "wharf rat sober deadhead table" at a jam band concert.) Underneath his easy smile, the twinkle in his eye, and his soft-spoken manner, Mike has a keen ability to gently sift through the chatter and denial and to help students begin to get a clearer picture of their relationship with alcohol and other drugs.

"Much of my work here is with students who have been referred to me because of problems involving alcohol or drugs. While some students may continue to work with me for years, I may see others for only a few sessions. Many students haven't exhibited an issue related to dangerous drinking, but the drinking age law makes their behavior illegal. I attempt to use this as an opportunity to talk with them about harm reduction, safety, and risk management. It's also an opportunity for me to build a safe relationship with the students so that they are more likely to ask for help if they ever need it for themselves or a friend.

"I don't think of our sessions as 'counseling' but as a conversation a student is having with a caring adult, who will also treat them as adults. Students prefer a conversation to counseling. They prefer to be talked with instead of talked to. I try to show them I am interested and supportive, rather than threatening. The students I work with usually sense that I like and respect them. Humor is also great for helping people feel comfortable. My goal, through our conversation, is to hold up a mirror for students to see themselves and their alcohol use more clearly.

"The behavior-change models I rely on are the Stages of Change Model and motivational interviewing. The Developmental Model of Recovery mirrors the stages of change. The way I work with students depends on what stage they are in. Many are in precontemplation or contemplation stages for changing their drinking behavior. Motivational interviewing works best in these cases.

"Alcohol use is complicated since it can be both beneficial and harmful. Some students come from families who consider drinking, even heavy drinking, 'normal' behavior. I acknowledge the utility of alcohol for enhancing social connections. When people drink together, they experience feelings of social connection. Parties provide a shared experiential base. Many students drink because they are just trying to fit in, to satisfy the universal need for belonging. Some students have not yet learned how to drink. And students' perceptions of social norms are often inaccurate. The stories they hear after the party are usually about heavy drinking, so they get the idea that all students drink heavily. They don't hear about the students who choose not to drink or have a few drinks. I try to give them more-accurate information about student drinking behavior. For example, many are surprised to learn that only a minority of students drinks excessively and that most students don't approve of drunken behavior.

"In our conversations, we explore the student's motivations for using alcohol. I ask, 'When you drink, what are you looking for?' Then we look at whether or not the drinking behavior is accomplishing these goals. So, for example, if a student was drinking because she wanted to have fun but ended up vomiting in the trashcan after the party, I ask her if that was fun. I try to guide the conversation in directions that help the student think about better ways to have fun or achieve whatever her purpose is, either by not drinking or practicing moderate drinking strategies that will help prevent harm.

"I emphasize that alcohol use is a choice. Students feel respected and empowered and thus more motivated to change their behavior. In our conversations, I guide them to the big question: 'Have you crossed the line from safe to dangerous drinking behavior?' I want students to ask themselves: 'Do I have a problem?' If you think you have a problem, you probably do. I want them to discover where they are on the use, abuse, addiction continuum.

"Many students want to know how they can help a friend with an alcohol or drug use problem. They can talk to the friend who has a problem. They can write themselves a script for the talk, listing concrete examples of the problem behaviors. They can offer support, even refer. 'Hey, I know this guy at the counseling center . . . .' If they observe the friend drinking too much, they can try sending a text to get the friend's attention or take the friend away from the party to go get a sandwich. They don't need to wait until the friend is wasted to get help."

up the fight-or-flight response. Tobacco products raise blood pressure and heart rate, activate LDL cholesterol particles to stick to the artery lining, and increase clotting rate. Cardiovascular disease may result in heart attack, stroke, and dementia.

- **Cancer:** Tobacco use increases risk of many types of cancer, including cancer of the mouth, throat, larynx, esophagus, lungs, and bladder.
- **Chronic Respiratory Disease:** Smoking tobacco products increases risk of emphysema, chronic bronchitis, and pneumonia. Smoking exacerbates upper-respiratory infections and symptoms of asthma.

In addition to these life-threatening risks, tobacco use is associated with many other negative health effects including sexual dysfunction and infertility. Women who smoke during pregnancy experience increased risks of spontaneous abortion, premature delivery, and low-birth-weight babies. People who use tobacco products have poorer circulation and experience slower recovery from surgeries as well as faster aging of the skin.

Understanding Addiction to Tobacco Products

Despite knowledge of the health risks of using tobacco products, about 20% of people in the United States are smokers. While smoking rates have declined since the 1960s, this rate of decline has slowed considerably in recent years. In the United States, about 1000 people younger than 18 and 1800 people 18 years old and over become smokers each day (Substance Abuse and Mental Health Administration, 2008).

It is likely that health and fitness professionals will work with clients who are trying to quit smoking or using other tobacco products. Understanding the perceived benefits of tobacco use and how these habits develop can help health and fitness professionals work sympathetically with clients who are trying to quit. Most tobacco users developed their habit when they were fairly young. They knew smoking could cause health problems down the road, but that road seemed very long and those health problems far away. It may have seemed more important at the time to bond with friends and conform to peer expectations. Perhaps tobacco products gave users a distinction and definition they needed back then.

Nicotine addiction develops very readily, so users quickly become physically dependent on tobacco. In addition, habits of use reinforce behavioral dependency. Users turn to tobacco products for stress relief, relaxation, or simply because it is a habit that accompanies homework, talking on the phone, taking a break, or spending time with friends.

Support for Tobacco-Use Cessation

No one knows why some people have little trouble quitting tobacco use while others struggle for years and make many attempts to quit before they are successful. Many factors are involved. One of the most important is how dependent one's body has become on nicotine. In general, the longer people have been tobacco users and the more frequently they use tobacco each day, the greater the chance that quitting will be difficult.

Clients' personal situations may affect how hard it is for them to quit. For example, if their close friends smoke and they are often in places and situations where people are smoking, it may be more challenging for them to kick the habit. If they smoke to take a break from work, they will need to find new ways to take a break and relax. People recovering from an addiction to alcohol or other drugs may find quitting especially difficult. If smoking has helped them through recovery from a more-serious addiction, they may be worried about relapse.

Some people may have a hard time quitting because nicotine withdrawal symptoms are especially troublesome for them. These symptoms include not only strong cravings for tobacco products but emotional symptoms as well, such as depression, anger, irritability, tension, and anxiety. Some people have difficulty concentrating and feel more restless than usual. Difficulty sleeping, increased hunger, and weight gain can also occur during nicotine withdrawal. Since negative feelings are the main reason people begin smoking again after they have tried to quit, it is very important for people who want to quit to figure out ways to reduce the stress of quitting. Strategies that may help clients to quit using tobacco products include the following:

- **Building social support.** Many people find that smoking-cessation programs are extremely helpful. Clients may be able to find a program through their workplace, health insurance, local health-care organizations, or community groups. The American Lung Association has designed a program offered both in groups and online called Freedom From Smoking (ALA, 2012). These programs help people design effective quit-smoking strategies. In addition, most people appreciate the help of family and friends. Smokers might try spending as much time as possible with people who support their intentions to quit.
- **Improving lifestyle to prevent fatigue, stress, and weight gain.** Relapse is most likely when people are feeling tired and stressed. Clients can fight fatigue by eating well and getting enough sleep. They should try to avoid snacking unless truly hungry. Some ex-smokers develop a tendency to replace cigarettes and other forms of tobacco use with chewing. If chewing helps, encourage clients to try crunchy vegetables or sugarless gum. They should drink at least four glasses of water a day to prevent fatigue from dehydration.
- **Use of medical support as necessary.** Nicotine-replacement products such as electronic cigarettes, nicotine patches, and nicotine gum dramatically decrease the risks associated with the use of tobacco products and can help people

overcome their behavioral addictions to tobacco use first and then gradually taper their reliance on nicotine. Some people find that they need antidepressants or other medications to help them overcome a tobacco-use habit.

- **Identification of behavior chains.** Health and fitness professionals can help clients identify their personal tobacco-use patterns. Smoking-cessation programs often begin by asking participants to monitor smoking behavior throughout the day. As they break down the antecedents and consequences of tobacco-use behaviors, clients can then avoid or come up with alternative responses for the situations that tend to trigger tobacco use. Those who have quit before can learn from previous attempts. They can anticipate situations and feelings that might lead to a relapse and think of ways to get through these times without resuming a life-threatening habit.

- **Exercise.** Studies have found that people who exercise regularly while quitting smoking have better success than nonexercisers (Ciccolo et al., 2011; Williams et al., 2010; What's the Evidence? 11-1). Exercise can relieve feelings of depression, anxiety, irritability, and tension. Exercise helps combat the negative health effects of smoking, especially by reducing risk for heart disease. Regular physical activity improves sleep quality and helps prevent or reduce the weight gain that sometimes occurs when people quit smoking.

WHAT'S THE EVIDENCE? 11-1

Resistance Training Strengthens Ability to Quit Smoking

Ciccolo, J. T., Dunsiger, S. I., Williams, D. M., Bartholomew, J. B., Jennings, E. G., Ussher, M. H., . . . Marcus, B. H. (2011). Resistance training as an aid to standard smoking cessation treatment: A pilot study. *Nicotine & Tobacco Research, 13*(8), 756-760.

◼ PURPOSE

Prior research had suggested that aerobic exercise may reduce many of the negative symptoms associated with nicotine withdrawal. Earlier research had also suggested that a single bout of resistance training was perceived by subjects to reduce nicotine cravings. The purpose of this study was to determine whether people who engaged in resistance training during a smoking-cessation treatment would be more successful in their efforts to quit smoking than control subjects. This project was a pilot study, which means that only a small group of volunteers was used, and one of the purposes of the study was to see whether the study methods were reliable and valid and would be feasible for a larger group.

◼ STUDY

Tobacco smokers interested in quitting served as subjects. Subjects were recruited through newspaper, Internet, and television advertisements and paid a small amount to participate. Twenty-five male and female smokers aged 18 to 65 completed the study. All subjects attended a 15- to 20-minute counseling session on how to quit smoking and received nicotine patches, with their nicotine dose matching prior cigarette use.

Subjects were randomly assigned to either a resistance training (RT) or contact control condition. People in the RT group participated in two 60-minute RT workouts per week for 12 weeks. Programs were individually designed for each subject, and workouts were supervised for safety; but each subject worked out alone. (This removed the potential effect of group social support.) Subjects in the contact control group watched one 25-minute video two times a week, alone in a room. Films covered various health-related topics. Subjects completed a variety of assessment measures, including smoking variables, body weight and composition, exercise level, and strength measures before the study began and again 3 months and 6 months later. Both groups had lost one or two subjects at the 3-month period when treatments stopped. At 6 months, about 62% of RT subjects and 50% of controls completed the final assessments.

As predicted, participants in the RT group were more successful in quitting smoking than control subjects. At 3 months, quit rates were 46% for the RT group and 17% for controls. At 6 months, quit rates were 16% and 8%, respectively. In addition, RT subjects on average lost a small amount of weight and body fat and gained strength, while control subjects on average gained a little weight and lost strength. While the small numbers completing the study limited statistical analysis, calculation of odds ratios and effect sizes predicted that in a larger group, these differences would be statistically significant.

◼ IMPLICATIONS

People trying to quit smoking should make exercise part of their smoking-cessation strategy. This study suggests that people who perform RT in addition to using nicotine patches are about twice as successful in quitting smoking as people who receive only the patches. In addition, participation in RT increases strength, improves body composition, and may prevent the weight gain that commonly occurs when people quit smoking.

■ *Several months later, Kim's supervisor Andrew expresses his concern about Eliza's exercise level. "She is spending two or more hours a day in classes or working out. I know she is always in your class. Should we be worried about her?" Kim agrees to check in with Eliza after class that evening.*

"I am so glad you are enjoying my class and working out in the fitness center," Kim begins. "And I am really glad you are still not smoking. Congratulations! But I hope you are not overtraining. I would hate to see you get injured. Tell me everything you are currently doing for exercise." Eliza proudly spells out her the details of her exercise schedule. Although she never has a complete rest day, on Sunday she and her husband go walking in the park, nothing too vigorous. "The exercise makes me feel great, and with each session I renew my commitment to not smoking." Kim determines that Eliza is performing a variety of activities, is not developing injuries, still works part time in the mornings, and seems to be enjoying life. She knows Eliza and Louis are even still married, despite the stress of quitting smoking together. She lets Andrew know that although Kim is exercising quite a bit, it is probably helping her to not resume smoking and doesn't seem to be causing any harm at this point in time. ■

Harmful Weight-Control Behaviors

Chapter 10 presented information on weight management and some of the issues health and fitness professionals may encounter when working with clients trying to manage weight and body composition. The chapter emphasized that health and fitness professionals should strive to take a positive approach to weight management and encourage clients to develop healthful lifestyles rather than focus solely on weight loss. One reason for an emphasis on the positive is that clients are more likely to be successful in the long run in keeping the weight off and preventing the health problems associated with excess body fat. Another important reason is to help clients avoid developing negative health behaviors in their quest for body composition improvement.

Unfortunately, weight-loss advice and efforts to reduce weight, often coupled with unrealistic body size ideals and a fear of fatness, can lead to the development of a wide range of pathogenic, or harmful, weight-control measures. The term pathogenic weight control refers to weight-control practices that can be harmful to physical and psychological health. Examples of pathogenic weight-control practices include using tobacco products and drugs to lose weight; following very unrealistic low-calorie eating plans that are likely to fail; engaging in detoxification programs that require fasting, enemas, and other treatments; using laxatives and diuretics to achieve weight loss; vomiting for the purpose of purging the body of excess energy intake; and engaging in excessive amounts of exercise.

A tendency to be overweight or obese and pathogenic weight-control measures, including disordered eating behaviors, intertwine in complex patterns that are often difficult to understand, let alone treat (Fig. 11-8). Problems with eating behavior and pathogenic weight-control measures are sometimes, although by no means always, associated with obesity. Obesity (real or perceived) or fear of obesity may lead some clients to behave in harmful ways. Ironically, many people eventually gain, rather than lose, weight from misguided weight-loss attempts. Other clients may develop disordered eating behaviors for reasons unrelated to obesity. This section will help readers understand and recognize pathogenic weight-control practices, help their clients recognize and change negative weight-control behaviors, and know when to refer clients for professional psychological support.

Body Dissatisfaction

Health and fitness professionals often hear clients (and coworkers) complain about their bodies. Most take it for granted that many of the people who seek their advice come on a mission of body improvement. Body dissatisfaction is part of the American way of life and has been for many years. Many health and fitness professionals are concerned about the prevalence and depth of the body dissatisfaction they see all around them and the pathogenic weight-control behaviors that are often the result.

Researchers who study body dissatisfaction have focused a great deal on people's concepts regarding perceptions of their physical appearance, a concept known as body image. Body image is the image people have of their bodies and includes not only how people see their physical appearance but also their judgment of

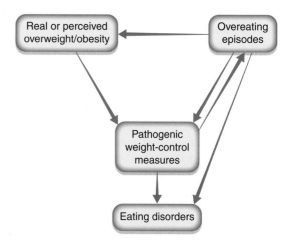

Figure 11-8. **Pathogenic weight control measures and obesity.**

what they see. This judgment includes how satisfied people are with their appearance as well as the emotions associated with this judgment. These emotions vary in intensity depending on the extent to which a person values appearance as a measure of self-worth. This means that people with similar degrees of "beauty" may have very different body images.

People judge themselves by comparing themselves with others. When they compare themselves with someone they feel is better, they judge themselves as inferior. When they compare themselves with someone they perceive as inferior, they feel better about themselves. Unfortunately, when it comes to body image, people often compare themselves with the bodies they see in the media, and they rarely find that their appearance meets this standard.

Body image contributes to a person's self-esteem. Some people place a great deal of importance on their appearance, and thus a poor body image may have a very negative impact on their self-esteem. Many writers have lamented the damage that results from negative body image, when women and men experience emotional distress that drives them to spend a great deal of time worrying about their appearance. This worry may prompt people to engage in risky behaviors as they attempt to change appearance, including pathogenic weight-control measures or steroid abuse. Eating disorders often begin with a negative body image that evolves into obsessions with food and weight. Experts have offered many explanations for the widespread body dissatisfaction found in many cultures:

- **Impossible standards of ideal appearance.** Every culture has standards of beauty. Throughout the ages and around the world, people have evaluated their appearance and that of others. A pleasing appearance has often been associated with higher status, better opportunities to attract a mate, and other positive qualities. Much of the widespread body dissatisfaction seen today can be attributed to the enormous disparity between current cultural beauty ideals (for women: very thin, yet with curves in the right places; for men: very fit and muscular) and people's actual bodies, with two-thirds of the population in the United States overweight. Female fashion models are often 20% below a healthful weight. Compare this with the fashion ideals of the 1940s. Marilyn Monroe was a healthy size 14, with a body more similar to that of most women at the time. A very small percentage of the population actually resembles the fashion ideals of today. For men, a cultural ideal of muscularity can drive a preoccupation with appearance and body image (Kanayama & Pope, 2011).
- **Body objectification.** Objectification means to regard something as an object. Body objectification refers to the practice of regarding the body, especially one's appearance, from an outsider's perspective. Most of the research on body objectification and body-image dissatisfaction focuses on females. Research has found that to enhance their social desirability and self-evaluation, girls and women tend to be very concerned with their appearance and often go to great lengths to increase their physical attractiveness (Breines, Crocker, & Garcia, 2008). Higher levels of body objectification are associated with lower levels of self-esteem and higher risk of depression in adolescence (Impett, Henson, Breines, Schooler, & Tolman, 2011). Studies have also found that higher levels of body objectification are associated with lower levels of intrinsic motivation, fewer experiences of flow states, and lower perceived levels of autonomy and vitality (Moradi & Yu-Ping, 2008).
- **Family behaviors and attitudes.** Research suggests parents' attitudes toward body size and eating influence children's satisfaction with their bodies (Agras, Bryson, Hammer, & Kraemer, 2007). This presents a challenging situation for parents and caregivers. Well-intentioned efforts to prevent obesity and promote a healthy lifestyle in children can backfire if too much effort to control their eating behavior and size is expended. Parents' dissatisfaction with their own bodies increases the likelihood that children will develop the same attitude. Perceived negative judgment from parents has also been linked to increased risk of disordered eating (Field et al., 2008).
- **A belief that self-control can give one the perfect body.** In reality, control of the body's appearance is limited. People cannot make their shoulders significantly broader, increase their height, or change their facial features (without the help of plastic surgery). What can be changed is weight, at least in theory, so weight becomes the focus of self-improvement efforts. Body weight becomes the target when people are dissatisfied with their looks and, sometimes, with themselves. Unfortunately, the idea that body weight is purely a function of self-control is misleading. Studies show that long-term weight loss is the exception rather than the rule. Yet the myth that with enough self-control a person can make huge changes in body weight persists, leading clients to experience guilt and frustration when their weight-control attempts don't give them an absolutely perfect body.
- **Living in a culture of first impressions.** Many people interact with large numbers of "new" people every day, especially in their work lives. People judge others based on how they dress, how they talk, how they move and what they look like.

Support Body-Image Resilience

Successful behavior changes are more likely to occur when a person feels strong and competent, rather than weak and ineffective. If body dissatisfaction is a problem and associated with low self-confidence, a client will have a harder time sticking to a behavior-change program than a client who feels confident. Clients with high body dissatisfaction could benefit from confronting and coming to terms with these negative feelings so that their plans to improve their lifestyles come from positions of strength. As discussed above, health and fitness professionals should refer clients with significant body-image problems for professional support.

People who need to lose some weight should focus on improving lifestyle rather than just on attaining a specific weight goal. Lifestyle is more controllable than weight. A healthy lifestyle will eventually help clients reach the best achievable weight, a weight they can maintain in good health. Encourage clients to develop their own style. Help them to make peace with their genes.

Body image sometimes improves with regular physical activity, as discussed in Chapter 3. Clients should be encouraged to exercise for positive reasons: to be healthy and feel good. Exercise builds self-confidence and appreciation for the body's power, endurance, and strength. Sports can help people appreciate their body's skill and agility. Exercise can help people relax and improve mood. When people engage in physical activity, they experience their bodies as the subject of the experience, not the object of someone else's appraisal.

Encourage clients to limit exposure to media and be active instead. The media inundate viewers with unrealistic "body models." People soak up these impressions at both conscious and subconscious levels. People with teens and preteens should teach them to analyze the messages they see in media advertisements and to view media critically. Health and fitness professionals can encourage clients to challenge beauty ideals.

Health and fitness professionals should be healthy body image role models. They should avoid conversations about how imperfect their bodies are or about the latest diet craze. They should never gossip about who needs to lose weight or build muscle and avoid making judgments based solely on a person's appearance. People with body-image resilience understand that the impression a person makes has a lot to do with posture, confidence, and personal style. They wear clothes they love that are comfortable and make them look and feel good.

Muscle Dysmorphia

The term muscle dysmorphia was coined by psychiatrist (and weight lifter) Harrison G. Pope, Jr., to described people abnormally preoccupied with the appearance of their muscles (Pope, Gruber, Choi, Olivardia, & Phillips, 1997). Before the creation of this term, bodybuilders themselves had recognized the existence of the disorder among their peers and referred to it as "bigorexia" and "reverse anorexia nervosa" (Kanayama & Pope, 2011). These terms were coined to capture the obsessive and compulsive eating and exercise behaviors observed in people with muscle dysmorphia, behaviors that resemble those seen in individuals with anorexia nervosa. But, rather than pursuing a smaller size, as seen with anorexia nervosa, people with "reverse anorexia nervosa" were trying to get bigger. People with muscle dysmorphia worry excessively that their muscles are not large enough and go to great lengths to increase muscle size. Not surprisingly, resistance training forms the heart of their efforts, which is why health and fitness professionals might see people with muscle dysmorphia in the fitness center.

What is an "abnormal preoccupation" and how do preoccupied lifters differ from the average fitness center member (and employee)? After all, many people who perform resistance training hope to improve their appearance, perhaps along with their health and athletic performance. Muscle dysmorphia is generally diagnosed when concern about one's muscularity becomes "distressing or impairing" and interferes with daily life or good health (Phillips et al., 2010; Murray, Rieger, Touyz, & De la Garza García Lic, 2010). People with muscle dysmorphia may have several of the following characteristics (Leone, Sedory, & Gray, 2005):

- **Devotion to daily resistance exercise, even when injured.** People with muscle dysmorphia are afraid to take even one day off, for fear their muscles will begin to atrophy. People with muscle dysmorphia obsess about exercise and can't take time off even when they develop symptoms of injury. They may feel unable to control exercise participation.
- **Profound dissatisfaction with their bodies.** People with muscle dysmorphia focus excessively on how they look. They may spend a great deal of time assessing their appearance in front of mirrors. They may wear baggy clothes and avoid situations that require exposing one's body, such as going to the beach. Many people with muscle dysmorphia may even avoid fitness centers, where they worry about others appraising their bodies, choosing to work out at home instead. People with this disorder may spend over 3 hours a day thinking about their muscularity.
- **Extremely rigid or ritualistic eating behaviors.** Most people with muscle dysmorphia may consume special diets to lose fat and build muscle. They often consume dietary supplements that claim to build muscle and burn fat.
- **Anabolic androgenic steroid use.** People with muscle dysmorphia may use steroids even though they understand the health risks involved.
- **Additional psychological disorders.** Many people with muscle dysmorphia also have eating disorders or mood disorders such as depression

and anxiety. Many also have other symptoms of obsessive-compulsive disorders.

Like other addicts, people with muscle dysmorphia spend a great deal of time on their addiction and may lose the ability to enjoy life. They may give up activities they previously enjoyed, reduce contact with friends and family, and even lose their jobs when all of their efforts go into their training programs. While muscle dysmorphia is rarely fatal, complications can develop from overtraining and from supplement and drug use. Muscle dysmorphia and disordered eating have been associated with a number of negative health behaviors in adolescent and young adult males and females, including increased risk of starting to use drugs and starting to binge drink frequently (Field et al., 2012). Health and fitness professionals who are worried about clients or friends should share their concern and refer them to experienced mental health-care providers.

Disordered Eating and Eating Disorders

Most health and fitness professionals are familiar with disordered eating behaviors. These disorders are generally variations on the themes of restricting, bingeing, and purging (Fig. 11-9). Like other addictions and negative health behaviors, disordered eating behaviors occur across a continuum that ranges in severity from

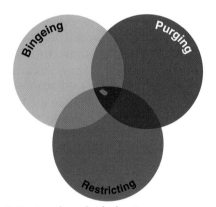

Figure 11-9. **Eating disorder behaviors.**

mild to life threatening (Fig. 11-10). Once disordered behaviors become severe, the symptoms qualify for a diagnosis of an eating disorder. The diagnostic criteria for the three most well-defined eating disorders are summarized in Box 11-5.

Anorexia nervosa (AN) is an eating disorder marked by an intense fear of gaining weight or becoming fat and severe food restriction leading to an abnormally low body weight. **Binge eating disorder** (BED) is characterized by recurrent episodes of eating very large volumes of food, while feeling a lack of control over one's ability to stop eating. People with **bulimia nervosa** (BM) perform binge eating along with harmful compensatory behaviors to prevent weight gain, including self-induced vomiting; misuse of laxatives, diuretics, and other drugs; fasting; or excessive exercise.

Eating disorders are very-serious mental illnesses. Experts estimate that mortality rates for these disorders are about 4% to 5% (Crow et al., 1999). Eating disorders may begin with some use of pathogenic weight-control behaviors focused on food and weight that can gradually become more severe over time. Eating disorders often begin as very-low-calorie diets as people attempt to lose weight. Successful losers may gain pride in their conquest over their hunger and appetite and feel a powerful sense of control over their lives. Anorexia nervosa may develop as controlling food and weight becomes the primary focus of a client's life. Clients with binge eating disorders consume large quantities of food when hunger and food cravings drive them to overeat. Binge eaters may also overeat in attempts to reduce feelings of anxiety and stress. People with bulimia follow binge eating with attempts to purge themselves of the extra calories.

But most people who occasionally practice disordered eating and other pathogenic weight-control behaviors do not develop full-blown eating disorders. Some of the factors associated with the development of eating disorders include:

- **Genetic predisposition.** One study of female-female sibling pairs compared rates of eating disorders in biologically related sisters with those of adopted pairs, not biologically related (Klump,

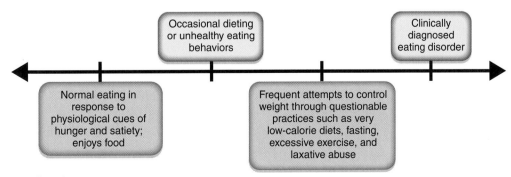

Figure 11-10. **Disordered eating continuum.**

Box 11-5. Diagnostic Criteria for Eating Disorders

Anorexia Nervosa

Severe restriction of food intake that causes significantly low body weight, that is, below the minimum of what would be expected for the person's age, sex, and health

Intense fear of gaining weight or becoming fat, or practicing harmful weight-control behaviors even though significantly underweight

Disturbance in the experience of one's body shape or weight or lack of acceptance that one's low weight is having serious negative health effects

Binge Eating Disorder

Recurrent episodes of binge eating characterized by eating abnormally large volumes of food in a discrete time period and experiencing a lack of control over food consumption

Binge eating episodes are characterized by three or more of the following:

- Eating more rapidly than normal
- Eating until uncomfortably full
- Binge eating in the absence of physical hunger
- Eating alone because of embarrassment about eating behavior
- Feeling depressed, guilty, or disgusted with oneself after binge eating
- Distress regarding binge eating behavior
- Binge eating occurs at least once a week for 3 months

Bulimia Nervosa

Recurrent binge eating, as described previously, with a feeling that one lacks control over eating behavior

Regular inappropriate compensatory behavior performed to prevent weight gain, such as self-induced vomiting; misuse of laxatives, diuretics, or other drugs; fasting; or excessive exercise

Binge eating and compensatory behaviors occur at least once a week for 3 months

Self-evaluation is overly influenced by one's perceptions of one's body weight and shape

Eating Disorder Not Otherwise Specified (EDNOS)

EDNOS is diagnosed when symptoms of eating disorders are present but do not meet the full diagnostic criteria of any specific category.

Source: American Psychiatric Association. (2013). *The Diagnostic and Statistical Manual of Mental Disorders,* 5th ed. Washington, DC: American Psychiatric Association.

observation suggests that genetics may influence the likelihood of developing an eating disorder.

- **Gender.** Females have much higher rates of eating disorders than males, comprising about 85% to 90% of those diagnosed with eating disorders (National Association of Anorexia Nervosa and Related Disorders, 2006). Girls and women may be more prone to the development of eating disorders because of cultural influences that cause them to link self-regard with their appearance. Negative body image is more common in females and may precipitate pathogenic weight-control behaviors that spiral out of control into eating disorders. An interesting longitudinal study found that compared with adolescent boys, adolescent girls were more likely to develop poor body image, depression, and disordered eating symptoms over a 2-year period (Ferreiro, Seoane, & Senra, 2011). It should be noted, however, that because males have a lower prevalence of eating disorders, it may be easier for these illnesses to be overlooked in them.

- **Anxiety disorders, depression, and substance-use disorders.** A majority of people diagnosed with an eating disorder also exhibit symptoms of other mental-health disorders, including anxiety disorders, depression, and substance-use disorders (Day et al., 2011; Konstantellou, Campbell, Eisler, Simic, & Treasure, 2011). Negative emotions may drive the development of eating-disorder behaviors, and the behaviors associated with their disorder may help people feel better, at least in the short run.

- **Cultural factors.** Eating disorders are primarily found in affluent countries that value a thin physique. Repeated exposure to media emphasizing unobtainable beauty ideals appears to influence body image, especially in vulnerable adolescents, but in adult women and men as well (Derenne & Beresin, 2006).

MOTIVATING CHANGE: Working With Clients With Disordered Eating Behaviors

All eating disorders involve food, but they are also behavior patterns that help people cope with stress and other personal issues. Clients with these complex psychological disorders require long-term support from knowledgeable, experienced professionals. You can encourage your clients with eating disorders to get professional help, but you can't just "talk some sense into them." In addition to referring clients with disordered eating for professional help, health and fitness professionals can do the following:

- **Model healthy behaviors.** Education is not always helpful. Ironically, talking to your clients about eating disorders can make things worse. Instead, model healthy attitudes: food is delicious and nutritious; food is fuel, and healthful eating supports exercise and sports performance. Model a balanced attitude about weight, as well. Healthy, strong bodies allow people to enjoy workouts and

Suisman, Burt, McGue, & Iacono, 2009). The chance that both sisters would have an eating disorder diagnosis was significantly greater for biological sibling pairs than adopted pairs. This

participate in challenging and rewarding activities. Focus on performance, not weight.

- **Pay attention.** Don't ignore eating disorders. They have the highest mortality rate of any psychological illness. Your feedback may help get your client into treatment.
- **Take a team approach.** Work with your supervisor and colleagues when you are worried about a client. Your workplace should have guidelines and procedures in place for referrals for eating disorders and other psychological problems.
- **Speak to your client in private.** Express your concern and cite specific, objective, observable behaviors that worry you. Encourage the client to meet with a counselor. Be ready with names and contact information. If your client is a minor, speak to his or her parents, as well.
- **Keep your distance.** Don't counsel your clients about eating disorders. Offer sympathy and a referral. Avoid discussions about food and weight. Your client needs help "changing the channel"; don't get drawn into the obsession.
- **Be patient.** Eating disorders are difficult to overcome, and recovery may take a long time. Be tolerant, respectful, and supportive. Your client is going through a very difficult time.
- **Learn about eating disorders.** For more information on how to help clients with eating disorders, consult helpful sources such as the National Eating Disorders Association (www.nationaleatingdisorders.org). Keep in mind, however, that referring someone with an eating disorder to websites can do more harm than good, as they may use the sites to "improve" their abilities to control food and weight (Mule & Sidelli, 2009). Chat rooms can create opportunities to talk with other disturbed people, reinforce pathogenic thoughts and behaviors, learn new disordered behaviors, and normalize eating-disorder behaviors.

Excessive Exercise

Most health and fitness professionals have many stories to tell about clients (and coworkers) who exercise too much. What may begin as a commitment to a healthy lifestyle can gradually develop into an unhealthy behavior pattern or even a full-blown addiction. Like addiction to work, Internet use, dieting, and other "positive" behaviors, addiction to exercise can be difficult to recognize. Many people engage in large volumes of exercise without causing harm to themselves or others, but others develop a compulsion to exercise that interferes with their health and/or daily life. Although little research has examined the prevalence of exercise addiction, experts estimate that it may affect about 3% of adults in the United States (Sussman, Lisha, & Griffiths, 2011). While exercise addiction is not included in the DSM-5 as a diagnosable mental disorder, exercise addiction fits the description of a behavioral addiction such as gambling (Berczik et al., 2012). Freimuth, Moniz, & Kim (2011) have summarized the symptoms of exercise addiction to show that these symptoms resemble descriptions of behavioral addictions:

- **Tolerance.** People addicted to exercise may find they need more exercise than they used to in order to achieve the desired effect, such as feelings of euphoria, reductions in anxiety, or feelings of accomplishment.
- **Withdrawal.** When people addicted to exercise are unable to exercise, they experience negative effects such as restlessness, irritability, anxiety, and problems sleeping.
- **Lack of control, lack of ability to follow through with intentions to change behavior.** People addicted to exercise may be unsuccessful in their attempts to decrease exercise volume. Even though they may have intentions to exercise less, they are unable to do this. They persist in excessive exercise despite knowledge that the exercise behaviors are harming physical or psychological health and/or interfering with interpersonal relationships.
- **Time spent on exercise and behaviors related to exercise.** A great deal of time is dedicated not only to exercise itself but also to preparation for and recovery from exercise activities.
- **Reduction in other activities.** People with exercise addiction usually decrease time spent on other activities, including activities related to work and social and recreational activities they used to enjoy.

Exercise addiction that occurs without other symptoms of eating disorders is known as primary exercise addiction. Excessive exercise often occurs as part of a larger constellation of disordered-eating behaviors. In this case, it is known as secondary exercise addiction. People with eating disorders may exercise excessively to purge calories and control weight, as described in the previous section.

Readers will remember from Chapter 3 that exercise is a mind-altering activity. Research in rats has shown that high levels of exercise can transform the dopamine reward circuitry in the brain and decrease the rewarding effects of other substances that usually produce a dopamine response (Adams, 2009). If this effect occurs in humans, and it is not clear that it does, this might suggest that people have to maintain high levels of intense exercise to optimize the reward circuitry of the mesolimbic dopamine reward system. Even if this research does not translate into human reality, it is still certainly true that physical exercise can be perceived as a very-rewarding activity that some people learn to turn to for positive experiences.

Health and fitness professionals should note that high volumes of exercise alone are not necessarily harmful (Johnston, Reilly, & Kremer, 2011). Athletes in training often exercise for hours a day, although most take at least one day of relative rest each week. Rather, the exercise addiction continuum resembles

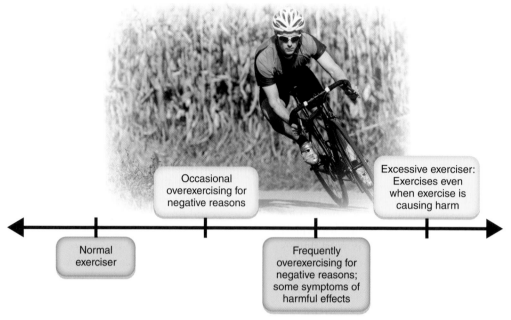

Occasional overexercising for negative reasons

Excessive exerciser: Exercises even when exercise is causing harm

Normal exerciser

Frequently overexercising for negative reasons; some symptoms of harmful effects

Figure 11-11. **Excessive exercise continuum.** Photograph © Thinkstock

the general addiction continuum (Fig. 11-11). Exercise becomes excessive and an activity of concern when it is causing, or likely to cause, harm. For example, swimmers may train for hours a day as they prepare for their competitive season. Swimmers training according to their team's protocol would not necessarily be suspected of exercising excessively. However, swimmers who perform high-volume training with their team, and, in addition, train on the days when they have been told to rest and recover, would be exercising excessively. This additional exercise qualifies as a negative health behavior, as it increases risk of overuse injuries and hurts athletic performance. In fact, the most-common harmful effect associated with excessive exercise is overuse injury, including stress fractures (Dalle Grave, 2009).

Another sign of excessive exercise is when people exercise even though they are injured and have been told to avoid aggravating the injury. Compare two runners, both with a stress fracture in the tibia (bone of the lower leg). One switches to cycling and swimming, as recommended by his orthopedist. The other continues to run, despite his physician's advice. The latter illustrates excessive exercise as a negative health behavior (Behavior Change in Action 11-1).

BEHAVIOR CHANGE IN ACTION 11-1

Clients Who Exercise Too Much

■ CHALLENGE
What should health and fitness professionals do when they observe someone exercising for prolonged periods most days of the week?

■ PLAN
Health and fitness professionals who work in a fitness center setting can't help but notice clients who spend a great deal of time working out. Sometimes everyone knows the client is an athlete in training for an upcoming competitive season, and everyone admires the athlete's drive and perseverance. Other times, the client is someone nobody knows. If clients with high levels of exercise are very thin, people who work at the fitness center as well as other clients are especially likely to wonder if they should intervene. If you are concerned about someone who appears to be exercising excessively, try the following.

■ TALK TO YOUR SUPERVISOR OR STAFF
If you are worried about a particular client, talk to your supervisor. If you are the supervisor, talk to the other people with whom you work. Do they see the same thing you are seeing or are you overreacting? Does someone know something about this person that explains the high exercise volume? Maybe she is already in treatment for some other problem, and exercising is helping her get through a rough time. Has someone else already intervened and

BEHAVIOR CHANGE IN ACTION 11-1–cont'd

expressed concern? It's important that you are all on the same wavelength and don't interfere with each other's efforts. Decide as a group whether or not you think this client is at risk for injury.

Are there policies at your workplace that you need to follow? For example, at a university fitness center, you may be told to call the dean of students or other offices if a student may have a health problem.

■ NEVER DISCUSS CLIENTS WITH OTHER CLIENTS
It is common for other clients to notice the person who exercises for hours a day and who appears to live at the fitness center. When other clients are concerned, acknowledge their concern but do not discuss the client in question. You might say something like, "I appreciate your concern, but I am not at liberty to discuss this situation." You might assure this person that you are doing all you can.

■ ARRANGE FOR ONE PERSON TO SPEAK WITH THE CLIENT IN QUESTION
If your supervisor or group agrees that the client may need help, decide who will speak with the client. The best person may be one of the health and fitness professionals who is acquainted with the client in some capacity. One person who develops a helpful relationship with the client will do more good than several strangers dropping critical remarks and questions.

■ EXPRESS YOUR CONCERN IN A SUPPORTIVE, TACTFUL MANNER
If you decide to talk to your overexercising client, be as tactful as possible. Could you offer her a free personal training session to discuss her fitness goals and exercise program? Tell her this session comes with her membership benefits. During this consultation, you could discuss her health and fitness goals to try to understand her reasons for exercising so much. This session might also be an opportunity to educate her in a professional manner about the importance of rest and recovery and the dangers of excessive exercise. You could also express your concern about her health and your worry that too much exercise could lead to injury or health problems.

Keep your focus on health, not weight. If she does have an eating disorder (and don't assume that she does), she will not see low body weight as a problem but as a good thing. Instead, mention specifics such as how she exercises every single day or how she exercises even when she is sick or injured.

■ CHECK MEDICAL CLEARANCE FORMS
Health professionals may not discriminate against clients with eating disorders, according to the Americans with Disabilities Act. However, such clients may be at risk for cardiovascular complications during exercise. When clients exhibit very-low body weight, blood pressure, or resting heart rate, ask them to check in with their health-care providers and update your medical clearance forms, just as you would for any other client at risk. Require a physician's consent form and check in with the physician if you are worried.

Motivation for exercise often differs for those who exercise excessively. While improving athletic performance may have formerly been an important goal, over time people addicted to exercise may exercise just because they must, even though performance is declining. Exercise becomes an end in and of itself, rather than a means to another more-important goal, such as good health or athletic performance.

■ *Kim returns to her work at the community center after a 2-week vacation. As she prepares for the evening dance exercise class, Hope and Eliza come dancing in the door. "We have some news for you!" Hope is practically jumping up and down. "Eliza is expecting!" Her baby is not due for 6 months, and her health-care providers have encouraged her to keep up with her exercise program for now. Nevertheless, Kim gives Eliza a list of signs that mean she should stop exercising and see her provider. As Eliza's due date approaches, Kim is relieved to observe her slowing down a bit and eventually*

transferring to the community center's class for pregnant women and new mothers. "I am so glad I was able to quit smoking," Eliza often says to Kim. "I will never forget all the support I have gotten from you and everyone here." ■

KEY TERMS

abuse
addiction
alcohol dehydrogenase
anorexia nervosa
binge eating disorder
body image
body objectification
bulimia nervosa
contingency management therapies

craving
detoxification
fetal alcohol spectrum disorders
harm reduction
hedonic hotspots
hepatocellular carcinoma
liver cirrhosis
mesolimbic dopaminergic pathway

KEY TERMS–cont'd

muscle dysmorphia	reward pathway	steatohepatitis	tolerance
nucleus accumbens	secondary exercise addiction	substance-related disorder	ventral tegmental area
pathogenic weight control	self-medication	substance-use disorder	withdrawal symptoms
primary exercise addiction	social control	substance dependence	
	steatosis	teratogen	

CRITICAL THINKING QUESTIONS

1. Apply the use, abuse, addiction continuum to use of the Internet. Describe controlled use, abuse, and addiction. What might these different stages look like? Apply this same question to texting.

2. Use an ecological perspective to describe factors that promote and prevent cigarette smoking. Include factors at the intrapersonal level, including a person's knowledge, values, beliefs and preferences; the interpersonal level, including close interpersonal relationships, such as family members and close friends; the organizational level, including influences such as a person's workplace, health-care systems, and recreational groups; the community level, including the built environment as well as neighbors; and the societal and cultural level, including larger social and cultural influences, such as government structures, public-health policies and programs, and economic structures.

3. Describe how lower levels of ECF might impact important variables in the Health Belief Model and the Theory of Planned Behavior Model. How might these observations be applied to addiction treatment in adolescents, whose brains have not yet matured in the ECF area?

4. Imagine a college student going through the stages of change for quitting binge drinking. Write descriptions for this person in each stage of change, from precontemplation through maintenance. What kind of behaviors might you observe at each stage?

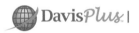 For additional resources log in to Davis*Plus* (http://davisplus.fadavis.com/ keyword "Brehm") and click on the Premium tab. (Don't have a *Plus*Code to access Premium Resources? Just click the Purchase Access button on the book's Davis*Plus* page.)

REFERENCES

Adams, J. (2009). Understanding exercise dependence. *Journal of Contemporary Psychotherapy, 39*(4), 231-240.

Agras, S. W., Bryson, S., Hammer, L. D., & Kraemer, H. C. (2007). Childhood risk factors for thin body preoccupation and social pressure to be thin. *Journal of the American Academy of Child & Adolescent Psychiatry, 46*(2), 171-178.

Alcoholics Anonymous. (2012). AA Timeline: Origins. www.aa.org/aatimeline/. Accessed 3/1/12.

Alcoholics Anonymous World Services, Inc. (2001). *The Big Book Online.* (4th ed.). www.aa.org/bigbookonline. Accessed 3/1/12.

Alfonso-Loeches, S., & Guerri, C. (2011). Molecular and behavioral aspects of the actions of alcohol on the adult and developing brain. *Critical Reviews in Clinical Laboratory Sciences, 48*(1), 19-47.

American Lung Association. (2012). Freedom From Smoking. www.lung.org/stop-smoking/how-to-quit/freedom-from-smoking. Accessed 4/11/12.

American Psychiatric Association. (2013). *The Diagnostic and Statistical Manual of Mental Disorders,* 5th ed. Washington, DC: American Psychiatric Association.

Amodeo, M., Lundgren, L., Cohen, A., Rose, D., Chassler, D., Beltràme, C., & D'Ippolito, M. (2011). Barriers to implementing evidence-based practices in addiction treatment programs: comparing staff reports on motivational interviewing, adolescent community reinforcement approach, assertive community treatment, and cognitive-behavioral therapy. *Evaluation and Program Planning, 3*(4), 382-389.

Bates, M. E., Pawlak, A. P., Tonigan, J. S., & Buckman, J. F. (2006). Cognitive impairment influences drinking outcome by altering therapeutic mechanism of change. *Psychology of Addictive Behaviors, 20,* 241-253.

Bava, S., & Tapert, S. F. (2010). Adolescent brain development and the risk for alcohol and other drug problems. *Neuropsychology Review, 20*(4), 398-413.

Berczik, K., Szabó, A., Griffiths, M. D., Kurimay, T., Kun, B., Urbán, R., & Demetrovics, Z. (2012). Exercise addiction: symptoms, diagnosis, epidemiology, and etiology. *Substance Use and Misuse, 47*(4), 403-417.

Berridge, K. C., & Kringelbach, M. L. (2013). Neuroscience of affect: brain mechanisms of pleasure and displeasure. *Current Opinion in Neurobiology, 23* (3), 294-303.

Blednov, Y. A., Ponomarev, I., Geil, C., Bergeson, S., Koob, G. F., & Harris, R. A. (2012). Neuroimmune regulation of alcohol consumption: behavioral validation of genes obtained from genomic studies. *Addiction Biology, 17*(1), 108-120.

Blume, A. N., & Marlatt, B. A. (2009). The role of executive cognitive functions in changing substance use: what we know and what we need to know. *Annals of Behavioral Medicine, 37*(2), 117-125.

Bohn, S. K., Ward, N. C., Hodgson, J. M., & Croft, K. D. (2012). Effects of tea and coffee on cardiovascular disease risk. *Food & Function, 3*(6), 575-591.

Bolton, J. M., Robinson, J., & Sareen, J. (2009). Self-medication of mood disorders with alcohol and drugs in the National Epidemiologic Survey on Alcohol and Related Conditions. *Journal of Affective Disorders, 115*(3), 367-375.

Brehm, J. W. (2000). Reactance. In: Kazdin, A. E. (ed.) *Encyclopedia of Psychology*, 10-12. Oxford: Oxford University Press.

Breines, J. G., Crocker, J., & Garcia, J. A. (2008). Self-objectification and well-being in women's daily lives. *Personality and Social Psychology Bulletin, 34*, 583-598.

Conrod, P. J., Castellanos-Ryan, N., & Strang, J. (2010). Brief, personality-targeted coping skills interventions and survival as a non-drug user over a 2-year period during adolescence. *Archives of General Psychiatry, 67*(1), 85-93.

Cooper, C., Atkinson, E. J., Wahner, H. W., O'Fallon, W. M., Riggs, B. L., Judd, H. L., & Melton, L. J. 3rd (2009). Is caffeine consumption a risk factor for osteoporosis? *Journal of Bone and Mineral Research, 7*(4), 465-471.

Crews, F. T., & Boettiger, C. A. (2009). Impulsivity, frontal lobes and risk for addiction. *Pharmacology, Biochemistry and Behavior, 93*(3), 237-247.

Crow, S. J., Peterson, C. B., Swanson, S. A., Raymond, N. C., Specker, S., Eckert, E. D., & Mitchell, J. E. (2009). Increased mortality in bulimia nervosa and other eating disorders. *American Journal of Psychiatry, 166*, 1342-1346.

Dalle Grave, R. (2009). Features and management of compulsive exercising in eating disorders. *The Physician and Sportsmedicine, 37*(3), 20-28.

Davis, L., Uezato, A., Newell, J. M., & Frazier, E. (2008). Major depression and comorbid substance use disorders. *Current Opinion in Psychiatry, 21*, 14-18.

Day, J., Schmidt, U., Collier, D., Perkins, S., Van den Eynde, F., Treasure, J., . . . Eisler, I. (2011). Risk factors, correlates, and markers in early onset bulimia nervosa and ED-NOS. *International Journal of Eating Disorders, 44*(4), 287-294.

Derenne, J. L., & Beresin, E. V. (2006). Body image, media, and eating disorders. *Academic Psychiatry, 30*(3), 257-261.

DiFranza, J., Wellman, R., & Savageau, J. (2012). Does progression through the stages of physical addiction indicate increasing overall addiction to tobacco? *Psychopharmacology, 219*(3), 815-822.

Douglas, K. R., Chan, G., Gelernter, J., Arias, A. J., Anton, R. F., Weiss, R. D., . . . Kranzler, H. R. (2010). Adverse childhood events as risk factors for substance dependence: partial mediation by mood and anxiety disorders. *Addictive Behaviors, 35*(1), 7-13.

Ettinger, R. H. (2011). *Psychopharmacology*. Boston, MA: Prentice Hall.

Ferreiro, F., Seoane, G., & Senra, C. (2011). A prospective study of risk factors for the development of depression and disordered eating in adolescents. *Journal of Clinical Child and Adolescent Psychology, 40*(3), 500-505.

Field, A. E., Javaras, K. M., Aneja, P., Kitos, N., Camargo, C. A., Jr., Taylor, C. B., & Laird, N. M. (2008). Family, peer, and media predictors of becoming eating disordered. *Archives of Pediatric and Adolescent Medicine, 162*(6), 574-579.

Field, A. E., Sonneville, K. R., Micali, N., Crosby, R. D., Swanson, S. A., Laird, N. M., . . . Horton, N. J. (2012). Prospective association of common eating disorders and adverse outcomes. *Pediatrics, 130*(2), e289-e295.

Foll, B. L., Gallo, A., Strat, Y. L., Lu, L., & Gorwood, P. (2009). Genetics of dopamine receptors and drug addiction: a comprehensive review. *Behavioural Pharmacology, 20*(1), 1-17.

Forbes, E. E., Ryan, N. D., Phillips, M. L., Manuck, S.B., Worthman, C. M., Moyles, D. L., . . . Dahl, R. E. (2010). Healthy adolescents' neural response to reward: association with puberty, positive affect, and depressive symptoms. *Journal of the American Academy of Child and Adolescent Psychiatry, 49*(2), 162-172.

Freimuth, M., Moniz, S., & Kim, S. R. (2011). Clarifying exercise addiction: Differential diagnosis, co-occurring disorders, and phases of addiction. *International Journal f Environmental Research and Public Health, 8*(10), 4069-4081.

Goldstein, A. (2009). *Addiction: From Biology to Drug Policy.* New York: Oxford University Press.

Goldstein, R. Z., & Volkow, N. D. (2011). Dysfunction of the prefrontal cortex in addiction: neuroimaging findings and clinical implications. *Nature Reviews Neuroscience, 12*(11), 652-669.

Goudriaan, A. E., Oosterlaan, J., de Beurs, E., & van den Brink, W. (2006). Neurocognitive functions in pathological gambling: a comparison with alcohol dependence, Tourette syndrome, and normal controls. *Addiction, 101*, 534-547.

Gross, M. (2010). Alcoholics Anonymous: still sober after 75 years. *American Journal of Public Health, 100*(12), 2361-2363.

Hall, W., Degenhardt, L., & Teesson, M. (2009). Understanding comorbidity between substance use, anxiety, and affective disorders: broadening the research base. *Addictive Behaviors, 34*(6-7), 526-530.

Hien, D. A., Huiping, J., Campbell, A. N. C., Hu, M.-C., Miele, G. M., Cohen, L. R., . . . Nunes, E.V. (2010). Do treatment improvements in PTSD severity affect substance use outcomes? A secondary analysis from a randomized clinical trial in NIDA's Clinical Trials Network. *American Journal of Psychiatry, 167*(1), 95-101.

Impett, E. A., Henson, J. M., Breines, J. G., Schooler, D., & Tolman, D. L. (2011). Embodiment feels better: girls' body objectification and well-being across adolescence. *Psychology of Women Quarterly, 35*(1), 46-58.

Johnston, O., Reilly, J., & Kremer, J. (2011). Excessive exercise: from quantitative categorization to a qualitative continuum approach. *European Eating Disorders Review, 19*(3), 237-248.

Kanayama, G., & Pope, H. G. Jr. (2011). Gods, men, and muscle dysmorphia. *Harvard Review of Psychiatry, 19*(2), 95-98.

Klump, K. L., Suisman, J. L., Burt, S. A., McGue, M., & Iacono, W. G. (2009). Genetic and environmental influences on disordered eating: an adoption study. *Journal of Abnormal Psychology, 118*(4), 797-805.

Konstantellou, A., Campbell, M., Eisler, I., Simic, M., & Treasure, J. (2011). Testing a cognitive model of generalized anxiety disorder in the eating disorders. *Journal of Anxiety Disorders, 25*(7), 864-869.

Leone, J. E., Sedory, E. J., & Gray, K. A. (2005). Recognition and treatment of muscle dysmorphia and related body image disorders. *Journal of Athletic Training, 40*(4), 352-359.

Leotti, L. A., Iyengar, S. S., & Ochsner, K. N. (2010). Born to choose: The origins and value of the need for control. *Trends in Cognitive Sciences, 14*(10), 457-463.

Lester, B. M., & Padbury, J. F. (2009). Third pathophysiology of prenatal cocaine exposure. *Developmental Neuroscience, 31*(1-2), 23-35.

Li, M. D., & Burmeister, M. (2009). New insights into the genetics of addiction. *Nature Reviews Genetics, 10*(4), 225-231.

Linden, D. J. (2011). *The Compass of Pleasure: How Our Brains Make Fatty Foods, Orgasm, Exercise, Marijuana, Generosity, Vodka, Learning, and Gambling Feel so Good.* New York: Viking.

Logic, M., Okun, M. A., & Publiese, J. A. (2009). Expanding the mediation model of the effects of health-related social control. *Journal of Applied Social Psychology, 39*(6), 1373-1396.

Lueth, N. A., Anderson, K. E., Harnack, L. J., Fulkerson, J. A., & Robien, K. (2008). Coffee and caffeine intake and the risk of ovarian cancer: the Iowa Women's Health Study. *Cancer Causes and Control, 19*(10), 1365-1372.

Marlatt, G. A., & Witkiewitz, K. (2010). Update on harm-reduction policy and intervention research. *Annual Review of Clinical Psychology, 6,* 591-606.

Miller, W. R., & Rollnick, S. (1991). *Motivational Interviewing: Preparing People to Change Addictive Behavior.* New York: Guilford Press.

Miller, W. R., & Rollnick, S. (2013). *Motivational Interviewing: Preparing People to Change, 3rd ed.* New York: Guilford Press.

Miller, W. R., & Rose, G. R. (2009). Toward a theory of motivational interviewing. *American Psychologist, 64*(6), 527-537.

Mochly-Rosen, D., & Zakhari, S. (2010). Focus on: the cardiovascular system: what did we learn from the French (paradox)? *Alcohol Research & Health, 3*(1-2), 76-86.

Mokdad, A. H., Marks, J. S., Stroup, D. F., & Gerberding, J. L. (2004). Actual causes of death in the United States, 2000. *Journal of the American Medical Association, 291*(10), 1238-1245.

Molina, P. E., Happel, K. I., Zhang, P., Kolls, J. K., & Nelson, S. (2010). Focus on: alcohol and the immune system. *Alcohol Research & Health, 33*(1-2), 97-108.

Moradi, B., & Yu-Ping, H. (2008). Objectification theory and psychology of women: a decade of advances and future directions. *Psychology of Women Quarterly, 32,* 377-398.

Mule, A., & Sidelli, L. (2009). Eating disorders on the Web: risks and resources. *Studies in Health Technology and Informatics, 144*(7), 8-12.

Murray, S. B., Rieger, E., Touyz, S. W., & De la Garza García Lic, Y. (2010). Muscle dysmorphia and the DSM-V conundrum: where does it belong? A review paper. *International Journal of Eating Disorders, 43*(6), 483-491.

National Association of Anorexia Nervosa and Related Disorders. (2006). Eating Disorders Statistics. www.anad.org/get-information/about-eating-disorders/eating-disorders-statistics/. Accessed 12/31/12.

National Institute on Alcohol Abuse and Alcoholism. (2005). Epidemiology of alcohol problems in the United States. http://pubs.niaaa.nih.gov/publications/Social/Module1Epidemiology/Module1.html. Accessed 12/21/12.

National Institute on Alcohol Abuse and Alcoholism. (2010). *Rethinking Drinking: Alcohol and Your Health.* Washington, DC: U.S. Department of Health and Human Services; April, 2010. NIH publication 10-3770. http://rethinkingdrinking.niaaa.nih.gov/. Accessed 12/31/12.

National Research Council/Institute of Medicine. (2007). *Ending the Tobacco Problem: A Blueprint for the Nation.* Washington, DC: National Academies Press.

Patel, S., & Rizzolo, D. (2012). When the patient asks: is caffeine safe during pregnancy? *Journal of the American Academy of Physicians Assistants, 25*(5), 69.

Paul, S. L., Blizzard, L., Patton, G. C., Dwyer, T., & Venn, A. (2008). Parental smoking and smoking experimentation in childhood increases the risk of becoming a smoker 20 years later: the childhood determinants of adult health study. *Addiction, 103*(5), 846-853.

Peele, S. (2004). *7 Tools to Beat Addiction.* New York: Three Rivers Press.

Phillips, K. A., Wilhelm, S., Koran, L. M., Didie, E. R., Fallon, B. A., Feusner, J., & Stein, D. J. (2010). Body dysmorphic disorder: Some key issues for DSM-V. *Depression and Anxiety, 27*(6), 573-591.

Pope, H. G., Jr., Gruber, A. J., Choi, P. Y., Olivardia, R., & Phillips, K. A. (1997). Muscle dysmorphia: an underrecognized form of body dysmorphic disorder. *Psychosomatics, 38,* 548-557.

Prochaska, J. O., & DiClemente, C. C. (1983). Stages and processes of self-change of smoking: Toward an integrative model of change. *Journal of Consulting and Clinical Psychology, 51*(3), 390-395.

Rivkees, S. A., & Wendler, C. C. (2012). Regulation of cardiovascular development by adenosine and adenosine-mediated embryo protection. *Arteriosclerosis, Thrombosis, and Vascular Biology, 32*(4), 851-855.

Rogers, C. R. (1959). A theory of therapy, personality, and interpersonal relationships as developed in the client-centered framework. In: Koch, S. (ed.). *Psychology: The Study of a Science.* New York: McGraw-Hill.

Rogers, C. R. (1980). *A Way of Being.* Boston, MA: Houghton Mifflin.

Schutte, K. K., Brennan, P. L., & Moos, R. H. (2009). Treated and untreated remission from problem drinking in late life: post-remission functioning and health-related quality of life. *Drug and Alcohol Dependence, 99*(1-3), 150-159.

Seitz, H. K., & Becker, P. (2007). Alcohol metabolism and cancer risk. *Alcohol Research & Health, 30*(1), 38-47.

Substance Abuse and Mental Health Administration. *Results from the 2008 National Survey on Drug Use & Health: Detailed Tables.* www.oas.samhsa.gov/nsduh/reports.htm#2k8. Accessed 4/11/12.

Sullivan, E. V., Harris, A., & Pfefferbaum, A. (2010). Alcohol's effects on brain and behavior. *Alcohol Research & Health, 33*(1-2), 127-143.

Sunitha, E. G., Ramalakshmi, K., & Rao, L. J. M. (2008). A perception on health benefits of coffee. *Critical Reviews in Food Science and Nutrition, 48*(5), 464-486.

Sussman, S., Lisha, N., & Griffiths, M. (2011). Prevalence of the addictions: a problem of the majority or the minority? *Evaluation and the Health Professions, 34*(1), 3-56.

Szabo, G., & Mandrekar, P. (2010). Focus on: alcohol and the liver. *Alcohol Research & Health, 33*(1-2), 87-96.

Thoits, P. A. (2010). Stress and health: Major findings and policy implications. *Journal of Health and Social Behavior, 51*(1 suppl), S41-S53.

Thomas, J. D., Warren, K. R., & Hewitt, B. G. (2010). Fetal alcohol spectrum disorders. *Alcohol Research & Health, 33*(1-2), 118-126.

Vonlaufen, A., Wilson, J. S., Pirola, R. C., & Apte, M. V. (2007). Role of alcohol metabolism in chronic pancreatitis. *Alcohol Research & Health, 30*(1), 48-54.

Wakefield, M. A., Loken, B., & Hornik, R. C. (2010). Use of mass media campaigns to change health behaviour. *Lancet, 376*(9748), 1261-1271.

White, W., & Miller, W. (2007). The use of confrontation in addiction treatment: History, science, and time for change. *Counselor, 8*(4), 12-30.

Williams, D. M., Whitely, J. A., Dunsiger, S., Jennings, E. G., Albrecht, A. E., Ussher, M. H., ... Marcus, B. H. (2010). Moderate intensity exercise as an adjunct to standard smoking cessation treatment for women: a pilot study. *Psychology of Addictive Behaviors, 24*(2), 349-354.

Witkiewitz, K., & Marlatt, G. A. (2010). Behavioral therapy across the spectrum. *Alcohol Research & Health, 33*(4), 313-319.

Zangeneh, M., Ala-leppilampi, K., Barmaki, M., & Peric, T. (2007). The potential role of physical exercise in addiction treatment and recovery: the social costs of substance misuse. *International Journal of Mental Health and Addiction, 5*(3), 210-218.

CHAPTER OUTLINE

LEARNING OBJECTIVES

After reading this chapter, you will be able to:

1. Explain the concept of illness representation.
2. Describe some of the most-common psychological effects of becoming a patient in a medical system.
3. Discuss some of the responses athletes may have to a serious injury and the factors that commonly affect this response.
4. Understand the complex nature of pain syndromes and explain why people with pain syndromes benefit from appropriate physical activity.

5. List the typical emotions people experience during the process of grieving.
6. Describe the importance of self-management for chronic health problems.
7. Explain several models that illustrate how people adjust psychologically to chronic health problems.
8. Discuss helpful strategies for promoting psychological adjustment to chronic health problems.

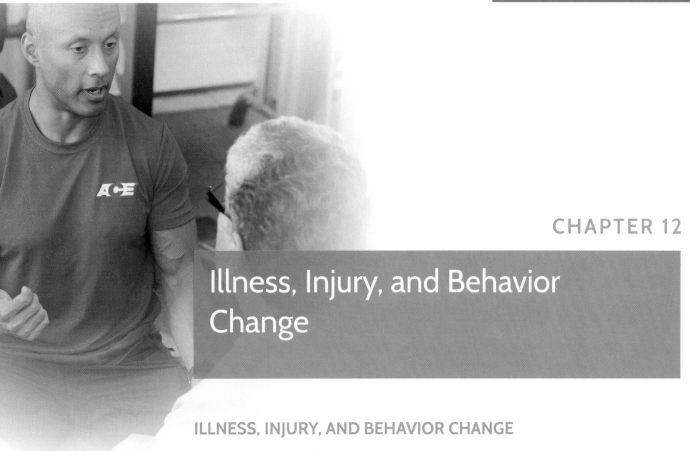

CHAPTER 12

Illness, Injury, and Behavior Change

ILLNESS, INJURY, AND BEHAVIOR CHANGE

■ *Mason and Grant are classmates in an undergraduate kinesiology program. They are both enrolled as interns in the same medical fitness facility for the school year. Clients at the facility generally began as rehabilitation patients following hospitalization for an illness or injury. Mason and Grant both help supervise the exercise programs of clients who have progressed enough to move from physical therapy to more of a personal training environment. Mason and Grant are looking forward to gaining experience with a wide variety of medical issues. Although Mason and Grant have had experience working in the university fitness center with beginning exercisers, neither has worked extensively with patients recently released from the hospital or rehabilitation center, and both are a little nervous about working with people who have fairly low levels of fitness and serious health problems. When Mason mentions his concerns, Grant reassures him. "We'll have instructions from the doctors and physical therapists to follow. And, basically, this is like basic exercise program design. You see what patients can do and ask them to do a little more." ■*

Health behaviors play important roles in both the development and treatment of injury and illness. Encouraging people to improve health behaviors to prevent or delay chronic illness forms the heart of the primary prevention efforts of many public-health programs. In addition, people diagnosed with injury or illness are often directed by medical professionals to alter health behaviors to speed recovery or to reduce injury or illness severity. The experiences of injury and illness occur in every life, and they strongly affect motivation and behavior. The topics of injury and illness have been woven into discussions throughout this book in a variety of contexts. This chapter explores these topics in more depth to help illuminate the experiences of coping with injury and illness and how these experiences influence the behavior-change process. The goal of this chapter is to broaden the health and fitness professional's understanding of how people perceive and respond to health challenges (Box 12-1).

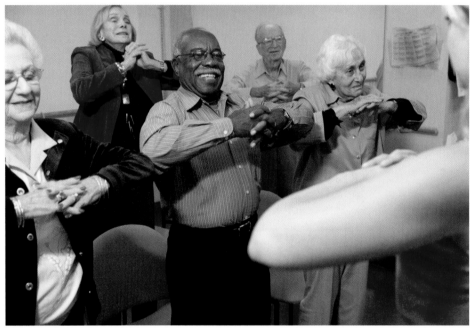

© Thinkstock

Box 12-1. Work in the Clinical Setting

Many health and fitness professionals work with patients in the clinical setting. Professionals may work in hospitals, outpatient clinics, and various types of rehabilitation centers. Some may work in assisted-living communities that provide medical fitness services. Many health and fitness professionals offer wellness as well as medical services in long-term care institutions. Some hospitals operate medical fitness centers, where patients perform rehabilitation therapy or exercise prescriptions as part of their medical treatment.

   Health and fitness professionals must adhere to scope-of-practice restrictions at all times, including when they are working in a clinical setting. Many professionals are qualified to recommend lifestyle behavior change to patients with a variety of illnesses, from heart disease and hypertension to arthritis and diabetes. Athletic trainers work with a wide variety of injuries. Professionals should be clear on what their trainings and certifications allow them to do and on the expectations of their employer. Professionals should be familiar with consensus standards and position papers available from respected professional organizations regarding behavior change for the health problems with which they work. For example, the American College of Sports Medicine and the American Diabetes Association have established guidelines on exercise recommendations for people with type 2 diabetes that serve as the standard of care for this population (Colberg, 2010).

   Job expectations in the clinical setting differ somewhat from those in health and fitness center settings for apparently healthy people. Some of these differences include the following.
   • **Position as part of a medical team:** Medical teams generally have established expectations regarding how communications among members occur as well as clearly defined roles for team members. Working as part of a medical team offers opportunities for assistance in formulating care guidelines for individual patients or discussing challenging situations that arise with people in treatment. Teamwork in the clinical setting works best when members share a common philosophy regarding the type of experience people receiving care will have and when members respect and value the work of all team members.

Box 12-1. Work in the Clinical Setting–cont'd

- **Challenging patient situations:** Patients in medical settings may present with complicated health situations, often with very serious health challenges. Health and fitness professionals must be skilled in assessing patients with a variety of health challenges and providing effective and safe guidance. They must be able to embody a positive attitude even with patients who are very ill and may never get better and to help patients cope, moment by moment, with the challenges they are facing.
- **Patients in early stages of change:** Although health and fitness professionals who work in a fitness or athletic training setting are likely to encounter people at least in the preparation stage of change, patients in a medical setting may not yet have committed to changing. They may have been issued orders to change, but they may feel overwhelmed and lack self-efficacy for performing the recommended behaviors.
- **Patients with very low fitness levels:** Behavior-change recommendations, including recommendations for physical activity, may need to accommodate very-low levels of physical fitness as well as other disabilities. Training in adapted physical education and rehabilitation can help professionals working with patient populations.

THE EXPERIENCE OF INJURY AND ILLNESS

Challenges to health take many forms. Some are generally easy to accommodate, whereas others require dramatic shifts in self-perception and expectations for daily life. People's responses to health threats are influenced both by the nature of the health problems they are encountering as well as their own perceptions of and ideas about health and their particular health problems.

The Dynamic Nature of Health Problems

In this chapter, the term "health problem" is used to encompass any health challenge, including injury and illness. Injury is generally considered to be harm to a body part caused by some sort of force, such as trauma or overuse. Illness usually refers to a state of poor health, often including symptoms indicating suboptimal function of an organ or physiological system. For example, hypertension may indicate problems with the kidney or the cardiovascular system. Injury and illness sometimes overlap, as when people with bone-density problems develop stress fractures. Both injuries and illnesses may be very short lived, with people making a speedy recovery and resuming normal life after a few days or weeks. An acute health problem refers to an injury or illness with a sudden onset that is fairly serious but relatively short lived. Other injuries and illnesses may last longer. Some injuries and illnesses may come and go or never entirely go away. For example, some back injuries may heal quite a bit but continue to be a source of some degree of discomfort or pain from time to time. They may require special exercises and accommodations to keep the pain at bay. Clients may be able to prevent pain by improving posture and body mechanics and avoiding activities that stress the injured area. Acute illness may develop into chronic illness. For example, a patient may develop phlebitis,

pain in the leg caused by a blood clot in a vein of the leg. Some cases of phlebitis resolve fairly quickly with treatment; in others the initial acute case of phlebitis develops into chronic problems with the leg veins.

Chronic illness and chronic disease mean the same thing and refer to illnesses that have no permanent cure, though symptoms may be managed through lifestyle or medical treatment. The Centers for Disease Control and Prevention (CDC) defines chronic diseases as "noncommunicable illnesses that are prolonged in duration, do not resolve spontaneously, and are rarely cured completely" (CDC, 2009). Many chronic illnesses last a lifetime, though the severity of the illness may change over time.

The effect that illnesses and injuries have on people varies considerably depending on the nature of the health problem. When injuries and illnesses are short lived and curable, their effect on the patient is obviously less likely to be traumatic than disabling health problems would be. It is more difficult to cope with injuries and illnesses that significantly interfere with people's performance of important roles. For example, injury that disrupts an athlete's sport participation generally has a very negative effect on that athlete's life. People may respond differently to illnesses that produce bothersome symptoms than to health problems that do not produce symptoms. For example, rheumatoid arthritis is accompanied by joint swelling and pain, so people with this disease usually must accommodate the illness by making many changes in their daily lives. On the other hand, type 2 diabetes may have few symptoms in its early stages and be easily ignored.

Common Sense Models of Illness and Injury

Each individual acquires specific beliefs about illness and injury and how people are supposed to respond to symptoms and diagnoses. A person's ideas about a particular health problem can be called an illness representation or schema. In other words, it is a sort of personal model that describes a given health problem and the factors related to it (Leventhal, Weinman, Leventhal, & Phillips, 2008). Leventhal and colleagues have described an individual's illness representation as a Common Sense Model of Illness. In other words, the model is perceived by the individual to be "common sense." The person's ideas about the health problem make sense to him or her, based on prior knowledge and personal experience as well as information from family, friends, acquaintances, media sources, and health-care providers (Health Psychology in Your Life 12-1). Common Sense Models include basic information about the illness, such as the following (Fig. 12-1):

- Identity of the illness or injury, usually with a name for the health problem
- The causes of the illness, including infectious agents, lifestyle factors, genetics, and other risk factors. People use their illness representation to try to understand why they have developed the health problem. For an injury, they try to understand how the injury occurred and why it happened to them.

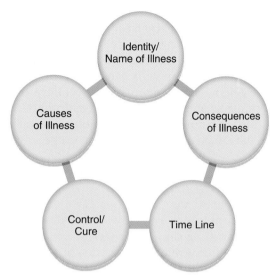

Figure 12-1. Common sense models of illness.

HEALTH PSYCHOLOGY IN YOUR LIFE 12-1.
Common Sense Models of the Common Cold

Everyone has experience with upper-respiratory infections called "colds." Think about your own Common Sense Model of this illness and answer the following questions. Then interview one or more friends, asking them the same questions. You might get especially interesting answers if you interview someone much older than you or someone who is from another state or country. How does your Common Sense Model of the common cold differ from the model of the person you interviewed?

1. Do you use another name for the common cold? If so, what do you call this illness?
2. What causes you to catch a cold? Is it caused by an infectious agent (germs)? What kind? Is your likelihood of catching a cold influenced by genetics? If so, what is the nature of this influence? List lifestyle factors that influence your risk of catching a cold, if any. List any other factors that cause colds for you.
3. What happens when you catch a cold? What symptoms do you get? How do you know you have a cold? How long does the cold last and how do the symptoms change over time?
4. How do you treat a cold when you catch one? List actions taken and remedies used to speed healing or control symptoms. Which treatments have been most helpful for you?

- The health problem's consequences and their severity
- The time line for the development of these consequences, including how long the illness is expected to last or how much time an injury will take to heal.
- Ideas about treatment, especially how the illness can be controlled or cured through treatments. People may have an understanding about their likelihood of recovery given various treatment paths. When people think about treatments, they may focus on biomedical alternatives, complementary and alternative treatments, family remedies, and other treatment approaches.

The Common Sense Model of illness has been applied in many situations, including athletic injury (van Wilgen, Kaptein, & Brink, 2010) and traumatic injury (Lee, Chaboyer, & Wallis, 2010), and it appears to offer a good description of how people construct an understanding of injuries as well as illnesses.

People's illness representations are affected by numerous variables, so the illness representation of a given individual varies from day to day, and even moment to moment (Petersen, van den Berg, Janssens, & Van den Bergh, 2011). For example, a negative mood state may lead to more anxiety about one's symptoms. Learning new information about an illness may alter symptom perception and decisions regarding whether and how to seek treatment. Social comparison influences how people perceive their symptoms. If an acquaintance has experienced a certain illness that began with a particular symptom, and a person is experiencing that symptom, he or she may be more inclined to worry that the symptom indicates the particular illness experienced by the acquaintance. A person's cultural expectations strongly influence symptom experience. Symptoms may be interpreted in different ways in different cultures or in different ways in the same culture at different times in history (Harrington, 2011).

People's illness representations may or may not agree with current scientific beliefs about the illness. Regardless, the representation shapes an individual's illness experience, including the perception and interpretation of symptoms; decisions about whether to consult someone for advice and, if so, whom to consult; and the person's understanding of information received from providers and others regarding the health problem. People's understanding of an illness or injury also eventually influences how and to what extent they follow treatment recommendations and adjust to the health problem.

Treatment and behavior-change interventions must address patients' inaccurate and unhelpful perceptions of illness and injury (Petrie & Weinman, 2012). A meta-analysis examining illness perceptions and patient outcomes found that several illness-representation variables predicted higher levels of psychological distress (Hagger & Orbell, 2003). These variables included higher perceived consequences, low perceptions of the illness being controllable or curable, and longer time-line perceptions. Several subsequent studies have also found that negative illness perceptions predict a greater likelihood of slower recovery and higher levels of disability (Galli, Ettlin, Palla, Ehlert, & Gaab, 2010; Kaptein et al., 2010). Researchers have wondered whether people with negative perceptions might simply have more-serious health problems, but studies have found that people's perceptions of illness severity are generally not strongly related to objective physical symptoms (Petrie & Weinman, 2012).

MOTIVATING CHANGE: Understand Clients' Common Sense Models of Illness and Injury

Understanding people's illness representations is important for anyone trying to motivate behavior change. Too often, when working with clients coping with illness or injury, health and fitness professionals slip into lecture mode. Health and fitness professionals must understand how the person sees the illness or injury and how the suggested behavior changes relate to the client's illness representation. For example, if clients believe the illness is primarily genetic or bad luck, they may think, "Why bother to exercise or change eating behaviors?" Professionals cannot assume clients see their health problems the same way as the professional does. Patients resist following treatment recommendations that don't make sense to them in terms of their personal illness representations.

How do you uncover a person's illness representation? Ask open questions and listen reflectively to be sure that you are understanding correctly. Discuss clients' misperceptions about behavior-change recommendations, giving information that is more accurate, yet also positive and hopeful. Let your conversation be guided by a client's readiness to change and discuss your advice.

The Psychology of Becoming a Patient

Clients generally turn into patients once they enter the health-care system. The word "client" usually refers to a person who is requesting services from a professional, whereas the word "patient" indicates a more-passive role, as in situations where symptoms have driven a person to seek medical care. A patient is typically seen as a receiver of care, whereas a client is more apt to be seen as a seeker of care. What's the difference? Once people see themselves in the patient role, their perceptions of themselves and their situation may change. People's illness representations exert a strong influence on how they perceive their role as patients and their response to injury or an illness diagnosis.

For many people, becoming a patient involves a shift of control and responsibility from oneself to providers and caregivers. This shift of control may also be enabled by health-care providers and caregivers who, often with the best of intentions, want to give patients direction and advice. Patients who develop an external locus of control regarding their health conditions generally exert less effort to manage their illness or injury, since they do not perceive personal effort to be helpful. Some research suggests that as health issues become more complex, patients are more likely to score higher on external locus of control. One study of 3212 community-dwelling older adults found that as the number of chronic conditions increased, subjects were more likely to show a more-external locus of control (Henninger, Whitson, Cohen, & Ariely, 2012).

As patients feel less in control of their health, they may experience a decline in self-efficacy regarding their ability to perform the actions recommended to treat or control their illnesses (Martin, Haskard-Zolnierek, & DiMatteo, 2010). Low self-efficacy reduces the likelihood that patients will comply with treatment recommendations, especially when difficulties arise. Barriers that interfere with behavior-change efforts are often very challenging and, especially combined with low self-efficacy, can easily derail patients' behavior-change plans. Barriers might consist of financial difficulties that limit one's ability to afford medications, transportation limitations that make it difficult to get to medical appointments or scheduling difficulties for people struggling to balance work, family responsibilities, and treatment recommendations.

It is important to note, however, that becoming a patient may also provide a person with opportunities for coping more effectively with health problems. Resources may become available for consultation with a variety of health-care providers (Fig. 12-2). People who maintain an active role in their care can make use of these opportunities to obtain good advice and treatment. When patients and health-care providers develop good relationships, patients usually report more satisfaction and better health outcomes (Martin et al., 2010).

"I didn't realize working in medical fitness would be so different from working in the athletic training room," Mason says to Grant after their first week at the medical fitness center. "Are you finding that? I mean, I was ready for the health issues to be different. But I wish I knew more about

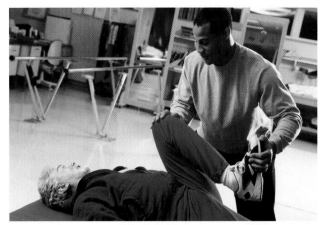

Figure 12-2. Patient working with physical therapist.
© Thinkstock

health psychology. Some of the patients are great, with great attitudes. They soak up every word I say, and you can see that nothing will get in the way of their recovery if they can help it! But some of the others are so timid and fearful. They've never exercised before, and they don't know where to begin. I'll have to be careful not to overwhelm them with information. Sometimes after they've been working with me, they just look more lost instead of more empowered." Grant acknowledges that this is a problem. "It's easy to talk and harder to listen. Remember the OARS skills we learned in our exercise psychology class? You've got to try to get into the clients' heads before you overload them with too much advice. When clients are getting health care, they tend to get buried in advice. Better to get them to accomplish something and feel good than talk too much."

The next day Mason is working for the second time with Howard, an elderly man recovering from a heart attack. Howard is fairly frail and has little confidence in his ability to be physically active, fearing another heart attack. Mason decides that instead of trying to convince Howard he can exercise safely, he will just assist Howard as he walks at a slow pace on the treadmill. As Howard walks, Mason can sense him starting to relax a bit. "I guess that is another good thing about not talking; I have a better sense of how the client is feeling." He praises Howard's accomplishment at the end of the session. Howard smiles and seems pleased with himself. "Maybe I am going to be OK after all," he says. ■

The Psychology of Sports Injury

Coping with injury can be especially challenging for athletes, who rely on a highly functioning body for their performance. Most health and fitness professionals have coped with injury and know how frustrating the experience can be. People tend to discuss injury as

something that happens to a part of the body, as a physical occurrence, with physical causes and physical symptoms. But the physical aspect of an injury is only a part of the story, just as an athlete's body is only part of the athlete. Every fitness professional knows that one's thoughts, feelings, and spirit all contribute to sport performance and are important parts of every athlete. Although the physical part of a person and of an injury is the most visible, it is important to consider the whole person when working with each client. Athletes are no exception.

Athletes' emotional responses to injury are as varied as athletes themselves, and it is impossible to devise one model that fits all. In general, whereas a small minority of athletes are relieved to have a reason to leave a sport, most athletes experience a wide range of intense, negative emotions following injury. Athletes usually feel some combination of frustration, anger, boredom, depression, fear, anxiety, confusion, and loneliness after injury. These negative emotions not only interfere with athletes' success in school, work, and personal relationships but also can interfere with athletes' determination to return to play and their adherence to their rehabilitation and fitness programs. Several factors influence an athlete's emotional response to injury.

- **Nature of the injury:** Obviously, the more serious the injury, the more the injury disrupts the athlete's sport participation and life in general. An injury may disrupt school or work because of medical appointments and mobility limitations. Pain and pain medications may cause difficulty concentrating. Work and stress pile up. Sometimes athletes may have trouble accomplishing simple tasks such as getting meals, cleaning, and doing laundry.

- **Perception of the injury:** An athlete's psychological response to injury is strongly influenced by his or her perception of the injury. Does the medical team seem concerned? What is the prognosis? Even apparently minor injuries may be very worrisome if the prognosis is uncertain or poor. Chronic injuries that don't seem to heal can also be problematic. Good athletic trainers and other health-care providers know that athletes need information, but they also need hope. When speaking with patients about their injuries, health and fitness professionals should be sure to always offer hope for recovery.

- **Meaning of sport participation in the athlete's life:** The more strongly people identify themselves with the role of athlete, and the more important sport is in their lives, the more they will suffer psychologically from sports injuries. Life without sport participation may feel boring or depressing, and athletes sidelined with injury may struggle with a changing sense of identity, especially when injuries are serious.

- **Athlete's personal situation:** Many personal factors influence an athlete's psychological response to a sport injury. The timing of the injury in terms of the sport season and in terms of the athlete's career is important. An athlete's personality and stress hardiness influence his or her response to injury. Athletes who feel strong positive social support from teammates, friends, and family tend to weather injury stress better.

Staying in shape is important to most athletes, whose physical condition is a large part of their self-concept. Being sidelined by injury is a pretty depressing experience, and watching oneself get out of shape can make this experience even more depressing. In addition, most athletes are used to high volumes of physical activity. Many athletes report feeling stressed and depressed when unable to train, experiencing withdrawal when their usual level of psychological benefit from physical activity declines. Cross training and physical therapy may help injured athletes experience at least some of the psychological benefits of exercise.

Most injuries require extensive rehabilitation. One might think that athletes would show excellent compliance with medical advice, but this is not always the case. Physical therapy can be tedious and time consuming and not nearly as enjoyable and rewarding as sport participation. Some research suggests that athletes who tend to use positive coping strategies and score high on hardiness characteristics are more likely to comply with rehabilitation instructions (Wadey, Evans, Hanton, & Neil, 2012).

When sport training and competition are no longer a part of an athlete's day, life may feel pretty empty (Podlog & Eklund, 2007). To create meaningful work, some injured athletes take on new roles for their team, serving as referees, managers, announcers, sports writers, or other assistants. Some volunteer their time at local schools and community centers, coaching youth sport teams. Many athletes become interested in the rehabilitation process and train for careers as athletic trainers, physical therapists, chiropractors, massage therapists, and other health-care providers who work with injured athletes. Injured athletes can also create meaningful work by expanding their involvement in activities unrelated to sport.

Self-Determination Theory (SDT) may be helpful for professionals working with injured athletes (Podlog, Dimmock, & Miller, 2011). Many of the concerns athletes experience fall into the three important domains of SDT. For example, many recovering athletes feel stressed by inadequate levels of competence and worry about recovering to preinjury skill level. The isolation athletes feel as they no longer compete with their teams is experienced as a loss of connection, or relatedness. And, for many recovering athletes, autonomy of motivation may feel violated as they experience pressure to return to sport from coaches, teammates, and others.

The Hospital Experience

People whose health situations require intensive care often receive this care in a hospital. Hospitals are designed to provide medical treatments such as surgeries and other higher-risk procedures designed to address injuries, illnesses, and other conditions, with the goal of reducing harm and promoting healing. Highly trained physicians and allied health professionals provide specialized care that epitomizes the best that biomedicine has to offer. For example, patients experiencing a stroke may receive drugs that break up a clot and lessen the brain damage caused by the stroke. People with acute appendicitis may receive life-saving surgery to eliminate the source of infection. Post-surgical care for treatment of injury and illness begins in the hospital and may then move to some form of rehabilitation center. Hospitals are often the site of dramatic life-saving procedures, but they are also home to last-ditch efforts that fail to provide relief and palliative care that relieves pain for patients whose health does not improve.

Becoming a hospital patient is often a challenging experience. Most readers have probably had a variety of experiences with hospitals, either as patients themselves or visiting friends and relatives who were hospitalized. How does being a patient feel? In general, people who are hospitalized for a health problem report feeling worried or even frightened about their health. They are often anxious about impending procedures, perhaps even fearing a life-threatening diagnosis or poor surgical outcome. Patients are informed of all the risks accompanying their medications and procedures, so there is plenty to worry about. Family members may be worried and tense, and the hospital environment may do little to help people relax.

Specialization is one of the strengths of biomedicine. But many hospital patients and their families feel frustrated by complex medical bureaucracies, where many different professionals treat different parts of the medical problem. Health-care providers may become experts in one body organ or system, and one patient may need a variety of specialists. Some health-care workers take blood, others administer the EKG, and still others provide respiratory therapy. Workers come and go because hospital work continues 24 hours a day. In some cases, patients may see dozens of different people each day. Often, the hospital environment can feel noisy, cold, and indifferent, as busy hospital staff struggle to keep up with the patients who need help and the piles of forms that need to be completed. The focus of hospital work tends to be on treating the bodily illness with less attention to the patient's emotional well-being. Patients and families may find it is depressing to be around a lot of sick people. The anxiety experienced by patients and hospital workers can be contagious.

Despite the life-saving advances in biomedicine, patients and clinicians alike express great concern regarding the quality of health care in most countries, including the United States. All agree that major changes in health-care systems, including hospitals, are called for to improve patient safety, patient satisfaction, clinical outcomes, and the work environment for all health-care workers. In 2001, the Institute of Medicine (2001) called for national efforts to improve health care in the United States. Much energy has been directed toward improving all aspects of health-care systems, including medical education, treatment protocols, and hospital organization and environments (Lukas et al., 2007). Although there is still much work to be done, a great deal has been accomplished to improve patient satisfaction with hospital care (Fryers, Young, & Rowland, 2012). Many hospitals have added programs aimed at improving the emotional wellness of both patients and staff. For example, many health-care systems are implementing better communication practices between clinicians and patients and between staff and patients' family members. Better patient and family education as well as better communication with patients and their families improve patient satisfaction as well as clinical outcomes (Comp, 2011). Hospitals are upgrading their physical environments to promote positive emotions by adding fountains, music, and gardens (Fig. 12-3; Franklin, 2012). Many hospitals are responding to patient interest in complementary and alternative therapies by providing programs in therapeutic touch and massage; stress-reduction therapies such as healing visualization and biofeedback experiences; education on health-promoting lifestyle behaviors; and better hospital menus and healthful meals. The importance of positive emotions for optimal healing and pain reduction has been widely acknowledged (Game Changers 12-1).

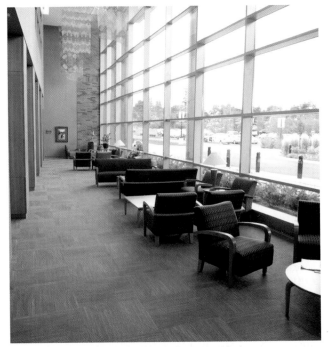

Figure 12-3. **Hospital lobby with natural light.** © Thinkstock

Game Changers 12-1. Norman Cousins: Laughter, Pain Reduction, and Healing

In 1976, Norman Cousins became one of the most unusual contributors to the medical research on pain with the publication of his article "Anatomy of an Illness (As Perceived by the Patient)" in the prestigious *New England Journal of Medicine*. Cousins' work was unusual in that he wrote from the perspective of a science writer and informed patient rather than as a physician or scientist. As an editor at the *Saturday Review* from 1940 to 1971, Cousins had developed a keen interest in medical science and the healing process, an interest he applied to himself when he became ill in 1964 with a painful connective tissue disorder known as ankylosing spondylitis. Ankylosing spondylitis is a type of arthritis, characterized by chronic inflammation between the vertebrae and between the spine and pelvic bones. Over time, the affected bones fuse together, creating more pain and limited mobility.

Medical specialists gave Cousins one in 500 odds of recovering from this extremely painful disorder. Determined to be that one in 500, Cousins conducted his own research on this little-understood disorder and with his physician's cooperation designed a maverick treatment program. Familiar with the current research in mind–body communication, and the field that would come to be known as psychoneuroimmunology, Cousins believed that stress had played an important role in the development of his illness. He reasoned, "If negative emotions produce negative chemical changes in the body, wouldn't the positive emotions produce positive chemical changes? Is it possible that love, hope, faith, laughter, confidence, and the will to live have therapeutic values?" (Cousins, 1991). Cultivating these positive emotions was a cornerstone of his treatment. Cousins checked himself out of the hospital and into a hotel where he could pursue his treatment program free of the hospital routine and its depressing environment.

Cousins found that he could muster positive emotions, but laughter was difficult to come by because he was in a great deal of pain. His solution was to view funny films and read humor books. He was elated to discover that "ten minutes of genuine belly laughter had an anesthetic effect and would give me at least two hours of pain-free sleep" (Cousins, 1991). His health slowly but surely improved over the next several weeks, and he was soon back with his family and at work.

Cousins went on to pursue his interest in positive emotions and health as a faculty member at UCLA, an experience from which he wrote his 1989 book, *Head First: The Biology of Hope*. His work has inspired scientific research on the physiology of laughter and positive emotions.

Source: Cousins, N. (1991). Anatomy of an illness (as perceived by the patient). In: Monat, A., & Lazarus, R. S. (eds.). *Stress and Coping*. New York: Columbia University Press.

Understanding Pain

Most of the time, pain is a helpful response that motivates people to correct or escape from a situation causing harm. For example, if a person sits in the same slumped position for too long, neck and shoulders start to ache, motivating the individual to get up, stretch, and change position. Pain that occurs with injury provides a similar motivation: people limit movement while the injury heals. Many illnesses, such as the flu, make one ache all over, which encourages people to stay in bed and receive the rest needed to cope with the illness.

But sometimes pain remains long after an injury has apparently healed. Sometimes pain develops with chronic conditions that may never heal, such as arthritis and fibromyalgia. People with chronic pain often avoid physical activity, since it hurts. But avoidance leads to weakness, as muscles and joint structures atrophy with disuse. Endurance, strength, and flexibility decline, which leads to further losses in functional capacity and, ironically, more pain. Weight gain and depression often accompany chronic pain.

To feel pain, nerves must send information to the brain, and the brain must interpret the information as pain. This is more complicated than it sounds. The perception of pain is different from the perception of visual or auditory information, where sensory receptors receive stimulation and then relay input to the brain. The perception of pain is the brain's interpretation of stimuli coming from inside the body, for example, from sensors of chemical, temperature, and pressure changes (Auvray, Myin, & Spence, 2010). The interpretation of these inputs is complex and involves many brain areas. Over time, neural pathways may reorganize in ways that modulate the processing of input to alter sensations of pain. Sometimes the brain interprets sensations as pain even when the inputs do not merit attention (Moseley & Flor, 2012). When it senses danger, the brain may amplify sensations that don't really warrant much attention. And the brain is not always in touch with reality. Emotional states such as fear, resentment, anger, and sadness may amplify feelings of pain. Similarly, the brain may decide certain sensations are harmless and not bother to "feel" them. Laughter, happiness, hopefulness, and other positive emotional states can help reduce pain intensity. Simply understanding what is causing pain can reduce the intensity of pain sensations (Butler & Moseley, 2003).

Researchers believe that chronic pain can be worsened by maladaptive, subconscious habits of perception, where certain nerve pathways have "learned" to amplify and interpret sensations as painful. The pain is very real, of course, but is caused only partly by tissue damage (including tight muscles, scar tissue, inflammation, and so forth) and partly by the brain's habitual patterns and conscious and subconscious expectations.

This is not to say that people can think their pain away. But they can learn to lessen the effect pain has on their lives by understanding their pain and coping as positively as possible with challenges. This process can be very difficult, but research suggests that pain education can be very helpful (Moseley, 2012). One double-blind randomized control trial found that education about pain physiology was associated with better pain control than a treatment offering education on pacing and self-management (Meeus, Nils, Van Oosterwijck, Van Alsenoy, & Truijen, 2010). A review of eight studies examining the effect of pain education on patients with chronic musculoskeletal pain found that such education reduced pain, disability, anxiety, and stress (Louw, Diener, Butler, & Puentedura, 2011). Subjects receiving pain education were less likely than control subjects to make their pain worse by catastrophizing, focusing on the worst possible outcomes for their situation. Pain education also improved physical function levels more than control conditions.

Physical activity is often prescribed for patients with pain syndromes. Activity improves circulation and the health of the muscles, joints, and bones. Joints respond positively to compression and the movement of fluid within the joint (Behavior Change in Action 12-1). Although movement can be difficult for people experiencing pain, it can prevent pain from becoming worse and slow the loss of joint function over time.

Coping With Death, Tragedy, and Grief

Sometimes the experience of injury and illness includes coping with death, tragedy, and grief. Until fairly recently in human history, death was a common, mostly unpredictable event and a part of everyday life. Dying was not just for the sick and elderly. People died in infancy, childhood, and adulthood. Sick people often died at home, and family members regularly witnessed death and dying. Cultures evolved rituals to help the dying accept their departure and bid farewell to friends and family and to help those left behind express their grief and begin to heal.

Nowadays death is a less-familiar occurrence, except to those who work in end-of-life care. Death in infancy, childhood, and young adulthood is less common than it once was. Relatives often die in hospitals or other health-care facilities with less involvement of family and friends. As participation in religious traditions has declined, people have fewer institutional systems to help them accept death and to grieve (Meier, 2010).

Many theorists have examined the process of grieving, both for people learning of a traumatic diagnosis and for those losing loved ones to death or other tragedies. One of the most well-known historical figures in this area is Elisabeth Kübler-Ross, whose book *On Death and Dying* brought the grieving process to the attention of both the medical community and the public (Kübler-Ross, 1969). Kübler-Ross worked with terminally ill patients and their families. She believed that grieving people go through the following five stages:

- **Denial:** Initially, people can't believe they are ill or that a loved one is terminally ill.

BEHAVIOR CHANGE IN ACTION 12-1

Motivating People Who Are Experiencing Pain

■ CHALLENGE
How do I motivate a client to exercise when physical activity is painful?

■ PLAN
The best approach is to educate the client about the nature of pain and the benefits of physical activity. Clients living with chronic pain will need to start slowly and increase exercise volume gradually so that physical activity makes them feel better, not worse.

■ UNDERSTAND THE CAUSES OF PAIN
Clients coping with chronic pain will need medical clearance and a diagnosis regarding the causes of their pain. You and your client must both understand what is causing the pain. Educate clients about the nature of pain and the benefits of exercise for pain reduction. Once clients understand that pain does not necessarily indicate harm, they will have more confidence in your recommendations and in their ability to become more active. Because many clients are afraid of causing themselves more pain, you must put their fears to rest. Fear increases perception of pain.

■ FOLLOW TREATMENT RECOMMENDATIONS REGARDING ACTIVITY AND PAIN CONTROL
Health-care professionals should provide you and your clients with clear guidelines about what types of activities are recommended and what if any particular movements should be avoided. Clients must feel confident that the activities in which they engage will do no harm. Providers may also recommend the use of ice, medication, and other treatments to control pain experienced in conjunction with physical activity.

■ SEEK ADVICE IF PAIN BECOMES WORSE
In general, clients should start with an amount and intensity of activity that does not cause pain to become worse, either during the activity or after. This may be as little as a few minutes of walking or physical therapy exercise. If clients experience an increase in pain, consult their providers about how to alter exercise recommendations.

■ BUILD CLIENT SELF-EFFICACY FOR PHYSICAL ACTIVITY
While the health and fitness professional can serve as a confident, supportive advisor, clients must monitor their own pain and take charge of activity levels. Clients must learn to become more active in their daily lives, without a coach present every minute of the day. As clients build self-efficacy, fear and pain will lessen. With consistent effort, exercise levels will improve slowly but surely, and clients will begin to feel more in charge of their lives.

■ CONNECT PHYSICAL ACTIVITY TO CLIENTS' GOALS
Increase client motivation for physical activity by connecting exercise to the achievement of important goals, such as independent living, participation in valued activities, or feeling less pain. Your goal is for clients to experience autonomous motivation for behavior change so they will stick to their treatment recommendations and stay active. Adding activity to the life of someone who is experiencing pain is often difficult but worth the effort as clients begin to take charge of their lives and make the most of their abilities, participating in the activities that give life meaning for them.

- **Anger:** People wonder why life is unfair and why the tragedy is happening to them, and they experience feelings of anger.
- **Bargaining:** People facing tragedy may then try to make a deal with a divine power, promising to take certain actions if they are allowed more time.
- **Depression:** Sad feelings develop as grief sets in.
- **Acceptance:** People eventually accept their circumstances when they realize change is not possible.

Many writers since Kübler-Ross have questioned her stage theory, arguing that not all people go through these stages in this order or even through all such

stages (Jacobs, 1993). Others have explored the human capacity to bounce back from tragedy and even grow from experiences of loss (Bonnano, 2004).

One study of bereaved people has generalized the emotions people experience following the loss of a loved one (Maciejewski, Zhang, Block, & Prigerson, 2007). This research categorized emotional experiences into the following groups.

- **Disbelief:** Similar to denial, people often experience disbelief when first receiving information about a catastrophe. Whether the event is a death, divorce, or even bad news about an injury for a competitive athlete, disbelief is typically the first response. Disbelief declines quickly as time goes by.

- **Yearning:** As the new information settles in, people may yearn for things to be different and are sad about the change in their life. They feel nostalgic for things that will remain undone and for people left behind. Feelings of yearning usually grow for several months after a tragedy but on average, begin to decline after about 4 months.
- **Anger:** Anger at the situation and life's unfairness tends to build for several months and begin to decline after 5 to 6 months.
- **Depression:** Feelings of sadness and loss usually grow for the first 6 months following the event and then slowly decline.
- **Acceptance:** Acceptance of the situation builds slowly and gradually over time. As grief proceeds and people endure and work through their feelings, they gradually reach a stage of acceptance where they try to make the most of what remains.

Health and fitness professionals working with people facing traumatic news and events should never make assumptions about stages of grief but should instead allow people to work through difficulties at their own pace. Some clients want to talk about the issues that they are facing, whereas others do not. Health and fitness professionals should follow the client's lead.

THE CHALLENGE OF CHRONIC HEALTH PROBLEMS

According to the CDC, approximately half of adults in the United States live with at least one chronic illness, the most common being heart disease, cancer, stroke, diabetes, and arthritis (CDC, 2009). Although adults are much more likely than children to develop chronic illnesses, the rates of chronic disease are also rising in children and adolescents. Over 7% of children and adolescents in the United States were living with a chronic illness in 2004, compared with fewer than 2% in the 1960s. The CDC estimates that about 75% of health-care costs in the United States are attributed to chronic illness.

About one-fourth of people with chronic illness experience significant limitation on daily function (CDC, 2009). Some injuries can also interfere significantly with daily function and cause disability. Disability refers to some type of impairment that limits normal function. Disabilities can be mental or physical and range from mild to severe in nature.

Self-Management and the Treatment of Chronic Health Problems

People living with chronic health problems almost always must become involved on a daily basis with managing their health issues. Self-management activities include taking medications as prescribed, following behavior-change recommendations for improving health markers, and adjusting to the limitations imposed by

the health problem. Suboptimal adherence to medical advice is associated with poorer clinical outcomes and higher health-care costs, as patients develop complications and seek treatment at emergency medical departments (Cantrell, Priest, Cook, Fincham, & Burch, 2011). Self-management recommendations can feel overwhelming and complex to patients as they struggle to take charge of their lives. Adherence to lifestyle-change recommendations appears to be especially low, with some experts estimating that only 15% to 25% of patients improve lifestyle behaviors such as diet and exercise after a chronic disease diagnosis (Dunbar-Jacob & Mortimer-Stephens, 2001). Health and fitness professionals play a vital role in helping people develop the skills and motivation to actively manage their health conditions through appropriate lifestyle change.

As the number of people living with chronic, lifelong conditions grows around the world, the need for continuing care far surpasses most countries' health-care resources (*The Economist*, 2012). Chronic health problems pose a challenge not only in high-income countries but in medium- and low-income countries as well. Noting that the effectiveness of standard health care for many chronic health problems is fairly low and the expense is very high, some experts are calling for a radical shift in health care to focus more on empowering patients to manage their own health conditions, especially in areas where resources for medical care are very limited. Researchers van Olmen and colleagues (2011) have suggested that self-management may be the most feasible approach to the treatment of chronic illness in low-income countries. Their concept of "full self-management" places patients at the center of their care, with support from peers and information networks and occasional contact with health-care providers. This type of self-management may very well be the only viable option in resource-poor areas of the world. In their research, van Olmen and colleagues have described their vision of people with chronic health problems being supported primarily by "expert peers"—lay people with knowledge of the care required for chronic conditions. Expert peers may be other people managing the same health condition, such as diabetes or tuberculosis. Smartphone technology could provide data, such as a person's blood pressure, to providers in any location and information to patients regarding their care. Such a health-care delivery model would require a radical shift in the structure of the health-care industry. It would hopefully include a stronger emphasis on lifestyle changes to prevent and manage chronic health problems.

Patient Compliance With Treatment Recommendations

In North America, people diagnosed with chronic health problems rarely rely totally on self-management but instead combine self-management with guidance from their health-care providers. When patients follow the directions given by health-care providers, this is known as patient compliance. Many factors are associated with patient compliance, just as many factors are associated with adherence to lifestyle behavior change in any setting.

Treatment of hypertension provides an interesting illustration of the complexity of patient compliance and the achievement of treatment goals, typically a blood pressure of <130/90 mm Hg. Treatment usually consists of a combination of behavior-change recommendations and medication. Often more than one type of medication is used to obtain a target blood pressure. Despite the fact that treatment can be very effective, a large number of people diagnosed with hypertension never achieve good blood pressure control. A great deal of research has explored this observation in an attempt to explain the factors responsible for success or failure and hopefully to devise suggestions for addressing factors that increase the risk of poor blood pressure control.

Some research has suggested that patients' personality factors may contribute to a lack of compliance with medical instructions for blood pressure control. For example, one research group in Spain studied 85 hypertensive patients seen in a hospital emergency department (Joyner-Grantham et al., 2009). This group found that patients with uncontrolled hypertension were more likely than patients with controlled hypertension to score higher on measures of hopelessness and in general failed to make the behavior changes and take the medications that could help control their blood pressure—a mind-set the investigators called patient inertia. Another study comparing personality traits for patients with controlled and uncontrolled hypertension found that those with uncontrolled hypertension showed higher scores on impulsiveness, depression, anger, and stress (Sanz et al., 2010). Investigators noted that the last three traits are known to contribute to hypertension, so it is unclear whether or not they help explain treatment compliance.

Some research suggests that better clinical practices and patient follow-up are needed (Huebschmann, Mizrahi, Soenksen, Beaty, & Denberg, 2012). Indeed, Huebschmann and colleagues refer to clinical inertia, a lack of clinically effective practices, as the root cause for the high number of patients who fail to achieve good blood pressure control. In their randomized controlled trial, patients who received more-thorough and comprehensive treatment attained better control.

Interesting work by health psychologists Christensen and colleagues (2010) suggests that the provider-patient context contributes to treatment compliance for hypertension and other chronic health problems. Specifically, Christensen's group has examined patient and physician scores on the Health Locus of Control (HLOC) questionnaire. This questionnaire assesses how strongly patients believe that chronic illness is related to factors under their control. In one study, Christensen's team enrolled 18 physicians and 246 of their patients diagnosed with both type 2 diabetes and hypertension. The researchers measured a number of variables, including diastolic blood pressure and whether or not patients refilled their medication prescriptions. Higher adherence to refilling medication prescriptions and slightly lower diastolic blood pressure were found in patients who scored similarly to their physicians on the HLOC questionnaire. In other words, whether both parties scored high or low on internal locus of control, patients in these dyads showed the best compliance. Patients who scored higher on the HLOC than their physicians showed only slightly lower compliance, suggesting that patient sense of control is still important. But it could also be that patients who have confidence in their physicians because they share similar beliefs with them have greater satisfaction with their physicians' treatment recommendations and are more likely to follow them. Other research suggests that nonphysician health-care providers may be somewhat more effective than physicians at achieving cardiovascular patient compliance for taking prescribed medications. Cutrona and colleagues reviewed 82 studies of interventions to increase patient compliance for taking prescribed medications for cardiovascular disease (Cutrona et al., 2010). They found that interventions conducted by providers who were not physicians tended to result in slightly higher patient compliance.

As explained in the first section of this chapter, illness representations play an important role in people's adherence to treatment recommendations, including adherence to behavior-change recommendations as well as compliance with directions regarding medication use. When lifestyle changes have been recommended, then patients' perceptions and beliefs about these behaviors and their effects on illness outcome become an important part of their illness representations (Sperry, 2009). For example, if patients with diabetes believe that eating behaviors will not have a significant effect on their blood sugar levels, then they will probably not change eating behaviors, even though their providers have stressed that such behaviors are important for managing blood sugar levels. A study of patients participating in a cardiac-rehabilitation program found a positive relationship between subjects' illness beliefs (believing that behavior makes a difference) and adherence to lifestyle behavior-change recommendations (Stafford, Jackson, & Berk, 2008). Lifestyle behavior change takes a great deal of effort, so patients must be very convinced that behavior-change efforts will pay off or they will decide not to bother. The same holds true for people's beliefs about medications. Their beliefs about their symptoms and illness and their beliefs about medication risks and benefits help predict their adherence to medication recommendations (Nicklas, Dunbar, & Wild, 2010).

As discussed in Chapter 4, SDT helps explain people's motivation to stick to behavior-change programs. Health and fitness professionals should always try to understand which goals and treatment outcomes are most important for their clients, as motivation is strongest for reaching important goals. Health-care providers may recommend treatment primarily to reduce symptoms and prevent disease progression. However, patients may be more motivated to follow treatment recommendations if they also address quality of life in the broadest sense of the term. An interesting research study that examined "outcomes that matter most" in a group of people with chronic illness found that the following were some of the most often cited desirable treatment outcomes (Zubialde, Mold, & Eubank, 2009).

- Participants expressed the desire to obtain a good understanding of their illness, along with learning how to live a "purpose-filled life" even though living with a chronic illness.
- Given the presence of chronic illness, patients still wanted to make the most of their physical and mental function.
- Subjects in this study generally hoped for a satisfying social life and good social function skills, including the ability to develop meaningful relationships and participate in rewarding activities.
- Patients valued feelings of hope and a sense of engagement in life.
- Patients told the investigators they still wished to live life to the fullest extent possible while adapting to the conditions imposed by their illness.

The results of this study emphasize the observation that while the management of physical symptoms and slowing disease progression are valued, the quality of daily life matters just as much to patients and clients. The researchers suggest that health-care providers should target this wider set of outcomes, or at least those meaningful to the individual patient, in order to achieve more-effective and meaningful patient care (Zubialde, Mold, & Eubank, 2009). The researchers also felt that SDT could help guide practitioners trying to capture these directions in their work, as striving to improve patients' autonomy, connection, and competence would help them move toward these important goals.

Additional research supports the idea that autonomous motivation in patients increases the likelihood of treatment adherence. An interesting study of adults recently diagnosed with type 2 diabetes examined factors related to treatment adherence in terms of dietary self-care (Nouwen, Ford, Balan, Twisk, & Ruggiero, 2011). Patients scoring higher on measures of autonomous motivation and sense of support for developing autonomous motivation for dietary change were more successful in changing their eating habits.

Nouwen and colleagues also examined several variables from social cognitive theory in relation to treatment adherence. Not surprisingly, these researchers found that higher self-efficacy for making dietary changes translated into better adherence to dietary-change recommendations. In addition, patients with the highest scores on self-evaluation also tended to have better adherence. Self-evaluation is a process in which people compare their current performance with a desired standard of performance or behavioral goal. In fact, Nouwen's group found that high scores on self-evaluation were more strongly related to successful dietary change than any other variable measured.

MOTIVATING CHANGE: Behavior-Change Skills in the Clinical Setting

One of the most-important functions of health and fitness professionals is to assist clients who seem ready to change with goal setting and self-evaluation. Professionals can help clients in several ways. First, they can help them clarify behavior-change goals. S.M.A.R.T. goals can guide the development of effective action plans and behavior change. Clearer goals also enable people to get a better evaluation of how they are currently doing in terms of their desired goals. Second, health and fitness professionals can help clients develop effective self-monitoring strategies, so clients get a more-accurate picture of their current behaviors. And third, health and fitness professionals can engage in productive conversations with clients as they work together to analyze what steps might be more helpful in applying the self-evaluation process to the development of behavior-change strategies. Although the behavior-change goals themselves may look a little different for people coping with health problems, behavior-change skills are useful for clients in almost any situation.

The Complexity of Adjustment to Chronic Health Problems

Adjustment to chronic illness and injury looks different in each client and often differs over time for any given individual. Chronic health problems influence the physical, psychological, and social realms of each person. Successful adjustment to chronic illness involves physical, emotional, cognitive, and behavioral adaptations (de Ridder, Geenen, Kuijer, & van Middendorp, 2008). Individuals must achieve adequate functional status, figuring out how to perform the activities of daily living, work, and other important tasks to the greatest extent possible. Life may look different after the diagnosis or development of a chronic health problem, and adjustment may take some time. Nevertheless, the majority of people diagnosed with chronic health problems do adjust. They show the same range of negative and positive emotions as everyone else (Fig. 12-4). People adapting to chronic health problems often show good emotional balance and participate in healthy relationships.

Longitudinal research on people's adjustment to various types of serious, chronic health problems has illustrated the complexity of the chronic illness experience (Stanton & Revenson, 2011). Because adjustment to chronic health problems varies considerably from person to person, health and fitness professionals should allow each patient to reveal his or her own story. Professionals should consider all levels of the ecological perspective as they try to understand each patient's illness experience.

Many factors at a patient's intrapersonal level influence adaptation to chronic illness, particularly the patient's illness representation, as discussed above. The

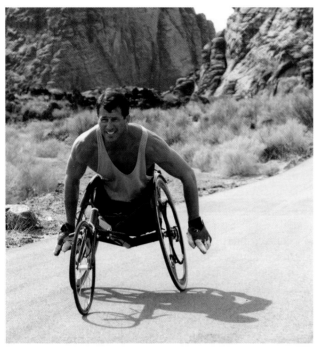

Figure 12-4. **Adapted physical activity.** © Thinkstock

patient's interpersonal relationships, organizational involvements, community, and culture in turn influence the illness representation, which is why looking at the big picture of a patient's life is important for understanding his or her adjustment to chronic health problems. Some of the variables that appear to be the most influential in determining patients' adaptation are shown in Figure 12-5.

Health Problems as Stressors

The psychophysiology of stress and coping presented in Chapter 6 can be applied to the situation of people coping with a health problem (Baldwin, Kellerman, & Christensen, 2010; Fig. 12-6). The illness or injury is a stressor. People perceive a health problem using the information they have from their providers, along with information obtained from family, friends, the Internet, and other resources. In addition, sociocultural ideas exert a strong influence on people's perceptions of health problems and on their coping expectations. As discussed in Chapter 6, simply feeling anxious about a health problem (even an imaginary one) initiates a full-blown psychophysiological stress response, activating the sympathetic nervous system and stress hormones and the many physiological and psychological changes subsequently influenced by these mind–body systems. Symptoms, a diagnosis, treatment recommendations, and the limitations imposed by a health problem can all feed into a person's stress appraisal and response. In general, the greater the demands imposed by a health problem, and the more it is perceived to exceed a person's coping resources, the more likely it is that the health problem will be seen as a significant stressor in that person's life.

People use both problem-focused and emotion-focused coping to deal with health problems. Problem-focused coping includes seeking medical advice for symptoms and exploring treatment options. It also includes other actions taken to address the stress of illness, such as changing one's work schedule, obtaining medicine, following

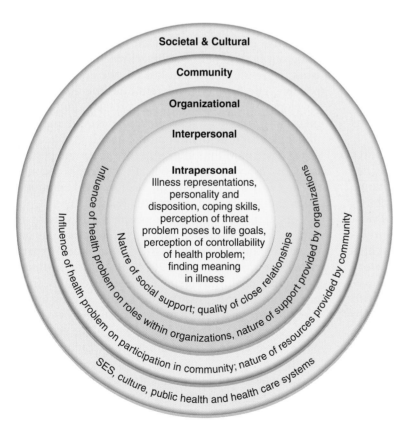

Figure 12-5. Adjustment to chronic health problems: An ecological perspective.

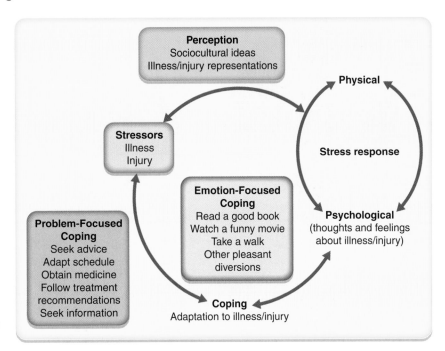

Figure 12-6. The stress cycle: Health problems as stressors.

treatment recommendations, and searching the Internet for more information about the problem. Emotion-focused coping does not address the illness itself but reduces feelings of stress. Emotion-focused coping includes strategies such as reading a good book, watching a movie, or taking a walk. Spending time with friends and engaging in hobbies are other examples of emotion-focused coping. People adjusting to health problems often change the way they view the problem, a process called cognitive reappraisal. **Cognitive reappraisal** means seeing the stressor in a new way that makes it seem less of a threat. Cognitive reappraisal is a type of emotion-focused coping.

To illustrate, consider how people might respond to learning that they have celiac disease (gluten intolerance). Problem-focused coping responses would include eliminating foods containing gluten from their home and learning more about sources of gluten and how to avoid them. Emotion-focused coping might include any sort of pleasant diversion or activity that reduces stress arousal. Demonstrating cognitive reappraisal, a person might think, "Gluten intolerance is not so bad. At least I now know what is causing my symptoms. I can learn to live with this."

Cognitive Adaptation Model

The **Cognitive Adaptation Model** helps explain the process of coping with chronic health problems. Psychologist Shelley Taylor created this model to explain how people cope with threatening situations, such as chronic health problems (Taylor, 1983; Taylor, Kemeny, Reed, Bower, & Gruenewald, 2000). According to this model, successful coping revolves around cognitive processes that lead to successful adaptation to one's new circumstances. Taylor and colleagues have been impressed over the years of their research with the remarkable ability

of people to cope with threatening situations in their lives, including serious health problems. Taylor began her research by interviewing women who had been diagnosed with breast cancer and built her original Cognitive Adaptation Model from these data (Taylor, 1983). Since that time, Taylor and her colleagues have looked at subjects coping with a variety of other serious health problems as well. Their research supports the idea that most people manage over time to adjust to severely disruptive events, including death of loved ones, traumatic accidents, and diagnoses of life-threatening illnesses. The Cognitive Adaptation Model proposes that successful coping involves three important issues related to the threat: finding meaning, mastery, and self-enhancement.

The first of these issues, finding meaning, refers to finding meaning both in the illness experience and in life in general (Fig. 12-7). When people are adjusting to a serious health problem, they often try to understand what caused the problem. For example, a cancer diagnosis usually prompts people to search for causes in their lifestyle or their environment or even for metaphysical explanations that grow out of cultural or spiritual belief systems. They may wonder about foods they have eaten, chemicals they have used, or water quality. In this search for meaning, people may never know what actually caused their problem, but the search appears to be important anyway. In fact, people may reach incorrect conclusions, but, unless such conclusions alter behavior in a harmful way, adjustment still occurs (Taylor et al., 2000). People who adjust successfully to health problems also tend to reevaluate the meaning of their own lives given the change in their health status. For some, priorities shift. For example, people might decide to spend fewer hours at work and more time with loved ones.

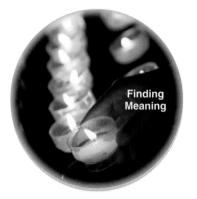
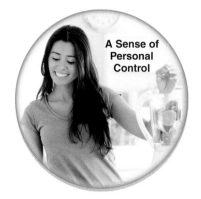
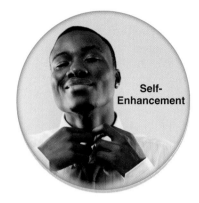

Figure 12-7. The Cognitive Adaptation Model. Photograph © Thinkstock

The second issue addressed by people showing successful psychological adjustment is to reestablish a sense of personal control, both over the health problem and over life in general. People look for actions they can take to reduce the severity of the problem or to at least lessen its negative effects. They look for ways to adapt their behaviors and change their thoughts and feelings to improve daily function. For example, people diagnosed with an illness might exercise control by changing their eating habits or other lifestyle behaviors or their work schedule. They might read information about controlling the problem or making other adjustments to improve quality of life. The issue of control echoes the idea from SDT that people are motivated to achieve competence and autonomy in their lives.

The last element of the Cognitive Adaptation Model is self-enhancement. Chronic health problems generally lead to negative emotions and even depression. Finding ways to feel better about oneself serves to counter these negative feelings and thus improve coping ability (de Ridder, Geenen, Kuijer, & van Middendorp, 2008). Self-enhancement strategies include comparing oneself to those less fortunate and valuing one's personal strengths. Self-enhancement processes may help increase a person's ability to experience hope and optimism—essential ingredients for emotional health.

Research examining the Cognitive Adaptation Model reveals an interesting observation: perception need not match reality for coping to be successful (Taylor et al., 2000). In fact, people often have mistaken beliefs about the causes of their illness, the degree of control they have over the progression of their disease, or how severe their injury is in comparison with other cases. For example, a woman with breast cancer may read about her disease and come up with a list of possible risk factors that set the scene for the development of her cancer. She may read on the Internet that stress contributes to cancer. In reality, the evidence supporting this link in breast cancer is fairly weak, but, nevertheless, the woman may feel satisfied that she has uncovered the reason for her illness. She may make several changes in her life to help her feel less stressed. She might read all kinds of unsubstantiated information about diet and

breast cancer, for example, and make many unnecessary changes in her eating behavior. Yet, she feels more in control of her situation and thus more successfully adapts to her diagnosis. She may create an image of herself as having a fairly mild form of the disease, of successfully beating the cancer, and achieving success at overcoming her cancer. She may adjust to living with her diagnosis, hopefully also following the course of treatment associated with the best possible outcome.

Self-Regulation Model of Illness

The Self-Regulation Model is a psychological model designed to explain goal-directed behavior and has been applied in many contexts, including to people's efforts to adjust to chronic health problems (Carver & Scheier, 2002). The Self-Regulation Model of illness grows out of common-sense models of illness, in that people's self-regulation efforts are connected to their illness representations. Self-regulation refers to people's capacity to change and control their behavior. People are generally motivated to self-regulate in order to reach important goals or to meet certain standards they value. Self-regulation means the same thing as self-control, as discussed in Chapter 5, with reference to behavior change.

Chronic health problems commonly interfere with people's progress toward important goals or achievement of valued standards. For example, chronic health problems may disrupt daily life and make it difficult for people to fulfill their perceived obligations as workers, parents, or friends. According to the Self-Regulation Model of illness, people feel stressed when they perceive barriers to be inhibiting goal achievement. In this context, successful coping requires an ability to reassess personal goals and plans for reaching them. Self-regulation is the process people use to make these cognitive and emotional adjustments. People must employ cognitive skills to reframe their expectations, setting more-realistic and achievable goals. Along with this cognitive self-regulation must come emotional adjustment as well; people need to accept the new situation and engage with their new goals (Baldwin, Kellerman, & Christensen, 2010).

Some researchers suggest that an optimistic outlook predicts better adjustment to chronic health problems, possibly through optimizing the self-regulation processes described (Baldwin, Kellerman, & Christensen, 2010). Optimal cognitive and emotional adjustment to health problems may be associated with positive behavioral changes that lead to more-effective disease or injury management. For example, patients recovering from myocardial infarction must reassess their goals and lifestyles to accommodate this change in health status. Once medical interventions are complete, patients usually need to continue taking medications and practicing lifestyle changes to prevent future heart problems. Prognosis for recovery improves for people who adhere to behavior-change recommendations, such as quitting smoking and improving exercise and eating habits. An optimistic outlook may give such patients hope that lifestyle makes a difference and thus energize cognitive and emotional adjustment to the new health situation. An optimistic outlook may also increase feelings of self-efficacy for behavior change. Such adjustment can then set the stage for effective behavior-change efforts and better health outcomes.

Depression, Anxiety, and Negative Emotions

Emotional health problems often add to the complexity of chronic illness. Mood disorders influence the way people perceive symptoms, seek care, interact with caregivers, and summon the energy to engage in self-management. Mood disorders and negative emotions sap the energy available for self-control and interfere with a person's ability to commit to behavior change and to follow through with self-care intentions. Depression increases mortality and morbidity rates for many illnesses.

Interesting research on the way mood disorders influence symptom perception suggests that depression and depressed mood increase the likelihood that people will recall more symptoms from the past, whereas anxiety and anxious mood increase the perception of current symptoms (Howren & Suls, 2011). Emotional states influence the way symptoms are appraised and reported and can be both helpful, as when self-awareness leads to seeking appropriate treatment, or harmful, as when too much rumination leads to imaginary symptoms (Wagner & Brown, 2012).

Depression in patients appears to influence the efforts of family and friends to offer social support. One study reported that although family and friends of depressed patients are willing to offer support, they experience significantly more difficulty discussing health issues with depressed patients than with patients without depression, and they encounter more barriers when trying to provide social support (Janevic, Rosland, Wiitala, Connell, & Piette, 2012). People with depression may intentionally or unintentionally "push others away," including caregivers, family, and friends.

Researchers have found that depression may increase risk of morbidity and mortality from a number of illnesses, including cardiovascular disease, arthritis, and diabetes (Karakus & Patton, 2011). The mind–body effects of depression may modulate this association. One study found that depressed heart disease patients had an 80% higher rate of mortality and that they also showed higher rates of other illnesses such as hypertension, which may have contributed to the higher mortality rates as well as poorer lifestyle behaviors, which may also have influenced mortality rates (Atlantis et al., 2012).

■ *"There sure are a lot of scared and lonely people who come here for treatment," Grant observes to Mason. "I wonder why all the work here is one on one. I mean, don't you think some group work would help these lonely clients feel less alone? Build social support? Connection? Do you think we should propose some group activities?" Mason agrees, and they decide to come up with a plan that they take to their internship supervisor. After several weeks of planning, they schedule some of the patients into two group exercise sessions each week. Patients begin together in a small group, complete their individualized exercise programs, and then come back together for a cool-down and 10 minutes of stretching. Howard, the elderly cardiac rehabilitation patient, is part of a small group with whom Mason is working. Having observed Howard's shyness, Mason takes him aside. "Howard, you have made some good progress on your walking program over the past 2 months. I am putting you on a treadmill next to that man, Jim, over there in the blue shirt. He is just getting started and is a little nervous about exercising. Don't tell him I put you there, but just talk to him when you have a chance and let him know getting started was not easy but that now you feel so much better."*

Howard works out next to Bill for several weeks. Mason observes the two talking together more and even laughing now and then. During the end of session stretch, Mason encourages the members of the group to share positive exercise experiences and accomplishments. He is pleased when Howard tells the group how his confidence in his abilities to climb stairs and perform other activities has grown with his fitness level. ■

PROMOTING PSYCHOLOGICAL ADJUSTMENT TO CHRONIC HEALTH PROBLEMS

Health and fitness professionals working with patients should do as much as possible to facilitate psychological adjustment to chronic health problems in order to help improve quality of life and support behavior-change efforts. Many factors are associated with resilience in people coping with chronic health problems (Fig. 12-8). Several strategies may help patients adjust psychologically to chronic health problems, including the following.

Help Patients Remain as Active and Involved as Possible

Illness is often accompanied by infection and/or inflammation. Cytokines released during these processes are believed to contribute to the psychological effects that accompany illness, such as weakness, difficulty concentrating, depressed mood, lethargy, and loss of appetite. This cluster of symptoms is known as sickness behavior and serves an adaptive purpose during acute illness, causing people to rest and recover. However, sickness behavior can become maladaptive for people experiencing chronic illness, as too much bed rest and inactivity can hasten physical decline and lead to greater levels of pain and disability. In the past, patients with pain were advised to rest; now they are generally told to participate in some level of physical activity appropriate for their fitness level and medical conditions. Tailored exercise therapy is effective for most chronic health problems (Smidt et al., 2005).

Patients should be encouraged to engage in useful and meaningful activities (Fig. 12-9). From the activities of daily living to participation in family, work, and community events, people benefit from involvement.

Such involvement can help reverse sickness behavior and enable patients to find motivation for participating in rehabilitation and treatment activities.

Support Culturally Appropriate Emotional Expression

Research on the importance of emotional expression suggests that at least for people from North American and Western European cultures, the suppression of emotion and avoidance of emotional processing and expression is associated with poorer adaptation to chronic health problems (Garssen, 2007). In Asian cultures, which are generally less emotionally expressive, nonexpressive styles of emotion regulation appear to be more adaptive. Culturally sensitive emotional regulation processes may therefore vary from person to person (de Ridder et al., 2008).

Nevertheless, several studies have found that for people from Western cultures, emotional-disclosure interventions improve adaptation to illness. Emotional disclosure may take the form of writing in a journal, talking to a close friend or family member, or even expressing emotions to a health and fitness professional. It is possible that acknowledging, expressing, and processing emotions helps patients to resolve negative emotional states and work toward a more positive outlook. Simply "venting," or expressing negative emotions in an uncontrolled fashion, does not appear to be adaptive

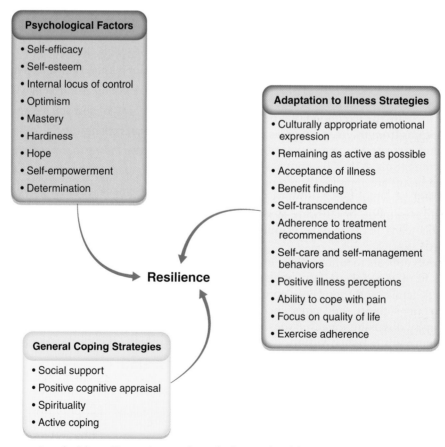

Figure 12-8. Factors associated with resilience in people with chronic health problems. © Thinkstock

(de Ridder et al., 2008). Chronic, negative emotional states may harm health and reduce adaptation by over-activating the sympathetic nervous system. Negative emotional states may also reduce motivation for behavior change and the energy required for self-control. The goal of emotional processing is to achieve some perspective on one's situation, adopt problem-solving strategies when feasible, and move toward psychophysiological balance.

Encourage Self-Management Behaviors

Self-management forms the heart of treatment for chronic injuries and illnesses. Optimal management of chronic health problems is associated with good psychological adjustment to new health status. It is possible that engaging in self-management behaviors gives people a greater sense of control over their lives. It is also possible that patients who are adjusting successfully have the energy to engage in self-management; in other words, because they are faring better emotionally, they have more self-control energy available for behavior change (de Ridder et al., 2008). Either way, coaching patients to engage in positive behavior change forms the core of the work provided by health and fitness professionals (What's the Evidence? 12-1).

Support Cognitive Adaptation and Benefit Finding

Patients who successfully adapt to chronic health problems often seek meaning in their experiences. Indeed,

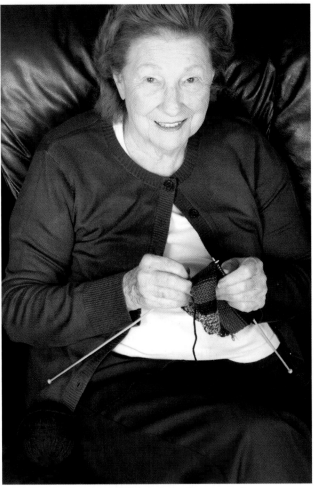
Figure 12-9. Meaningful activity enhances adjustment to chronic health problems. © Thinkstock

WHAT'S THE EVIDENCE? 12-1

Promoting Exercise Adherence in Rehabilitation Settings
Fleig, L., Lippke, S., Pomp, S., & Schwarzer, R. (2011). Intervention effects of exercise self-regulation on physical exercise and eating fruits and vegetables: a longitudinal study in orthopedic and cardiac rehabilitation. *Preventive Medicine, 53*(3), 182–187.

■ PURPOSE
The first purpose of this research project was to examine the mechanisms by which an exercise self-regulation program affected exercise behavior in orthopedic- and cardiac-rehabilitation settings. The second goal was to see whether the experimental group showed any changes in fruit and vegetable intake, even though dietary choices were not part of the intervention. The investigators hypothesized that self-regulation behaviors taught in an exercise context might be applied by subjects to other health behaviors. They also suggested that as exercise becomes more of a habit and less self-regulation is required to engage in physical activity behaviors, more self-regulation energy is available for other behaviors, such as making desirable dietary choices.

■ STUDY
Patients prescribed physical exercise as part of a rehabilitation program following orthopedic or cardiac treatment were solicited to participate in the experiment. Volunteers were assigned to an exercise self-regulation intervention or a control group, in addition to receiving standard therapeutic treatments, such as physical therapy. The self-regulation intervention consisted of two instructional sessions delivered online to encourage subjects to participate in regular exercise after their discharge from the rehabilitation program. One session was delivered at the beginning of the rehabilitation program, the other at the end. The first program taught skills in goal setting, evaluating goal importance, making action plans, and recalling positive exercise experiences, and it took participants about 36 minutes to complete. The second intervention, which occurred about 3 weeks later, focused on making action plans, thinking

Continued

WHAT'S THE EVIDENCE? 12-1–cont'd

about positive exercise experiences, and using an action control record sheet to monitor exercise behavior at home. This session took subjects an average of 25 minutes to complete. Subjects in the control group only completed an online questionnaire at the beginning and end of their programs. All subjects received a final questionnaire assessment 6 weeks after discharge.

This project evaluated subjects' scores on self-regulatory variables called action planning and action control. Action planning describes self-regulatory strategies that involve mentally planning behaviors to perform in specific situations to accomplish behavior-change goals. Action control refers to self-control strategies actually used in specific situations, such as self-monitoring behaviors and comparing these behaviors with one's behavioral goals. The researchers also examined subjects' perceived satisfaction with exercise outcomes and exercise habit strength. Exercise habit strength measures how much people feel they exercise because it is a habit rather than something that requires a great deal of planning and self-control.

The researchers found that subjects in the intervention group had a greater increase in exercise participation, exercise habit strength, and fruit and vegetable intake than those in the control group. Increases in exercise behavior were related to changes in measures of action control and positive exercise experience but not to changes in action planning. (Because action planning was part of the standard rehabilitation program, both groups received training in this, which might explain why no differences were found between groups on this variable.) Changes in fruit and vegetable intake were related to an increase in exercise habit strength.

■ IMPLICATIONS

Teaching self-regulatory skills may help promote an increase in physical activity. Encouraging the recall of positive experiences with physical activity may also contribute to better exercise adherence. Helping clients make exercise a habit may lead to improvements in other health behaviors, such as dietary choices, as well.

people experiencing health problems commonly report positive as well as negative outcomes. The process of perceiving positive changes following exposure to adversity has been called benefit finding. Commonly reported positive outcomes include an increased appreciation for life, clearer sense of purpose, reassessment of life priorities, and better personal relationships (Barclay-Goddard, King, Dubouloz, & Schwartz, 2012; Ehde, 2010; Sato, Yamazaki, Sakita, & Bryce, 2008; Tartaro et al., 2005). Some research suggests that facing adversity and experiencing suffering even leads to self-transcendence for some (Iwamoto, Yamawaki, & Sato, 2011).

An interesting review of 52 articles on resilience in the physically ill generated a list of factors associated with resilience (Stewart & Yuen, 2011). Stewart and Yuen's review confirmed the importance of the factors discussed previously in this section and are included in Fig. 12-8. Most of these factors echo similar observations in the apparently healthy population and in people facing other forms of adversity, underscoring the notion that health and fitness professionals should use the same strengths-promoting strategies in all clients, whether healthy or coping with chronic health problems (Leddy, 2006). In her writing on applying positive psychology in rehabilitation settings, Dawn Ehde notes that over half of the people who face adversity in the form of chronic illness or disability do bounce back and adapt to their new situations (Ehde, 2010). Ehde notes that negative emotions are probably part of the adjustment process and that helping professionals should not confuse normal sadness and grief with depression.

For most people facing adversity, negative emotions come and go, alternating with positive emotions, and do not seriously interfere with functioning.

MOTIVATING CHANGE: Helping Patients Build Positive Emotions

Health and fitness professionals should strive to help every client build the positive emotional experiences that help motivate behavior change. Professionals should develop good working relationships with clients and help clients incorporate enjoyable activities into their lives. Time spent experiencing positive emotions seems to be more important than the intensity of the positive emotions. Even people with very limited abilities experience pleasure. Often simple experiences, such as sitting outdoors in nice weather, taking a drive in a car, reading a good book, or enjoying a favorite food make people feel good. Maximizing quality of life must be woven into behavior-change recommendations.

BEHAVIOR CHANGE FOR PEOPLE EXPERIENCING HEALTH PROBLEMS

The behavior-change models and applications discussed in Chapters 4 and 5 apply to patients experiencing health problems. Health and fitness professionals should use an ecological perspective to get a picture of the many variables influencing a given client's situation. They should assess clients' readiness to change and help them weigh the pros and cons of behavior change, hopefully motivating them to form a decision to adopt helpful behaviors. Professionals can help patients set goals and devise realistic action plans. Health and fitness professionals can help patients cultivate social support, build self-efficacy for behavior change, and develop behavior-change skills. Patients can learn how to cope with lapses and adjust expectations as changes in health occur.

Applying Behavior-Change Models

All of the behavior-change models and strategies discussed in this book have been extensively applied to a variety of patient populations and in rehabilitation settings for people coping with illness and injury. As discussed in previous chapters, the process of changing behavior looks different for each person and for a given person over time. Two landmarks in this process appear to be making a decision to change and implementing an action plan for change. Health and fitness professionals should assess each patient for readiness to change on each behavior-change recommendation, set priorities with patients, and help patients find autonomous motivation to follow treatment recommendations.

Most treatment plans will involve some recommendations regarding physical activity (Health Psychology at Work 12-1). Physical activity can help build feelings of self-confidence as level of physical function improves. Improvement in physical activity may also help people adopt other healthy behaviors. An interesting study of patients in orthopedic- and cardiac-rehabilitation programs described above found that patients who developed an exercise habit and had positive feelings about exercise were more likely to also increase fruit and vegetable intake (Fleig, Lippke, Pomp, & Schwarzer, 2011b).

Psychological Benefits of Exercise

The psychological benefits of exercise discussed in Chapter 3 extend to both apparently healthy and clinical populations. Appropriate physical activity not only improves physical function but enhances psychological function and quality of life as well. The mechanisms of these actions in people living with chronic illness or injury appear to be the same as those for healthy people. In addition, participating in physical activity may give patients a sense of control in lives that otherwise seem ruled by their health problems. Beginning an exercise

---

HEALTH PSYCHOLOGY AT WORK 12-1. Working With Clients Who Have Health Challenges Can Be Rewarding Work

Helene Parker holds a bachelor's degree in Exercise Science from Smith College and an American College of Sports Medicine personal training certification. She manages a personal training facility in New York City, trains clients in their homes, and instructs group exercise classes. She has helped people who have conditions ranging from sarcopenia to complicated migraine syndrome to torn ligaments improve their quality of life and regain function.

"My philosophy as a personal trainer is never to have a 'normal' client. Every individual has fears, injuries, health problems, goals, and preferences that are unique to them. Even from day to day, the same client will differ based on his or her own life.

"Most of us take for granted things as simple as walking down the street. One of my clients had trouble doing even that due to her complicated migraine syndrome, which seriously decreased her balance abilities, and also weakness from letting the syndrome prevent her from ever being physically active. When we started working together, she had never been able to pick up her 3-year-old grandson. After 3 months of working in her living room with resistance bands and calisthenics exercises, she started carrying her own groceries—and picked up her grandson for the first time.

"Success stories like this one are what make working with people with limitations so rewarding. These clients may not look like supermodels, athletes, or bodybuilders (who does?), but they will make more important gains, physically and psychologically. Many people are proud of their achievements not only in the gym setting but also for what these achievements mean in their daily lives. These results and this pride are important to utilize as positive motivation for clients. I make a huge deal when a client gets an exercise they've been struggling with right.

"Another wonderful motivating tool is to have a carrot to dangle. I had a 74-year-old client with extreme kyphosis, sarcopenia, and arthritis. He hated exercising but loved to be stretched. I always knew that I could get him to do an exercise that he particularly disliked by promising extra stretching time. Eventually, people will begin to notice that they can climb stairs without being winded, run without knee pain, wake up with less stiffness in their back, have less arthritis pain, be in a better mood. Then they won't need as much encouragement, because they already know what they're getting out of it. My 74-year-old client kept telling me that he wished he had discovered 'fitness' sooner! He was not the only one who gained pride from our relationship."

program is a good antidote to the helpless, hopeless feelings that can arise from the experience of being a medical patient. Instead of focusing on the disease, health and fitness professionals can maximize the positive force of exercise by focusing on the whole person, the active person working to regain strength and ability and to improve quality of life (Behavior Change in Action 12-2). Positive exercise experiences in turn encourage further participation in physical activity (Fleig, Lippke, Pomp, & Schwarzer, 2011a). Researchers have examined the psychological benefits of physical activity for many common health problems. Some of the more-common problems that health and fitness professionals may find themselves working with include cardiovascular disease, chronic obstructive pulmonary disease (COPD), and cancer.

BEHAVIOR CHANGE IN ACTION 12-2

Implementing Physical Activity Recommendations With Patient Populations

■ CHALLENGE

Many people with health problems need so much help it is hard to know where to start. What are the most-important guidelines to keep in mind for professionals beginning work with a new client who has health problems?

■ PLAN

Focus on building a good connection with clients, helping clients find autonomous motivation for behavior change, and increasing client self-efficacy for behavior change.

■ DEVELOP GOOD COMMUNICATION WITH YOUR CLIENTS

Before you begin handing out an exercise program or other behavior-change recommendations, spend some time getting to know your new clients. What is happening in their lives? What are they hoping to achieve in their exercise rehabilitation programs? Do they seem ready to commit to a program of regular physical activity? Or have they been dragged in by a family member or friend? Clients who have not yet committed themselves mentally to an exercise program are unlikely to have much success. Educate these clients about the importance of the exercise program and try to get them inspired to begin. People often respond to medical authorities: remind them that their doctor is expecting them to exercise.

Good communication also ensures that clients have a clear understanding of what they are supposed to do and why they are supposed to do it. Keep instructions simple and write everything down. Give clients handouts on how exercise will help them with their problems. People who believe their exercise programs are important and effective develop a stronger commitment to regular physical activity.

■ DEVELOP GOOD COMMUNICATION WITH YOUR MEDICAL TEAM

You need good communication with your medical team so that you understand the exercise limitations of your clients and the exercise goals that have been established. In addition, your observations may help other members of the medical team. Fitness professionals sometimes find, for example, that a client is not receiving adequate treatment for a medical problem, such as depression or pain. Encourage your clients to check in with their doctors and let the doctors know what you have found.

■ HELP CLIENTS SET QUALITY-OF-LIFE GOALS

Fitness goals must be meaningful to each individual client. Clients in the clinical setting are more likely to be focused on improving their physical and emotional health and on reducing symptoms. They may place more value on functional goals, such as being able to climb a set of stairs, than fitness goals such as increasing aerobic endurance. What would motivate your client to exercise regularly? Gaining the ability to carry groceries or lift a grandchild? Take a walk with family members or friends? Be sure to tailor your exercise recommendations to these important goals.

■ ALLAY FEARS AND CREATE A LOW-RISK EXERCISE PROGRAM

Many clients with health problems do not exercise because they fear injury. Having already lost some functional capacity or physical ability because of their health problems, they worry about losing more. Discuss clients' fears and reassure them that exercise will help them become stronger and *less* prone to injury. And, of course, be sure the exercise program is as safe as possible.

■ ENCOURAGE CLIENTS TO BUILD SOCIAL SUPPORT

Clients feel encouraged when they see others like themselves exercising. Group exercise can be very effective when group members encourage each other along. Group support builds over time as members exercise together.

BEHAVIOR CHANGE IN ACTION 12-2–cont'd

In the clinical setting, you are likely to find friends and family members involved in your clients' exercise programs. Spouses and adult children may be providing transportation and care. Family members and friends can provide helpful support to your client, so involve them as much as possible. You may even wish to include them in meetings with your client if you (and the client) feel their presence is helpful.

BUILD SELF-EFFICACY WITH INSTANT SUCCESS

Structure exercise programs to provide instant success. Find out what your clients are doing now and ask them to do a little bit more. Teach one or two new skills at a time and build slowly. Let clients feel successful, even though progress may be very slow.

Cardiovascular Disease and Chronic Obstructive Pulmonary Disease

Just as exercise helps prevent cardiovascular disease, so does it help restore this system to health. The number of people surviving heart attacks has increased greatly over the past several decades. The number undergoing operations to improve blood flow to the heart, such as bypass surgery and angioplasty, has increased dramatically as well. Cardiac-rehabilitation programs provide lifestyle and medical support that helps patients recover from cardiovascular disease.

Patients without complications usually begin simple arm and leg exercises 1 or 2 days after heart attack or heart surgery and may begin walking for several minutes at a time. Walking time and frequency are gradually increased, and patients begin climbing stairs. Health workers monitor heart rate and blood pressure frequently to be sure the patient's heart is responding well to the activity.

As recovery continues, patients may perform an exercise stress test to check for heart rate and rhythm abnormalities and chest pain during exercise. From test results, patients may be given target exercise heart rate zones. These zones represent exercise intensities that will be both beneficial and safe, when the heart is getting plenty of blood flow and thus oxygen, and is not experiencing excessive stress.

After leaving the hospital, patients sometimes enroll in medically supervised exercise programs designed for people recovering from heart attack or heart surgery. Unfortunately, many people do not have access to such programs, due to geographical, financial, time, motivational, or other limitations. Some doctors may neglect to emphasize the importance of rehabilitation, so patients may not make it a priority in their lives. Some patients are given instruction and are then told to exercise on their own. They may use heart-rate monitors that can send recorded signals via telephone to healthcare providers, or they may simply monitor exercise intensity and warning signs on their own, checking in periodically with their health-care providers.

Although regular exercise is the cornerstone of cardiac-rehabilitation programs, these programs should also include multiple strategies to aggressively reduce risk for subsequent cardiovascular events, such as heart attack and stroke, and to encourage regression of the plaque that has built up in the arteries. Good programs provide support for quitting smoking, developing heart-healthy eating behaviors, and exercising regularly. When necessary, medications to control blood pressure and blood lipids are prescribed. Patients may also have access to a variety of therapies for reducing stress and coping with the depression, anxiety, and grieving that often follow a heart disease diagnosis.

Similar rehabilitation programs are available for patients with chronic heart failure and COPD. Even though health status in patients with these disorders may decline over time, rehabilitation programs that include physical activity can hopefully slow the decline, improve functional capacity, and increase quality of life. Such programs offer many psychological benefits, including reductions in symptoms of depression and anxiety (Yohannes, Willgoss, Baldwin, & Connolly, 2010).

Recovery from cardiovascular and chronic pulmonary diseases is often a challenge. Exercise helps people overcome the fear of exertion and gives them confidence in performing the physical activities that are part of daily life. Supervised exercise programs can provide peer support and build self-efficacy for physical activity (Worcester & Le Grande, 2008). Exercise not only improves physical function, but it helps people with cardiovascular and pulmonary diseases become active participants in their recovery and in life.

Cancer

Exercise can help cancer patients in different ways depending upon the client's stage of treatment. A cancer diagnosis may be followed by some type of surgery if there is a tumor and if the tumor can be removed. Cancer patients often receive some sort of therapy before and/or after surgery, if surgery occurs, such as radiation therapy or chemotherapy, designed to kill cancer cells.

Physical therapy usually begins a day or two after surgery, to restore range of motion (ROM) and aid healing of the affected area. This type of exercise is best administered by a physical therapist familiar with post-op patients. As recovery continues, strength exercise and mild cardiovascular exercise may be added to ROM exercises to help patients recover functional ability. The goal of physical therapy at this time is to help patients return home with the ability to perform the tasks of daily living.

People vary considerably in their responses to chemotherapy and other treatments. Some people feel so sick that anything but very minimal activity may be out of the question. Other people are well enough to participate in mild-to-moderate levels of physical activity during their treatment programs. Many people continue to live at home and even go to work during these types of treatment.

Recent research has documented many benefits of physical activity for people undergoing various cancer treatments (Spence, Heesch, & Brown, 2010). Exercise of mild-to-moderate intensity often helps reduce feelings of fatigue, one of the most problematic side effects of treatment. Regular physical activity helps people regain daily function more quickly. People are able to do more, sooner, and thus get back into activities they previously enjoyed.

Muscle loss and wasting often occur during cancer treatment, and strength exercise can help lessen this effect. Perhaps the most important benefit of physical activity is improved mood. Exercise helps reduce feelings of anxiety, stress, and depression and to improve body image and self-esteem. It improves sleep quality, especially important since insomnia is a common and debilitating side effect of treatment. Any combination of these effects means improved quality of life during what can be an extremely painful and exhausting time (Ferrer, Huedo-Medina, Johnson, Ryan, & Pescatello, 2011).

■ *Mason and Grant are giving a presentation to their class-mates on their internship experiences at the medical fitness center. They are especially proud of the group work they helped to start and present several case studies of patients who seemed to benefit from increased levels of physical activity and social support. Mason describes Howard's progress from fear of activity to confident reintegration into independent living in his retirement community. Howard had progressed from a very-low fitness level and exercise self-efficacy to walking 2 miles in the late afternoon every day. "I'll never forget our handshake, Howard's grip strong and sure, as I said goodbye after our last session together. This was a man who seemed to have forgotten how to smile at the beginning of my internship. After 6 months, he was much more confident and relaxed and seemed to be enjoying life again. While I was proud of his fitness improvements, I was most proud that our work improved Howard's quality of life."* ■

KEY TERMS

acute	Common Sense Model of Illness
benefit finding	
chronic disease	disability
chronic illness	illness
clinical inertia	illness representation
Cognitive Adaptation Model	injury
cognitive reappraisal	patient inertia
	sickness behavior

CRITICAL THINKING QUESTIONS

1. Review the Health Belief Model from Chapter 4. How might knowledge of a client's illness representation help you apply the Health Belief Model to helping him or her form an intention to change a health behavior? Discuss how an illness representation gives you information about the following variables in the Health Belief Model: perceived susceptibility to illness, perceived seriousness of illness, and perceived benefits of a health behavior.

2. Think about an injury or illness that you personally experienced. Illustrate the factors in the Stress Cycle Model (Fig. 12-6) from this experience. Describe the stressor, your physical and psychological response to the injury or illness, and your coping strategies. Include both problem-focused and emotion-focused strategies that you used to cope with the stressor.

3. Imagine a patient like Howard, described in this chapter's scenario, and describe what movement through the stages of change might look like for him or her. Describe how a cardiac-rehabilitation patient might progress from contemplation (assume health providers have prescribed exercise, so the patient is at least thinking about exercising), to preparation, and to action. Describe the processes of change and how they might apply in this imaginary situation.

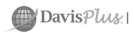

REFERENCES

Atlantis, E., Shi, Z., Penninx, B. J. W. H., Wittert, G. A., Taylor, A. & Almeida, O.P. (2012). Chronic medical conditions mediate the association between depression and cardiovascular disease mortality. *Social Psychiatry and Psychiatric Epidemiology, 47*(4): 615-625.

Auvray, M., Myin, E., & Spence, C. (2010). The sensory-discriminative and affective-motivational aspects of pain. *Neuroscience & Biobehavioral Reviews, 34*(2): 214-223.

Baldwin, A. S., Kellerman, Q. D., & Christensen, A. J. (2010). Coping with chronic illness. In: Suls, J. M., Davidson, K. W., & Kaplan, R. M. (eds.). *Handbook of Health Psychology and Behavioral Medicine.* New York: Guilford Press.

Barclay-Goddard, R., King, J., Dubouloz, C. J., & Schwartz, C. E. (2012). Building on transformative learning and response shift theory to investigate health-related quality of life changes over time in individuals with chronic health conditions and disability. *Archives of Physical Medicine and Rehabilitation, 93*(2): 214-220.

Bonnano, G. A. (2004). Loss, trauma, and human resilience: Have we underestimated the human capacity to thrive after extremely aversive events? *American Psychologist, 59*(1): 20-28.

Butler, D. S., & Moseley, G. L. (2003). *Explain Pain.* Adelaide, Australia: Noigroup Publications.

Cantrell, C. R., Priest, J. L., Cook, C. L., Fincham, J., & Burch, S.P. (2011). Adherence to treatment guidelines and therapeutic regimens: a U.S. claims–based benchmark of a commercial population. *Population Health Management, 14* (1): 33-41.

Carver, C. S., & Scheier, M. R. (2002). Coping processes and adjustment to chronic illness. In: Christensen, A. J., & Antoni, M. H. (eds.). *Chronic Physical Disorders: Behavioral Medicine's Perspective.* Oxford: Blackwell.

Carver, C. S., & Vargas, S. (2011). Stress, coping, and health. In: Friedman, H. S. (ed.). *The Oxford Handbook of Health Psychology.* New York: Oxford University Press.

Centers for Disease Control and Prevention, U.S. Department of Health and Human Services. (2009). Chronic diseases: the power to prevent, the call to control. At a glance 2009. www.cdc.gov/chronicdisease/resources/publications/AAG/chronic.htm. Accessed 8/16/12.

Christensen, A. J., Howren, M. B., Hillis, S. L., Kaboli, P., Carter, B. L., Cvengros, J. A., . . . Rosenthal, G. E. (2010). Patient and physician beliefs about control over health: association of symmetrical beliefs with medication regimen adherence. *Journal of General Internal Medicine, 25*(5): 397-402.

Colberg, S. R., Sigal, R. J., Fernhall, B., Regensteiner, J. G., Blissmer, B. J., Rubin, R. R., . . . Braun, B. (2010). Exercise and type 2 diabetes: the American College of Sports Medicine and the American Diabetes Association. Joint position statement. *Diabetes Care, 33*(12): e147-e167.

Comp, D. (2011). Improving parent satisfaction by sharing the inpatient daily plan of care: an evidence review with implications for practice and research. *Pediatric Nursing, 37*(5): 237-242.

Cousins, N. (1991). Anatomy of an illness (as perceived by the patient). In: Monat, A., & Lazarus, R. S. (eds.). *Stress and Coping.* New York: Columbia University Press.

Cutrona, S. L., Choudhry, N. K., Stedman, M., Servi, A., Liberman, J. N., Brennan, T., . . . Shrank, W. H. (2011). Physician effectiveness in interventions to improve cardiovascular medication adherence: a systematic review. *Journal of General Internal Medicine, 25*(10): 1090-1096.

de Ridder, D., Geenen, R., Kuijer, R., & van Middendorp, H. (2008). Psychological adjustment to chronic disease. *Lancet, 372,* 1371-1378.

Dunbar-Jacob, J., & Mortimer-Stephens, M. K. (2001). Treatment adherence in chronic disease. *Journal of Clinical Epidemiology, 54*(Suppl 1): S57-S60.

Economist, The. (2012). The future of medicine. Squeezing out the doctor: the role of physicians at the centre of health care is under pressure. *The Economist, 403*(8787): 29-32.

Ehde, D. M. (2010). Application of positive psychology to rehabilitation psychology. In: Frank, R. G., Rosenthal, M., & Caplan, B. (eds.) *Handbook of Rehabilitation Psychology.* (2nd ed.). Washington, DC: American Psychological Association.

Ferrer, R. A., Huedo-Medina, T. B., Johnson, B. T., Ryan, S., & Pescatello, L. S. (2011). Exercise interventions for cancer survivors: a meta-analysis of quality of life outcomes. *Annals of Behavioral Medicine, 41,* 32-47.

Fleig, L., Lippke, S., Pomp, S., & Schwarzer, R. (2011a). Exercise maintenance after rehabilitation: how exercise can make a difference. *Psychology of Sport and Exercise, 12,* 293-299.

Fleig, L., Lippke, S., Pomp, S., & Schwarzer, R. (2011b). Intervention effects of exercise self-regulation on physical exercise and eating fruits and vegetables: a longitudinal study in orthopedic and cardiac rehabilitation. *Preventive Medicine, 53*(3): 182-187.

Franklin, D. (2012). Nature that nurtures. *Scientific American, 306*(3): 24-25.

Fryers, M., Young, L., & Rowland, P. (2012). Creating and sustaining a collaborative model of care. *Healthcare Management Forum, 25*(1): 20-25.

Galli, U., Ettlin, D. A., Palla, S., Ehlert, U., & Gaab, J. (2010). Do illness perceptions predict pain-related disability and mood in chronic orofacial pain patients? A 6-month follow-up study. *European Journal of Pain, 14,* 550-558.

Garssen, B. (2007). Repression: finding our way in a maze of concepts. *Journal of Behavioral Medicine, 30,*471-481.

Hagger, M. S., & Orbell, S. (2003). A meta-analytic review of the common-sense model of illness representations. *Psychology & Health, 18*(2): 141-184.

Harrington, A. (2011). "Bodies behaving badly: what we learn from the history of mind–body medicine, and why we should care." Lecture given at Smith College, Northampton, MA, December 7.

Henninger, D. E., Whitson, H. E., Cohen, H. J., & Ariely, D. (2012). Higher medical morbidity burden is associated with external locus of control. *Journal of the American Geriatrics Society, 60*(4): 751-755.

Howren, M. B., & Suls, J. (2011). The symptom perception hypothesis revised: depression and anxiety play different roles in concurrent and retrospective physical symptom reporting. *Journal of Personality and Social Psychology, 100*(1): 182-195.

Huebschmann, A. G., Mizrahi, T., Soenksen, A., Beaty, B. L., & Denberg, T. D. (2012). Reducing clinical inertia in hypertension treatment: a pragmatic randomized controlled trial. *Journal of Clinical Hypertension (Greenwich, Conn.), 14*(5): 322-329.

Institute of Medicine. (2001). *Crossing the Quality Chasm: A New Health Care System for the 21st Century.* Washington, DC: National Academy Press.

Iwamoto, R., Yamawaki, N., & Sato, T. (2011). Increased self-transcendence in patients with intractable diseases. *Psychiatry and Clinical Neurosciences, 65*(7): 638-647.

Jacobs, S. (1993). *Pathological Grief: Maladaptation to Loss.* Washington, DC: American Psychiatric Press.

Janevic, M. R., Rosland, A. M., Wiitala, W., Connell, C. M., & Piette, J. D. (2012). Providing support to relatives and friends managing both chronic physical illness and depression: the views of a national sample of U.S. adults. *Patient Education and Counseling, 89*(1): 191-198.

Joyner-Grantham, J., Mount, D. L., McCorkle, O. D., Simmons, D. R., Ferrario, C. M., & Cline, D. M. (2009). Self-reported influences of hopelessness, health literacy, lifestyle action, and patient inertia on blood pressure control in a hypertensive emergency department population. *American Journal of Medical Science, 338*(5): 368-372.

Kaptein, A. A., Bijsterbosch, J., Scharloo, M., Hampson, S. E., Kroon, H. M., & Kloppenburg, M. (2010). Using the common sense model of illness perceptions to examine osteoarthritis change: a 6-year longitudinal study. *Health Psychology, 29*(1): 56-64.

Karakus, M. C., & Patton, L. C. (2011). Depression and the onset of chronic illness in older adults: a 12-year prospective study. *Journal of Behavioral Health Services & Research, 38*(3): 373-382.

Kübler-Ross, E. (1969). *On Death and Dying*. New York: Simon & Schuster.

Leddy, S. K. (2006). *Health Promotion: Mobilizing Strengths to Enhance Health, Wellness, and Well-being*. Philadelphia, PA: F.A. Davis Company.

Lee, B. O., Chaboyer, W., & Wallis, M. (2010). Illness representations in patients with traumatic injury: a longitudinal study. *Journal of Clinical Nursing, 19*(3-4): 556-563.

Leventhal, H., Weinman, J., Leventhal, E. A., & Phillips, L. A. (2008). Health psychology: the search for pathways between behavior and health. *Annual Review of Psychology, 59*, 477-505.

Louw, A., Diener, I., Butler, D. S., & Puentedura, E. J. (2011). The effect of neuroscience education on pain, disability, anxiety, and stress in chronic musculoskeletal pain. *Archives of Physical Medicine and Rehabilitation, 92*(12): 2041-2056.

Lukas, C. V., Holmes, S. K., Cohen, A. B., Restuccia, J., Cramer, I. E., Shwartz, M., & Charns, M. P. (2007). Transformational change in health care systems: an organizational model. *Health Care Management Review, 32*(4): 309-320.

Maciejewski, P. K., Zhang, B., Block, S. D., & Prigerson, H. G. (2007). An empirical examination of the stage theory of grief. *JAMA, 297*(7): 716-723.

Martin, L. R., Haskard-Zolnierek, K. B., & DiMatteo, M. R. (2010). *Health Behavior Change and Treatment Adherence*. New York: Oxford University Press.

Meeus, M., Nils, J., Van Oosterwijck, J., Van Alsenoy, V., & Truijen, S. (2010). Pain physiology education improves pain beliefs in patients with chronic fatigue syndrome compared with pacing and self-management education: a double-blind randomized controlled trial. *Archives of Physical Medicine and Rehabilitation, 91*(8): 1153-1159.

Meier, D. E. (2010). The development, status, and future of palliative care. In: Meier, D. E., Isaacs, S. L., & Hughes, R. (eds.). *Palliative Care: Transforming the Care of Serious Illness*. New York: Wiley.

Mokdad, A. H., Marks, J. S., Stroup, D. F., & Gerberding, J. L. (2004). Actual causes of death in the United States, 2000. *JAMA, 291*(10): 1238-1245.

Moseley, G. L. (2012). Teaching people about pain: why do we keep beating around the bush? *Pain Management, 2*(1): 1-3.

Moseley, G. L., & Flor, H. (2012). Targeting cortical representations in the treatment of chronic pain: a review. *Neurorehabilitation and Neural Repair, 26*(6): 646-652.

Nicklas, L. B., Dunbar, M., & Wild, M. (2010). Adherence to pharmacological treatment of non-malignant chronic pain: the role of illness perceptions and medication beliefs. *Psychology & Health, 25*(5): 601-615.

Nouwen, A., Ford, T., Balan, A. T., Twisk, J., & Ruggiero, L. (2011). Longitudinal motivational predictors of dietary self-care and diabetes control in adults with newly diagnosed type 2 diabetes mellitus. *Health Psychology, 30*(6): 771-779.

Petersen, S., van den Berg, R. A., Janssens, T., & Van den Bergh, O. (2011). Illness and symptom perception: a theoretical approach towards an integrative measurement model. *Clinical Psychology Review, 31*(3): 428-439.

Petrie, K. J., & Weinman, J. (2012). Patients' perceptions of their illness: the dynamo of volition in health care. *Current Directions in Psychological Science, 21*(1): 60-65.

Podlog, L., & Eklund, R. C. (2007). The psychosocial aspects of a return to sport following serious injury: a review of the literature from a self-determination perspective. *Psychology of Sport and Exercise, 8*(4): 535-566.

Podlog, L., Dimmock, J., & Miller, J. (2011). A review of return to sport concerns following injury rehabilitation: practitioner strategies for enhancing recovery outcomes. *Physical Therapy in Sport, 12*(1): 36-42.

Sanz, J., Garcia-Vera, M. P., Espinosa, R., Fortún, M., Magán, I., & Segura, J. (2010). Psychological factors associated with poor hypertension control: differences in personality and stress between patients with controlled and uncontrolled hypertension. *Psychological Reports, 107*(3): 923-938.

Sato, M., Yamazaki, Y., Sakita, M., & Bryce, T. J. (2008). Benefit-finding among people with rheumatoid arthritis in Japan. *Nursing & Health Sciences, 10*(1): 51-58.

Smidt, N., de Vet, H. C., Bouter, L. M., Dekker, J., Arendzen, J. H., de Bie, R. A., . . . Exercise Therapy Group. (2005). Effectiveness of exercise therapy: a best-evidence summary of systematic reviews. *Australian Journal of Physiotherapy, 51*(2): 71-85.

Spence, R. R., Heesch, K. C., & Brown, W. J. (2010). Exercise and cancer rehabilitation: a systematic review. *Cancer Treatment Reviews, 36*(2): 185-194.

Sperry, L. (2009). Lifestyle convictions and illness perceptions as predictors of treatment compliance and noncompliance. *Journal of Individual Psychology, 65*(3): 298-304.

Stafford, L., Jackson, H. J., & Berk, M. (2008). Illness beliefs about heart disease and adherence to secondary prevention regimens. *Psychosomatic Medicine, 70*(8): 942-948.

Stanton, A. L., & Revenson, T. A. (2011). Adjustment to chronic illness: Progress and promise in research. In: Friedman, H. S. *The Oxford Handbook of Health Psychology*. New York: Oxford University Press.

Stewart, D. E., & Yuen, T. (2011). A systematic review of resilience in the physically ill. *Psychosomatics, 52*(3): 199-209.

Tartaro, J., Roberts, J., Nosarti, C., Crayford, T., Luecken, L., & David, A. (2005). Who benefits? Distress, adjustment and benefit-finding among breast cancer survivors. *Journal of Psychosocial Oncology, 23*(2-3): 45-64.

Taylor, S. E. (1983). Adjustment to threatening events: a theory of cognitive adaptation. *American Psychologist, 38*(11): 1161-1173.

Taylor, W. E., Kemeny, M. E., Reed, G. M., Bower, J. E., & Gruenewald, T. L. (2000). Psychological resources, positive illusions, and health. *American Psychologist, 55*(1): 99-109.

van Olmen, J., Ku, G. M., Bermejo, R., Kegels, G., Hermann, K., Van Damme, W. (2011). The growing caseload of chronic life-long conditions calls for a move towards full self-management in low-income countries. *Global Health, 7*(1): 38.

van Wilgen, C. P., Kaptein, A. A., & Brink, M. S. (2010). Illness perceptions and mood states are associated with injury-related outcomes in athletes. *Disability and Rehabilitation, 32*(19): 1576-1585.

Wadey, R., Evans, L., Hanton, S., & Neil, R. (2012). An examination of hardiness throughout the sport injury process. *British Journal of Health Psychology, 17*(1): 103-128.

Wagner, S. A., & Brown, S. L. (2012). Associations between hypochondriacal symptoms and illness appraisals, and their moderation by self-focused attention. *Journal of Applied Social Psychology, 42*(1): 195-212.

Worcester, M. U. C., & Le Grande, M. R. (2008). The role of cardiac rehabilitation in influencing psychological outcomes. *Stress & Health, 24*(3): 267-277.

Yohannes, A. M., Willgoss, T. G., Baldwin, R. C., & Connolly, M. J. (2010). Depression and anxiety in chronic heart failure and chronic obstructive pulmonary disease: prevalence, relevance, clinical implications and management principles. *International Journal of Geriatric Psychiatry, 25*(12): 1209-1221.

Zubialde, J. P., Mold, J., & Eubank, D. (2009). Outcomes that matter in chronic illness: a taxonomy informed by self-determination and adult-learning theory. *Families, Systems, & Health, 27*(3): 193-200.

absorptive cells cells lining the surface of fingerlike projections extending from the inner surface of the small intestine that take in small compounds from the digestive tract and break them down further, preparing them for absorption into the bloodstream

abstinence violation effect the behavior of people who resume a behavior they are trying to avoid after a period of abstinence; the resumption of the behavior is triggered by a single episode of failing to follow the new planned behavior, such as failing to follow a prescribed diet

abuse use of a substance or performance of a behavior that hurts or endangers the user or those around him or her

accelerometer an instrument that provides an indication of exercise volume by measuring changes in the speed of movement

acquired immunity the immune system's ability to recognize and attack pathogens, developed over time from prior exposure to these pathogens

action (stage of change) one of the six stages of change in the Transtheoretical Model in which the behavior change is in progress; however, the new behavior has not yet lasted 6 months

action plan a plan that spells out the where, when, and how details of behavior-change recommendations

activation energy level (in reference to mood), with deactivated meaning low energy level and activated meaning high energy level

active static stretching a form of flexibility training in which a muscle group is placed in a stretching position, and the opposing muscle group is isometrically contracted

acute an adjective describing something with a sudden onset that is relatively short lived, such as an illness

acute stress response the immediate psychophysiological reaction to a stressor

adaptive coping responses coping strategies that produce desirable long-term results

addiction the compulsive use of a substance or performance of an activity even if it is causing or is likely to cause harm

adiponectin a substance secreted by fat cells that increases the responsiveness of the body's cells to insulin

adiposopathy the hypertrophy of visceral adipocytes, associated with many negative health effects

adrenal cortex the outside layer of the adrenal gland

adrenal glands glands that sit on top of the kidneys, with an outside layer called the adrenal cortex and an inner portion called the adrenal medulla

adrenal medulla the inner portion of the adrenal gland

adrenocorticotrophic hormone (ACTH) a hormone secreted by the pituitary gland that acts on the adrenal cortex, stimulating it to release two families of hormones called glucocorticoids and mineralocorticoids

aerobic exercise activities that involve movement of the large muscle groups at a moderately vigorous level, leading to a sustained elevation in metabolic rate

affect the perceived positive or negative nature of moods and emotions of an individual

afferent nervous system the branch of the nervous system that consists of the nerve cells that receive information from the external and internal environments and conducts this information to the brain

affirmations statements that reinforce a client's strengths and accomplishments or indicate that progress is being made

agoraphobia a type of anxiety disorder characterized by fear of being in situations from which one cannot escape if a panic attack strikes, such as in public situations or in transportation situations (on airplanes, trains, buses, etc.)

alcohol dehydrogenase a key enzyme responsible for breaking down alcohol

aldosterone a mineralocorticoid that causes the kidneys to retain sodium and water

alveoli (alveolus, singular) the tiny air sacs of the lungs in which the exchange of oxygen and carbon dioxide between the blood and the air occurs

Alzheimer's disease the most-common cause of dementia, marked by abnormal clumps of protein deposits in the brain

ambivalence the state of having simultaneously both positive and negative thoughts and feelings about something, such as a behavior

amenorrhea the absence of menstrual periods

amino acids the building blocks of proteins

amotivation a word to describe a motivational state in which there is no motivation whatsoever

amygdala the area of the brain that plays important roles in memory formation and in the association of memory with emotion

anaerobic energy production pathways that do not require the immediate presence of oxygen

anaerobic exercise high-intensity exercise that utilizes anaerobic energy production pathways

anal sphincter a band of muscle whose function is to control elimination of feces

anandamide an endogenous cannabinoid neurotransmitter similar in structure to the active ingredient in marijuana

anaphylaxis a severe reaction to an allergen; symptoms include difficulty swallowing or breathing, itching, swelling, nausea and vomiting, and anxiety and confusion

anorexia nervosa (AN) an eating disorder marked by an intense fear of gaining weight or becoming fat as well as severe food restriction leading to an abnormally low body weight

antecedent a component of a behavior chain; an action that occurs prior to and triggers a behavior of interest

anthropometry measures that describe physical characteristics of a person

antioxidants molecules that neutralize the harmful chemicals produced as a byproduct of energy metabolism or from the intake of pollutants

anxiety feelings of worry, self-doubt, and fearful uncertainty about the future

anxiety hyperventilation a condition that occurs in response to anxiety in which breathing becomes very fast and interferes with the normal regulation of blood gas concentrations, resulting in dizziness, shortness of breath, pounding heart, and even fainting

anxiolytic anxiety reducing

appetite the psychological desire to eat

arteries the blood vessels carrying oxygen-rich blood from the heart to the body

arterioles smaller arteries

arthritis a group of disorders involving the joints

atherosclerosis an artery disease in which, over time, the lining of the arteries becomes thickened with the deposition of fatty deposits that interfere with arterial function; also known as "hardening of the arteries"

atrophy the shrinking or wasting away of a body organ or tissue, often used with reference to loss of muscle tissue

attitudes people's thoughts and feelings about the positive and negative aspects of a behavior or situation

attentional control the process of deciding what, among the wide array of stimuli coming into the brain through the sensory organs and other parts of the brain, are the most important things that need one's focus

attributions explanations people have for why things happen

autoimmune response a condition characterized by the immune system mistakenly attacking the cells of the body of which it is a part

autonomic nervous system (ANS) the branch of the nervous system that sends information between the central nervous system and the nonmusculoskeletal systems such as the circulatory system, respiratory system, digestive system, and endocrine system

autonomous motivation the feeling that one's behavior is of one's own free will, in accordance with one's personal wishes

autonomy the feeling of having the ability to make choices about behavior according to one's own wishes

B lymphocytes immune cells that identify invaders the body has previously been exposed to, producing antibodies that mark the invaders for destruction

ballistic stretching a form of flexibility training that utilizes a bouncing movement of the body to rapidly place intermittent force on the muscle group being stretched

bariatric surgery surgery designed to facilitate weight loss in which the digestive system, typically the stomach and/or small intestine, is surgically altered in ways that discourage overeating or reduce the absorption of calories from a meal

basal metabolic rate (BMR) basic energy expenditure while a person is awake but resting and lying down

behavior the way something acts, or behaves

behavior chain behaviors that are commonly linked together

behavior-change skills techniques that are useful for helping people change behavior

behavioral-learning theory theories that consider the rewards and punishments people (and animals) learn to associate with certain behaviors and how these associations shape behavior

behaviorism a movement in psychology focusing on observable phenomena, primarily behavior

benefit finding a process of perceiving positive changes following exposure to adversity

bile a substance manufactured by the liver that helps to emulsify (break into smaller particles) the fats in the food being digested

bioelectrical impedance analysis (BIA) a body-composition test based on the fact that fat tissue conducts electricity more slowly than nonfat tissue, which contains quite a bit of water; BIA equipment sends a weak electric current through the body, and the speed of the current reflects relative fatness

biomechanics the physics of movement

biomedical model of health a model of health that focuses on the physical causes and symptoms of disease and other health problems

binge eating disorder (BED) an eating disorder marked by recurrent episodes of eating very large volumes of food while feeling a lack of control over one's ability to stop eating

biopsychosocial model of health a model of health that focuses on the biological, psychological, and social components of health

bipolar disorder a disorder diagnosed when depressive symptoms alternate with periods of extremely elevated mood (mania)

blood sugar the level of glucose in the blood

body composition an estimate of the percentage of the body composed of fat tissue

body image the way in which an individual views his or her own body; the subjective evaluations of one's own physical appearance

body objectification the practice of regarding one's body, especially one's appearance, from an outsider's perspective

brain a dense concentration of nerve cells contained in the skull, which serves as the primary organ of the central nervous system

brainstem the deepest area of the brain that contains structures that automatically regulate essential life functions such as breathing, heart action, and digestion through the sympathetic and parasympathetic branches of the autonomic nervous system

brain-derived neurotrophic factor (BDNF) a protein associated with the formation of new brain cells

brown adipose tissue (BAT) a special type of fat that contains a higher density of capillaries and mitochondria than white fat

bulimia nervosa (BN) an eating disorder marked by frequent episodes of binge eating along with harmful compensatory behaviors to prevent weight gain

burnout the feeling that one does not have the resources to cope with what are perceived as excessive demands and thus feeling unable to continue in one's roles

bursa (plural, bursae) a saclike structure filled with fluid that helps reduce friction near a joint

bursitis inflammation of one or more bursae

C-reactive protein (CRP) a protein produced by the liver, whose blood level provides a reflection of a person's level of systemic inflammation

cancer a group of diseases that are characterized by uncontrolled cell growth

capillaries the smallest blood vessels

carbohydrates a large group of organic molecules that include starches, sugars, cellulose, and other types of fibers

carcinogens substances or radiation that initiates or promotes the development of cancer

cardiorespiratory system the respiratory and cardiovascular systems, which work together to supply all body cells with oxygen and nutrients and to take away the waste products of cellular metabolism

cardiovascular system a physiological system that includes the heart, blood vessels, and blood

cardiovascular exercise activities that involve movement of the large muscle groups at a moderately vigorous level, leading to a sustained elevation in metabolic rate; same as aerobic exercise

cartilage smooth tissue that covers the ends of bones where the bones come together at joints; reduces friction, facilitates movement, and protects the ends of the bones

case–control studies a type of correlational research commonly used by epidemiologists and medical researchers in which naturally occurring disease patterns are observed. In case–control studies, researchers examine people with the variable of interest, such as a certain disease. They then select a comparable group of people without the disease as the "control" group. The researchers try to match the control group to the other group on as many variables as possible, including age, gender, socioeconomic status, and so forth. The groups are then compared on a number of variables of interest to the researchers.

catecholamines a group of chemicals that function as hormones or neurotransmitters; includes epinephrine, norepinephrine, and dopamine

celiac disease a digestive disease activated by the presence of a protein called gluten that is found in wheat, rye, and barley, that triggers the immune system to attack the cells lining the small intestine

cell membrane a membrane surrounding the cell, composed primarily of fats and proteins

central nervous system branch of the nervous system that contains the brain and spinal cord

central obesity excess fat storage in the torso

cerclage a procedure in which the cervix is closed with stitches to treat a condition in which, during pregnancy, the cervix is in danger of opening prematurely, leading to a preterm delivery

cerebellum the area of the brain that aids in the regulation of movement

cerebral cortex the outer layer of the brain

cerebrum the largest brain area, consisting of two halves or hemispheres; controls and coordinates behavior and mental activities

change talk statements from clients that suggest they are, at that moment, thinking favorably about positive behavior change

chromosomes long chains of genetic material, including DNA, found in the nucleus of cells

chromatin a structure that contains DNA and other proteins in the chromosomes; influences operation of the DNA

chronic disease same as chronic illness

chronic illness illnesses that have no permanent cure, although symptoms can be managed through lifestyle changes or medical treatment

chronic lower-respiratory disease chronic diseases of the lungs

chronic obstructive pulmonary disease (COPD) the most-severe type of chronic lower-respiratory disease; involves persistent obstruction of airflow and includes emphysema and chronic bronchitis

chronic stress response repeated, long-term activation of a stress response

chronic traumatic encephalopathy (CTE) a brain disorder characterized by abnormal clumps of tau protein in the brain, resulting from a history of multiple concussions

circadian rhythm a pattern of physiological and behavioral function observed in living things that corresponds to an approximately 24-hour cycle, often influenced by the light-dark cycle of day and night

circumference the distance around a particular body part, such as the waist, hips, and upper arm

classical conditioning a learning process in animals and people in which a previously neutral stimulus is paired with naturally occurring connections between another stimulus and response. For example, a dog will naturally begin to salivate when food is presented. If a bell is repeatedly rung when food is presented, eventually the dog will learn to salivate when the bell is rung, even if no food is presented.

client-centered a behavior-change treatment philosophy that puts the client first, wherein the helping professional listens carefully to understand a client's questions and concerns and at times gives clients a choice in treatment plans

clinical inertia a state of medical practice characterized by a lack of clinically effective treatments and failure to put into practice more-effective treatment strategies

closed questions questions that elicit only brief answers, such as yes or no, and are less helpful than open questions for gathering information on specific topics

Cognitive Adaptation Model a model based on the idea that coping successfully with adversity, such as serious illness or injury, revolves around cognitive processes that lead to adaptation to one's new circumstances

cognitive-behavioral approaches behavior-change strategies that examine how people's thinking and emotional states are linked to their behavior

cognitive reappraisal seeing a stressor, such as a health problem, in a new way that makes it seem less of a threat

cognitive restructuring replacing automatic thought patterns that lead to negative emotions and unwanted behaviors with more-productive thinking

colon the last section of the digestive system that absorbs some water and a few minerals and then passes the waste to the rectum; also known as the large intestine

Common Sense Model of Illness a person's ideas about a health problem that are informed by prior knowledge and personal experience

compact bone tissue a type of bone tissue characterized by a dense network of bone cells with few spaces

competence one's feelings about ability to function in different situations; related to self-efficacy

complement a complex network of over 30 proteins in the immune system that work together and with immune cells to disable pathogens

complete proteins foods that contain all nine essential amino acids

complex carbohydrates large molecules of carbohydrate, including starches and some types of dietary fibers

concussion a brain injury that occurs as a result of shaking or hitting forces

connection the feeling of belonging to a particular group or place

consequences a component of the behavior chain; the outcome following a behavior of interest

contemplation (stage of change) one of the six stages of change in the Transtheoretical Model in which the client is beginning to think about making a change within the next 6 months

contingency management therapies use of operant conditioning principles to shape behavior, usually through the use of rewards that clients can achieve by exhibiting desirable behaviors

control group a group of subjects in a study that is compared with the treatment group(s) to observe the influence of a variable of interest. The control group typically receives a placebo treatment rather than the value of the variable thought to exert a predicted effect.

controlled motivation a type of motivation that causes an individual to perform a certain behavior because he or she is pressured to do so from external forces

coping strategies employed to deal with a source of stress or feelings of stress

coping planning devising strategies for dealing with potential barriers that might interfere with behavior-change plans

coping skills behaviors used by people to deal with difficult situations or stressors

coronary heart disease heart disease caused by insufficient circulation to the heart, which occurs because the coronary arteries have become narrowed or blocked by artery disease

correlation a statistical calculation that represents how strongly two or more variables are related to one another

corticosterone a glucocorticoid hormone released by the adrenal cortex in response to a stressor; similar to cortisol, except with no anti-inflammatory action

corticotropin-releasing hormone (CRH) a hormone secreted by the hypothalamus that stimulates the pituitary gland to release the hormone adrenocorticotropic hormone (ACTH)

cortisol a glucocorticoid hormone released by the adrenal cortex in response to a stressor; exerts an anti-inflammatory action

cortisone a glucocorticoid hormone released by the adrenal cortex in response to a stressor

counterconditioning a strategy than involves planning a new response to a problematic stimulus

craving a strong and usually uncomfortable drive to consume a given substance or participate in a given behavior

cross-stressor adaptation hypothesis an observation that those with higher fitness levels have a lower physiological response to laboratory stressors

cultural awareness recognition of external signs that indicate another person may be from a different cultural background

cultural competence possessing the knowledge and skills necessary to interact with people from other cultures in culturally appropriate ways

cultural sensitivity awareness of other people's cultural differences, accompanied by behavior that attempts not to offend others

cytokines small proteins released by immune cells that allow these cells to communicate with other immune cells and a variety of cells and tissues

decisional balance the idea that as people move through the stages of change, the way they feel about the behavior will change, and the balance of positive and negative thoughts associated with the behavior may shift in ways that lead to a decision to change

dementia a group of nervous system disorders marked by memory impairment and also by an extreme decline in mental abilities such as judgment and abstract thinking as well as changes in personality

density weight per unit volume

deoxyribonucleic acid (DNA) genetic material that serves as a master plan for all proteins the body needs to make

dependent variable the outcome variable of interest in an experiment that is thought to be influenced by or related to another variable, called the independent variable

depression a mood disorder marked by feelings of sadness, guilt, loss, hopelessness, and low energy level, along with physical symptoms such as change in appetite or sleep habits

detoxification the initial stage of abstinence from an addictive substance, during which the person addicted may experience a number of physical and psychological withdrawal effects

diabetes a disorder marked by poor blood sugar regulation, resulting in elevated levels of resting blood sugar

dichotomous thinking an irrational thought pattern that offers only two possible categorizations, such as foods being either "good" or "bad" or that a person is either "on the diet" or "off the diet"

diencephalon a region of the brain that is primarily made up of the thalamus, hypothalamus, and pineal gland

dietary fiber structures that come primarily from plants and are not broken down by the digestive system

dietary restraint a type of self-control related to regulating food intake

disability a type of physical, mental, or emotional impairment that limits normal function

disaccharides simple carbohydrates that contain two small sugar units

disinhibited eating a lack of dietary restraint, where people feel unable to control how much they eat

diverse an adjective describing groups of people (or other things) that are different from each other on various dimensions, such as cultural background, age, ethnicity, sport background, gender identity, health status, economic status, and other qualities

diverticulitis a digestive disorder characterized by inflammation and infection in the colon caused by trapped particles of feces

docosahexaenoic acid (DHA) a long-chain, omega-3 fatty acid associated with beneficial health effects, found in fish oils

double-blind study a scientific experiment in which neither the experimenters running the tests nor the participants themselves know who is receiving the experimental or placebo treatment

dual-energy x-ray absorptiometry a technology that uses two x-ray energies to measure bone density and body composition, used to assess body composition primarily in research settings

dualism the notion that the body and mind are separate entities

dynamic stretching flexibility training that involves slow movement from one stretching position to another

dynapenia the loss of muscle strength and power that occurs with aging

dysthymic disorder a chronic, less-intense form of depression; less disabling than major depression; causes a person to feel unwell or to function at less-than-optimal levels; also known as dysthymia

ecological perspective a view of health and health behaviors that considers health behaviors as a function of individuals and the environments in which they live, including the people, organizations, communities, and cultural and societal forces around them

efferent nervous system the branch of the nervous system that carries messages between the brain and the rest of the body

eicosapentaenoic acid (EPA) a long-chain omega-3 fatty acid associated with beneficial health effects, found in fish oils

embolus a blood clot that moves through the bloodstream until it becomes lodged and blocks circulation

emotion short-lived feelings experienced in response to a specific stimulus, including one's thoughts

emotion-focused coping measures that do not directly change or eliminate the source of stress but instead are focused on changing the way the person feels and reducing the stress response

emphysema a disease condition of the lungs characterized by the progressive destruction of the alveoli and eventually the collapse of the respiratory bronchioles

emulsify to break large globules of fat into smaller particles in order to increase the surface area of the fat exposed to digestive enzymes

endocannabinoids a family of endogenous cannabinoid compounds

endogenous produced within the body

endorphins short for "endogenous morphine"; neurotransmitter molecules found in the central nervous system that are similar in structure to exogenous opiates (e.g., opium and morphine) and exert opiate-like effects, including pain reduction

energy balance the relationship between energy taken in (eaten) and energy expended (burned)

energy density calories per unit weight of food

enteric nervous system a branch of the nervous system that governs the function of the gastrointestinal system

environmental reengineering changing surroundings in ways that promote (or at least do not inhibit) desirable behaviors

epidemiology the study of patterns of health and disease within groups of people and the factors associated with disease patterns

epigenetics the study of the mechanisms by which genes are expressed and the many factors that influence genetic expression

epinephrine a hormone that mimics the action of the sympathetic nervous system by increasing heart rate (HR) and the contractile force of the heart, increasing blood pressure, dilating the airways, and increasing the airflow to the lungs

epiphanies sudden insights, revelations, or understandings

ergometer a stationary piece of exercise equipment on which researchers can apply a very precise workload

esophagus a muscular, tube-shaped organ that carries food from the mouth to the stomach

essential amino acids amino acids that must be obtained from the diet

essential body fat the minimal amount of body fat required for normal functioning

essential fatty acids fatty acids that must be provided by the diet

ethnicity cultural background, defined by factors such as language, country of origin, religion, family ethnic identification, or other cultural categories

euphoria feelings of intense happiness or well-being

eumenorrhea normal menstrual cycle

eustress stressors and situations that evoke the stress response but are experienced as positive

executive function processes that are involved in future-oriented behavior, such as planning, multitasking, setting priorities, and coping with distractions

exercise a type of physical activity performed with the intention of improving physical fitness and/or sport performance

exercise adherence sticking to an exercise program

exercise duration how long an exercise activity lasts, typically measured in seconds, minutes, and hours

exercise frequency how often an exercise activity is performed, typically measured in sessions per day, week, or month

exercise intensity the level of physical exertion experienced by a person performing an exercise activity

exercise mode the type of physical activity performed, such as cycling, swimming, or running

exercise physiology the study of the physiological response of the body to physical activity in health and disease

exercise psychology the study of the psychological factors related to the performance of exercise and physical activity

exercise volume total quantity of exercise performed; often expressed in units of energy expenditure, such as kJ or kcals

exocrine organs glands that release hormones to their target organs via ducts

expectancies the values people place on their expectations

expectations what people think is going to happen in a given situation, such as when beginning an exercise program

external regulation behaviors that occur as a result of outside pressures

extrinsic motivation the pursuit of an activity to achieve a desired outcome as opposed to engaging in the activity because it is inherently enjoyable

faith-placed programs behavior-change programs that provide spiritual reinforcement for behavior change, take place in a religious setting, and are organized and run with significant involvement of a faith group

false hope theory a theory that describes how people with unrealistically high expectations are motivated to make resolutions to change but are then likely to relapse once their expectations are unmet

fast-twitch glycolytic (FG) muscle fibers (type IIB) a muscle fiber type that is larger than slow-twitch oxidative fibers and is capable of producing more force faster; relies on anaerobic energy systems to produce energy quickly

fast-twitch oxidative-glycolytic (FOG) muscle fibers (type IIA) an intermediate muscle fiber type that contracts quickly but has greater endurance than the fast-twitch glycolytic muscle fibers; can produce energy from both anaerobic and aerobic pathways

fat-free mass (FFM) the portion of the body composed of tissue other than fat

fat mass (FM) the portion of the body composed of fat tissue

female athlete triad a syndrome affecting females that includes three concurrent conditions: disordered eating, amenorrhea, and osteoporosis

fetal alcohol spectrum disorders a wide range of physical, behavioral, and cognitive abnormalities caused by exposure to alcohol during fetal development

fitness general good health and physical condition

flexibility the range of motion (ROM) around a joint

flexibility training the performance of activities designed to increase flexibility (the ROM around joints)

flow an enjoyable state of consciousness characterized by feeling totally engaged and at one with an activity

food allergy an immune system allergic response that occurs soon after the ingestion of a specific food

food intolerance a condition in which the ingestion of a certain food or food component creates uncomfortable digestive symptoms, such as bloating or diarrhea

food sensitivity a condition in which people find that certain foods "disagree" with them, causing difficulty digesting the food or a stomachache after that food has been eaten; similar to but less severe than a food intolerance

the French paradox the observation that even though French cuisine is high in fat and calories, the French people generally have much lower rates of obesity and heart disease than people in the United States

fructose a monosaccharide that is a component of sucrose and occurs naturally in other sugars, including the sugars found in fruits

functional connectivity a term describing the coordination of various cognitive processes in order to accomplish complex cognitive tasks

functional fitness training exercise training that employs motor skills such as agility, balance, and coordination in exercises designed to improve daily functional ability and reduce risk of falling and fear of falling in older adults and those with limited fitness

functional magnetic resonance imaging (fMRI) an imaging technique that measures blood flow to the different areas of the brain, mapping which areas become active under certain conditions

gall bladder an organ that stores the bile manufactured by the liver and secretes the bile into the small intestine when the presence of fat is detected

gastrin a hormone produced by specialized cells in the stomach that helps to regulate the production and secretion of stomach acid

gastroesophageal reflux disease (GERD) a disorder in which acidic stomach contents back up into the esophagus, causing pain, irritation, and erosion of the esophageal lining

generalized anxiety disorder a mood disorder characterized by frequent experiences of fear; excessive fear about a variety of situations; and feeling unable to control feelings of fear

genes units of DNA that lie in specific locations on the chromosomes; associated with inherited traits in living organisms

ghrelin a hormone that stimulates feelings of hunger and the drive to eat

gingivitis a gum disease characterized by inflammation and bleeding of gum tissue

glands groups of specialized hormone-producing cells

glucagon a hormone released by the pancreas that signals the liver to break down glycogen and release glucose into the bloodstream

glucocorticoids a class of steroid hormones released from the adrenal cortex involved in the metabolism of carbohydrates, fats, and proteins and in helping to regulate energy production

glucose a monosaccharide that is the primary source of energy for the body

gluten a protein found in wheat, rye, and barley

glycemic index a measure of how quickly the carbohydrate in food is digested and absorbed into the bloodstream as glucose

glycemic load the glycemic index of a food multiplied by its grams of carbohydrate, then divided by 100; compared to glycemic index, glycemic load is a better measure of a given food's actual impact on blood sugar

glycogen a form of starch manufactured by animals, including humans, consisting of large chains of glucose; stored primarily in the liver and in skeletal muscles

goal intentions decisions to work toward a goal

Golgi complex a cellular organelle that receives most of the proteins processed by the rough endoplasmic reticulum for further processing and makes molecules that will be secreted by its cell

gonadotropin-inhibiting hormone (GnIH) a hormone that inhibits reproductive function

gonadotropin-releasing hormone (GnRH) a hormone that drives the reproductive system in both sexes

green exercise physical activities that incorporate elements of nature into their environment, especially outdoor exercise

hardiness a model of resilience or stress resistance characterized by control, commitment, and challenge

harm reduction a guiding goal of many behavior-change efforts, acknowledging that total abstinence from a substance or behavior by everyone in the target audience may be an unrealistic goal; therefore, efforts are made to at least reduce the harm accrued by use of the substance or participation in that behavior

health "a state of complete physical, mental and social well-being and not merely the absence of disease or infirmity" (as defined by the World Health Organization)

health behavior related to or affecting health; same as health-related behavior

Health Belief Model a model that describes how people's ideas and underlying emotions about illnesses, prevention, and treatment may influence health behaviors and decisions about health behaviors. The Health Belief Model has at least four variables that help to explain how people make decisions about behavior change: perceived susceptibility to illness, perceived seriousness of illness, perceived benefits of a health behavior, and perceived barriers to a health behavior (see Fig. 4-4). The first two variables involve the individual's beliefs about a health threat. The second two variables reflect the individual's beliefs about the health behavior that could reduce the threat.

health locus of control the extent to which individuals feel that their health is either under their own control or controlled by outside forces, including other people or chance

health promotion activities and programs designed to change behaviors in ways that are likely to lead to better health outcomes

health psychology an area of psychology concerned with the interactions of thoughts, emotions, and behavior with health and illness conditions and experiences

health-related behavior behavior related to or affecting health; same as health behavior

heartburn a condition that occurs when the sphincter located between the esophagus and the stomach relaxes and allows the acidic contents of the stomach to enter the esophagus and produce a burning sensation

hedonic hotspots groups of neurons that help to produce sensations of pleasure when stimulated

hemoconcentration the increased concentration of blood that results as fluid is removed from the circulatory system

hemoglobin the substance responsible for binding oxygen and carbon dioxide in the red blood cells

hemorrhagic stroke when a blood vessel in the brain bursts and disrupts normal circulation

hepatocellular carcinoma liver cancer

high-density lipoprotein (HDL) one variety of lipoproteins, large compounds that carry cholesterol and fat in the bloodstream; higher HDL levels are associated with lower risk of artery disease

hippocampus an area of the brain that plays important roles in memory formation

holistic health a concept of health stating that health involves more than the physical body; it encompasses not only body, mind, and community but other realms of life as well, including spiritual well-being

homeostasis the ability of organisms to maintain the stability of variables such as body temperature, blood glucose level, and water balance

hormone a chemical produced by the endocrine system that conveys messages by binding to receptors located on the membranes of target cells

humanism a movement in the development of the field of psychology that focuses on and emphasizes the conscious experience of human beings. The humanist psychologists believe that behavior is more than a conditioned response shaped by reward and punishment and that human beings possess free will and the ability to make decisions. Carl Rogers and Abraham Maslow are two of the best-known humanist psychologists.

hunger the biological drive to eat

hydrochloric acid a chemical manufactured and secreted by special cells in the stomach lining that creates the extremely acidic environment in the stomach that aids in the digestion of food

hydrogenation a process used by food product manufacturers to make fatty acids in foods more saturated, leading to greater stability and a longer shelf life

hydrometry a method of estimating body composition from calculation of total body water, based on the observation that water content differs for fat and fat-free mass. The higher the water content for a given body size, the greater the relative amount of fat-free mass.

hydrostatic weighing a method of estimating body composition by calculating body density from the weight of a person in water; same as underwater weighing

hypertension high blood pressure, a condition diagnosed when the resting pressure inside the arteries is too high according to diagnostic criteria

hypertrophy a process in which an organ, such as a muscle, experiences an increase in size

hypothalamic-pituitary-adrenal (HPA) axis a communication pathway comprised of hormonal messages sent from the hypothalamus to the pituitary gland and then from the pituitary gland to the adrenal cortex

hypothalamus an important control center for many physiological functions; controls the autonomic nervous system, regulates the pituitary gland, and secretes several hormones and other chemical factors

hypothesis a prediction made in a scientific study before data are collected, describing the expected relationship among two or more variables of interest

identified regulation self-management that occurs when people identify with the goal or value of the behavior, especially when the goal achieved by the behavior in question is valued; a type of motivation

illness a state of poor health, often including symptoms indicating suboptimal function of an organ or physiological system

illness representation a person's ideas about a particular health problem

immune system a network of cells spread throughout the body that carry on extensive communication to coordinate proteins, cells, tissues, and organs in various parts of the body; coordinates the body's efforts to protect itself against pathogens

implementation intentions commitment to a specific action plan or plans for behavior change

incomplete proteins protein foods lacking one or more essential amino acids

independent variable the variable of interest in an experiment that is thought to influence or be related to another variable, called the dependent variable

induced menopause cessation of the menstrual cycle that occurs when the ovaries are removed surgically or are inhibited from producing hormones through the use of medication

inflammation a response mounted by the immune system in response to an injury; symptoms include redness and swelling, caused by increased blood flow and the migration of phagocytes to the injured area

inflammatory bowel disease (IBD) a group of disorders characterized by the inflammation of the colon with symptoms such as abdominal pain, and blood (produced by bleeding ulcers present on the colon) and mucus in the stools

injury harm to a body part caused by a force such as trauma or overuse

innate immunity the mechanisms by which the body protects itself from pathogens, such as the barriers provided by the skin and mucous membranes that keep out pathogens; its mechanisms act against all pathogens, rather than a specific variety of pathogen

innervated to have nerve input from

insomnia the inability to get an adequate amount of good quality sleep

insulin a hormone released by the pancreas which reduces blood glucose levels by signaling cells to take up glucose from the blood

insulin resistant the inability of cells to respond appropriately to the hormone insulin, as observed in type 2 diabetes mellitus

integrated regulation a type of motivation characterized by the goal or value of a behavior becoming a part of an individual's personal values, resulting in the adjustment of behavior to pursue the goal (thus a form of autonomous motivation); the behavior has become integrated into a person's self-concept

interferons proteins that spread into neighboring cells, stimulating them to produce proteins that block the process of viral replication, thus limiting damage from invading viruses

interval training a form of exercise in which short bursts of high-intensity anaerobic exercise are combined with longer periods of aerobic exercise or rest that allow the muscles time to recover

intervertebral discs fibrocartilaginous structures with a soft, shock-absorbing interior

intramuscular triglycerides (IMTG) fat found in muscle tissue

intrinsic motivation the pursuit of an activity because it is inherently interesting or enjoyable

introjected regulation motivation that results when people feel obliged to perform a particular behavior, not from a personal desire to perform it

irisin a myokine that initiates the change of white adipose tissue to brown adipose tissue

irritable bowel syndrome (IBS) a digestive disorder of the lower intestinal tract marked by pain and irregular bowel movements

ischemic stroke brain damage caused by a lack of blood flow to a region of the brain, caused by a blockage in an artery, typically associated with artery disease

islets of Langerhans specialized regions of the pancreas that produce hormones, including insulin and glucagon

joint a point of connection between bones or, in some cases, between bones and cartilage

joint capsule a fibrous structure attached to the bones of a joint that completely encloses the joint and whose lining generates synovial fluid, a thin, viscous fluid that lubricates the joint structures

lactose intolerance a food intolerance in which people lack or have low levels of the enzyme lactase, which is required to break down the milk sugar lactose

learned helplessness a psychological state in which people have come to believe that they are helpless in, or have no power or control over, certain situations

learning style differences variations in the way people process and retain new information

leptin a hormone that informs the body, including the brain, about total fat stores and helps regulate other bodily functions

leukocytes immune cells that circulate throughout the body in the blood vessels and lymphatic system, also known as white blood cells; these cells help the immune system protect the body from pathogens

ligaments strong, fibrous tissue structures that connect bones to each other and help form joints

limbic system the area of the brain that lies above and around the brainstem and is involved with motivation, emotion, and memory; includes part of the cerebral cortex as well as other areas, such as the hippocampus and the amygdala

liver cirrhosis the replacement of healthy liver tissue with collagen scar tissue, thus leading to a decline in liver function

locus of control the extent to which people think things happen for internal versus external reasons

loving kindness meditation a type of meditation designed to evoke feelings of compassionate, positive regard for others

low-density lipoprotein (LDL) one variety of lipoproteins, large compounds that carry cholesterol and fat in the bloodstream; higher LDL levels are associated with higher risk of artery disease

lymphatic system the physiological system that contains high concentrations of immune cells that guard the body from infection

lymphocytes one group of leukocytes that fall into two categories: the B lymphocytes and the T lymphocytes

macrominerals minerals such as calcium, phosphorus, and magnesium, which are needed in relatively large quantities (compared to other minerals) to sustain normal bodily function

maintenance (stage of change) one of the six stages of change in which the client is actively engaged in the continuation of a behavior change; the new behavior has lasted longer than 6 months

major depressive disorder a mood disorder diagnosed when a person shows at least five depression symptoms as defined by clinical criteria, symptoms have continued for at least 2 weeks, and the person has experienced a change in ability to function in daily life

maladaptive coping responses coping responses that may produce desirable short-term results but cause more stress or health problems in the future

mastery experience a situation in which a person feels successful at performing, or mastering, a given task

maximal heart rate the highest number of beats per minute a person's or animal's heart can achieve during maximal activity

medial prefrontal cortex (MPFC) the area of the brain believed to exert inhibitory control over the amygdala, in order to help people appropriately regulate their emotional responsiveness

melatonin a hormone produced by the pineal gland that increases with exposure to darkness, enhances sleep, and helps to regulate the body's biological clock

menopause the cessation of the menstrual cycle in women that occurs when the ovaries decrease their production of the sex hormones estrogen and progesterone

menopause transition the years leading up to menopause, during which symptoms such as irregular menstrual cycles, hot flashes, and mood swings may develop; also known as perimenopause

mesolimbic dopaminergic pathway the reward pathway involving dopamine located in the central portion of the brain's limbic system

MET the abbreviation for metabolic equivalent, a measure of exercise intensity that allows for comparison of people of different sizes; one MET is equivalent to the number of calories burned at rest

meta-analysis statistical procedure that combines the data from several studies into one large analysis to get a clearer picture of the relationship between two or more variables

metabolic rate the energy expenditure required to sustain metabolism in a given period of time, usually expressed as calories or kilojoules per hour

metabolism the entire collection of biochemical processes that occur in the body, many of which require energy

microbiome the total collection of microbes living in a defined environment. The human microbione refers to the collection of microbes that live in and on the human body. These microbes include bacteria, viruses, and other single-cell organisms.

microbiota a group of microbes, microscopic living organisms

migraine headache a type of head pain caused by pressure and pain precipitated by vascular changes that lead to increased blood volume in the blood vessels of the head

mindful eating a present-moment, nonjudgmental awareness of the physical and emotional experience of eating

mineralocorticoids a class of steroid hormones released from the adrenal cortex involved with maintaining electrolyte balance

mitochondria specialized energy-producing organelles contained in cells

model a representation, usually a simplification, of a subject of interest

monosaccharides small sugar units, two of which combine to form a disaccharide

monounsaturated fatty acids fatty acids with one carbon-carbon double bond

mood a lasting emotional state

morbidity illness

mortality death

motivational interviewing a treatment philosophy and a set of strategies to help people increase their own internal drive to change

motor learning the process of motor skill acquisition and performance

motor neurons the neurons that carry messages to the skeletal muscles

motor unit one motor neuron plus the muscle fibers that it innervates

multifactorial characterized by many factors contributing to the development of a phenomenon, such as an illness

muscle dysmorphia an abnormal preoccupation with the appearance of ones muscles

muscle fibers specialized cells containing proteins that slide into one another to produce a shortening of the cell that results in muscular contraction

musculoskeletal system the physiological system comprised of the bones, muscles, and joint structures

myocardial infarction a heart attack, usually caused when blockage occurs in an artery of the heart

myokines peptide molecules released by the muscles that communicate with cells in other parts of the body

natural menopause menopause that occurs when the ovaries naturally decrease their sex hormone production as women age

negative energy balance a physiological state in which more energy is expended than taken in

nervous system one of the physiological systems that connect the body and mind, composed of the central nervous system and the peripheral nervous system; made up of nervous tissue that transmits impulses that enable communication between cells

nervous tissue collections of specialized cells that support communication between nerve cells and communication between the brain and the rest of the body

net endogenous acid production (NEAP) a factor that reflects how the digestion of foods affects the body's acid-base balance

neurogenesis formation of new neurons from stem cells or precursor cells

neuroglia cells that support and nourish the neurons, maintaining a good environment for neuron function

neuromotor exercise training exercise training that employs motor skills such as agility, balance, and coordination in exercises designed to improve daily functional ability and, in people with limited fitness, reduce risk of falling and fear of falling; also known as functional fitness training

neuromuscular exercise training same as neuromotor exercise training and functional fitness training

neurons cells designed to communicate with one another by sending electrical signals to adjacent neurons. Neurons are capable of activating muscles, other organs, and glands; carrying information from the sensory organs, such as the eyes and ears, to the brain; and carrying out psychological functions such as thinking and remembering.

neuroscience a specialized area of study of the structure and function of the brain and nervous system

neurotransmitters special chemicals released by communicating neurons which travel across the minute space between the two cells (synaptic cleft); they enable one cell to influence the behavior of the adjacent cell receiving the neurotransmitter

nitric oxide (NO) a compound that performs a variety of helpful roles in the body and is important for the normal function of arteries

nitric oxide synthase an enzyme that stimulates the lining of arteries to manufacture nitric oxide

nocebo effect an effect that occurs when people develop negative outcomes to a treatment because they believe a negative outcome will result, after a clinician or researcher has suggested such outcomes might occur

nonalcoholic fatty liver disease a disorder in which excess fatty deposits occur in the liver with little or no intake of alcohol

nonessential amino acids amino acids that can be manufactured by the body

nonexercise activity thermogenesis (NEAT) physical activities that expend energy but do not fall into the categories of sleeping, eating, or exercise

norepinephrine a hormone that mimics the action of the sympathetic nervous system by increasing HR and contractile force of the heart, increasing blood pressure, dilating the airways, and increasing breathing rate and airflow to the lungs

normal-weight obesity a condition of normal body mass index occurring with a lack of muscle size and strength and excess adipose tissue that is accompanied by the same health risks as standard obesity

nucleus an organelle that contains the cell's genetic material

nucleus accumbens a group of neurons in the limbic system that receives projections from the ventral tegmental area; stimulation of this area is associated with feelings of pleasure

nutrient a substance in food that is required for growth and maintenance of the body or has the chemical bonds that supply the energy that is captured and used by the cells for fuel

nutrient density the nutritive value per calorie of a given food

nutrition the process of nourishing the body with food; the study of this process

oligomenorrhea a condition in which a female has fewer than the normal number of menstrual periods or abnormally light menstrual blood flow but some menstrual cycle activity

omega-3 fatty acids fatty acids with a carbon-carbon double bond located at the third carbon from the methyl end of the fatty acid

omega-6 fatty acids fatty acids with a carbon-carbon double bond found at the sixth carbon from the methyl end of the fatty acid

open questions questions that invite clients to provide more information, tell their stories, and paint a broader picture of issues under discussion; also called open-ended questions

operant conditioning a learning situation in which voluntary behavior is shaped by punishments and rewards delivered after a behavior occurs

opiates drugs derived from the poppy flower or synthetically produced drugs similar in structure to natural opiates, including opium, heroin, morphine, and cocaine

organ a functional group of tissues, such as the stomach, brain, and so forth

organelles specialized structures inside each cell

orthorexia a higher-than-normal concern with dietary perfection

osteoarthritis a disorder that affects the cartilage that covers the ends of the bones in a joint

osteoblasts specialized bone cells that build new bone and eventually become bone cells (osteocytes) in the bony matrix

osteoclasts specialized bone cells that help break down bone tissue to enhance the remodeling of the bones in response to the forces being placed on them and to release minerals into the bloodstream

osteocytes bone cells

osteons arrangements of different types of bone cells around a central canal occupied by blood and lymphatic vessels and nerves, which supply the bone with nutrients and deliver hormones and peptide messengers that help to direct bone activity

osteoporosis a disease characterized by progressive loss of bone mineral

outcome expectancies what people think will happen if they engage in a given behavior

oxytocin a hormone released from the pituitary gland that raises blood pressure by contracting arteries; also associated with feelings of emotional closeness

pancreas an organ located near the junction of the stomach and small intestine that secretes sodium bicarbonate, digestive enzymes, and hormones that regulate blood sugar level

pancreatitis inflammation of the pancreas

panic disorder a psychological disorder characterized by the experience of panic attacks, which are short, intense periods of fear, marked by a strong fight-or-flight response, with a rapid, pounding HR, and often sweating, trembling, and nausea

parasympathetic nervous system (PNS) the branch of the autonomic nervous system associated with the optimal activity of resting functions, including digestion and reproduction

passive static stretching a form of flexibility training that involves holding a stretching position for 10 seconds or more, gradually increasing the stretch placed on the muscle group

pathogenic capable of causing harm

pathogenic weight control weight-control practices that can be harmful to physical and psychological health

pathogens invaders such as viruses, bacteria, fungi, and other agents that can cause harm to an organism

patient-centered treatment a treatment philosophy that puts the patient first in which the helping professional listens carefully to understand a patient's questions and concerns and at times gives patients a choice in treatment plans

patient inertia a situation characterized by a patient's failure to make behavior changes that may aid in recovery, often associated with feelings of hopelessness and low self-efficacy for following treatment recommendations

pedometer a device that provides an indication of exercise volume by counting the number of steps taken within a period of time

peer review process a process used by academic journals in which scientific experts in the subject area scrutinize an article or research report to be sure the authors measured what they thought they were measuring, that the statistical methods were used appropriately, and that the conclusions are sound. Results of a study are not accepted by the scientific community until the report of the findings has gone through the peer review process and been accepted for publication.

perceived behavioral control similar to self-efficacy; people's beliefs about their own ability to engage in a specific task or behavior

perimenopause the years leading up to menopause, during which symptoms such as irregular menstrual cycles, hot flashes, and mood swings may develop

peripheral nervous system the branch of the nervous system consisting of the nerves that spread from the spinal cord to all parts of the body

peripheral resistance the amount of resistance to blood flow in the arterial system; increases when arteries constrict, thus reducing the area through which the blood is flowing

peristalsis the slow wave contractions produced by the smooth muscles of the digestive system that move food along the gastrointestinal tract

personality the distinctive qualities of character that can be used to describe individuals' patterns of thinking and behavior

phagocytes a group of leukocytes that attack and break down invading organisms

phobia a type of anxiety disorder marked by excessive fear of something not regarded by most people as worthy of excessive fear, such as spiders, exams, or snakes

physical activity any bodily movement, especially movement involving large muscle groups, and elevated energy expenditure

pineal gland a gland located deep in the brain that secretes the hormone melatonin

pituitary gland a gland located in the middle of the base of the brain, which releases a number of important hormones that help to regulate key bodily processes; often called "the master gland"

placebo a dummy condition that closely matches the treatment condition but lacks the ingredient believed to be exerting an effect

placebo effect when subjects in a study may demonstrate changes in the dependent variable simply because they are getting attention or expecting an effect

placenta previa during pregnancy, a medical condition in which the placenta is located near or on top of the cervix, often leading to bleeding and preterm labor

planning fallacy the natural tendency of people to underestimate the time, money, and energy required to accomplish their goals

plaque the material that accumulates in and upon the artery lining from the process of atherosclerosis

plasma the liquid portion of the blood

platelets components of the blood that facilitate the blood-clotting process

polyunsaturated fatty acids fatty acids that have more than one carbon-carbon double bond

positive energy balance a situation in which more energy is consumed than expended

positive reappraisal changing the way a stressor is viewed to make it appear less stressful

postmenopausal an adjective describing women who have already gone through the menopause transition

postsynaptic neuron the neuron on the side of a synapse that is receiving the neurotransmitter

postural muscles muscles of the lower and upper back, shoulders, neck, and face that enable the body to remain upright when sitting, standing, and moving

poverty-obesity paradox the observation that despite having fewer resources, people living with the conditions created by poverty in the richer countries have higher rates of obesity

preconscious processes memories and feelings that people may not currently be aware of but that they can remember and which can influence their thoughts and feelings

precontemplation (stage of change) stage in which clients are not ready to change or even thinking about changing their behavior

premenopausal an adjective describing women who have not yet reached menopause

preparation (stage of change) one of the six stages of change in which the client is making small attempts at behavior change and plans to make a full change within the next 30 days

presynaptic neuron the neuron on the side of a synapse that is releasing the neurotransmitter

primary exercise addiction exercise addiction that occurs without other symptoms of eating disorders

primary prevention a way of addressing health behaviors before people become ill

probiotics beneficial bacteria often found in the gastrointestinal tract

problem-focused coping strategies implemented during times of stress that are designed to change or eliminate the source of stress or to deal with the problem directly

product goal a goal that involves a measurable change in a physical parameter, such as weight or strength

process goal a goal that can be reached by simply performing a given activity, such as completing an exercise session or not smoking on a given day

processes of change activities and events that contribute to successful behavior modification

progressive relaxation a relaxation technique designed by Edmund Jacobson that involves alternately tensing and relaxing each muscle group, one group at a time, to induce feelings of relaxation

proprioceptive neuromuscular facilitation (PNF) a form of flexibility training with many variations, most of which involve first isometrically contracting the muscle group to be stretched and then following the contraction with a static stretch for the same muscle group; sometimes called contract-relax stretching. Force is applied to enhance the stretch either by the person stretching or another person trained in this method.

proprioceptors receptors that send information about the internal environment and the body's position in space to the central nervous system

prospective a type of research study that gathers data about variables in the present time and continues collecting data over time

protein compounds composed of amino acids

psychology the scientific study of the mind and particularly thoughts, emotions, and behavior

psychoneuroimmunology a field that studies the interrelationships of the immune system, the nervous system, and the endocrine system as they serve as communication networks in the maintenance of health

psychophysiology the study of physiology as it relates to thoughts, emotions, and behaviors

psychosomatic having both mental (psycho) and physical (somatic) causes

punch-drunk syndrome the term for boxers who show cognitive decline

punishment conditioning applied to behaviors that an individual wants to decrease in frequency

precontemplation one of the six stages of change in which the client is not ready to change and is not even thinking about making any kind of change in the near future

qualitative research methods research that typically collects and analyzes non-numerical data on a small group of participants. Researchers may interview people extensively, asking open-ended questions to probe deeply into why they think, feel, or act in certain ways. Even though statistical analyses are not usually performed, researchers using qualitative methods still strive for empirical rigor by combing their data in established ways for patterns and themes.

quality of life an individual's state of well-being as perceived subjectively by that person

race groups defined by physically visible differences that are biologically inherited, such as skin color and type of hair

random assignment a process of assigning subjects in an experimental study to treatment groups in which each subject has the same chance of getting into a given group

rapport a relationship based on mutual understanding and trust

rating of perceived exertion (RPE) a subjective perception of an individual's effort, often measured using the Borg Scale

readiness how willing and prepared a person is to change a given behavior

receptor sites molecular sites in the cell membrane to which signaling molecules may bind

recruitment a term pinpointing which motor units are activated (caused to contract) by the nervous system

rectum the terminal portion of the colon that receives digestive waste and stores it until elimination

red bone marrow tissue that produces red blood cells, white blood cells, and platelets

reflective listening active listening combined with verbal and nonverbal responses to indicate interest and understanding and to encourage the speaker to continue

reflexive unconscious and automatic responses that occur with classical conditioning

registered dietitian a licensed professional who specializes in nutrition and health

reinforcement conditioning applied to behaviors an individual wants to increase in frequency

relapse a condition in which a person resumes unwanted behavior patterns that he or she has been attempting to change

relaxation response the feeling of relaxation that occurs with parasympathetic nervous system activation; also refers to a relaxation technique developed by Herbert Benson that involves repeating a soothing word with each exhalation in order to induce feelings of relaxation

religion a set of beliefs, values, and practices related to belief in a higher power and usually based on the teachings of a spiritual leader

repetitions (reps) the number of times a given exercise is performed

resilience a state of successful adaptation to stressful events and circumstances

respiratory system the physiological system composed of the organs that provide for the exchange of oxygen and carbon dioxide

resting metabolic rate (RMR) energy expenditure at rest measured with subject in a seated position

reticular formation (RF) a major communication pathway between the brain and the rest of the body that runs through the middle of the brainstem up into the diencephalon

retrospective a type of research study that gathers data about variables that occurred in the past, relying on people's memory of the value of these variables (which is not always accurate)

reward pathway the anatomic locations and biochemical events that make up the mind-body's experience of pleasure

rheumatoid arthritis an autoimmune condition in which immune cells attack the joint lining, producing inflammation and pain

ribosome an organelle that makes proteins needed by the cell and for specialized functions

risk factors variables that help to predict the likelihood of an event or the development of a health problem

rough endoplasmic reticulum an organelle that sorts and processes proteins with other substances to make larger molecules such as neurotransmitters

saliva a watery fluid secreted by the salivary glands that moistens food, making it easier to swallow

sarcopenia a loss of muscle mass

sarcopenic obesity excess body fat accompanied by a loss of lean body mass

satiety feeling like one has had enough to eat

saturated fatty acids fatty acids in which the bonds between carbon atoms are all single

scaling rating a variable on a numerical scale, such as a scale from 1 to 10

scientific method the process of observing, thinking logically, predicting relationships, experimenting to test ideas, measuring variables, evaluating data, and drawing conclusions about the relationships among variables of interest

screen use the time spent viewing or using electronic devices such as televisions, computers, cell phones, and video games

seasonal affective disorder (SAD) a type of depression that typically occurs during the winter months

secondary exercise addiction excessive exercise that occurs as part of a larger constellation of disordered eating behaviors

secondary screening a way of addressing health behaviors early in an illness when the problem is most treatable

self-concept the way in which an individual perceives or defines himself or herself

self-confidence the extent to which an individual feels likely to perform well in a given situation

self-control the control people exert over their thoughts, feelings, and behaviors; similar to self-regulation

Self-Determination Theory a theory described by Edward Deci and Richard Ryan that discusses autonomy, competence, and connection as the three primary factors that guide human development and influence motivation

self-disclosure sharing personal thoughts and experiences and, in the process, revealing more about oneself

self-efficacy the degree to which an individual believes that she or he can successfully perform a task or behavior

self-esteem an individual's evaluation and judgment about his or her self-concept

self-management managing one's thoughts, feelings, and behaviors

self-medication use of drugs, alcohol, or tobacco to reduce emotional distress

self-monitoring behavior-change methods in which clients keep records of their activities and progress as related to behavioral change

self-regulation the control people exert over their thoughts, feelings, and behaviors; similar to self-control

set one series of exercises

sex-specific fat adipose tissue stores found in females, related primarily to reproductive functions and found mostly in the breasts, hips, and thighs

shaping a plan to reinforce the new, desired behavior by adjusting a behavior chain

sickness behavior a cluster of symptoms that accompany illness, including weakness, difficulty concentrating, depressed mood, lethargy, and loss of appetite, which serve an adaptive purpose during an acute illness or injury, leading individuals to rest and recover, but which can be maladaptive for people trying to cope with chronic illness or injury

simple carbohydrates relatively small molecules of carbohydrate, including the disaccharides, found naturally in fruits, vegetables, and milk

skinfold thickness the thickness of the skin and layer of subcutaneous fat as it is pulled away from the underlying muscle

slow-twitch oxidative (SO) muscle fiber (type I) a muscle fiber type that is recruited for aerobic exercise, activity requiring a sustained elevation of metabolic rate and muscle contraction. These muscle fibers are somewhat slower in contractile speed, somewhat lower in force production, but more resistant to fatigue than other types; they rely on oxygen to produce energy.

smooth endoplasmic reticulum an organelle that makes fatty acids and hormones such as estrogen and testosterone

social control efforts to motivate other people to change their behavior

social psychology a field of study in which psychologists investigate how people form relationships with one another and behave in groups

social support any behavior on the part of other people that helps a person achieve his or her goals and objectives

sociology the study of social structure and function

somatic nervous system a branch of the efferent nervous system that sends impulses from the central nervous system to skeletal muscles

sphincter a tight band of muscle that can open and close. For example, the lower esophageal sphincter, located between the esophagus and the stomach, opens to allow food to pass into the stomach and then closes to prevent stomach contents from backing up into the esophagus.

spinal cord a thick band of nervous tissue that is contained within the spinal column

spirituality the concern with the nature of spirit or soul, the intangible and immaterial essence of a person

spongy bone tissue (trabecular bone tissue) bone tissue that is less dense than cortical bone tissue, containing large spaces between columns of bone tissue

sport a physical activity that is performed according to rules and customs

sport psychology the psychology of athletes and sport performance

Stages of Change stages described in models that propose that individuals go through several phases as they attempt to change behavior. The most commonly used Stages of Change Model is the Transtheoretical Model, which includes six stages of change.

state anxiety heightened worry that arises for a short period of time but then resolves

steatohepatitis liver disease characterized by inflammation and the accumulation of fat

steatosis fatty liver

stimulus control behavior-change techniques based on the observation that for each person, certain factors trigger automatic responses, and by changing the factors (the stimuli), behavior changes as well; used especially for reducing negative behaviors

strength how much force muscles can exert against an object

strength training exercise performed to increase muscle strength

stress a feeling of anxiety and tension that occurs when people feel that the demands being placed on them exceed their abilities and resources for coping

stress management the use of a variety of techniques that can enhance one's ability to cope with stress

stress reactivity the nature and strength of an individual's stress response

stressor any demand or challenge that causes a stress response

stretching exercise that pushes joints to the edge of their ROM and improves flexibility

subcutaneous fat tissue found under the skin

subjective norms people's beliefs about what they think others typically do as well as what they think others want them to do

substance-related disorder a problem involving the use of substances (such as drugs, alcohol, and tobacco products) and associated difficulties, such as coping with withdrawal symptoms or emotional health problems, related to the substance

substance-use disorder problems with substance dependence and abuse; a type of substance-related disorder

substance dependence compulsive use of chemicals such as drugs, tobacco, and alcohol

sucrose a disaccharide that is composed of one glucose molecule bonded with one fructose molecule

sympathetic nervous system (SNS) branch of the autonomic nervous system that is activated when the body needs to move or is experiencing the stress response

sympathomimetic something that mimics the action of the sympathetic nervous system

synapse the place where two neurons communicate

synaptic cleft the minute space between two neurons

synovial fluid a thin, viscous fluid that lubricates the joint structures

synovial joint a type of joint that allows for the greatest ROM; composed of the ends of two bones, the ligaments connecting them, the muscles and tendons that help to form the joint and produce movement at the joint, and the joint capsule that surrounds the ends of the bones (see Figure 2-15)

system a group of organs that work together to accomplish a specific task, such as digestion (the digestive system)

T lymphocytes lymphocytes that attack pathogens that the B lymphocytes have identified as invaders

tau protein a protein that normally serves to support nerve cells in the brain; however, abnormal clumps of the protein indicate pathology

telomerase an enzyme that helps to restore telomere length

telomeres strands of repetitive DNA sequences that are found on the ends of chromosomes

tendonitis inflammation of one or more tendons

tendons layers of connective tissue that join together at the ends of the muscle and insert into the bone

tension headache head pain caused by excess muscle tension in the forehead, face, jaw, and neck, often brought on by stress

teratogen a substance that disrupts fetal development, causing irreversible damage

termination (stage of change) a proposed stage of change in which the individual continues the behavior change indefinitely and in which the old, unwanted behavior is terminated

tertiary treatments interventions that address health behaviors after people become ill or injured

thalamus a region of the brain that integrates and relays sensory information to the cerebral cortex

theory an explanation for things that scientists have observed

Theory of Planned Behavior theory proposing that a person's attitudes, subjective norms, and perceived behavioral control influence behavioral intentions

thermic effect of exercise (TEE) the calories used during exercise

thermic effect of food (TEF) the energy required for the processes of digestion and absorption

thrombus a blood clot that forms within a blood vessel or in one of the chambers of the heart

thyrotropic hormone a hormone released from the pituitary gland that stimulates the thyroid gland to release thyroxin

thyrotropic hormone-releasing factor a hormone released by the hypothalamus that stimulates the pituitary gland to release thyrotropic hormone

thyroxin a hormone released from the thyroid gland that increases blood fat and sugar levels, breathing rate, HR, and blood pressure

tolerance requiring increased amounts of a substance to produce a given effect

total body water (TBW) the amount of water that is contained in a person's body, estimated by giving some form of tracer that diffuses into all water compartments. A sample of water, such as saliva, is taken, and TBW is extrapolated from the tracer amount in the sample. TBW measurements can provide an estimate of body composition.

trabecular bone tissue (spongy bone tissue) bone tissue that is less dense than cortical bone tissue, containing large spaces between columns of bone tissue

trace minerals minerals needed by the body in small amounts, e.g., zinc, iron, and copper

trachea the tube-shaped organ that carries air to the lungs

trait anxiety heightened worry that is considered a part of an individual's personality profile and is a fairly common and enduring characteristic of that person

trait self-control the level of an individual's ability to regulate emotions and behaviors

trans fatty acids fatty acids that contain a type of carbon-carbon double bond that causes the fatty acid to take a shape that is similar to the shape of saturated fatty acids; commonly produced during the process of hydrogenation and associated with higher risk of artery disease

Transtheoretical Model a model of behavior change proposed by James O. Prochaska and colleagues that draws from many theories and describes behavior change as a process that goes through stages and is facilitated by a number of cognitive and behavioral processes, known as the processes of change

type I muscle fibers (slow-twitch oxidative [SO] muscle fiber) a muscle fiber type that is recruited for aerobic exercise, activity requiring a sustained elevation of metabolic rate and muscle contraction. These muscle fibers are somewhat slower in contractile speed and somewhat lower in force production, but more resistant to fatigue than other types; they rely on oxygen to produce energy.

type IIA muscle fibers (fast-twitch oxidative-glycolytic [FOG] fiber) an intermediate muscle fiber type that contracts quickly but has greater endurance than the fast-twitch glycolytic fibers; can produce energy from both anaerobic and aerobic pathways

type IIB muscle fibers (fast-twitch glycolytic [FG] muscle fiber) a muscle fiber type that is larger than slow-twitch oxidative fibers and capable of producing more force faster; relies on anaerobic energy systems to produce energy quickly

type 2 diabetes a type of diabetes that begins with a problem in the body's response to the hormone insulin, which signals receptors on the cell membranes to take up sugar from the blood

Type A behavior pattern (TABP) a cluster of traits including a hard-driving competitiveness, hostility, a sense of time urgency, and a concern with achievement and acquisition of objects

Type D personality a cluster of distressed behavior traits, such as anxiety, irritability, and insecurity, that puts individuals at greater risk of heart disease

ulcer an open sore that develops from a cut in the lining of the stomach or other organ

underwater weighing a method of estimating body composition by calculating body density from the weight of a person in water; same as hydrostatic weighing

unsaturated fatty acids fatty acids with at least one carbon-carbon double bond

valence how positive an emotional state feels to a person; ranges from unpleasant to pleasant

variable something that varies, that can take on two or more values

vascular dementia dementia caused by inadequate blood supply to the brain

vasopressin hormone released from the pituitary gland that raises blood pressure by contracting arteries

vegan a diet that does not include animal products

veins vessels that eventually return the blood to the right atrium of the heart

ventral tegmental area (VTA) area in the limbic system of the brain that is part of the mesolimbic system

venules little veins

vertebrae (singular vertebra) the column of 26 bones that form the spinal column

vertebral column the spine

vertebral compression fracture fracture of the vertebrae responsible for the dowager's hump sometimes seen in older adults

viscera the abdominal organs, including the liver, stomach, intestines, and kidneys

visceral adipose tissue (VAT) fat stored around the abdominal organs, including the liver, stomach, intestines, and kidneys

visceral obesity a type of obesity characterized by deposition of excess visceral adipose tissue

volume of oxygen consumed (VO_2) the amount of oxygen taken in by the body to produce energy

water-insoluble fiber a type of dietary fiber that adds bulk to feces and speeds its passage through the gastrointestinal tract

water-soluble fiber a type of dietary fiber that attracts water and forms a gel-like mixture in the digestive tract, which slows stomach emptying

wellness a dynamic state of well-being in which people strive to maximize their well-being in all areas of life, from physical, emotional, and spiritual health to occupational, economic, and environmental health

white blood cells also known as leukocytes, these cells are part of the immune system and help to protect the body from pathogens

withdrawal symptoms signs and symptoms experienced by users when the substance to which they are addicted is not used

yellow bone marrow tissue found inside the bones that is composed primarily of adipocytes

INDEX

Note: Page numbers followed by f refer to figures, page numbers followed by t refer to tables, and page numbers followed by b refer to boxes.